Nurse's Pocket Guide

Diagnoses, Interventions,
and Rationales

Nurse's Pocket Guide

Diagnoses, Interventions, and Rationales

NINTH EDITION

Marilynn E. Doenges, RN, BSN, MA

Clinical Specialist—Adult Psychiatric/Mental Health, Retired
Adjunct Faculty
Beth-El College of Nursing and Health Sciences CU-Springs
Colorado Springs, Colorado

Mary Frances Moorhouse, RN, BSN, CRRN, CLNC

Nurse Consultant
TNT-RN Enterprises
Adjunct Faculty
Pikes Peak Community College
Colorado Springs, Colorado

Alice C. Murr, RN, BSN

Telephone Triage Nurse
Legal Nurse Consultant
Colorado Springs, Colorado

 F.A. Davis Company • Philadelphia

F.A. Davis Company
1915 Arch Street
Philadelphia, PA 19103
www. fadavis.com

Printed in Canada

Last digit indicates print number: 10 9 8 7 6 5 4 3

Publisher: Robert G. Martone
Cover Design: Joan Wendt

As new scientific information becomes available through basic and clinical research, recommended treatments and drug therapies undergo changes. The author(s) and publisher have done everything possible to make this book accurate, up to date, and in accord with accepted standards at the time of publication. The authors, editors, and publisher are not responsible for errors or omissions or for consequences from application of the book, and make no warranty, expressed or implied, in regard to the contents of the book. Any practice described in this book should be applied by the reader in accordance with professional standards of care used in regard to the unique circumstances that may apply in each situation. The reader is advised always to check product information (package inserts) for changes and new information regarding dose and contraindications before administering any drug. Caution is especially urged when using new or infrequently ordered drugs.

ISBN 0-8036-1179-X

Contributor

Sheila Marquez
Executive Director
Vice President/Chief Operating Officer
The Colorado SIDS Program, Inc.
Denver, Colorado

Dedication

This book is dedicated to:

Our families, who helped with the mundane activities of daily living that allowed us to write this book and who provide us with love and encouragement in all our endeavors.

Our friends, who support us in our writing, put up with our memory lapses, and love us still.

Bob Martone, Publisher, Nursing, who asks questions that stimulate thought and discussion, and who maintains good humor throughout.

The F.A. Davis production staff, who coordinated and expedited the project through the printing process, meeting unreal deadlines, and sending pages to us with bated breath.

Robert H. Craven, Jr., and the F.A. Davis family.

And last and most important:
The nurses we are writing for, to those who have found the previous editions of the Pocket Guide helpful, and to other nurses who are looking for help to provide quality nursing care in a period of transition and change, we say, "Nursing Diagnosis is the way."

ACKNOWLEDGMENTS

A special acknowledgment to Marilynn's friend, the late Diane Camillone, who provoked an awareness of the role of the patient and continues to influence our thoughts about the importance of quality nursing care, and to our late colleague, Mary Jeffries, who introduced us to nursing diagnosis.

To our colleagues in NANDA who continue to formulate and refine nursing diagnoses to provide nursing with the tools to enhance and promote the growth of the profession.

> Marilynn E. Doenges
> Mary Frances Moorhouse
> Alice C. Murr

Contents

Health Conditions and Client Concerns with Associated Nursing Diagnoses appear on pages 603-720.

For each nursing diagnosis, the following information is provided:
Taxonomy II, Domain, Class, Code, Year Submitted

Diagnostic Division
Definition
Related/Risk Factors, Defining Characteristics:
    Subjective/Objective
    Desired Outcomes/Evaluation Criteria
    Actions/Interventions
    Nursing Priorities
    Documentation Focus
    Sample Nursing Outcomes & Interventions Classifications
      (NOC/NIC)

How to Use the Nurse's Pocket Guide

The American Nurses Association (ANA) Social Policy Statement of 1980 was the first to define nursing as the diagnosis and treatment of human responses to actual and potential health problems. This definition, when combined with the ANA Standards of Practice, has provided impetus and support for the use of nursing diagnosis. Defining nursing and its effect on client care supports the growing awareness that nursing care is a key factor in client survival and in the maintenance, rehabilitative, and preventive aspects of healthcare. Changes and new developments in healthcare delivery in the last decade have given rise to the need for a common framework of communication to ensure continuity of care for the client moving between multiple healthcare settings and providers. Evaluation and documentation of care are important parts of this process.

This book is designed to aid the practitioner and student nurse in identifying interventions commonly associated with specific nursing diagnoses as proposed by NANDA International (formerly the North American Nursing Diagnosis Association). These interventions are the activities needed to implement and document care provided to the individual client and can be used in varied settings from acute to community/home care.

Chapters 1 and 2 present brief discussions of the nursing process, data collection, and care plan construction. Chapter 3 contains the Diagnostic Divisions, Assessment Tool, a sample plan of care, and corresponding documentation/charting examples. For more in-depth information and inclusive plans of care related to specific medical/psychiatric conditions (with rationale and the application of the diagnoses), the nurse is referred to the larger works, all published by the F.A. Davis Company: *Nursing Care Plans: Guidelines for Planning and Documenting Patient Care*, ed. 6 (Doenges, Moorhouse, Geissler-Murr, 2002); *Psychiatric Care Plans: Guidelines for Planning and Documenting Client Care*, ed. 3 (Doenges, Townsend, Moorhouse, 1998); and *Maternal/Newborn Plans of Care: Guidelines for Planning and Documenting Client Care*, ed. 3 (Doenges, Moorhouse, 1999).

Nursing diagnoses are listed alphabetically in Chapter 4 for ease of reference and include the diagnoses accepted for use by

NANDA through 2003. Each approved diagnosis includes its definition and information divided into the NANDA categories of Related or Risk Factors and Defining Characteristics. Related/Risk Factors information reflects causative or contributing factors that can be useful for determining whether the diagnosis is applicable to a particular client. Defining Characteristics (signs and symptoms or cues) are listed as subjective and/or objective and are used to confirm actual diagnoses, aid in formulating outcomes, and provide additional data for choosing appropriate interventions. The authors have not deleted or altered NANDA's listings; however, on occasion, they have added to their definitions and suggested additional criteria to provide clarification and direction. These additions are denoted with brackets [ ].

With the development and acceptance of Taxonomy II following the biennial conference in 2000, significant changes were made to better reflect the content of the diagnoses within the taxonomy. It is designed to reduce miscalculations, errors, and redundancies. The framework has been changed from the Human Response Patterns and is organized in Domains only and Classes, with 13 domains, 105 classes, and 167 diagnoses. Although clinicians will use the actual diagnoses, understanding the taxonomic structure will help the nurse to find the desired information quickly. Taxonomy II is designed to be multiaxial with 7 axes (see Appendix 2). An axis is defined as a dimension of the human response that is considered in the diagnostic process. Sometimes an axis may be included in the diagnostic concept, such as ineffective community coping in which the unit of care (e.g., community) is named. Some are implicit, such as activity intolerance in which the individual is the unit of care. Sometimes an axis may not be pertinent to a particular diagnosis and will not be a part of the nursing diagnosis label or code. For example, the time axis may not be relevant to each diagnostic situation. The Taxonomic Domain and Class are noted under each nursing diagnosis heading. An Axis 6 descriptor is included in each nursing diagnosis label.

The ANA, in conjunction with NANDA, proposed that specific nursing diagnoses currently approved and structured according to Taxonomy I Revised be included in the International Classification of Diseases (ICD) within the section "Family of Health-Related Classifications." While the World Health Organization did not accept this initial proposal because of lack of documentation of the usefulness of nursing diagnoses at the international level, the NANDA list has been accepted by SNOMED (Systemized Nomenclature of Medicine) for inclusion in its international coding system and is included in the Unified Medical Language System of the National Library of

Medicine. Today, researchers from around the world are validating nursing diagnoses in support for resubmission and acceptance in future additions of ICD.

The authors have chosen to categorize the list of nursing diagnoses approved for clinical use and testing into Diagnostic Divisions, which is the framework for an assessment tool (Chapter 3) designed to assist the nurse to readily identify an appropriate nursing diagnosis from data collected during the assessment process. The Diagnostic Division label is included following the Taxonomic label under each nursing diagnosis heading.

Desired Outcomes/Evaluation Criteria are identified to assist the nurse in formulating individual client outcomes and to support the evaluation process.

Interventions in this pocket guide are primarily directed to adult care settings (although general age span considerations are included) and are listed according to nursing priorities. Some interventions require collaborative or interdependent orders (e.g., medical, psychiatric), and the nurse will need to determine when this is necessary and take the appropriate action. Although all defining characteristics are listed, interventions that address specialty areas outside the scope of this book are not routinely presented (e.g., obstetrics/gynecology/pediatrics) except for diagnoses that are infancy-oriented, such as Breastfeeding, ineffective; Infant Behavior, disorganized; and Parent/Infant/Child Attachment, risk for impaired. For example, when addressing deficient Fluid Volume, isotonic (hemorrhage), the nurse is directed to stop blood loss; however, specific direction to perform fundal massage is not listed.

The inclusion of Documentation Focus suggestions is to remind the nurse of the importance and necessity of recording the steps of the nursing process.

Finally, in recognition of the ongoing work of numerous researchers over the past 15 years, the authors have referenced the Nursing Interventions and Outcomes labels developed by the Iowa Intervention Projects (Bulechek & McCloskey; Johnson, Mass, & Moorhead). These groups have been classifying nursing interventions and outcomes to predict resource requirements and measure outcomes, thereby meeting the needs of a standardized language that can be coded for computer and reimbursement purposes. As an introduction to this work in progress, sample NIC and NOC labels have been included under the heading Sample Nursing Interventions & Outcomes Classifications at the conclusion of each nursing diagnosis section. The reader is referred to the various publications by Joanne C. McCloskey and Marion Johnson for more in-depth information.

Chapter 5 presents over 400 disorders/health conditions reflecting all specialty areas, with associated nursing diagnoses written as client diagnostic statements that include the "related to" and "evidenced by" components. This section will facilitate and help validate the assessment and problem/need identification steps of the nursing process.

As noted, with few exceptions, we have presented NANDA's recommendations as formulated. We support the belief that practicing nurses and researchers need to study, use, and evaluate the diagnoses as presented. Nurses can be creative as they use the standardized language, redefining and sharing information as the diagnoses are used with individual patients. As new nursing diagnoses are developed, it is important that the data they encompass are added to the current database. As part of the process by clinicians, educators, and researchers across practice specialties and academic settings to define, test, and refine nursing diagnosis, nurses are encouraged to share insights and ideas with NANDA at the following address: NANDA International, 1211 Locust Street, Philadelphia, PA 19107, USA; e-mail: nanda@rmpinc.com.

CHAPTER 1

The Nursing Process

Many years ago, the nursing profession identified a problem-solving process that "combines the most desirable elements of the art of nursing with the most relevant elements of systems theory, using the scientific method" (Shore, 1988). The term *nursing process* was introduced in the 1950s and has gained national acceptance as the basis for providing effective nursing care. It is now included in the conceptual framework of all nursing curricula and is accepted in the legal definition of nursing in the nurse practice acts of most states. This nursing process is central to nursing actions in any setting, because it is an efficient method of organizing thought processes for clinical decision making and problem solving.

Use of the nursing process requires the skills of (1) assessment (systematic collection of data relating to clients and their needs), (2) problem/need identification (analysis of data), (3) planning (setting goals, choice of solutions), (4) implementation (putting the plan into action), and (5) evaluation (assessing the effectiveness of the plan and changing the plan as indicated by the current needs). Although these skills are presented as separate, individual activities, they are interrelated and form a continuous circle of thought and action.

To use this process, the nurse must demonstrate fundamental abilities of knowledge, creativity, adaptability, commitment, trust, and leadership. In addition, intelligence and interpersonal and technical skills are important. Because decision making is crucial to each step of the process, the following assumptions are important for the nurse to consider:

- The client is a human being who has worth and dignity.
- There are basic human needs that must be met, and when they are not, problems arise, requiring interventions by another person until and if the individual can resume responsibility for self.
- The client has a right to quality health and nursing care delivered with interest, compassion, competence, and a focus on wellness and prevention of illness.
- The therapeutic nurse-client relationship is important in this process.

Nurses have struggled for years to define nursing by identifying the parameters of nursing with the goal of attaining professional status. To this end, nurses meet, discuss, and conduct research (in both the national and international arenas) to identify and label client problems and responses that fall within the scope of nursing practice. Changes in healthcare delivery and reimbursement methods, the advent of health maintenance organizations (HMOs), and alternative healthcare settings (home health, extended-care facilities, and the like) continue to increase the need for a commonality of communication to ensure continuity of care for the client who moves from one setting/area to another. Evaluation and improvement of provided services are an important part of this process, and both providers and users of care benefit from accurate documentation of the care provided and the client's response.

The use of nursing diagnosis (ND) provides nurses with a common language for identifying client needs, aids in the choice of nursing interventions, and provides guidance for evaluation. It promotes improved communication among nurses, shifts, units, other healthcare providers, and alternative care settings. This language further provides a base for clinicians, educators, and researchers to document, validate, and/or alter the process. The American Nurses Association (ANA) Social Policy Statements (1980/1995) and the ANA Standards of Practice (1973/1991) have provided impetus and support for the use of nursing diagnosis in the practice setting.

Currently, there are differing definitions of nursing diagnosis. NANDA International (formerly The North American Nursing Diagnosis Association) has accepted the following definition:

> Nursing diagnosis is a clinical judgment about individual, family, or community responses to actual and potential health problems/life processes. Nursing diagnoses provide the basis for selection of nursing interventions to achieve outcomes for which the nurse is accountable.

Although it continues to evolve, the current NANDA list provides diagnostic labels and information for appropriate use. Nurses need to become familiar with the parameters of the diagnoses, identifying strengths and weaknesses, thus promoting research and further development. Although nursing practice is more than nursing diagnosis, the use of standardized nursing language can help to define and to refine the profession. Also, NDs can be used within many existing conceptual frameworks because they are a generic approach adaptable to all.

Whereas nursing actions were once based on variables such as signs and symptoms, diagnostic tests, and medical diagnoses, NDs are a uniform way of identifying, focusing on, and dealing with specific client problems/needs. The accurate nursing diagnosis of a client need can set a standard for nursing practice, thus leading to improved care delivery.

Nursing and medicine are interrelated and have implications for each other. This interrelationship includes the exchange of data, the sharing of ideas/thinking, and the development of plans of care that include all data pertinent to the individual client as well as the family/significant other(s) (SO[s]). This relationship also extends to all disciplines that have contact with the individual/family. Although nurses work within the medical and psychosocial domains, nursing's phenomena of concern are the patterns of human response, not disease processes. Therefore, nursing diagnoses usually do not parallel or mimic medical/psychiatric diagnoses but do involve independent nursing activities as well as collaborative roles and actions. Thus, the written plan of care contains more than actions initiated by medical orders. It contains a combination of the orders and plans of care of all involved disciplines. The nurse is responsible for seeing that these different activities are pulled together into a functional plan to provide holistic care for the individual/family.

Summary

In using ND as an integral part of the nursing process, the nursing profession has identified a body of knowledge that contributes to the prevention of illness as well as to the maintenance and/or restoration of health (or relief of pain and discomfort when a return to health is not possible). Because the nursing process is the basis of all nursing actions, it is the essence of nursing. The process is flexible and yet sufficiently structured so as to provide the base for nursing actions. It can be applied in any healthcare or educational setting, in any theoretical or conceptual framework, and within the context of any nursing philosophy.

Subsequent chapters help the nurse apply the nursing process to become more familiar with the current NANDA-approved list of NDs, their definitions, related/risk factors (etiology), and defining characteristics. Coupled with desired outcomes and the most commonly used interventions, the nurse can write, implement, and document an individualized plan of care.

CHAPTER 2

Application of the Nursing Process

Because of their hectic schedules, many nurses believe that time spent writing plans of care is time taken away from client care. Plans of care have been viewed as "busy work" to satisfy accreditation requirements or the whims of supervisors. In reality, however, quality client care must be planned and coordinated. Properly written and used plans of care can provide direction and continuity of care by facilitating communication among nurses and other caregivers. They also provide guidelines for documentation and a tool for evaluating the care provided.

The components of a plan of care are based on the nursing process. Creating a plan of care begins with the collection of data (assessment). The client database consists of subjective and objective information encompassing the various concerns reflected in the current NANDA International (formerly the North American Nursing Diagnosis Association) list of nursing diagnoses (NDs) (Table 2–1). Subjective data are those that are reported by the client (and SOs) in the individual's own words. This information includes the individual's perceptions and what he or she wants to share. It is important to accept what is reported because the client is the "expert" in this area. Objective data are those that are observed or described (quantitatively or qualitatively) and include diagnostic testing and physical examination findings. Analysis of the collected data leads to the identification of problems or areas of concern/need. These problems or needs are expressed as NDs.

A nursing diagnosis is a decision about a need/problem that requires nursing intervention and management. The need may be anything that interferes with the quality of life the client is used to and/or desires. It includes concerns of the client, SOs, and/or nurse. The ND focuses attention on a physical or behavioral response, either a current need or a problem at risk for developing. When the ND label is combined with the individual's specific related/risk factors and defining characteristics (as appropriate), a client diagnostic statement is created. This provides direction for nursing care, and its affective tone can

Table 2–1. NURSING DIAGNOSES

Accepted for Use and Research (2003–2004)

---

*New to the 2nd NANDA/NIC/NOC (NNN) Conference.

Information that appears in brackets has been added by the authors to clarify and enhance the use of NDs.

Please also see the NANDA diagnoses grouped according to Gordon's Functional Health Patterns on the inside front cover.

(*Continued*)

Table 2–1. NURSING DIAGNOSES (CONTINUED)

---

*New to the 2nd NANDA/NIC/NOC (NNN) Conference.

Information that appears in brackets has been added by the authors to clarify and enhance the use of NDs.

Please also see the NANDA diagnoses grouped according to Gordon's Functional Health Patterns on the inside front cover.

Table 2-1. NURSING DIAGNOSES

Infection, risk for   307–310
Injury, risk for   310–313
Injury, risk for perioperative positioning   313–316
Intracranial Adaptive Capacity, decreased   316–319

Knowledge, deficient [Learning Need] (specify)   319–323
*Knowledge (specify), readiness for enhanced   323–325

Loneliness, risk for   326–328

Memory, impaired   328–331
Mobility, impaired bed   331–333
Mobility, impaired physical   333–337
Mobility, impaired wheelchair   337–339

+Nausea   339–343
Noncompliance [Adherence, ineffective] [specify]   343–347
Nutrition: imbalanced, less than body requirements   347–352
Nutrition: imbalanced, more than body requirements   352–355
Nutrition: imbalanced, risk for more than body requirements
   356–358
*Nutrition, readiness for enhanced   359–362

Oral Mucous Membrane, impaired   362–365

Pain, acute   365–369
Pain, chronic   370–374
Parental Role Conflict   374–377
Parenting, impaired   377–381
*Parenting, readiness for enhanced   381–385
Parenting, risk for impaired   385–387
Peripheral Neurovascular Dysfunction, risk for   387–390
Personal Identity, disturbed   390–393
Poisoning, risk for   393–396
Post-Trauma Syndrome [specify stage]   396–401
Post-Trauma Syndrome, risk for   402–404
Powerlessness [specify level]   404–408
Powerlessness, risk for   408–410
Protection, ineffective   411–412

Rape-Trauma Syndrome   412–417
Rape-Trauma Syndrome: compound reaction   413

+Revised NDs.
*New to the 2nd NANDA/NIC/NOC (NNN) Conference.
Information that appears in brackets has been added by the authors
to clarify and enhance the use of NDs.
Please also see the NANDA diagnoses grouped according to
Gordon's Functional Health Patterns on the inside front cover.

(Continued)

Table 2–1. NURSING DIAGNOSES *(CONTINUED)*

Rape-Trauma Syndrome: silent reaction   413
Relocation Stress Syndrome   417–420
Relocation Stress Syndrome, risk for   421–422
Role Performance, ineffective   422–425

Self-Care Deficit: bathing/hygiene   425–430
Self-Care Deficit: dressing/grooming   425–430
Self-Care Deficit: feeding   425–430
Self-Care Deficit: toileting   425–430
*Self-Concept, readiness for enhanced   430–433
Self-Esteem, chronic low   433–437
Self-Esteem, situational low   437–440
Self-Esteem, risk for situational low   440–441
Self-Mutilation   442–445
Self-Mutilation, risk for   445–449
Sensory Perception, disturbed (specify: visual, auditory, kinesthetic,
   gustatory, tactile, olfactory)   449–454
Sexual Dysfunction   454–458
Sexuality Pattern, ineffective   458–461
Skin Integrity, impaired   461–465
Skin Integrity, risk for impaired   465–468
Sleep Deprivation   468–472
Sleep Pattern, disturbed   472–477
*Sleep, readiness for enhanced   477–480
Social Interaction, impaired   480–484
Social Isolation   484–487
Sorrow, chronic   487–489
+Spiritual Distress   490–494
Spiritual Distress, risk for   494–497
+Spiritual Well-Being, readiness for enhanced   497–500
Suffocation, risk for   500–503
Suicide, risk for   503–507
Surgical Recovery, delayed   507–510
Swallowing, impaired   510–515

Therapeutic Regimen Management: community, ineffective   515–517
Therapeutic Regimen Management: effective   517–519
Therapeutic Regimen Management: family, ineffective   520–522
Therapeutic Regimen Management: ineffective   522–525
*Therapeutic Regimen Management: readiness for enhanced
   525–527
Thermoregulation, ineffective   527–529
Thought Processes, disturbed   529–533

+Revised NDs.

*New to the 2nd NANDA/NIC/NOC (NNN) Conference.

Please also see the NANDA diagnoses grouped according to
Gordon's Functional Health Patterns on the inside front cover.

Table 2–1. NURSING DIAGNOSES

Tissue Integrity, impaired   533–537
Tissue Perfusion, ineffective (specify type: renal, cerebral, cardiopul-
    monary, gastrointestinal, peripheral)   537–544
Transfer Ability, impaired   544–546
Trauma, risk for   547–551

Unilateral Neglect   551–554
Urinary Elimination, impaired   554–558
*Urinary Elimination, readiness for enhanced   558–561
Urinary Incontinence, functional   561–564
Urinary Incontinence, reflex   564–566
Urinary Incontinence, stress   567–569
Urinary Incontinence, total   570–572
Urinary Incontinence, urge   572–575
Urinary Incontinence, risk for urge   576–578
Urinary Retention [acute/chronic]   578–581

Ventilation, impaired spontaneous   581–586
Ventilatory Weaning Response, dysfunctional   586–590
Violence, [actual/] risk for other-directed   590–591
Violence, [actual/] risk for self-directed   591–596

Walking, impaired   597–599
Wandering [specify sporadic or continuous]   599–602

*New to the 2nd NANDA/NIC/NOC (NNN) Conference.
Information that appears in brackets has been added by the authors
to clarify and enhance the use of NDs.
Please also see the NANDA diagnoses grouped according to
Gordon's Functional Health Patterns on the inside front cover.

shape expectations of the client's response and/or influence the nurse's behavior toward the client.

The key to accurate diagnosis is collection and analysis of data. In Chapter 3, the NDs have been categorized into divisions (Diagnostic Divisions: Nursing Diagnoses Organized According to a Nursing Focus, Section 2) and an assessment tool designed to assist the nurse to identify appropriate NDs as the data are collected. Nurses may feel at risk in committing themselves to documenting a nursing diagnosis for fear they might be wrong. However, unlike medical diagnoses, NDs can change as the client progresses through various stages of illness/maladaptation to resolution of the condition/situation.

Desired outcomes are formulated to give direction to, as well as to evaluate, the care provided. These outcomes emerge from the diagnostic statement and are what the client hopes to achieve. They serve as the guidelines to evaluate progress toward resolution of needs/problems, providing impetus for revising the plan as appropriate. In this book, outcomes are stated in general terms to permit the practitioner to individualize them by adding timelines and other data according to specific client circumstances. Outcome terminology needs to be concise, realistic, measurable, and stated in words the client can understand. Beginning the outcome statement with an action verb provides measurable direction, for example, "Verbalizes relationship between diabetes mellitus and circulatory changes in feet within 2 days" or "Correctly performs procedure of home glucose monitoring within 48 hours."

Interventions are the action steps taken to achieve desired outcomes and, because they are communicated to others, they must be clearly stated. A solid nursing knowledge base is vital to this process because the rationale for interventions needs to be sound and feasible with the intention of providing effective individualized care. The actions may be independent or collaborative and may encompass specific orders from nursing, medicine, and other disciplines. Written interventions that guide ongoing client care need to be dated and signed. To facilitate the planning process, specific nursing priorities have been identified in this text to provide a general ranking of interventions. This ranking would be altered according to individual client situations. The seasoned practitioner may choose to use these as broad-based interventions. The student or beginning practitioner may need to develop a more detailed plan of care by including the appropriate interventions listed under each nursing priority. Finally, as each client usually has a perception of individual needs or problems he or she faces and an expectation of what could be done about the situation, the plan of care must be congruent with the client's reality or it will fail.

The plan of care documents client care in areas of accountability, quality assurance, and liability. The nurse needs to plan care with the client, because both are accountable for that care and for achieving the desired outcomes.

Summary

Healthcare providers have a responsibility for planning with the client and family for continuation of care to the eventual outcome of an optimal state of wellness or a dignified death. Planning, setting goals, and choosing appropriate interventions are essential to the construction of a plan of care as well as to delivery of quality nursing care. These nursing activities comprise the planning phase of the nursing process and are documented in the plan of care for a particular client. As a part of the client's permanent record, the plan of care not only provides a means for the nurse who is actively caring for the client to be aware of the client's needs (NDs), goals, and actions to be taken, but it also substantiates the care provided for review by third-party payors and accreditation agencies, while meeting legal requirements.

CHAPTER 3

Putting Theory into Practice: Sample Assessment Tools, Plan of Care, and Documentation

The client assessment is the foundation on which identification of individual needs, responses, and problems is based. To facilitate the steps of assessment and diagnosis in the nursing process, an assessment tool (Assessment Tools for Choosing Nursing Diagnoses, Section 1) has been constructed using a nursing focus instead of the medical approach of "review of systems." This has the advantage of identifying and validating nursing diagnoses (NDs) as opposed to medical diagnoses.

To achieve this nursing focus, we have grouped the NANDA International (formerly the North American Nursing Diagnosis Association) NDs into related categories titled Diagnostic Divisions (Section 2), which reflect a blending of theories, primarily Maslow's Hierarchy of Needs and a self-care philosophy. These divisions serve as the framework or outline for data collection/clustering that focuses attention on the nurse's phenomena of concern—the human responses to actual and potential health problems—and directs the nurse to the most likely corresponding NDs.

Because the divisions are based on human responses and needs and not specific "systems," information may be recorded in more than one area. For this reason, the nurse is encouraged to keep an open mind, to pursue all leads, and to collect as much data as possible before choosing the ND label that best reflects the client's situation. For example, when the nurse identifies the cue of restlessness in a client, the nurse may infer that the client is anxious, assuming that the restlessness is psychologically based and overlooking the possibility that it is physiologically based.

From the specific data recorded in the database, an individualized client diagnostic statement can be formulated using the problem, etiology, signs/symptoms (PES) format to accurately represent the client's situation. For example, the diagnostic statement may read, "deficient Knowledge regarding diabetic care, related to misinterpretation of information and/or lack of recall, evidenced by inaccurate follow-through of instructions and failure to recognize signs and symptoms of hyperglycemia."

Desired client outcomes are identified to facilitate choosing appropriate interventions and to serve as evaluators of both nursing care and client response. These outcomes also form the framework for documentation.

Interventions are designed to specify the action of the nurse, the client, and/or SOs. Interventions need to promote the client's movement toward health/independence in addition to achievement of physiologic stability. This requires involvement of the client in his or her own care, including participation in decisions about care activities and projected outcomes.

Section 3, "Client Situation and Prototype Plan of Care," contains a sample plan of care formulated on data collected in the nursing model assessment tool. Individualized client diagnostic statements and desired client outcomes (with timelines added to reflect anticipated length of stay and individual client/nurse expectations) have been identified. Interventions have been chosen based on concerns/needs identified by the client and nurse during data collection, as well as by physician orders.

Although not normally included in a written plan of care, rationales are included in this sample for the purpose of explaining or clarifying the choice of interventions to enhance the nurse's learning.

Finally, to complete the learning experience, samples of documentation based on the client situation are presented in Section 4, "Documentation Techniques." The plan of care provides documentation of the planning process and serves as a framework/outline for charting of administered care. The primary nurse needs to periodically review the client's progress and the effectiveness of the treatment plan. Persons then are able to read the notes and have a clear picture of what occurred with the client in order to make appropriate judgments regarding client management. The best way to ensure the clarity of progress notes is through the use of descriptive (or observational) statements. Observations of client behavior and response to therapy provide invaluable information. Through this communication, it can be determined if the client's current desired outcomes or interventions need to be eliminated or altered and if the development of new outcomes or interventions is warranted. Progress notes are an integral component of the overall medical record and should include all significant events that occur in the daily life of the client. They reflect implementation of the treatment plan and document that appropriate actions have been carried out, precautions taken, and so forth. It is important that both the implementation of interventions and progress toward the desired outcomes be documented. The notes need to be written in a clear and objective fashion, specific as to date and time, and signed by the person making the entry.

Use of clear documentation helps the nurse to individualize client care. Providing a picture of what has happened and is happening promotes continuity of care and facilitates evaluation. This reinforces each person's accountability and responsibility for using nursing process to provide individually appropriate and cost-effective client care.

SECTION 1

ASSESSMENT TOOLS FOR CHOOSING NURSING DIAGNOSES

This is a suggested guide/tool to create a database reflecting a nursing focus. Although the Diagnostic Divisions are alphabetized here for ease of presentation, they can be prioritized or rearranged in any manner to meet individual needs. In addition, the assessment tool can be adapted to meet the needs of specific client populations. Excerpts of assessment tools adapted for psychiatric and obstetric settings are included at the end of this section.

ADULT MEDICAL/SURGICAL ASSESSMENT TOOL

General Information

Name: _____
Age: _____ DOB: _____ Gender: _____ Race: _____
Admission Date: _____ Time: _____ From: _____
Source of Information: _____
Reliability (1–4 with 4 = very reliable): _____

Activity/Rest

SUBJECTIVE (REPORTS)

Occupation: _____ Usual activities: _____
Leisure time activities/hobbies: _____
Limitations imposed by condition: _____
Sleep: Hours: _____ Naps: _____ Aids: _____
   Insomnia: _____ Related to: _____
   Rested on awakening: _____
   Excessive grogginess: _____
Feelings of boredom/dissatisfaction: _____

OBJECTIVE (EXHIBITS)

Observed response to activity: Cardiovascular: _____
Respiratory: _____
Mental status (i.e., withdrawn/lethargic) _____
Neuro/muscular assessment:
   Muscle mass/tone: _____
   Posture: _____ Tremors: _____
   ROM: _____ Strength: _____ Deformity: _____

Circulation

SUBJECTIVE (REPORTS)

History of:
   Hypertension: _____ Heart trouble: _____
   Rheumatic fever: _____ Ankle/leg edema: _____
   Phlebitis: _____ Slow healing: _____
   Claudication: _____
   Dysreflexia: _____
   Bleeding tendencies/episodes: _____
   Palpitations: _____ Syncope: _____
Extremities: Numbness: _____ Tingling: _____
Cough/hemoptysis: _____
Change in frequency/amount of urine: _____

OBJECTIVE (EXHIBITS)

BP: R and L: Lying/sitting/standing: _____
    Pulse pressure: _____ Auscultatory gap: _____
Pulses (palpation): Carotid: _____ Temporal: _____
    Jugular: _____ Radial: _____ Femoral: _____
    Popliteal: _____ Post-tibial: _____ Dorsalis pedis: _____
Cardiac (palpation): Thrill: _____ Heaves: _____
Heart sounds: Rate: _____ Rhythm: _____ Quality: _____
    Friction rub: _____ Murmur: _____
Vascular bruit: _____ Jugular vein distention: _____
Breath sounds: _____
Extremities: Temperature: _____ Color: _____
    Capillary refill: _____
    Homans' sign: _____ Varicosities: _____
    Nail abnormalities: _____ Edema: _____
    Distribution/quality of hair: _____
    Trophic skin changes: _____
Color: General: _____
    Mucous membranes: _____ Lips: _____
    Nailbeds: _____ Conjunctiva: _____ Sclera: _____
Diaphoresis: _____

Ego Integrity

SUBJECTIVE (REPORTS)

Stress factors: _____
Ways of handling stress: _____
Financial concerns: _____
Relationship status: _____
Cultural factors/ethnic ties: _____
Religion: _____ Practicing: _____
Lifestyle: _____ Recent changes: _____
Sense of connectedness/harmony with self: _____
Feelings of: Helplessness: _____ Hopelessness: _____
    Powerlessness: _____

OBJECTIVE (EXHIBITS)

Emotional status (check those that apply):
    Calm: _____ Anxious: _____ Angry: _____
    Withdrawn: _____ Fearful: _____ Irritable: _____
    Restive: _____ Euphoric: _____
Observed physiologic response(s): _____
Changes in energy field:
    Temperature: _____ Color: _____ Distribution: _____
    Movement: _____
    Sounds: _____

Elimination

SUBJECTIVE (REPORTS)

Usual bowel pattern: _____

Laxative use: _____

Character of stool: _____ Last BM: _____

Diarrhea: _____ Constipation: _____

History of bleeding: _____ Hemorrhoids: _____

Usual voiding pattern: _____

   Incontinence/when: _____ Urgency: _____

   Frequency: _____ Retention: _____

Character of urine: _____

Pain/burning/difficulty voiding: _____

History of kidney/bladder disease: _____

   Diuretic use: _____

OBJECTIVE (EXHIBITS)

Abdomen: Tender: _____ Soft/firm: _____

   Palpable mass: _____ Size/girth: _____

   Bowel sounds: Location: _____ Type: _____

Hemorrhoids: _____ Stool guaiac: _____

Bladder palpable: _____ Overflow voiding: _____

CVA tenderness: _____

Food/Fluid

SUBJECTIVE (REPORTS)

Usual diet (type): _____

Cultural/religious restrictions: _____

Carbohydrate/protein/fat intake: g/d _____

Vitamin/food supplement use: _____

Food preferences: _____ Prohibitions: _____

No. of meals daily: _____

Dietary pattern/content: B: _____ L: _____ D: _____

Last meal/intake: _____

Loss of appetite: _____ Nausea/vomiting: _____

Heartburn/indigestion: _____

   Related to: _____ Relieved by: _____

Allergy/food intolerance: _____

Mastication/swallowing problems: _____

   Dentures: _____

Usual weight: _____ Changes in weight: _____

Diuretic use: _____

OBJECTIVE (EXHIBITS)

Current weight: _____ Height: _____ Body build: _____

Skin turgor: _____ Mucous membranes moist/dry: _____

Breath sounds: Crackles: _____ Wheezes: _____

Edema: General: _____ Dependent: _____
   Periorbital: _____ Ascites: _____
Jugular vein distention: _____
Thyroid enlarged: _____
Condition of teeth/gums: _____
   Appearance of tongue: _____
   Mucous membranes: _____ Halitosis: _____
Bowel sounds: _____
Hernia/masses: _____
Urine S/A or Chemstix: _____
Serum glucose (glucometer): _____

Hygiene

SUBJECTIVE (REPORTS)

Activities of daily living: Independent/dependent (level):
   Mobility: _____ Feeding: _____
   Hygiene: _____ Dressing/grooming: _____ Toileting: _____
Preferred time of personal care/bath: _____
Equipment/prosthetic devices required: _____
Assistance required: _____
   provided by: _____

OBJECTIVE (EXHIBITS)

General appearance: _____
Manner of dress: _____ Personal habits: _____
   Body odor: _____ Condition of scalp: _____
   Presence of vermin: _____

Neurosensory

SUBJECTIVE (REPORTS)

Fainting spells/dizziness: _____
Headaches: Location: _____ Frequency: _____
Tingling/numbness/weakness (location): _____
Stroke/brain injury (residual effects): _____
Seizures: Type: _____ Aura: _____
   Frequency: _____ Postictal state: _____
   How controlled: _____
Eyes: Vision loss: _____ Last examination: _____
   Glaucoma: _____ Cataract: _____
Ears: Hearing loss: _____ Last examination: _____
Sense of smell: _____ Epistaxis: _____

OBJECTIVE (EXHIBITS)

Mental status (note duration of change):
   Oriented/disoriented: Time: _____ Place: _____
   Person: _____ Situation: _____

Check all that apply:
Alert: _____ Drowsy: _____ Lethargic: _____
Stuporous: _____ Comatose: _____
Cooperative: _____ Combative: _____
Delusions: _____ Hallucinations: _____
Affect (describe): _____
Memory: Recent: _____ Remote: _____
Glasses: _____ Contacts: _____ Hearing aids: _____
Pupil: Shape: _____ Size/reaction: R/L: _____
Facial droop: _____ Swallowing: _____
Handgrasp/release, R/L: _____
Posturing: _____
Deep tendon reflexes: _____ Paralysis: _____

Pain/Discomfort

SUBJECTIVE (REPORTS)

Primary focus: _____ Location: _____
Intensity (0–10 with 10 = most severe): _____
Frequency: _____ Quality: _____
Duration: _____ Radiation: _____
Precipitating/aggravating factors: _____
How relieved: _____
Associated symptoms: _____
Effect on activities: _____
Relationships: _____
Additional focus: _____

OBJECTIVE (EXHIBITS)

Facial grimacing: _____ Guarding affected area: _____
Posturing: _____ Behaviors: _____
Emotional response: _____ Narrowed focus: _____
Change in BP: _____ Pulse: _____

Respiration

SUBJECTIVE (REPORTS)

Dyspnea/related to: _____
Cough/sputum: _____
History of: Bronchitis: _____ Asthma: _____
Tuberculosis: _____ Emphysema: _____
Recurrent pneumonia: _____
Exposure to noxious fumes: _____
Smoker: _____ pk/day: _____ No. of pk-yrs: _____
Use of respiratory aids: _____ Oxygen: _____

OBJECTIVE (EXHIBITS)

Respiratory: Rate: _____ Depth: _____ Symmetry: _____
Use of accessory muscles: _____ Nasal flaring: _____
Fremitus: _____
Breath sounds: _____ Egophony: _____
Cyanosis: _____ Clubbing of fingers: _____
Sputum characteristics: _____
Mentation/restlessness: _____

Safety

SUBJECTIVE (REPORTS)

Allergies/sensitivity: _____ Reaction: _____
Exposure to infectious diseases: _____
Immunization history: _____
Previous alteration of immune system: _____
   Cause: _____
History of sexually transmitted disease (date/type): _____
   Testing: _____ High-risk behaviors: _____
Blood transfusion/number: _____ When: _____
   Reaction: _____ Describe: _____
Geographic areas lived in/visited: _____
Seat belt/helmet use: _____
Workplace safety/health issues: _____
History of accidental injuries: _____
   Fractures/dislocations: _____
Arthritis/unstable joints: _____
Back problems: _____
Changes in moles: _____ Enlarged nodes: _____
Delayed healing: _____
Cognitive limitations: _____
   Impaired vision/hearing: _____
Prosthesis: _____ Ambulatory devices: _____

OBJECTIVE (EXHIBITS)

Temperature: _____ Diaphoresis: _____
Skin integrity (mark location on diagram): _____
   Scars: _____ Rashes: _____ Lacerations: _____
   Ulcerations: _____ Ecchymoses: _____ Blisters: _____
   Burns (degree/percent): _____
   Drainage: _____
General strength: _____ Muscle tone: _____
   Gait: _____ ROM: _____
   Paresthesia/paralysis: _____
Results of cultures: _____ Immune system testing: _____
Tuberculosis testing: _____

Sexuality (Component of Ego Integrity and Social Interactions)

SUBJECTIVE (REPORTS)

Sexually active: _____ Use of condoms: _____
Birth control method: _____
Sexual concerns/difficulties: _____
Recent change in frequency/interest: _____

OBJECTIVE (EXHIBITS)

Comfort level with subject matter: _____

FEMALE: SUBJECTIVE (REPORTS)

Age at menarche: _____ Length of cycle: _____
    Duration: _____ No. of pads used/day: _____
    Last menstrual period: _____ Pregnant now: _____
Bleeding between periods: _____
Menopause: _____ Vaginal lubrication: _____
Vaginal discharge: _____
Surgeries: _____
Hormonal therapy/calcium use: _____
Practices breast self-examination: _____
Last mammogram: _____ Pap smear: _____

OBJECTIVE (EXHIBITS)

Breast examination: _____
Genital warts/lesions: _____ Discharge: _____

MALE: SUBJECTIVE (REPORTS)

Penile discharge: _____ Prostate disorder: _____
Circumcised: _____ Vasectomy: _____

Practice self-examination: Breast: _____ Testicles: _____
Last proctoscopic/prostate examination: _____

OBJECTIVE (EXHIBITS)

Breast: _____ Penis: _____ Testicles: _____
Genital warts/lesions: _____ Discharge: _____

Social Interactions

SUBJECTIVE (REPORTS)

Marital status: _____ Years in relationship: _____
Perception of relationship: _____
  Living with: _____
  Concerns/stresses: _____
Extended family: _____
  Other support person(s): _____
Role within family structure: _____
Perception of relationships with family members: _____
Feelings of: Mistrust: _____ Rejection: _____
  Unhappiness: _____
  Loneliness/isolation: _____
Problems related to illness/condition: _____
Problems with communication: _____
Genogram: _____

OBJECTIVE (EXHIBITS)

Speech: Clear: _____ Slurred: _____
  Unintelligible: _____ Aphasic: _____
  Unusual speech pattern/impairment: _____
  Use of speech/communication aids: _____
  Laryngectomy present: _____
Verbal/nonverbal communication with family/SO(s): _____
  Family interaction (behavioral) pattern _____

Teaching/Learning

SUBJECTIVE (REPORTS)

Dominant language (specify): _____ Second language: _____
  Literate: _____ Education level: _____
  Learning disabilities (specify): _____
  Cognitive limitations: _____
Where born: _____ If immigrant, how long in this
  country? _____
Health and illness beliefs/practices/customs: _____

Which family member makes healthcare decisions/
   is spokeperson: _____

Presence of Advance Directives: _____

   Durable Medical Power of Attorney: _____

Special healthcare concerns (e.g., impact of religious/
cultural practices): _____

Health goals: _____

Familial risk factors (indicate relationship):

   Diabetes: _____ Thyroid (specify): _____

   Tuberculosis: _____ Heart disease: _____

   Strokes: _____ High BP: _____

   Epilepsy: _____ Kidney disease: _____

   Cancer: _____ Mental illness: _____

   Other: _____

Prescribed medications:

   Drug: _____

   Dose: _____ Times (circle last dose): _____

   Take regularly: _____ Purpose: _____

   Side effects/problems: _____

Nonprescription drugs: OTC drugs: _____

   Street drugs: _____ Tobacco: _____

   Smokeless tobacco: _____

   Alcohol (amount/frequency): _____

Use of herbal supplements (specify): _____

Admitting diagnosis per provider: _____

Reason per client: _____

History of current complaint: _____

Client expectations of this hospitalization: _____

Previous illnesses and/or hospitalizations/surgeries: _____

Evidence of failure to improve: _____

Last complete physical examination: _____

Discharge Plan Considerations

DRG-projected mean length of stay: _____

Date information obtained: _____

Anticipated date of discharge: _____

Resources available: Persons: _____

   Financial: _____ Community: _____

   Support groups: _____

   Socialization: _____

Areas that may require alteration/assistance:

   Food preparation: _____ Shopping: _____

   Transportation: _____ Ambulation: _____

   Medication/IV therapy: _____ Treatments: _____

   Wound care: _____ Supplies: _____

   Self-care (specify): _____

Homemaker/maintenance (specify): _____
Physical layout of home (specify): _____
Anticipated changes in living situation after discharge: _____
Living facility other than home (specify): _____
Referrals (date, source, services):
Social services: _____ Rehab services: _____
Dietary: _____ Home care: _____
Resp/O_2: _____ Equipment: _____
Supplies: _____
Other: _____

EXCERPT FROM PSYCHIATRIC ASSESSMENT TOOL

Ego Integrity

SUBJECTIVE (REPORTS)

What kind of person are you (positive/negative, etc.)? _____

What do you think of your body? _____

How would you rate your self-esteem (1–10 with
10 = highest)? _____

What are your problematic moods? Depressed: _____

    Guilty: _____ Sad: _____

    Unreal: _____ Ups/downs: _____

    Apathetic: _____ Detached: _____

    Separated from the world: _____

Are you a nervous person? _____

Are your feelings easily hurt? _____

Report of stress factors: _____

Previous patterns of handling stress: _____

Financial concerns: _____

Relationship status: _____

Work history/military service: _____

Cultural factors: _____

Religion: _____ Practicing: _____

Lifestyle: _____ Recent changes: _____

Significant losses/changes (date): _____

Stages of grief/manifestations of loss: _____

Feelings of: Helplessness: _____

    Hopelessness: _____ Powerlessness: _____

OBJECTIVE (EXHIBITS)

Emotional status (check those that apply):

    Calm: ___ Friendly: ___ Cooperative: ___ Evasive: ___

    Anxious: _____ Angry/hostile: _____ Withdrawn: _____

    Fearful: ___ Irritable: ___ Restive: ___ Passive: _____

    Dependent: _____ Euphoric: _____ Other (specify): _____

Defense mechanisms:

    Projection: _____ Denial: _____ Undoing: _____

    Rationalization: _____ Repression: _____

    Passive-aggressive: _____ Sublimation: _____

    Intellectualization: _____ Somatization: _____

    Regression: _____ Identification: _____

    Introjection: _____ Reaction formation: _____

    Isolation: _____ Displacement: _____ Substitution: _____

Consistency of behavior:

    Verbal: _____ Nonverbal: _____

Characteristics of speech: _____
    Slow/rapid/volume: _____ Pressured: _____
    Impairments: _____ Aphasia: _____
Motor activity/behaviors: _____ Posturing: _____
Restless: _____ Under/overactive: _____
Stereotypic: _____ Tics/tremors: _____
Gait patterns: _____ Coping strategies: _____
Observed physiologic response(s): _____

Neurosensory

SUBJECTIVE (REPORTS)

Dreamlike states: _____ Walking in sleep: _____
    Automatic writing: _____
Believe/feel you are another person: _____
Perception different than others: _____
Ability to follow directions: _____
    Perform calculations: _____
    Accomplish ADLs: _____
Fainting spells/dizziness: _____
    Blackouts: _____
Seizures: _____

OBJECTIVE (EXHIBITS)

Mental status (note duration of change): _____
Oriented/disoriented: Time: _____
Place: _____ Person: _____
Check all that apply:
    Alert: ____ Drowsy: ____ Lethargic: ____ Stuporous: ____
    Comatose: _____ Cooperative: _____ Combative: _____
    Delusions: ____ Hallucinations: ____ Affect (describe): ____
Memory: Immediate: _____ Recent: _____ Remote: _____
Comprehension: _____
Thought processes (assessed through speech): Patterns of
    speech (e.g., spontaneous/sudden silences): _____
    Content: _____ Change in topic: _____
    Delusions: _____ Hallucinations: _____ Illusions: _____
    Rate or flow: _____
    Clear, logical progression: _____
    Expression: _____
    Flight of ideas: _____
    Ability to concentrate: _____ Attention span: _____
Mood: _____
    Affect: _____ Appropriateness: _____ Intensity: _____
    Range: _____
Insight: _____ Misperceptions: _____

Attention/calculation skills: _____
 Judgment: _____
 Ability to follow directions: _____
 Problem solving: _____
Impulse control: Aggression: ___ Hostility: ___ Affection: ___
Sexual feelings: _____

EXCERPT FROM PRENATAL ASSESSMENT TOOL

Safety

SUBJECTIVE (REPORTS)

Allergies/sensitivity: _____
  Reaction: _____
Previous alteration of immune system: _____
  Cause: _____
History of sexually transmitted diseases/gynecologic
  infections (date/type): _____ Testing: _____
High-risk behaviors: _____
Blood transfusion/number: _____ When: _____
  Reaction: _____ Describe: _____
Childhood diseases: _____
  Immunization history: _____
Recent exposure to German measles: _____
  Other viral infections: _____ X ray/radiation: _____
  House pets: _____
Previous ob/gyn problems: PIH: _____ Kidney: _____
  Hemorrhage: _____ Cardiac: _____
  Diabetes: _____ Infection/UTI: _____
  ABO/Rh sensitivity: _____ Uterine surgery: _____
  Anemia: _____
Length of time since last pregnancy: _____
  Type of previous delivery: _____
Health status of living children: _____
History of accidental injuries: _____
  Fractures/dislocations: _____ Physical abuse: _____
Arthritis/unstable joints: _____
  Back problems: _____
Changes in moles: _____ Enlarged nodes: _____
Impaired vision: _____ Hearing: _____
Prosthesis: _____ Ambulatory devices: _____

OBJECTIVE (EXHIBITS)

Temperature: _____ Diaphoresis: _____
  Skin integrity: _____ Scars: _____
  Rashes: _____ Sores: _____ Ecchymoses: _____
  Vaginal warts/lesions: _____
General strength: _____ Muscle tone: _____
  Gait: _____ ROM: _____ Paresthesia/paralysis: _____
Fetal: Heart rate: _____ Location: _____
  Method of auscultation: _____ Fundal height: _____
  Estimated gestation: _____
  Movement: _____ Ballottement: _____

Results of fetal testing: Date: _____ Test: _____ Result: _____
Results of cultures, cervical/rectal: _____ Immune system
   testing:_____
Blood type: Maternal: _____ Paternal: _____
Screenings: Serology: _____ Syphilis: _____ Sickle Cell: _____
   Rubella: _____ Hepatitis: _____ HIV: _____ AFP: _____

Sexuality (Component of Ego Integrity and Social Interactions)

SUBJECTIVE (REPORTS)

Sexual concerns: _____
Menarche: _____ Length of cycle: _____
   Duration: _____
First day of last menstrual period: _____
   Amount: _____
   Bleeding/cramping since LMP: _____
   Vaginal discharge: _____
Client's belief of when conception occurred: _____
Estimated date of delivery: _____
Practices breast self-examination (Y/N): _____
Last Pap smear: _____ Results: _____
Recent contraceptive method: _____
OB history (GPTPAL): Gravida: _____ Para: _____
   Term: _____ Preterm: _____ Abortions: _____
   Living: _____ Multiple births: _____
Delivery history: Year: _____ Place of delivery: _____
   Length of gestation: _____ Length of labor: _____
   Type of delivery: _____
   Born (alive or dead): _____
   Weight: _____ Apgar scores: _____
Complications (maternal/fetal): _____

OBJECTIVE (EXHIBITS)

Pelvic: Vulva: _____ Perineum: _____
   Vagina: _____ Cervix: _____
   Uterus: _____ Adnexal: _____
   Diagonal conjugate: _____
   Transverse diameter: _____ Outlet (cm): _____
   Shape of sacrum: _____ Arch: _____
   Coccyx: _____ SS Notch: _____
   Ischial spines: _____
   Adequacy of inlet: _____
   Mid: _____ Outlet: _____
Prognosis for delivery: _____
Breast examination: _____ Nipples: _____
Pregnancy test: _____ Serology test (date): _____
Pap smear date/results: _____

EXCERPT FROM INTRAPARTAL ASSESSMENT TOOL

Pain/Discomfort

SUBJECTIVE (REPORTS)

Uterine contractions began: _____
    Became regular: _____ Character: _____
    Frequency: _____ Duration: _____
Location of contractile pain:
    Front: _____ Sacral area: _____
    Degree of discomfort: Mild: _____ Moderate: _____
    Severe: _____
How relieved: Breathing/relaxation techniques: _____
    Positioning: _____ Sacral rubs: _____
    Effleurage: _____

OBJECTIVE (EXHIBITS)

Facial expression: _____ Narrowed focus: _____
    Body movement: _____
Change in blood pressure: _____ Pulse: _____

Safety

SUBJECTIVE (REPORTS)

Allergies/Sensitivity: _____
    Reaction (specify): _____
History of STD (date/type): _____
Month of first prenatal visit: _____
Previous/current obstetric problems/treatment:
    PIH: _____ Kidney: _____ Hemorrhage: _____
    Cardiac: _____ Diabetes: _____
    Infection/UTI: _____ ABO/Rh sensitivity: _____
    Uterine surgery: _____ Anemia: _____
Length of time since last pregnancy: _____
Type of previous delivery: _____
Health status of living children: _____
Blood transfusion: _____ When: _____
    Reaction (describe): _____
Maternal stature/build: _____
Fractures/dislocations: _____
Pelvis: _____
Arthritis/Unstable joints: _____
Spinal problems/deformity: Kyphosis: _____
    Scoliosis: _____ Trauma: _____
    Surgery: _____
Prosthesis/ambulatory devices: _____

Temperature: _____

Skin integrity: _____ Rashes: _____

   Sores: _____ Bruises: _____ Scars: _____

Paresthesia/Paralysis: _____

Fetal status: Heart rate: _____ Location: _____

   Method of auscultation: _____

   Fundal height: _____ Estimated gestation: _____

   Activity/movement: _____

   Fetal assessment testing (Y/N): _____

   Date: _____ Test: _____ Results: _____

Labor status: Cervical dilation: _____ Effacement: _____

   Fetal descent: _____ Engagement: _____

   Presentation: _____ Lie: _____

   Position: _____

Membranes: Intact: _____ Ruptured/time: _____

   Nitrazine test: _____ Amount of drainage: _____

   Character: _____

Blood type/Rh: Maternal: _____ Paternal: _____

Screens: Sickle cell: _____ Rubella: _____

   Hepatitis: _____ HIV: _____ Tuberculosis: _____

Serology: Syphilis: Pos _____ Neg _____

Cervical/rectal culture: Pos _____ Neg _____

Vaginal warts/lesions: _____

Perineal varicosities: _____

SECTION 2

DIAGNOSTIC DIVISIONS: NURSING DIAGNOSES ORGANIZED ACCORDING TO A NURSING FOCUS

After data are collected and areas of concern/need identified, the nurse is directed to the Diagnostic Divisions to review the list of nursing diagnoses that fall within the individual categories. This will assist the nurse in choosing the specific diagnostic label to accurately describe the data. Then, with the addition of etiology or related/risk factors (when known) and signs and symptoms or cues (defining characteristics), the client diagnostic statement emerges.

ACTIVITY/REST—Ability to engage in necessary/desired activities of life (work and leisure) and to obtain adequate sleep/rest

CIRCULATION—Ability to transport oxygen and nutrients necessary to meet cellular needs

EGO INTEGRITY—Ability to develop and use skills and behaviors to integrate and manage life experiences

ELIMINATION—Ability to excrete waste products

Information that appears in brackets has been added by the authors to clarify and enhance the use of NDs.

Please also see the NANDA diagnoses grouped according to Gordon's Functional Health Patterns on the inside front cover.

FOOD/FLUID—Ability to maintain intake of and utilize nutrients and liquids to meet physiologic needs

HYGIENE—Ability to perform activities of daily living

NEUROSENSORY—Ability to perceive, integrate, and respond to internal and external cues

Information that appears in brackets has been added by the authors to clarify and enhance the use of NDs.

Please also see the NANDA diagnoses grouped according to Gordon's Functional Health Patterns on the inside front cover.

Confusion, acute   147–150
Confusion, chronic   150–153
Infant Behavior, disorganized   295–301
Infant Behavior, readiness for enhanced organized   301–303
Infant Behavior, risk for disorganized   303–304
Memory, impaired   328–331
Peripheral Neurovascular Dysfunction, risk for   387–390
Sensory Perception, disturbed (specify: visual, auditory, kines-
    thetic, gustatory, tactile, olfactory)   449–454
Thought Processes, disturbed   529–533
Unilateral Neglect   551–554

PAIN/DISCOMFORT—Ability to control internal/external
environment to maintain comfort

Pain, acute   365–369
Pain, chronic   370–374

RESPIRATION—Ability to provide and use oxygen to meet
physiologic needs

Airway Clearance, ineffective   69–72
Aspiration, risk for   86–89
Breathing Pattern, ineffective   117–121
Gas Exchange, impaired   256–260
Ventilation, impaired spontaneous   581–586
Ventilatory Weaning Response, dysfunctional   586–590

SAFETY—Ability to provide safe, growth-promoting environment

Allergy Response, latex   73–75
Allergy Response, risk for latex   76–78
Body Temperature, risk for imbalanced   102–104
Death Syndrome, risk for sudden infant   185–189
Environmental Interpretation Syndrome, impaired   211–214
Falls, risk for   217–221
Health Maintenance, ineffective   275–278
Home Maintenance, impaired   281–283
Hyperthermia   287–290
Hypothermia   291–295
Infection, risk for   307–310
Injury, risk for   310–313
Injury, risk for perioperative positioning   313–316
Mobility, impaired physical   333–337
Poisoning, risk for   393–396
Protection, ineffective   411–412
Self-Mutilation   442–445
Self-Mutilation, risk for   445–449

SEXUALITY—[Component of Ego Integrity and Social Interaction] Ability to meet requirements/characteristics of male/female role

SOCIAL INTERACTION—Ability to establish and maintain relationships

Information that appears in brackets has been added by the authors to clarify and enhance the use of NDs.

Please also see the NANDA diagnoses grouped according to Gordon's Functional Health Patterns on the inside front cover.

TEACHING/LEARNING—Ability to incorporate and use information to achieve healthy lifestyle/optimal wellness

Information that appears in brackets has been added by the authors to clarify and enhance the use of NDs.

Please also see the NANDA diagnoses grouped according to Gordon's Functional Health Patterns on the inside front cover.

CLIENT SITUATION AND PROTOTYPE PLAN OF CARE

Client Situation

Mr. R.S., a type 2 diabetic client (noninsulin-dependent) for 5 years, presented to his physician's office with a nonhealing ulcer of 3 weeks' duration on his left foot. Screening studies done in the doctor's office revealed blood glucose of 356/fingerstick and urine Chemstix of 2%. Because of distance from medical provider and lack of local community services, he is admitted to the hospital.

ADMITTING PHYSICIAN'S ORDERS

Culture/sensitivity and Gram's stain of foot ulcer
Random blood glucose on admission and fingerstick BG qid
CBC, electrolytes, serum lipid profile, glycosylated Hb in AM
Chest x ray and ECG in AM
Diabeta 10 mg, PO bid
Glucophage 500 mg, PO qd to start—will increase gradually
Humulin N 10 U SC q AM and HS. Begin insulin instruction for postdischarge self-care if necessary
Dicloxacillin 500 mg PO q6h, start after culture obtained
Darvocet-N 100 mg PO q4h prn pain
Diet—2400 calories, 3 meals with 2 snacks
Up in chair ad lib with feet elevated
Foot cradle for bed
Irrigate lesion L foot with NS tid, then cover with wet to dry sterile dressing
Vital signs qid

CLIENT ASSESSMENT DATABASE

Name: R.S. Informant: Client
Reliability (Scale 1–4): 3
Age: 69   DOB: 5/3/31   Race: Caucasian   Gender: M
Adm. date: 6/28/2000   Time: 7 PM   From: home

Activity/Rest

SUBJECTIVE (REPORTS)

Occupation: farmer
Usual activities/hobbies: reading, playing cards. "Don't have

time to do much. Anyway, I'm too tired most of the time to do anything after the chores."

Limitations imposed by illness: "Have to watch what I order if I eat out."

Sleep: Hours: 6 to 8 h/night   Naps: no   Aids: no

Insomnia: "Not unless I drink coffee after supper."

Usually feels rested when awakens at 4:30 AM

OBJECTIVE (EXHIBITS)

Observed response to activity: limps, favors L foot when walking

Mental status: alert/active

Neuro/muscular assessment: Muscle mass/tone: bilaterally equal/firm   Posture: erect

ROM: full   Strength: equal 4 extremities/(favors L foot currently)

Circulation

SUBJECTIVE (REPORTS)

History of slow healing: lesion L foot, 3 weeks' duration

Extremities: Numbness/tingling: "My feet feel cold and tingly like sharp pins poking the bottom of my feet when I walk the quarter mile to the mailbox."

Cough/character of sputum: occ./white

Change in frequency/amount of urine: yes/voiding more lately

OBJECTIVE (EXHIBITS)

Peripheral pulses: radials 3+; popliteal, dorsalis, post-tibial/pedal, all 1+

BP: R: Lying: 146/90   Sitting: 140/86   Standing: 138/90
    L: Lying: 142/88   Sitting: 138/88   Standing: 138/84

Pulse: Apical: 86   Radial: 86   Quality: strong
    Rhythm: regular

Chest auscultation: few wheezes clear with cough, no murmurs/rubs

Jugular vein distention: 0

Extremities:
    Temperature: feet cool bilaterally/legs warm
    Color: Skin: legs pale
    Capillary refill: slow both feet (approx. 5 seconds)
    Homans' sign: 0
    Varicosities: few enlarged superficial veins both calves
    Nails: toenails thickened, yellow, brittle

Distribution and quality of hair: coarse hair to midcalf, none on ankles/toes

Color:

General: ruddy face/arms

Mucous membranes/lips: pink

Nailbeds: blanch well

Conjunctiva and sclera: white

Ego Integrity

SUBJECTIVE (REPORTS)

Report of stress factors: "Normal farmer's problems: weather, pests, bankers, etc."

Ways of handling stress: "I get busy with the chores and talk things over with my livestock. They listen pretty good."

Financial concerns: no insurance; needs to hire someone to do chores while here

Relationship status: married

Cultural factors: rural/agrarian, eastern European descent, "American," no ethnic ties

Religion: Protestant/practicing

Lifestyle: middle class/self-sufficient farmer

Recent changes: no

Feelings: "I'm in control of most things, except the weather and this diabetes now."

Concerned re possible therapy change "from pills to shots."

OBJECTIVE (EXHIBITS)

Emotional status: generally calm, appears frustrated at times

Observed physiologic response(s): occasionally sighs deeply/frowns, fidgeting with coin, shoulders tense/shrugs shoulders, throws up hands

Elimination

SUBJECTIVE (REPORTS)

Usual bowel pattern: almost every PM

Last BM: last night   Character of stool: firm/brown

Bleeding: 0   Hemorrhoids: 0   Constipation: occ.

Laxative used: hot prune juice on occ.

Urinary: no problems   Character of urine: pale yellow

OBJECTIVE (EXHIBITS)

Abdomen tender: no   Soft/firm: soft   Palpable mass: none

Bowel sounds: active all 4 quads

Food/Fluid

Usual diet (type): 2400 calorie (occ. "cheats" with dessert; "My wife watches it pretty closely.")

No. of meals daily: 3/1 snack

Dietary pattern:

B: fruit juice/toast/ham/decaf coffee

L: meat/potatoes/veg/fruit/milk

D: meat sandwich/soup/fruit/decaf coffee

Snack: milk/crackers at HS. Usual beverage: skim milk, 2 to 3 cups decaf coffee, drinks "lots of water"—several quarts

Last meal/intake: Dinner: roast beef sandwich, vegetable soup, pear with cheese, decaf coffee

Loss of appetite: "Never, but lately I don't feel as hungry as usual."

Nausea/Vomiting: 0   Food allergies: none

Heartburn/food intolerance: cabbage causes gas, coffee after supper causes heartburn

Mastication/swallowing problems: no

Dentures: partial upper plate—fits well

Usual weight: 175 lb   Recent changes: has lost about 5 lb this month

Diuretic therapy: no

Wt: 171 lb   Ht: 5 ft 10 in   Build: stocky

Skin turgor: good/leathery

Appearance of tongue: midline, pink

Mucous membranes: pink, intact

Condition of teeth/gums: good, no irritation/bleeding noted

Breath sounds: few wheezes cleared with cough

Bowel sounds: active all 4 quads

Urine Chemstix: 2%   Fingerstick: 356 (Dr. office) 450 adm, random BG drawn on adm

Hygiene

Activities of daily living: independent in all areas

Preferred time of bath: PM

General appearance: clean, shaven, short-cut hair; hands rough and dry; skin on feet dry, cracked and scaly

Scalp and eyebrows: scaly white patches
No body odor

Neurosensory

SUBJECTIVE (REPORTS)

Headache: "Occasionally behind my eyes when I worry too much."
Tingling/numbness: feet, once or twice a week (as noted)
Eyes: Vision loss, farsighted, "Seems a little blurry now"
    Examination: 2 yr ago
Ears: Hearing loss R: "Some" L: no (has not been tested)
Nose: Epistaxis: 0   Sense of smell: "No problem"

OBJECTIVE (EXHIBITS)

Mental status: alert, oriented to time, place, person, situation
Affect: concerned   Memory: Remote/Recent: clear and intact
Speech: clear/coherent, appropriate
Pupil reaction: PERLA/small
Glasses: reading   Hearing aid: no
Handgrip/release: strong/equal

Pain/Discomfort

SUBJECTIVE (REPORTS)

Primary problem focus: Location: medial aspect, heel of L foot
    Intensity (0–10): 4 to 5   Quality: dull ache with occ. sharp
    stabbing sensation
Frequency/duration: "Seems like all the time."   Radiation: no
Precipitating factors: shoes, walking   How relieved: ASA, not
    helping
Other complaints: sometimes has back pain following chores/
    heavy lifting, relieved by ASA/liniment rubdown

OBJECTIVE (EXHIBITS)

Facial grimacing: when lesion border palpated
Guarding affected area: pulls foot away
Narrowed focus: no
Emotional response: tense, irritated

Respiration

SUBJECTIVE (REPORTS)

Dyspnea: 0   Cough: occ. morning cough, white sputum
Emphysema: 0   Bronchitis: 0   Asthma: 0   Tuberculosis: 0

Smoker: filters pk/day: $^1/_2$ No. pk-yrs: 25+
Use of respiratory aids: 0

OBJECTIVE (EXHIBITS)

Respiratory rate: 22   Depth: good   Symmetry: equal, bilateral
Auscultation: few wheezes, clear with cough
Cyanosis: 0   Clubbing of fingers: 0
Sputum characteristics: none to observe
Mentation/restlessness: alert/oriented/relaxed

Safety

SUBJECTIVE (REPORTS)

Allergies: 0   Blood transfusions: 0
Sexually transmitted disease: none
Fractures/dislocations: L clavicle, 1966, fell getting off tractor
Arthritis/unstable joints: "I think I've got some in my knees."
Back problems: occ. lower back pain
Vision impaired: requires glasses for reading
Hearing impaired: slightly (R), compensates by turning "good
    ear" toward speaker

OBJECTIVE (EXHIBITS)

Temperature: 99.4°F (37.4°C) tympanic
Skin integrity: impaired L foot   Scars: R inguinal, surgical
Rashes: 0   Bruises: 0   Lacerations: 0   Blisters: 0
Ulcerations: medial aspect L heel, 2.5-cm diameter, approx.
    3 mm deep, draining small amount cream-color/pink-tinged
    matter, no odor noted
Strength (general): equal all extremities   Muscle tone: firm
ROM: good   Gait: favors L foot   Paresthesia/paralysis: 0

Sexuality: Male

SUBJECTIVE (REPORTS)

Sexually active: yes   Use of condoms: no (monogomous)
Recent changes in frequency/interest: "I've been too tired lately."
Penile discharge: 0   Prostate disorder: 0   Vasectomy: 0
Last proctoscopic examination: 2 yr ago   Prostate examina-
    tion: 1 yr ago
Practice self-examination: Breast/testicles: No
Problems/complaints: "I don't have any problems, but you'd
    have to ask my wife if there are any complaints."

OBJECTIVE (EXHIBITS)

Examination: Breast: no masses   Testicles: deferred
    Prostate: deferred

Social Interactions

SUBJECTIVE (REPORTS)

Marital status: married 45 yr   Living with: wife
Report of problems: none
Extended family: 1 daughter lives in town (30 miles away); 1 daughter married/grandson, living out of state
Other: several couples, he and wife play cards/socialize with 2 to 3 times/mo
Role: works farm alone; husband/father/grandfather
Report of problems related to illness/condition: none until now
Coping behaviors: "My wife and I have always talked things out. You know the 11th commandment is 'Thou shalt not go to bed angry.'"

OBJECTIVE (EXHIBITS)

Speech: clear, intelligible
Verbal/nonverbal communication with family/SO(s): speaks quietly with wife, looking her in the eye; relaxed posture
Family interaction patterns: wife sitting at bedside, relaxed, both reading paper, making occasional comments to each other

Teaching/Learning

SUBJECTIVE (REPORTS)

Dominant language: English   Second language: 0
    Literate: yes
Education level: 2-yr college
Health and illness/beliefs/practices/customs: "I take care of the minor problems and see the doctor only when something's broken."
Presence of Advance Directives: yes—wife to bring in
    Durable Medical Power of Attorney: wife
Familial risk factors/relationship:
    Diabetes: maternal uncle
    Tuberculosis: brother died, age 27
    Heart disease: father died, age 78, heart attack
    Strokes: mother died, age 81
    High BP: mother
Prescribed medications:
    Drug: Diabeta Dose: 10 mg bid
    Schedule: 8 AM/6 PM, last dose 6 PM today
    Purpose: control diabetes
    Takes medications regularly? yes
Home urine/glucose monitoring: "Stopped several months ago when I ran out of TesTape. It was always negative, anyway."
Nonprescription (OTC) drugs: occ. ASA

Use of alcohol (amount/frequency): socially, occ. beer

Tobacco: $^1/_2$ pk/day

Admitting diagnosis (physician): hyperglycemia with nonhealing lesion L foot

Reason for hospitalization (client): "Sore on foot and the doctor is concerned about my blood sugar, and says I'm supposed to learn this fingerstick test now."

History of current complaint: "Three weeks ago I got a blister on my foot from breaking in my new boots. It got sore so I lanced it but it isn't getting any better."

Client's expectations of this hospitalization: "Clear up this infection and control my diabetes."

Other relevant illness and/or previous hospitalizations/surgeries: 1969, R inguinal hernia repair

Evidence of failure to improve: lesion L foot, 3 wk

Last physical examination: complete 1 yr ago, office follow-up 3 mo ago

Discharge Considerations (as of 6/28)

Anticipated discharge: 7/1/00 (3 days)

Resources: self, wife   Financial: "If this doesn't take too long to heal, we got some savings to cover things."

Community supports: diabetic support group (has not participated)

Anticipated lifestyle changes: become more involved in management of condition

Assistance needed: may require farm help for several days

Teaching: learn new medication regimen and wound care; review diet; encourage smoking cessation

Referral: Supplies: Downtown Pharmacy or AARP

Equipment: Glucometer-AARP

Follow-up: primary care provider 1 wk after discharge to evaluate wound healing and potential need for additional changes in diabetic regimen

PLAN OF CARE FOR CLIENT WITH DIABETES MELLITUS

Client Diagnostic Statement:

impaired Skin Integrity related to pressure, altered metabolic state, circulatory impairment and decreased sensation, as evidenced by draining wound L foot.

Outcome: Blood Glucose Control (NOC) Indicators: Client Will:

Demonstrate correction of metabolic state as evidenced by FBS less than 120 mg/dL within 36 hr (6/30 0700).

Outcome: Wound Healing: Secondary Intention (NOC) Indicators: Client Will:

Be free of purulent drainage within 48 hr (6/30 1900).
Display signs of healing with wound edges clean/pink within 60 hr (discharge) (7/1 0700).

ACTIONS/ INTERVENTIONS	RATIONALE
Wound Care (NIC)	
Irrigate wound with room temperature sterile NS tid.	Cleans wound without harming delicate tissues.
Assess wound with each dressing change. Obtain wound tracing on adm and at discharge.	Provides information about effectiveness of therapy and identifies additional needs.
Apply wet to dry sterile dressing. Use paper tape.	Keeps wound clean/minimizes cross contamination. Adhesive tape may be abrasive to fragile tissues.
Infection Control (NIC)	
Follow wound precautions.	Use of gloves and proper handling of contaminated dressings reduces likelihood of spread of infection.
Obtain sterile specimen of wound drainage on admission.	Culture/sensitivity identifies pathogens and therapy of choice.

(Continued on the following page)

ACTIONS/ INTERVENTIONS

RATIONALE

Administer dicloxacillin 500 mg PO q6h, starting 10 PM. Observe for signs of hypersensitivity (i.e., pruritus, urticaria, rash).

Treatment of infection/prevention of complications. Food interferes with drug absorption, requiring scheduling around meals.
Although no prior history of penicillin reaction, it may occur at any time.

Administer antidiabetic medications: 10 U Humulin N insulin SC q AM/HS after fingerstick BG; Diabeta 10 mg PO bid; Glucophage 500 mg PO qd. Note onset of side effects.

Treats underlying metabolic dysfunction, reducing hyperglycemia and promoting healing. Glucophage lowers serum glucose levels by improving insulin sensitivity, increasing glucose utilization in the muscles. By using in conjunction with Diabeta, client may be able to discontinue insulin once target dosage is achieved (e.g., 2000 mg/day). Increase of 1 tablet per week is necessary to limit side effects of diarrhea, abdominal cramping, vomiting, possibly leading to dehydration and prerenal azotemia.

Client Diagnostic Statement:

acute Pain related to physical agent (open wound L foot), as evidenced by verbal report of pain and guarding behavior.

Outcome: Pain Control (NOC) Indicators: Client Will:

Report pain is minimized/relieved within 1 hr of analgesic administration (ongoing).
Report absence or control of pain by discharge (7/1).

Outcome: Pain Disruptive Effects (NOC) Indicators: Client Will:

Ambulate normally, full weight bearing by discharge (7/1).

ACTIONS/ INTERVENTIONS

RATIONALE

Pain Management (NIC)

Determine pain character-
istics through client's
description.

Establishes baseline for assessing improvement/changes.

Place foot cradle on bed,
encourage use of loose-
fitting slipper when up.

Avoids direct pressure to area
of injury, which could result
in vasoconstriction/increased
pain.

Administer Darvocet-N 100
mg PO q4h as needed.
Document effectiveness.

Provides relief of discomfort
when unrelieved by other
measures.

Client Diagnostic Statement:

ineffective peripheral Tissue Perfusion related to decreased arterial flow evidenced by decreased pulses, pale/cool feet; thick,
brittle nails; numbness/tingling of feet "when walks $1/4$ mile."

Outcome: Knowledge: Diabetes Management (NOC) Indicators: Client Will:

Verbalize understanding of relationship between chronic
disease (diabetes mellitus) and circulatory changes within 48
hr (6/30 1900).

Demonstrate awareness of safety factors/proper foot care
within 48 hr (6/30 1900).

Maintain adequate level of hydration to maximize perfusion, as
evidenced by balanced intake/output, moist skin/mucous
membranes, adequate capillary refill less than 4 seconds
(ongoing).

ACTIONS/ INTERVENTIONS

RATIONALE

**Circulatory Care: Arterial
Insufficiency** (NIC)

Elevate feet when up in
chair. Avoid long
periods with feet
dependent.

Minimizes interruption of
blood flow, reduces venous
pooling.

(Continued on the following page)

ACTIONS/ INTERVENTIONS	RATIONALE
Assess for signs of dehydration. Monitor intake/output. Encourage oral fluids.	Glycosuria may result in dehydration with consequent reduction of circulating volume and further impairment of peripheral circulation.
Instruct client to avoid constricting clothing/socks and ill-fitting shoes.	Compromised circulation and decreased pain sensation may precipitate or aggravate tissue breakdown.
Reinforce safety precautions regarding use of heating pads, hot water bottles/soaks.	Heat increases metabolic demands on compromised tissues. Vascular insufficiency alters pain sensation, increasing risk of injury.
Recommend cessation of smoking.	Vascular constriction associated with smoking and diabetes impairs peripheral circulation.
Discuss complications of disease that result from vascular changes (i.e., ulceration, gangrene, muscle or bony structure changes).	Although proper control of diabetes mellitus may not prevent complications, severity of effect may be minimized. Diabetic foot complications are the leading cause of nontraumatic lower extremity amputations. **Note:** Skin dry, cracked, scaly; feet cool; pain when walking a distance suggest mild to moderate vascular disease (autonomic neuropathy) that can limit response to infection, impair wound healing, and increase risk of bony deformities.
Review proper foot care as outlined in teaching plan.	Altered perfusion of lower extremities may lead to serious/persistent complications at the cellular level.

Client Diagnostic Statement:

Learning Need regarding diabetic condition related to misinterpretation of information and/or lack of recall as evidenced by inaccurate follow-through of instructions regarding home glucose monitoring and foot care, and failure to recognize signs/symptoms of hyperglycemia.

Outcome: Knowledge: Diabetes Management (NOC) Indicators: Client Will:

Perform procedure of home glucose monitoring correctly within 36 hr (6/30 0700).

Verbalize basic understanding of disease process and treatment within 38 hr (6/30 0900).

Explain reasons for actions within 28 hr (6/30 0900).

Perform insulin administration correctly within 60 hr (7/1 0700).

ACTIONS/ INTERVENTIONS	RATIONALE
Teaching: Disease Process (NIC)	
Determine client's level of knowledge, priorities of learning needs, desire/need for including wife in instruction.	Establishes baseline and direction for teaching/planning. Involvement of wife, if desired, will provide additional resource for recall/understanding and may enhance client's follow through.
Provide teaching guide, "Understanding Your Diabetes," 6/29 AM. Show film "Living with Diabetes" 6/29 4 PM, when wife is visiting. Include in group teaching session 6/30 AM. Review information and obtain feedback from client/wife.	Provides different methods for accessing/reinforcing information and enhances opportunity for learning/understanding.
Discuss factors related to/ altering diabetic control (e.g., stress, illness, exercise).	Drug therapy/diet may need to be altered in response to both short-term and long-term stressors.
Review signs/symptoms of hyperglycemia (e.g., fatigue, nausea/vomiting, polyuria/polydipsia). Discuss how to prevent and evaluate this situation and when to seek medical care. Have client identify appropriate interventions.	Recognition/understanding of these signs/symptoms and timely intervention will aid client in avoiding recurrences and preventing complications.

(Continued on the following page)

ACTIONS/ INTERVENTIONS	RATIONALE
Review and provide information about necessity for routine examination of feet and proper foot care (e.g., daily inspection for injuries, pressure areas, corns, calluses; proper nail cutting; daily washing, application of good moisturizing lotion [e.g., Eucerin, Keri, Nivea] bid). Recommend wearing loose-fitting socks and properly fitting shoes (break new shoes in gradually) and avoiding going barefoot. If foot injury/skin break occurs, wash with soap/dermal cleanser and water, cover with sterile dressing, inspect wound and change dressing daily; report redness, swelling, or presence of drainage.	Reduces risk of tissue injury, promotes understanding and prevention of stasis ulcer formation and wound healing difficulties.
Instruct regarding prescribed insulin therapy:	May be a temporary treatment of hyperglycemia with infection or may be permanent replacement of oral hypoglycemic agent.
Humulin N Insulin, SC;	Intermediate-acting insulin generally lasts 18–28 hr, with peak effect 6–12 hr.
Keep vial in current use at room temperature (if used within 30 days);	Cold insulin is poorly absorbed.
Store extra vials in refrigerator;	Refrigeration prevents wide fluctuations in temperature, prolonging the drug shelf life.

Information that appears in brackets has been added by the authors to clarify and enhance the use of NDs.

Please also see the NANDA diagnoses grouped according to Gordon's Functional Health Patterns on the inside front cover.

ACTIONS/ INTERVENTIONS	RATIONALE
Roll bottle and invert to mix, or shake gently, avoiding bubbles;	Vigorous shaking may create foam, which can interfere with accurate dose withdrawal and may damage the insulin molecule. **Note:** New research suggests that shaking the vial may be more effective in mixing suspension.
Choice of injection sites (e.g., across lower abdomen in Z pattern).	Provides for steady absorption of medication. Site is easily visualized and accessible by client, and Z pattern minimizes tissue damage.
Demonstrate, then observe client drawing insulin into syringe, reading syringe markings, and administering dose. Assess for accuracy.	May require several instruction sessions and practice before client/wife feel comfortable drawing up and injecting medication.
Instruct in signs/symptoms of insulin reaction/hypoglycemia (i.e., fatigue, nausea, headache, hunger, sweating, irritability, shakiness, anxiety, difficulty concentrating).	Knowing what to watch for and appropriate treatment (such as $^1/_2$ cup of grape juice for immediate response and snack within $^1/_2$ hr [e.g., 1 slice bread with peanut butter or cheese, fruit, and slice of cheese for sustained effect]) may prevent/minimize complications.
Review "Sick Day Rules" (e.g., call the doctor if too sick to eat normally/stay active), take insulin as ordered. Keep record as noted in Sick Day Guide.	Understanding of necessary actions in the event of mild/severe illness promotes competent self-care and reduces risk of hyper/hypoglycemia.

Information that appears in brackets has been added by the authors to clarify and enhance the use of NDs.

Please also see the NANDA diagnoses grouped according to Gordon's Functional Health Patterns on the inside front cover.

(Continued on the following page)

ACTIONS/ INTERVENTIONS	RATIONALE
Instruct client/wife in finger-stick glucose monitoring to be done QID until stable, then bid rotating times (e.g., FBS, before dinner; before lunch and HS). Observe return demonstrations of the procedure.	Fingerstick monitoring provides accurate and timely information regarding diabetic status. Return demonstration verifies correct learning.
Recommend client maintain record/log of fingerstick testing, antidiabetic medication, and insulin dosage/site, unusual physiological response, dietary intake. Outline desired goals (e.g., FBS 80–110, premeal 80–130).	Provides accurate record for review by caregivers for assessment of therapy effectiveness/needs.
Schedule consultation with dietitian to restructure meal plan and evaluate food choices.	Calories are unchanged on new orders but have been redistributed to 3 meals and 2 snacks. Dietary choices (e.g., increased vitamin C) may enhance healing.
Discuss other healthcare issues such as smoking habits, self-monitoring for cancer (breasts/testicles), and reporting changes in general well-being.	Encourages client involvement, awareness, and responsibility for own health; promotes wellness. **Note:** Smoking tends to increase client's resistance to insulin.

SECTION 4

DOCUMENTATION TECHNIQUES: SOAP AND FOCUS CHARTING®

Several charting formats are currently used for documentation. These include block notes, with a single entry covering an entire shift (e.g., 7 AM to 3 PM); narrative timed notes (e.g., "8:30 AM, ate breakfast well"); and the problem-oriented medical record system (POMR or PORS) using SOAP/SOAPIER approach, to name a few. The latter can provide thorough documentation; however, the SOAP/SOAPIER charting system was designed by physicians for episodic care and requires that the entries be tied to a problem identified from a problem list. (See Example 1.)

The Focus Charting® system (see Example 2) has been designed by nurses for documentation of frequent/repetitive care and to encourage viewing the client from a positive rather than a negative (problem only) perspective. Charting is focused on client and nursing concerns, with the focal point of client status and the associated nursing care. A Focus is usually a client problem/concern or nursing diagnosis but is not a medical diagnosis or a nursing task/treatment (e.g., wound care, indwelling catheter insertion, tube feeding).

Recording of assessment, interventions, and evaluation using Data, Action, and Response (DAR) categories facilitates tracking what is happening to the client at any given moment. Thus, the four components of this charting system are:

(1) **Focus**: Nursing diagnosis, client problem/concern, signs/symptoms of potential importance (e.g., fever, dysrhythmia, edema), a significant event or change in status or specific standards of care/agency policy.
(2) **Data**: Subjective/objective information describing and/or supporting the Focus.
(3) **Action**: Immediate/future nursing actions based on assessment and consistent with/complementary to the goals and nursing action recorded in the client plan of care.
(4) **Response**: Describes the effects of interventions and whether the goal was met.

The following charting examples are based on the data within the client situation of Mr. R.S. in Chapter 3, Section 3, pages 39–46.

Example 1. SAMPLE SOAP/IER CHARTING FOR PROTOTYPE PLAN OF CARE

S = SUBJECTIVE I = IMPLEMENTATION O = OBJECTIVE			
E = EVALUATION A = ANALYSIS R = REVISION P = PLAN			

DATE	TIME	NUMBER/ PROBLEM*	NOTE
6/30/00	1600	No. 1 (impaired Skin Integrity)	S: "That hurts" (when tissue surrounding wound palpated).
			O: Scant amount serous drainage on dressing. Wound borders pink. No odor present.
			A: Wound shows early signs of healing, free of infection.
			P: Continue skin care per plan of care.

To document more of the nursing process, some institutions have added the following: Implementation, Evaluation, and Revision (if plan was ineffective).

			I: NS soaks as ordered. Applied sterile wet dressing with paper tape.
			E: Wound clean, no drainage present.
			R: None required. Signed: E. Moore, RN
6/28/00	2100	No. 2 (acute Pain)	S: "Dull, throbbing pain in left foot." States there is no radiation to other areas.
			O: Muscles tense. Moving about bed, appears uncomfortable.
			A: Persistent pain.
			P: Foot cradle placed on bed. Signed: M. Siskin, RN
	2200		E: Reports pain relieved. Appears relaxed. Signed: M. Siskin, RN

S = SUBJECTIVE	I = IMPLEMENTATION	O = OBJECTIVE
E = EVALUATION	A = ANALYSIS	R = REVISION P = PLAN

DATE	TIME	NUMBER/ PROBLEM*	NOTE
6/30/00	1100	No. 3 (Learning Need, Diabetic Care)	S: "My wife and I have some questions and concerns we wish to discuss." O: Copy of list of questions attached to teaching plan. A: R. S. and wife need review of information and practice for insulin administration. P: Attended group teaching session with wife and read "Understanding Your Diabetes." To meet with dietitian. I: R. S. demonstrated insulin administration techniques for wife to observe. Procedure handout sheet for future reference provided to couple. Scheduled meeting for them with dietitian at 1300 today to discuss remaining questions. E: R. S. more confident in demonstration, performed activity correctly without hesitation or hand tremors. R. S. explained steps of procedure and reasons for actions to wife. Couple identified resources to contact if questions/problems arise. Signed: B. Briner, RN

*As noted on Plan of Care.

**Example 2. SAMPLE OF FOCUS CHARTING®
FOR PROTOTYPE PLAN OF CARE**

D = Data   A = Action   R = Response

DATE	TIME	FOCUS®	
6/30/00	1600	Skin integrity L foot	D: Scant amount serous drainage on dressing, wound borders pink, no odor present, denies discomfort except with direct palpation of surrounding tissue.
			A: NS soak as ordered. Sterile wet dressing applied with paper tape.
			R: Wound clean—no drainage present. Signed: E. Moore, RN
6/28/00	2100	Pain L foot	D: Reports dull/throbbing ache L foot—no radiation. Muscles tense, restless in bed.
			A: Foot cradle placed on bed. Darvocet-N 100 mg given PO. Signed: M. Siskin, RN
	2200	Pain L foot	R: Reports pain relieved. Appears relaxed. Signed: M. Siskin, RN
6/30/00	1100	Learning Need, Diabetic Teaching	D: Attended group teaching session with wife. Both have read "Understanding Your Diabetes."
			A: Reviewed list of questions/ concerns from R. S. and wife. (Copy attached to teaching plan.) R. S. demonstrated insulin administration technique for wife to observe.
			Procedure handout sheet for future reference provided to couple.
			Meeting scheduled with dietian for 1300 today to discuss remaining questions.

D = DATA	**A** = ACTION	**R** = RESPONSE

DATE	**TIME**	**FOCUS®**	
			R: R. S. more confident in demonstration, performed activity correctly without hesitation or hand tremors. He explained steps of procedure and reasons for actions to wife. Couple identified resources to contact if questions/problems arise.

The following is an example of documentation of a client need/concern that currently does not require identification as a client problem (nursing diagnosis) or inclusion in the plan of care and therefore is not easily documented in the SOAP format:

6/29/00	2020	Gastric distress	D: Awakened from light sleep by "indigestion/burning sensation." Places hand over epigastric area. Skin warm/dry, color pink, vital signs unchanged.
			A: Given Mylanta 30 ml PO. Head of bed elevated approximately 15 degrees.
			R: Reports pain relieved. Appears relaxed, resting quietly. Signed: E. Moore, RN

Source: FOCUS Charting®, Susan Lampe, RN, MS: Creative Nursing Management, Inc., 614 East Grant Street, Minneapolis, MN 55404.

CHAPTER 4

Nursing Diagnoses in Alphabetical Order

Activity Intolerance [specify level]

Taxonomy II: Activity/Rest—Class 4
Cardiovascular/Pulmonary Responses (00092)
[Diagnostic Division: Activity/Rest]
Submitted 1982

Definition: Insufficient physiological or psychological energy to endure or complete required or desired daily activities

Related Factors

Generalized weakness
Sedentary lifestyle
Bedrest or immobility
Imbalance between oxygen supply and demand
[Cognitive deficits/emotional status; secondary to underlying disease process/depression]
[Pain, vertigo, extreme stress]

Defining Characteristics

SUBJECTIVE

Report of fatigue or weakness
Exertional discomfort or dyspnea
[Verbalizes no desire and/or lack of interest in activity]

OBJECTIVE

Abnormal heart rate or blood pressure response to activity
Electrocardiographic changes reflecting dysrhythmias or ischemia
[Pallor, cyanosis]

Functional Level Classification (Gordon, 1987):

Level I: Walk, regular pace, on level indefinitely; one flight or more but more short of breath than normally

Information that appears in brackets has been added by the authors to clarify and enhance the use of nursing diagnoses.

Level II: Walk one city block [or] 500 ft on level; climb one flight slowly without stopping

Level III: Walk no more than 50 ft on level without stopping; unable to climb one flight of stairs without stopping

Level IV: Dyspnea and fatigue at rest

Desired Outcomes/Evaluation Criteria—Client Will:

- Identify negative factors affecting activity tolerance and eliminate or reduce their effects when possible.
- Use identified techniques to enhance activity tolerance.
- Participate willingly in necessary/desired activities.
- Report measurable increase in activity tolerance.
- Demonstrate a decrease in physiologic signs of intolerance (e.g., pulse, respirations, and blood pressure remain within client's normal range).

Actions/Interventions

NURSING PRIORITY NO. 1. To identify causative/precipitating factors:

- Note presence of factors contributing to fatigue (e.g., acute or chronic illness, heart failure, hypothyroidism, cancer, and cancer therapies, etc.).
- Evaluate current limitations/degree of deficit in light of usual status. (**Provides comparative baseline.**)
- Note client reports of weakness, fatigue, pain, difficulty accomplishing tasks, and/or insomnia.
- Assess cardiopulmonary response to physical activity, including vital signs before, during, and after activity. Note progression/accelerating degree of fatigue.
- Ascertain ability to stand and move about and degree of assistance necessary/use of equipment.
- Identify activity needs versus desires (e.g., is barely able to walk upstairs but would like to play racquetball).
- Assess emotional/psychologic factors affecting the current situation (**e.g., stress and/or depression may be increasing the effects of an illness, or depression might be the result of being forced into inactivity**).
- Note treatment-related factors, such as side effects/interactions of medications.

NURSING PRIORITY NO. 2. To assist client to deal with contributing factors and manage activities within individual limits:

- Monitor vital/cognitive signs, watching for changes in blood pressure, heart and respiratory rate; note skin pallor and/or cyanosis, and presence of confusion.
- Adjust activities **to prevent overexertion.** Reduce intensity

level or discontinue activities that cause undesired physiologic changes.

- Provide/monitor response to supplemental oxygen and medications and changes in treatment regimen.
- Increase exercise/activity levels gradually; teach methods **to conserve energy,** such as stopping to rest for 3 minutes during a 10-minute walk, sitting down instead of standing to brush hair.
- Plan care with rest periods between activities **to reduce fatigue.**
- Provide positive atmosphere, while acknowledging difficulty of the situation for the client. (**Helps to minimize frustration, rechannel energy.**)
- Encourage expression of feelings contributing to/resulting from condition.
- Involve client/SO(s) in planning of activities as much as possible.
- Assist with activities and provide/monitor client's use of assistive devices (crutches, walker, wheelchair, oxygen tank, etc.) **to protect client from injury.**
- Promote comfort measures and provide for relief of pain **to enhance ability to participate in activities.** (Refer to ND Pain, acute or Pain, chronic.)
- Provide referral to other disciplines as indicated (e.g., exercise physiologist, psychologic counseling/therapy, occupational/physical therapists, and recreation/leisure specialists) **to develop individually appropriate therapeutic regimens.**

NURSING PRIORITY NO. **3.** To promote wellness (Teaching/ Discharge Considerations):

- Plan for maximal activity within the client's ability.
- Review expectations of client/SO(s)/providers **to establish individual goals.** Explore conflicts/differences **to reach agreement for the most effective plan.**
- Instruct client/SO(s) in monitoring response to activity and in recognizing signs/symptoms that **indicate need to alter activity level.**
- Plan for progressive increase of activity level as client tolerates.
- Give client information that provides evidence of daily/ weekly progress **to sustain motivation.**
- Assist client to learn and demonstrate appropriate safety measures **to prevent injuries.**
- Provide information about the effect of lifestyle and overall health factors on activity tolerance (e.g., nutrition, adequate fluid intake, mental health status).
- Encourage client to maintain positive attitude; suggest use of

relaxation techniques, such as visualization/guided imagery as appropriate, **to enhance sense of well-being.**
- Encourage participation in recreation/social activities and hobbies appropriate for situation. (Refer to ND Diversional Activity, deficient.)

Documentation Focus

ASSESSMENT/REASSESSMENT

- Level of activity as noted in Functional Level Classification.
- Causative/precipitating factors.
- Client reports of difficulty/change.

PLANNING

- Plan of care and who is involved in planning.

IMPLEMENTATION/EVALUATION

- Response to interventions/teaching and actions performed.
- Implemented changes to plan of care based on Assessment/ Reassessment findings.
- Teaching plan and response/understanding of teaching plan.
- Attainment/progress toward desired outcome(s).

DISCHARGE PLANNING

- Referrals to other resources.
- Long-term needs and who is responsible for actions.

SAMPLE NURSING OUTCOMES & INTERVENTIONS CLASSIFICATIONS (NOC/NIC)

NOC—Activity Tolerance
NIC—Energy Management

Activity Intolerance, risk for

Taxonomy II: Activity/Rest—Class 4
Cardiovascular/Pulmonary Response (00094)
[Diagnostic Division: Activity/Rest]
Submitted 1982

Definition: At risk of experiencing insufficient physiological or psychological energy to endure or complete required or desired daily activities

Risk Factors

History of previous intolerance
Presence of circulatory/respiratory problems

Information that appears in brackets has been added by the authors to clarify and enhance the use of nursing diagnoses.

Deconditioned status

Inexperience with the activity

[Diagnosis of progressive disease state/debilitating condition, such as cancer, multiple sclerosis—MS, extensive surgical procedures]

[Verbalized reluctance/inability to perform expected activity]

NOTE: A risk diagnosis is not evidenced by signs and symptoms, as the problem has not occurred and nursing interventions are directed at prevention.

Desired Outcomes/Evaluation Criteria—Client Will:

- Verbalize understanding of potential loss of ability in relation to existing condition.
- Participate in conditioning/rehabilitation program to enhance ability to perform.
- Identify alternative ways to maintain desired activity level (e.g., if weather is bad, walking in a shopping mall could be an option).
- Identify conditions/symptoms that require medical reevaluation.

Actions/Interventions

NURSING PRIORITY NO. 1. To assess factors affecting current situation:

- Identify factors that could block/affect desired level of activity (e.g., age, arthritis, climate, or weather).
- Note presence of medical diagnosis and/or therapeutic regimen **that has potential for interfering with client's ability to perform at a desired level of activity.**
- Determine baseline activity level and physical condition. **(Provides opportunity to track changes.)**

NURSING PRIORITY NO. 2. To develop/investigate alternative ways to remain active within the limits of the disabling condition/situation:

- Implement physical therapy/exercise program in conjunction with the client and other team members (e.g., physical and/or occupational therapist, exercise/rehabilitation physiologist). **Coordination of program enhances likelihood of success.**
- Promote/implement conditioning program and support inclusion in exercise/activity groups **to prevent/limit deterioration.**

- Instruct client in unfamiliar activities and in alternate ways of doing familiar activities **to conserve energy and promote safety.**

NURSING PRIORITY NO. **3.** To promote wellness (Teaching/ Discharge Considerations):

- Discuss relationship of illness/debilitating condition to inability to perform desired activity(ies).
- Provide information regarding potential interferences to activity.
- Assist client/SO(s) with planning for changes that may become necessary.
- Identify and discuss symptoms for which client needs to seek medical assistance/evaluation **providing for timely intervention.**
- Refer to appropriate sources for assistance and/or equipment as needed **to sustain activity level.**

Documentation Focus

ASSESSMENT/REASSESSMENT

- Identified/potential risk factors for individual.
- Current level of activity tolerance and blocks to activity.

PLANNING

- Treatment options, including physical therapy/exercise program, other assistive therapies, and devices.
- Lifestyle changes that are planned, who is to be responsible for each action, and monitoring methods.

IMPLEMENTATION/EVALUATION

- Responses to interventions/teaching and actions performed.
- Attainment/progress toward desired outcome(s).
- Modification of plan of care.

DISCHARGE PLANNING

- Referrals for medical assistance/evaluation.

SAMPLE NURSING OUTCOMES & INTERVENTIONS CLASSIFICATIONS (NOC/NIC)

NOC—Endurance
NIC—Energy Management

Adjustment, impaired

Taxonomy II: Coping/Stress Tolerance—Class 2 Coping Responses (00070)
[Diagnostic Division: Ego Integrity]
Submitted 1986; Nursing Diagnosis Extension and Classification (NDEC) Revision 1998

Definition: Inability to modify lifestyle/behavior in a manner consistent with a change in health status

Related Factors

Disability or health status requiring change in lifestyle
Multiple stressors; intense emotional state
Low state of optimism; negative attitudes toward health behavior; lack of motivation to change behaviors
Failure to intend to change behavior
Absence of social support for changed beliefs and practices
[Physical and/or learning disability]

Defining Characteristics

SUBJECTIVE

Denial of health status change
Failure to achieve optimal sense of control

OBJECTIVE

Failure to take actions that would prevent further health problems
Demonstration of nonacceptance of health status change

Desired Outcomes/Evaluation Criteria—Client Will:

- Demonstrate increasing interest/participation in self-care.
- Develop ability to assume responsibility for personal needs when possible.
- Identify stress situations leading to impaired adjustment and specific actions for dealing with them.
- Initiate lifestyle changes that will permit adaptation to present life situations.
- Identify and use appropriate support systems.

Actions/Interventions

NURSING PRIORITY NO. 1. To assess degree of impaired function:

- Perform a physical and/or psychosocial assessment **to determine the extent of the limitation(s) of the present condition.**
- Listen to the client's perception of inability/reluctance to adapt to situations that are occurring at present.

Information that appears in brackets has been added by the authors to clarify and enhance the use of nursing diagnoses.

- Survey (with the client) past and present significant support systems (e.g., family, church, groups, and organizations) **to identify helpful resources.**
- Explore the expressions of emotions signifying impaired adjustment by client/SO(s) (e.g., overwhelming anxiety, fear, anger, worry, passive and/or active denial).
- Note child's interaction with parent/care provider (**development of coping behaviors is limited at this age, and primary care providers provide support for the child and serve as role models**).
- Determine whether child displays problems with school performance, withdraws from family/peers, or demonstrates aggressive behavior toward others/self.

NURSING PRIORITY NO. 2. To identify the causative/contributing factors relating to the impaired adjustment:

- Listen to client's perception of the factors leading to the present impairment, noting onset, duration, presence/absence of physical complaints, social withdrawal.
- Review previous life situations and role changes with client **to determine coping skills used.**
- Determine lack of/inability to use available resources.
- Review available documentation and resources to determine actual life experiences (e.g., medical records, statements by SO[s], consultants' notes). **In situations of great stress, physical and/or emotional, the client may not accurately assess occurrences leading to the present situation.**

NURSING PRIORITY NO. 3. To assist client in coping/dealing with impairment:

- Organize a team conference (including client and ancillary services) **to focus on contributing factors of impaired adjustment and plan for management of the situation.**
- Acknowledge client's efforts to adjust: "Have done your best." **Lessens feelings of blame/guilt and defensive response.** Share information with adolescent's peers when illness/injury affects body image (**peers are primary support for this age group**).
- Explain disease process/causative factors and prognosis as appropriate and promote questioning **to enhance understanding.**
- Provide an open environment encouraging communication **so that expression of feelings concerning impaired function can be dealt with realistically.**
- Use therapeutic communication skills (Active-listening, acknowledgment, silence, I-statements).
- Discuss/evaluate resources that have been useful to the client in adapting to changes in other life situations (e.g., vocational

rehabilitation, employment experiences, psychosocial support services).
- Develop a plan of action with client **to meet immediate needs** (e.g., physical safety and hygiene, emotional support of professionals and SO[s]) and assist in implementation of the plan. **Provides a starting point to deal with current situation for moving ahead with plan and for evaluation of progress.**
- Explore previously used coping skills and application to current situation. Refine/develop new strategies as appropriate.
- Identify and problem-solve with the client frustration in daily care. (**Focusing on the smaller factors of concern gives the individual the ability to perceive the impaired function from a less-threatening perspective, one-step-at-a-time concept.**)
- Involve SO(s) in long-range planning for emotional, psychological, physical, and social needs.

NURSING PRIORITY NO. 4. To promote wellness (Teaching/Discharge Considerations):

- Identify strengths the client perceives in present life situation. Keep focus on the present, **as unknowns of the future may be too overwhelming.**
- Refer to other resources in the long-range plan of care (e.g., occupational therapy, vocational rehabilitation) as indicated.
- Assist client/SO(s) to see appropriate alternatives and potential changes in locus of control.
- Assist SO(s) to learn methods of managing present needs. (Refer to NDs specific to client's deficits.)
- Pace and time learning sessions **to meet client's needs.** Provide feedback during and after learning experiences (e.g., self-cathetcrization, range-of-motion exercises, wound care, therapeutic communication) **to enhance retention, skill, and confidence.**

Documentation Focus

ASSESSMENT/REASSESSMENT

- Reasons for/degree of impairment.
- Client's/SO's perception of the situation.
- Effect of behavior on health status/condition.

PLANNING

- Plan for adjustments and interventions for achieving the plan and who is involved.
- Teaching plan.

- Client responses to the interventions/teaching and actions performed.
- Attainment/progress toward desired outcome(s).
- Modifications to plan of care.

DISCHARGE PLANNING

- Resources that are available for the client and SO(s) and referrals that are made.

SAMPLE NURSING OUTCOMES
& INTERVENTIONS CLASSIFICATIONS (NOC/NIC)

NOC—Acceptance: Health Status
NIC—Coping Enhancement

Airway Clearance, ineffective

Taxonomy II: Safety/Protection—Class 2 Physical Injury
(00031)
[Diagnostic Division: Respiration]
Submitted 1980; Revised 1996, and Nursing Diagnosis
Extension and Classification (NDEC) 1998

Definition: Inability to clear secretions or obstructions
from the respiratory tract to maintain a clear airway

Related Factors

ENVIRONMENTAL

Smoking; second-hand smoke; smoke inhalation

OBSTRUCTED AIRWAY

Retained secretions; secretions in the bronchi; exudate in the alveoli;
excessive mucus; airway spasm; foreign body in airway; presence of
artificial airway

PHYSIOLOGICAL

Chronic obstructive pulmonary disease (COPD); asthma; allergic
airways; hyperplasia of the bronchial walls; neuromuscular dysfunction; infection

Defining Characteristics

SUBJECTIVE

Dyspnea

Information that appears in brackets has been added by the authors
to clarify and enhance the use of nursing diagnoses.

OBJECTIVE

Diminished or adventitious breath sounds (rales, crackles, rhonchi, wheezes)
Cough, ineffective or absent; sputum
Changes in respiratory rate and rhythm
Difficulty vocalizing
Wide-eyed; restlessness
Orthopnea
Cyanosis

Desired Outcomes/Evaluation Criteria—Client Will:

- Maintain airway patency.
- Expectorate/clear secretions readily.
- Demonstrate absence/reduction of congestion with breath sounds clear, respirations noiseless, improved oxygen exchange (e.g., absence of cyanosis, ABG results within client norms).
- Verbalize understanding of cause(s) and therapeutic management regimen.
- Demonstrate behaviors to improve or maintain clear airway.
- Identify potential complications and how to initiate appropriate preventive or corrective actions.

Actions/Interventions

NURSING PRIORITY NO. 1. To maintain adequate, patent airway:

- Position head midline with flexion appropriate for age/condition to open or maintain open airway in at-rest or compromised individual.
- Assist with appropriate testing (e.g., pulmonary function/sleep studies) to identify causative/precipitating factors.
- Suction naso/tracheal/oral prn to clear airway when secretions are blocking airway.
- Elevate head of the bed/change position every 2 hours and prn to take advantage of gravity decreasing pressure on the diaphragm and enhancing drainage of/ventilation to different lung segments (pulmonary toilet).
- Monitor infant/child for feeding intolerance, abdominal distention, and emotional stressors that may compromise airway.
- Insert oral airway as appropriate to maintain anatomic position of tongue and natural airway.
- Assist with procedures (e.g., bronchoscopy, tracheostomy) to clear/maintain open airway.

- Keep environment allergen free (e.g., dust, feather pillows, smoke) according to individual situation.

NURSING PRIORITY NO. 2. To mobilize secretions:

- Encourage deep-breathing and coughing exercises; splint chest/incision to maximize effort.
- Administer analgesics to improve cough when pain is inhibiting effort. (Caution: Overmedication can depress respirations and cough effort.)
- Give expectorants/bronchodilators as ordered.
- Increase fluid intake to at least 2000 mL/day within level of cardiac tolerance (may require IV) to help liquify secretions. Monitor for signs/symptoms of congestive heart failure (crackles, edema, weight gain).
- Encourage/provide warm versus cold liquids as appropriate.
- Provide supplemental humidification, if needed (ultrasonic nebulizer, room humidifier).
- Perform/assist client with postural drainage and percussion as indicated if not contraindicated by condition, such as asthma.
- Assist with respiratory treatments (intermittent positive-pressure breathing—IPPB, incentive spirometer).
- Support reduction/cessation of smoking to improve lung function.
- Discourage use of oil-based products around nose to prevent aspiration into lungs.

NURSING PRIORITY NO. 3. To assess changes, note complications:

- Auscultate breath sounds and assess air movement to ascertain status and note progress.
- Monitor vital signs, noting blood pressure/pulse changes.
- Observe for signs of respiratory distress (increased rate, restlessness/anxiety, use of accessory muscles for breathing).
- Evaluate changes in sleep pattern, noting insomnia or daytime somnolence.
- Document response to drug therapy and/or development of adverse side effects or interactions with antimicrobials, steroids, expectorants, bronchodilators.
- Observe for signs/symptoms of infection (e.g., increased dyspnea with onset of fever, change in sputum color, amount, or character) to identify infectious process/promote timely intervention. Obtain sputum specimen, preferably before antimicrobial therapy is initiated, to verify appropriateness of therapy.
- Monitor/document serial chest x-rays/ABGs/pulse oximetry readings.
- Observe for improvement in symptoms.

NURSING PRIORITY NO. 4. To promote wellness (Teaching/Discharge Considerations):

- Assess client's knowledge of contributing causes, treatment plan, specific medications, and therapeutic procedures.
- Provide information about the necessity of raising and expectorating secretions versus swallowing them, **to examine and report changes in color and amount.**
- Demonstrate pursed-lip or diaphragmatic breathing techniques, if indicated.
- Include breathing exercises, effective cough, use of adjunct devices (e.g., IPPB or incentive spirometer) in preoperative teaching.
- Provide opportunities for rest; limit activities to level of respiratory tolerance. (**Prevents/lessens fatigue.**)
- Refer to appropriate support groups (e.g., stop-smoking clinic, COPD exercise group, weight reduction).
- Instruct in use of nocturnal positive pressure air flow **for treatment of sleep apnea.**

Documentation Focus

ASSESSMENT/REASSESSMENT

- Related Factors for individual client.
- Breath sounds, presence/character of secretions, use of accessory muscles for breathing.
- Character of cough/sputum.

PLANNING

- Plan of care and who is involved in planning.
- Teaching plan.

IMPLEMENTATION/EVALUATION

- Client's response to interventions/teaching and actions performed.
- Attainment/progress toward desired outcome(s).
- Modifications to plan of care.

DISCHARGE PLANNING

- Long-term needs and who is responsible for actions to be taken.
- Specific referrals made.

SAMPLE NURSING OUTCOMES & INTERVENTIONS CLASSIFICATION (NOC/NIC)

NOC—Respiratory Status: Airway Patency
NIC—Airway Management

Allergy Response, latex

Taxonomy II: Safety/Protection—Class 5 Defensive
Processes (00041)
[Diagnostic Division: Safety]
Submitted 1998

Definition: An allergic response to natural latex rubber
products

Related Factors

No immune mechanism response [although this is true of irritant and
allergic contact dermatitis, type I/immediate reaction is a true allergic response]

Defining Characteristics

Type I reactions [hypersensitivity; IgE-mediated reaction]: immediate
reaction (<1 hour) to latex proteins (can be life threatening);
contact urticaria progressing to generalized symptoms; edema of the
lips, tongue, uvula, and/or throat; shortness of breath, tightness in
chest, wheezing, bronchospasm leading to respiratory arrest;
hypotension, syncope, cardiac arrest. May also include: Orofacial
characteristics—edema of sclera or eyelids; erythema and/or itching
of the eyes; tearing of the eyes; nasal congestion, itching, and/or
erythema; rhinorrhea; facial erythema; facial itching; oral itching;
Gastrointestinal characteristics—abdominal pain; nausea;
Generalized characteristics—flushing; general discomfort; generalized edema; increasing complaint of total body warmth; restlessness
Type IV reactions [chemical and delayed-type hypersensitivity]:
delayed onset (hours); eczema; irritation; reaction to additives (e.g.,
thiurams, carbamates) causes discomfort; redness
Irritant [contact dermatitis] reactions: erythema; [dry, crusty, hard
bumps] chapped or cracked skin; blisters

Desired Outcomes/Evaluation
Criteria—Client Will:

- Be free of signs of hypersensitive response.
- Verbalize understanding of individual risks/responsibilities in
  avoiding exposure.
- Identify signs/symptoms requiring prompt intervention.

Actions/Interventions

NURSING PRIORITY NO. **1.** To assess contributing factors:

- Identify persons in high-risk categories (e.g., those with
  history of allergies, eczema, and other dermatitis); those
  routinely exposed to latex products: healthcare workers,

Information that appears in brackets has been added by the authors
to clarify and enhance the use of nursing diagnoses.

police/firefighters, emergency medical technicians (EMTs), food handlers (restaurant, grocery stores, cafeterias), hairdressers, cleaning staff, factory workers in plants that manufacture latex-containing products; those with neural tube defects (e.g., spina bifida) or congenital urologic conditions requiring frequent surgeries and/or catheterizations (e.g., extrophy of the bladder).

• History of recent exposure, for example, blowing up balloons (this might be an acute reaction to the powder); use of condoms (may affect either partner).

• Note presence of positive skin-prick test (SPT). (**Sensitive indicator of IgE sensitivity reflecting immune system activation/type I reaction.**)

• Perform challenge/patch test, if appropriate, placing gloves to skin for 15 minutes (**appearance of hives, itching, reddened areas indicates sensitivity**) or assist with/note response to radioallergosorbent test (RAST). **This is the only safe test for the client with a history of type I reaction.**

NURSING PRIORITY NO. 2. To take measures to reduce/limit allergic response/avoid exposure to allergens:

• Ascertain client's current symptoms, noting reports of rash, hives, itching, eye symptoms, edema, diarrhea, nausea, feeling of faintness.

• Assess skin (usually hands but may be anywhere) for dry, crusty, hard bumps, horizontal cracks caused by irritation from chemicals used in/on the latex item (e.g., powder in gloves, condoms, etc.).

• Assist with treatment of contact dermatitis/type IV reaction (most common response) (e.g., wash affected skin with mild soap and water, possible application of topical steroid ointment, avoidance of latex). Inform client that the most common cause is latex gloves, but that many other products contain latex and could aggravate condition.

• Monitor closely for signs of systemic reactions **because type IV response can lead to/progress to type I anaphylaxis.** Be watchful for onset of difficulty breathing, wheezing, hypotension, tachycardia, dysrhythmias (**indicative of anaphylactic reaction and can lead to cardiac arrest**).

• Administer treatment as appropriate if type I reaction occurs, including antihistamines, epinephrine, IV fluids, corticosteroids, and oxygen mechanical ventilation, if indicated.

• Post latex precaution signs and document allergy to latex in client's file. Encourage client to wear medical ID bracelet and to inform care providers.

• Survey and routinely monitor client's environment for latex-containing products and remove.

NURSING PRIORITY NO. 3. To promote wellness (Teaching/Learning):

- Emphasize the critical importance of taking immediate action for type I reaction.
- Instruct client/family/SO about signs of reaction and emergency treatment. **Promotes awareness of problem and facilitates timely intervention.**
- Provide work-site review/recommendations to prevent exposure.
- Ascertain that latex-safe products are available, including equipment supplies, such as rubber gloves, PCV IV tubing, latex-free tape, thermometers, electrodes, oxygen cannulas, even pencil erasers and rubber bands as appropriate.
- Refer to resources (e.g., *Latex Allergy News*, National Institute for Occupational Safety and Health—NIOSH) **for further information and assistance.**

Documentation Focus

ASSESSMENT/REASSESSMENT

- Assessment findings/pertinent history of contact with latex products/frequency of exposure.
- Type/extent of symptomatology.

PLANNING

- Plan of care and interventions and who is involved in planning.
- Teaching plan.

IMPLEMENTATION/EVALUATION

- Response to interventions/teaching and actions performed.
- Attainment/progress toward desired outcome(s).
- Modifications to plan of care.

DISCHARGE PLANNING

- Discharge needs/referrals made, additional resources available.

SAMPLE NURSING OUTCOMES & INTERVENTIONS CLASSIFICATIONS (NOC/NIC)

NOC—Immune Hypersensitivity Control
NIC—Latex Precautions

Allergy Response, risk for latex

Taxonomy II: Safety/Protection—Class 5 Defensive
Processes (00042)
[Diagnostic Division: Safety]
Submitted 1998

Definition: At risk for allergic response to natural latex
rubber products

Risk Factors

History of reactions to latex (e.g., balloons, condoms, gloves); allergies
to bananas, avocados, tropical fruits, kiwi, chestnuts, poinsettia
plants

History of allergies and asthma

Professions with daily exposure to latex (e.g., medicine, nursing,
dentistry)

Conditions associated with continuous or intermittent catheterization

Multiple surgical procedures, especially from infancy (e.g., spina
bifida)

> NOTE: A risk diagnosis is not evidenced by signs and symptoms, as
> the problem has not occurred and nursing interventions are
> directed at prevention.

Desired Outcomes/Evaluation Criteria—Client Will:

- Identify and correct potential risk factors in the environment.
- Demonstrate appropriate lifestyle changes to reduce risk of
  exposure.
- Identify resources to assist in promoting a safe environment.
- Recognize need for/seek assistance to limit response/compli-
  cations.

Actions/Interventions

NURSING PRIORITY NO. **1.** To assess causative/contributing
factors:

- Identify persons in high-risk categories (e.g., those with positive history of allergies, eczema, and other dermatitis); those
  routinely exposed to latex products: healthcare workers,
  police/firefighters, EMTs, food handlers, hairdressers, cleaning staff, factory workers in plants that manufacture latex-
  containing products; those with neural tube defects (e.g.,
  spina bifida) or congenital urologic conditions requiring
  frequent surgeries and/or catheterizations.

Information that appears in brackets has been added by the authors
to clarify and enhance the use of nursing diagnoses.

- Ascertain if client could be exposed through catheters, IV tubing, dental/other procedures in healthcare setting. **Recent information indicates that latex is found in thousands of medical supplies.**

NURSING PRIORITY NO. 2. To assist in correcting factors that could lead to latex allergy:

- Discuss necessity of avoiding latex exposure. Recommend/ assist client/family to survey environment and remove any medical or household products containing latex.
- Substitute nonlatex products, such as natural rubber gloves, PCV IV tubing, latex-free tape, thermometers, electrodes, oxygen cannulas, and so forth.
- Obtain lists of latex-free products and supplies for client/care provider.
- Ascertain that facilities have established policies and procedures to address safety and reduce risk to workers and clients.
- Promote good skin care, for example, handwashing immediately after glove removal (**reduces effects of latex in powder in gloves**).

NURSING PRIORITY NO. 3. To promote wellness (Teaching/ Discharge Considerations):

- Instruct client/care providers about potential for and possible progression of reaction.
- Identify measures to take if reactions occur and ways to avoid exposure to latex products.
- Refer to allergist **for testing as appropriate.** Perform challenge/patch test with gloves to skin (**appearance of hives, itching, reddened areas indicates sensitivity**).

Documentation Focus

ASSESSMENT/REASSESSMENT

- Assessment findings/pertinent history of contact with latex products/frequency of exposure.

PLANNING

- Plan of care, interventions, and who is involved in planning.
- Teaching plan.

IMPLEMENTATION/EVALUATION

- Response to interventions/teaching and actions performed.

DISCHARGE PLANNING

- Discharge needs/referrals made.

SAMPLE NURSING OUTCOMES & INTERVENTIONS CLASSIFICATIONS (NOC/NIC)

NOC—Immune Hypersensitivity Control
NIC—Latex Precautions

Anxiety [specify level: mild, moderate, severe, panic]

Taxonomy II: Coping/Stress Tolerance—Class 2 Coping Responses (00146)
[Diagnostic Division: Ego Integrity]
Submitted 1973; Revised 1982, and 1998 (by small group work 1996)

Definition: Vague uneasy feeling of discomfort or dread accompanied by an autonomic response (the source often nonspecific or unknown to the individual); a feeling of apprehension caused by anticipation of danger. It is an altering signal that warns of impending danger and enables the individual to take measures to deal with threat

Related Factors

Unconscious conflict about essential [beliefs]/goals and values of life
Situational/maturational crises
Stress
Familial association/heredity
Interpersonal transmission/contagion
Threat to self-concept [perceived or actual]; [unconscious conflict]
Threat of death [perceived or actual]
Threat to or change in health status [progressive/debilitating disease, terminal illness], interaction patterns, role function/status, environment [safety], economic status
Unmet needs
Exposure to toxins
Substance abuse
[Positive or negative self-talk]
[Physiological factors, such as hyperthyroidism, pheochromocytoma, drug therapy, including steroids, and so on]

Defining Characteristics

SUBJECTIVE

Behavioral
Expressed concerns due to change in life events
Affective
Regretful; scared; rattled; distressed; apprehension; uncertainty; fearful; feelings of inadequacy; anxious; jittery; [sense of impending doom]; [hopelessness]

Information that appears in brackets has been added by the authors to clarify and enhance the use of nursing diagnoses.

Cognitive
Fear of unspecific consequences; awareness of physiological symptoms
Physiological
Shakiness; worried; regretful; dry mouth (s); tingling in extremities
   (p); heart pounding (s); nausea (p); abdominal pain (p); diarrhea
   (p); urinary hesitancy (p); urinary frequency (p); faintness (p);
   weakness (s); decreased pulse (p); respiratory difficulties (s); fatigue
   (p); sleep disturbance (p); [chest, back, neck pain]

OBJECTIVE

Behavioral
Poor eye contact; glancing about; scanning and vigilance; extraneous
   movement (e.g., foot shuffling, hand/arm movements); fidgeting;
   restlessness; diminished productivity; [crying/tearfulness];
   [pacing/purposeless activity]; [immobility]
Affective
Increased wariness; focus on self; irritability; overexcited; anguish;
   painful and persistent increased helplessness
Physiological
Voice quivering; trembling/hand tremors; increased tension; facial
   tension; increased pulse; increased perspiration; cardiovascular
   excitation (s); facial flushing (s); superficial vasoconstriction (s);
   increased blood pressure (s); twitching (s); increased reflexes (s);
   urinary urgency (p); decreased blood pressure (p); insomnia;
   anorexia (s); increased respiration (s)
Cognitive
Preoccupation; impaired attention; difficulty concentrating; forgetfulness; diminished ability to problem-solve; diminished learning ability; rumination; tendency to blame others; blocking of thought;
   confusion; decreased perceptual field

Desired Outcomes/Evaluation Criteria—Client Will:

- Appear relaxed and report anxiety is reduced to a manageable
  level.
- Verbalize awareness of feelings of anxiety.
- Identify healthy ways to deal with and express anxiety.
- Demonstrate problem-solving skills.
- Use resources/support systems effectively.

Actions/Interventions

NURSING PRIORITY NO. 1. To assess level of anxiety:

- Review familial/physiologic factors, current prescribed
  medications, and recent drug history (e.g., genetic depressive
  factors, history of thyroid problems, metabolic imbalances,

---

p = parasympathetic nervous system; s = sympathetic nervous
   system

pulmonary disease, anemia, dysrhythmias; use of steroids, thyroid, appetite control medications; and substance abuse).

- Identify client's perception of the threat represented by the situation.
- Monitor physical responses; for example, palpitations/rapid pulse, repetitive movements, pacing.
- Observe behavior indicative of level of anxiety (the nurse needs to be aware of own feelings of anxiety or uneasiness, **which can be a clue to the client's level of anxiety**):

Mild:

Alert, more aware of environment, attention focused on environment and immediate events.

Restless, irritable, wakeful, reports of insomnia.

Motivated to deal with existing problems in this state.

Moderate:

Perception narrower, concentration increased and able to ignore distractions in dealing with problem(s).

Voice quivers or changes pitch.

Trembling, increased pulse/respirations.

Severe:

Range of perception is reduced; anxiety interferes with effective functioning.

Preoccupied with feelings of discomfort/sense of impending doom.

Increased pulse/respirations with reports of dizziness, tingling sensations, headache, and so on.

Panic:

Ability to concentrate is disrupted; behavior is disintegrated; the client distorts the situation and does not have realistic perceptions of what is happening. The individual may be experiencing terror or confusion or be unable to speak or move (paralyzed with fear).

- Note use of drugs (alcohol), insomnia or excessive sleeping, limited/avoidance of interactions with others, **which may be behavioral indicators of use of withdrawal to deal with problems.**
- Be aware of defense mechanisms being used (client may be in denial, regression, and so forth) **that interfere with ability to deal with problem.**
- Identify coping skills the individual is using currently, such as anger, daydreaming, forgetfulness, eating, smoking, lack of problem-solving.
- Review coping skills used in past **to determine those that might be helpful in current circumstances.**

NURSING PRIORITY NO. 2. To assist client to identify feelings and begin to deal with problems:

- Establish a therapeutic relationship, conveying empathy and unconditional positive regard.
- Be available to client for listening and talking.
- Encourage client to acknowledge and to express feelings, for

example, crying (sadness), laughing (fear, denial), swearing (fear, anger).

- Assist client to develop self-awareness of verbal and nonverbal behaviors.
- Clarify meaning of feelings/actions by providing feedback and checking meaning with the client.
- Acknowledge anxiety/fear. Do not deny or reassure client that everything will be all right.
- Provide accurate information about the situation. **Helps client to identify what is reality based.**
- Be truthful with child, avoid bribing, and provide physical contact (e.g., hugging, rocking) **to soothe fears and provide assurance.**
- Provide comfort measures (e.g., calm/quiet environment, soft music, warm bath, back rub).
- Modify procedures as possible (e.g., substitute oral for intramuscular medications, combine blood draws/use fingerstick method) **to limit degree of stress, avoid overwhelming child.**
- Manage environmental factors, such as harsh lighting and high traffic flow, which may be confusing/stressful to older individuals.
- Accept client as is. (**The client may need to be where he or she is at this point in time, such as in denial after receiving the diagnosis of a terminal illness.**)
- Allow the behavior to belong to the client; do not respond personally **because this may escalate the situation.**
- Assist client to use anxiety for coping with the situation, if helpful. (**Moderate anxiety heightens awareness and permits the client to focus on dealing with problems.**)

Panic State

- Stay with client, maintaining a calm, confident manner.
- Speak in brief statements using simple words.
- Provide for nonthreatening, consistent environment/atmosphere. Minimize stimuli. Monitor visitors and interactions **to lessen effect of transmission of feelings.**
- Set limits on inappropriate behavior and help client to develop acceptable ways of dealing with anxiety. **Note:** Staff may need to provide safe controls/environment until client regains control.
- Gradually increase activities/involvement with others as anxiety is decreased.
- Use cognitive therapy **to focus on/correct faulty catastrophic interpretations of physical symptoms.**
- Give antianxiety medications (antianxiety agents/sedatives) as ordered.

NURSING PRIORITY NO. 3. To promote wellness (Teaching/Discharge Considerations):

- Assist client to learn precipitating factors and new methods of coping with disabling anxiety.
- Review happenings, thoughts, and feelings preceding the anxiety attack.
- Identify things the client has done previously to cope successfully when feeling nervous/anxious.
- List helpful resources/people, including available "hotline" or crisis managers **to provide ongoing/timely support.**
- Encourage client to develop an exercise/activity program; **may be helpful in reducing level of anxiety by relieving tension.**
- Assist in developing skills (e.g., awareness of negative thoughts, saying "Stop," and substituting a positive thought) **to eliminate negative self-talk. Mild phobias seem to respond better to behavioral therapy.**
- Review strategies, such as role playing, use of visualizations to practice anticipated events, prayer/meditation; **useful for dealing with anxiety-provoking situations.**
- Review medication regimen and possible interactions, especially with over-the-counter drugs/alcohol and so forth. Discuss appropriate drug substitutions, changes in dosage or time of dose **to lessen side effects.**
- Refer to physician for drug management program/alteration of prescription regimen. (**Drugs often causing symptoms of anxiety include aminophylline/theophylline, anticholinergics, dopamine, levodopa, salicylates, steroids.**)
- Refer to individual and/or group therapy as appropriate **to deal with chronic anxiety states.**

Documentation Focus

ASSESSMENT/REASSESSMENT

- Level of anxiety and precipitating/aggravating factors.
- Description of feelings (expressed and displayed).
- Awareness/ability to recognize and express feelings.
- Related substance use, if present.

PLANNING

- Treatment plan and individual responsibility for specific activities.
- Teaching plan.

IMPLEMENTATION/EVALUATION

- Client involvement and response to interventions/teaching and actions performed.

- Attainment/progress toward desired outcome(s).
- Modifications to plan of care.

DISCHARGE PLANNING

- Referrals and follow-up plan.
- Specific referrals made.

SAMPLE NURSING OUTCOMES
& INTERVENTIONS CLASSIFICATIONS (NOC/NIC)

NOC—Anxiety Control
NIC—Anxiety Reduction

Anxiety, death

Taxonomy II: Coping/Stress Tolerance—Class 2 Coping
Response (00147)
[Diagnostic Division: Ego Integrity]
Submitted 1998

Definition: Apprehension, worry, or fear related to
death or dying

Related Factors

To be developed

Defining Characteristics

SUBJECTIVE

Fear of: developing a terminal illness; the process of dying; loss of
physical and/or mental abilities when dying; premature death
because it prevents the accomplishment of important life goals;
leaving family alone after death; delayed demise
Negative death images or unpleasant thoughts about any event related
to death or dying; anticipated pain related to dying
Powerlessness over issues related to dying; total loss of control over
any aspect of one's own death
Worrying about: the impact of one's own death on SOs; being the
cause of other's grief and suffering
Concerns of overworking the caregiver as terminal illness incapacitates
self; about meeting one's creator or feeling doubtful about the existence of God or higher being
Denial of one's own mortality or impending death

OBJECTIVE

Deep sadness
(Refer to ND Grieving, anticipatory.)

Information that appears in brackets has been added by the authors
to clarify and enhance the use of nursing diagnoses.

Desired Outcomes/Evaluation Criteria—Client Will:

- Identify and express feelings (e.g., sadness, guilt, fear) freely/effectively.
- Look toward/plan for the future one day at a time.
- Formulate a plan dealing with individual concerns and eventualities of dying.

Actions/Interventions

NURSING PRIORITY NO. 1. To assess causative/contributing factors:

- Determine how client sees self in usual lifestyle role functioning and perception and meaning of anticipated loss to him or her and SO(s).
- Ascertain current knowledge of situation **to identify misconceptions, lack of information, other pertinent issues.**
- Determine client's role in family constellation. Observe patterns of communication in family and response of family/SO to client's situation and concerns. **In addition to identifying areas of need/concern, also reveals strengths useful in addressing the concerns.**
- Assess impact of client reports of subjective experiences and past experience with death (or exposure to death), for example, witnessed violent death or as a child viewed body in casket, and so on.
- Identify cultural factors/expectations and impact on current situation/feelings.
- Note physical/mental condition, complexity of therapeutic regimen.
- Determine ability to manage own self-care, end-of-life and other affairs, awareness/use of available resources.
- Observe behavior indicative of the level of anxiety present (mild to panic) **as it affects client's/SO's ability to process information/participate in activities.**
- Identify coping skills currently used and how effective they are. Be aware of defense mechanisms being used by the client.
- Note use of drugs (including alcohol), presence of insomnia, excessive sleeping, avoidance of interactions with others.
- Note client's religious/spiritual orientation, involvement in religious/church activities, presence of conflicts regarding spiritual beliefs.
- Listen to client/SO reports/expressions of anger/concern, alienation from God, belief that impending death is a punishment for wrongdoing, and so on.
- Determine sense of futility, feelings of hopelessness, helpless-

ness, lack of motivation to help self. **May indicate presence of depression and need for intervention.**
- Active-listen comments regarding sense of isolation.
- Listen for expressions of inability to find meaning in life or suicidal ideation.

NURSING PRIORITY NO. 2. To assist client to deal with situation:

- Provide open and trusting relationship.
- Use therapeutic communication skills of Active-listening, silence, acknowledgment. Respect client desire/request not to talk. Provide hope within parameters of the individual situation.
- Encourage expressions of feelings (anger, fear, sadness, etc.). Acknowledge anxiety/fear. Do not deny or reassure client that everything will be all right. Be honest when answering questions/providing information. **Enhances trust and therapeutic relationship.**
- Provide information about normalcy of feelings and individual grief reaction.
- Make time for nonjudgmental discussion of philosophic issues/questions about spiritual impact of illness/situation.
- Review past life experiences of loss and use of coping skills, noting client strengths and successes.
- Provide calm, peaceful setting and privacy as appropriate. **Promotes relaxation and ability to deal with situation.**
- Assist client to engage in spiritual growth activities, experience prayer/meditation and forgiveness to heal past hurts. Provide information that anger with God is a normal part of the grieving process. **Reduces feelings of guilt/conflict, allowing client to move forward toward resolution.**
- Refer to therapists, spiritual advisors, counselors **to facilitate grief work.**
- Refer to community agencies/resources **to assist client/SO for planning for eventualities (legal issues, funeral plans, etc.).**

NURSING PRIORITY NO. 3. To promote independence:

- Support client's efforts to develop realistic steps to put plans into action.
- Direct client's thoughts beyond present state to enjoyment of each day and the future when appropriate.
- Provide opportunities for client to make simple decisions. **Enhances sense of control.**
- Develop individual plan using client's locus of control **to assist client/family through the process.**
- Treat expressed decisions and desires with respect and convey to others as appropriate.
- Assist with completion of Advance Directives and cardiopulmonary resuscitation (CPR) instructions.

Documentation Focus

ASSESSMENT/REASSESSMENT

- Assessment findings, including client's fears and signs/symptoms being exhibited.
- Responses/actions of family/SO(s).
- Availability/use of resources.

PLANNING

- Plan of care and who is involved in planning.

IMPLEMENTATION/EVALUATION

- Client's response to interventions/teaching and actions performed.
- Attainment/progress toward desired outcome(s).
- Modifications to plan of care.

DISCHARGE PLANNING

- Identified needs and who is responsible for actions to be taken.
- Specific referrals made.

SAMPLE NURSING OUTCOMES & INTERVENTIONS CLASSIFICATIONS (NOC/NIC)

NOC—Fear Control
NIC—Dying Care

Aspiration, risk for

Taxonomy II: Safety/Protection—Class 2 Physical Injury (00039)
[Diagnostic Division: Respiration]
Submitted 1988

Definition: At risk for entry of gastrointestinal secretions, oropharyngeal secretions, or [exogenous food] solids or fluids into tracheobronchial passages [due to dysfunction or absence of normal protective mechanisms]

Risk Factors

Reduced level of consciousness
Depressed cough and gag reflexes
Impaired swallowing [owing to inability of the epiglottis and true vocal cords to move to close off trachea]
Facial/oral/neck surgery or trauma; wired jaws
Situation hindering elevation of upper body [weakness, paralysis]

Information that appears in brackets has been added by the authors to clarify and enhance the use of nursing diagnoses.

Incomplete lower esophageal sphincter [hiatal hernia or other esophageal disease affecting stomach valve function], delayed gastric emptying, decreased gastrointestinal motility, increased intragastric pressure, increased gastric residual

Presence of tracheostomy or endotracheal (ET) tube; [inadequate or overinflation of tracheostomy/ET tube cuff]

[Presence of] gastrointestinal tubes; tube feedings/medication administration

---

NOTE: A risk diagnosis is not evidenced by signs and symptoms, as the problem has not occurred and nursing interventions are directed at prevention.

Desired Outcomes/Evaluation Criteria—Client Will:

- Experience no aspiration as evidenced by noiseless respirations, clear breath sounds; clear, odorless secretions.
- Identify causative/risk factors.
- Demonstrate techniques to prevent and/or correct aspiration.

Actions/Interventions

NURSING PRIORITY NO. **1.** To assess causative/contributing factors:

- Note level of consciousness/awareness of surroundings, cognitive impairment.
- Evaluate presence of neuromuscular weakness, noting muscle groups involved, degree of impairment, and whether they are of an acute or progressive nature (e.g., Guillain-Barré, amyotrophic lateral sclerosis—ALS).
- Assess amount and consistency of respiratory secretions and strength of gag/cough reflex.
- Observe for neck and facial edema, for example, client with head/neck surgery, tracheal/bronchial injury (upper torso burns, inhalation/chemical injury).
- Note administration of enteral feedings, being aware of potential for regurgitation and/or misplacement of tube.
- Ascertain lifestyle habits, for instance, use of alcohol, tobacco, and other drugs; **can affect awareness and muscles of gag/ swallow.**

NURSING PRIORITY NO. **2.** To assist in correcting factors that can lead to aspiration:

- Monitor use of oxygen masks in clients at risk for vomiting. Refrain from using oxygen masks for comatose individuals.
- Keep wire cutters/scissors with client at all times when jaws are wired/banded **to facilitate clearing airway in emergency situations.**

- Maintain operational suction equipment at bedside/chairside.
- Suction (oral cavity, nose, and ET/tracheostomy tube) as needed **to clear secretions.** Avoid triggering gag mechanism when performing suction or mouth care.
- Assist with postural drainage **to mobilize thickened secretions that may interfere with swallowing.**
- Auscultate lung sounds frequently (especially in client who is coughing frequently or not coughing at all; ventilator client being tube-fed) **to determine presence of secretions/silent aspiration.**
- Elevate client to highest or best possible position for eating and drinking and during tube feedings.
- Feed slowly, instruct client to chew slowly and thoroughly.
- Give semisolid foods; avoid pureed foods (**increased risk of aspiration**) and mucus-producing foods (milk). Use soft foods that stick together/form a bolus (e.g., casseroles, puddings, stews) **to aid swallowing effort.**
- Provide very warm or very cold liquids (**activates temperature receptors in the mouth that help to stimulate swallowing**). Add thickening agent to liquids as appropriate.
- Avoid washing solids down with liquids.
- Ascertain that feeding tube is in correct position. Measure residuals when appropriate **to prevent overfeeding.** Add food coloring to feeding **to identify regurgitation.**
- Determine best position for infant/child (e.g., with the head of bed elevated 30 degrees and infant propped on right side after feeding **because upper airway patency is facilitated by upright position and turning to right side decreases likelihood of drainage into trachea**).
- Provide oral medications in elixir form or crush, if appropriate.
- Refer to speech therapist for **exercises to strengthen muscles and techniques to enhance swallowing.**

NURSING PRIORITY NO. 3. To promote wellness (Teaching/Discharge Considerations):

- Review individual risk/potentiating factors.
- Provide information about the effects of aspiration on the lungs.
- Instruct in safety concerns when feeding oral or tube feeding. Refer to ND Swallowing, impaired.
- Train client to suction self or train family members in suction techniques (especially if client has constant or copious oral secretions) **to enhance safety/self-sufficiency.**
- Instruct individual/family member to avoid/limit activities that increase intra-abdominal pressure (straining, strenuous exercise, tight/constrictive clothing), **which may slow digestion/increase risk of regurgitation.**

Documentation Focus

ASSESSMENT/REASSESSMENT

- Assessment findings/conditions that could lead to problems of aspiration.
- Verification of tube placement, observations of physical findings.

PLANNING

- Interventions to prevent aspiration or reduce risk factors and who is involved in the planning.
- Teaching plan.

IMPLEMENTATION/EVALUATION

- Client's responses to interventions/teaching and actions performed.
- Foods/fluids client handles with ease/difficulty.
- Amount/frequency of intake.
- Attainment/progress toward desired outcome(s).
- Modifications to plan of care.

DISCHARGE PLANNING

- Long-term needs and who is responsible for actions to be taken.

SAMPLE NURSING OUTCOMES & INTERVENTIONS CLASSIFICATIONS (NOC/NIC)

NOC—Risk Control
NIC—Aspiration Precautions

Attachment, risk for impaired parent/infant/child

Taxonomy II: Role Relationships—Class 2 Family Relationships (00058)
[Diagnostic Division: Social Interaction]
Submitted 1994

Definition: Disruption of the interactive process between parent/SO and infant that fosters the development of a protective and nurturing reciprocal relationship

Risk Factors

Inability of parents to meet the personal needs
Anxiety associated with the parent role

Information that appears in brackets has been added by the authors to clarify and enhance the use of nursing diagnoses.

Substance abuse

Premature infant; ill infant/child who is unable to effectively initiate
   parental contact due to altered behavioral organization

Separation; physical barriers

Lack of privacy

[Parents who themselves experienced altered attachment]

[Uncertainty of paternity; conception as a result of rape/sexual
   abuse]

[Difficult pregnancy and/or birth (actual or perceived)]

> NOTE: A risk diagnosis is not evidenced by signs and symptoms, as
> the problem has not occurred and nursing interventions are
> directed at prevention.

Desired Outcomes/Evaluation Criteria—Parent Will:

- Identify and prioritize family strengths and needs.
- Exhibit nurturant and protective behaviors toward child.
- Identify and use resources to meet needs of family members.
- Demonstrate techniques to enhance behavioral organization
  of the infant/child.
- Engage in mutually satisfying interactions with child.

Actions/Interventions

NURSING PRIORITY NO. 1. To identify causative/contributing
factors:

- Interview parents, noting their perception of situation, individual concerns.
- Assess parent/child interactions.
- Ascertain availability/use of resources to include extended
  family, support groups, and financial.
- Evaluate parents' ability to provide protective environment,
  participate in reciprocal relationship.

NURSING PRIORITY NO. 2. To enhance behavioral organization
of infant/child:

- Identify infant's strengths and vulnerabilities. **Each child is
  born with his or her own temperament that affects interactions with caregivers.**
- Educate parents regarding child growth and development,
  addressing parental perceptions. **Helps clarify realistic expectations.**
- Assist parents in modifying the environment **to provide
  appropriate stimulation.**
- Model caregiving techniques that best support behavioral
  organization.
- Respond consistently with nurturance to infant/child.

NURSING PRIORITY NO. 3. To enhance best functioning of parents:

- Develop therapeutic nurse-client relationship. Provide a consistently warm, nurturant, and nonjudgmental environment.
- Assist parents in identifying and prioritizing family strengths and needs. **Promotes positive attitude by looking at what they already do well and using those skills to address needs.**
- Support and guide parents in process of assessing resources.
- Involve parents in activities with the infant/child that they can accomplish successfully. **Enhances self-concept.**
- Recognize and provide positive feedback for nurturant and protective parenting behaviors. **Reinforces continuation of desired behaviors.**
- Minimize number of professionals on team with whom parents must have contact **to foster trust in relationships.**

NURSING PRIORITY NO. 4. To support parent/child attachment during separation:

- Provide parents with telephone contact as appropriate.
- Establish a routine time for daily phone calls/initiate calls as indicated. **Provides sense of consistency and control; allows for planning of other activities.**
- Invite parents to use Ronald McDonald House or provide them with a listing of a variety of local accommodations, restaurants when child is hospitalized out of town.
- Arrange for parents to receive photos, progress reports from the child.
- Suggest parents provide a photo and/or audiotape of themselves for the child.
- Consider use of contract with parents **to clearly communicate expectations of both family and staff.**
- Suggest parents keep a journal of infant/child progress.
- Provide "homelike" environment for situations requiring supervision of visits.

NURSING PRIORITY NO. 5. To promote wellness (Teaching/ Discharge Considerations):

- Refer to addiction counseling/treatment, individual counseling, or family therapies as indicated.
- Identify services for transportation, financial resources, housing, and so forth.
- Develop support systems appropriate to situation (e.g., extended family, friends, social worker).
- Explore community resources (e.g., church affiliations, volunteer groups, day/respite care).

Documentation Focus

ASSESSMENT/REASSESSMENT

- Identified behaviors of both parents and child.
- Specific risk factors, individual perceptions/concerns.
- Interactions between parent and child.

PLANNING

- Plan of care and who is involved in planning.
- Teaching plan.

IMPLEMENTATION/EVALUATION

- Parents'/child's responses to interventions/teaching and actions performed.
- Attainment/progress toward desired outcomes.
- Modifications to plan of care.

DISCHARGE PLANNING

- Long-term needs and who is responsible.
- Plan for home visits to support parents and to ensure infant/child safety and well-being.
- Specific referrals made.

SAMPLE NURSING OUTCOMES & INTERVENTIONS CLASSIFICATIONS (NOC/NIC)

NOC—Parenting
NIC—Attachment Promotion

Autonomic Dysreflexia

Taxonomy II: Coping/Stress Tolerance—Class 3
Neurobehavioral Stress (00009)
[Diagnostic Division: Circulation]
Submitted 1988

Definition: Life-threatening, uninhibited sympathetic response of the nervous system to a noxious stimulus after a spinal cord injury [SCI] at T7 or above

Related Factors

Bladder or bowel distention; [catheter insertion, obstruction, irrigation]
Skin irritation
Lack of client and caregiver knowledge
[Sexual excitation]
[Environmental temperature extremes]

Information that appears in brackets has been added by the authors to clarify and enhance the use of nursing diagnoses.

Defining Characteristics

SUBJECTIVE

Headache (a diffuse pain in different portions of the head and not
confined to any nerve distribution area)

Paresthesia, chilling, blurred vision, chest pain, metallic taste in mouth,
nasal congestion

OBJECTIVE

Paroxysmal hypertension (sudden periodic elevated blood pressure in
which systolic pressure >140 mm Hg and diastolic >90 mm Hg)

Bradycardia or tachycardia (heart rate <60 or >100 beats per minute,
respectively)

Diaphoresis (above the injury), red splotches on skin (above the
injury), pallor (below the injury)

Horner's syndrome (contraction of the pupil, partial ptosis of the
eyelid, enophthalmos and sometimes loss of sweating over the
affected side of the face); conjunctival congestion

Pilomotor reflex (gooseflesh formation when skin is cooled)

Desired Outcomes/Evaluation Criteria—Client/Caregiver Will:

- Identify risk factors.
- Recognize signs/symptoms of syndrome.
- Demonstrate corrective techniques.
- Experience no episodes of dysreflexia or will seek medical
  intervention in a timely manner.

Actions/Interventions

NURSING PRIORITY NO. 1. To assess precipitating risk factors:

- Monitor for bladder distention, presence of bladder spasms/
  stones or infection.
- Assess for bowel distention, fecal impaction, problems with
  bowel management program.
- Observe skin/tissue pressure areas, especially following
  prolonged sitting.
- Remove client from and/or instruct to avoid environmental
  temperature extremes/drafts.
- Monitor closely during procedures/diagnostics that manipulate bladder or bowel.

NURSING PRIORITY NO. 2. To provide for early detection and
immediate intervention:

- Investigate associated complaints/symptoms (e.g., severe
  headache, chest pains, blurred vision, facial flushing, nausea,
  metallic taste, Horner's syndrome).
- Correct/eliminate causative stimulus (e.g., distended bladder/
  bowel, skin pressure/irritation, temperature extremes).

- Elevate head of bed to 45-degree angle or place in sitting position **to lower blood pressure.**
- Monitor vital signs frequently during acute episode. Continue to monitor blood pressure at intervals after symptoms subside **to evaluate effectiveness of interventions.**
- Administer medications as required **to block excessive autonomic nerve transmission, normalize heart rate, and reduce hypertension.** Administer and carefully adjust dosage of antihypertensive medications for child. (**Assists in preventing seizures and maintaining blood pressure within desired range.**)
- Apply local anesthetic ointment to rectum; remove impaction after symptoms subside **to remove causative problem without causing additional symptoms.**

NURSING PRIORITY NO. 3. To promote wellness (Teaching/Discharge Considerations):

- Discuss warning signs and how to avoid onset of syndrome with client/SO(s).
- Instruct client/caregivers in bowel and bladder care, prevention of skin breakdown, care of existing skin breaks, prevention of infection.
- Instruct family member/healthcare provider in blood pressure monitoring during acute episodes.
- Review proper use/administration of medication if indicated.
- Assist client/family in identifying emergency referrals (e.g., physician, rehabilitation nurse/home care supervisor). Place phone number(s) in prominent place.
- Refer to ND Autonomic Dysreflexia, risk for.

Documentation Focus

ASSESSMENT/REASSESSMENT

- Individual findings, noting previous episodes, precipitating factors, and individual signs/symptoms.

PLANNING

- Plan of care and who is involved in planning.
- Teaching plan.

IMPLEMENTATION/EVALUATION

- Client's responses to interventions and actions performed, understanding of teaching.
- Attainment/progress toward desired outcome(s).
- Modifications to plan of care.

DISCHARGE PLANNING

• Long-term needs and who is responsible for actions to be taken.

SAMPLE NURSING OUTCOMES
& INTERVENTIONS CLASSIFICATIONS (NOC/NIC)

NOC—Neurological Status: Autonomic
NIC—Dysreflexia Management

Autonomic Dysreflexia, risk for

Taxonomy II: Coping/Stress Tolerance—Class 3
Neurobehavioral Stress (00010)
[Diagnostic Division: Circulation]
Nursing Diagnosis Extension and Classification (NDEC)
Submission 1998/Revised 2000

Definition: At risk for life-threatening, uninhibited response of the sympathetic nervous system post spinal shock, in an individual with a spinal cord injury [SCI] or lesion at T6 or above (has been demonstrated in clients with injuries at T7 and T8)

Risk Factors

MUSCULO-SKELETAL—INTEGUMENTARY STIMULI

Cutaneous stimulations (e.g., pressure ulcer, ingrown toenail, dressing, burns, rash); sunburns; wounds
Pressure over bony prominences or genitalia; range-of-motion exercises; spasms
Fractures; heterotrophic bone

GASTROINTESTINAL STIMULI

Constipation; difficult passage of feces; fecal impaction; bowel distention; hemorrhoids
Digital stimulation; suppositories; enemas
Gastrointestinal system pathology; esophageal reflux; gastric ulcers; gallstones

UROLOGIC STIMULI

Bladder distention/spasm
Detrusor sphincter dyssynergia
Instrumentation or surgery; calculi
Urinary tract infection; cystitis; urethritis; epididymitis

REGULATORY STIMULI

Temperature fluctuations; extreme environmental temperatures

Information that appears in brackets has been added by the authors to clarify and enhance the use of nursing diagnoses.

SITUATIONAL STIMULI

Positioning; surgical procedure
Constrictive clothing (e.g., straps, stockings, shoes)
Drug reactions (e.g., decongestants, sympathomimetics, vasoconstrictors, narcotic withdrawal)

NEUROLOGICAL STIMULI

Painful or irritating stimuli below the level of injury

CARDIAC/PULMONARY STIMULI

Pulmonary emboli; deep vein thrombosis

REPRODUCTIVE [AND SEXUALITY] STIMULI

Sexual intercourse; ejaculation
Menstruation; pregnancy; labor and delivery; ovarian cyst

> NOTE: A risk diagnosis is not evidenced by signs and symptoms, as the problem has not occurred and nursing interventions are directed at prevention.

Desired Outcomes/Evaluation Criteria—Client Will:

- Identify risk factors present.
- Demonstrate preventive/corrective techniques.
- Be free of episodes of dysreflexia.

Actions/Interventions

NURSING PRIORITY NO. 1. To assess risk factors present:

- Monitor for potential precipitating factors, including urologic (e.g., bladder distention, urinary tract infections, kidney stones); gastrointestinal (bowel overdistention, hemorrhoids, digital stimulation); cutaneous (e.g., pressure ulcers, extreme external temperatures, dressing changes); reproductive (e.g., sexual activity, menstruation, pregnancy/delivery); and miscellaneous (e.g., pulmonary emboli, drug reaction, deep vein thrombosis).

NURSING PRIORITY NO. 2. To prevent occurrence:

- Monitor vital signs, noting changes in blood pressure, heart rate, and temperature, especially during times of physical stress **to identify trends and intervene in a timely manner.**
- Instruct in preventive interventions (e.g., routine bowel care, appropriate padding for skin and tissue care, proper positioning, temperature control).
- Instruct all care providers in safe and necessary bowel and bladder care, and immediate and long-term care for the

prevention of skin stress/breakdown. **These problems are associated most frequently with dysreflexia.**

- Administer antihypertensive medications when at-risk client is placed on routine "maintenance dose," **as might occur when noxious stimuli cannot be removed (presence of chronic sacral pressure sore, fracture, or acute postoperative pain).**
- Refer to ND Autonomic Dysreflexia.

NURSING PRIORITY NO. 3. To promote wellness (Teaching/Discharge Considerations):

- Discuss warning signs of autonomic dysreflexia with client/caregiver (i.e., congestion, anxiety, visual changes, metallic taste in mouth, increased blood pressure/acute hypertension, severe pounding headache, diaphoresis and flushing above the level of SCI, bradycardia, cardiac irregularities). **Early signs can develop rapidly (in minutes), requiring quick intervention.**
- Review proper use/administration of medication if preventive medications are anticipated.
- Assist client/family in identifying emergency referrals (e.g., healthcare provider number in prominent place).

Documentation Focus

ASSESSMENT/REASSESSMENT

- Individual findings, noting previous episodes, precipitating factors, and individual signs/symptoms.

PLANNING

- Plan of care and who is involved in planning.
- Teaching plan.

IMPLEMENTATION/EVALUATION

- Client's responses to interventions and actions performed, understanding of teaching.
- Attainment/progress toward desired outcome(s).
- Modifications to plan of care.

DISCHARGE PLANNING

- Long-term needs and who is responsible for actions to be taken.

SAMPLE NURSING OUTCOMES & INTERVENTIONS CLASSIFICATIONS (NOC/NIC)

NOC—Risk Control
NIC—Dysreflexia Management

Body Image, disturbed

Taxonomy II: Self-Perception—Class 3 Body Image
(00118)
[Diagnostic Division: Ego Integrity]
Submitted 1973; Revised 1998 (by small group work
1996)

Definition: Confusion [and/or dissatisfaction] in mental
picture of one's physical self

Related Factors

Biophysical illness; trauma or injury; surgery; [mutilation, pregnancy];
   illness treatment [change caused by biochemical agents (drugs),
   dependence on machine]
Psychosocial
Cultural or spiritual
Cognitive/perceptual; developmental changes
[Significance of body part or functioning with regard to age, sex,
   developmental level, or basic human needs]
[Maturational changes]

Defining Characteristics

SUBJECTIVE

Verbalization of feelings/perceptions that reflect an altered view of
   one's body in appearance, structure, or function; change in life style
Fear of rejection or of reaction by others
Focus on past strength, function, or appearance
Negative feelings about body (e.g., feelings of helplessness, hopeless-
   ness, or powerlessness); [depersonalization/grandiosity]
Preoccupation with change or loss
Refusal to verify actual change
Emphasis on remaining strengths, heightened achievement
Personalization of part or loss by name
Depersonalization of part or loss by impersonal pronouns

OBJECTIVE

Missing body part
Actual change in structure and/or function
Nonverbal response to actual or perceived change in structure and/or
   function; behaviors of avoidance, monitoring, or acknowledgment
   of one's body
Not looking at/not touching body part
Trauma to nonfunctioning part
Change in ability to estimate spatial relationship of body to environ-
   ment
Extension of body boundary to incorporate environmental objects
Hiding or overexposing body part (intentional or unintentional)

Information that appears in brackets has been added by the authors
to clarify and enhance the use of nursing diagnoses.

Change in social involvement
[Aggression; low frustration tolerance level]

Desired Outcomes/Evaluation Criteria—Client Will:

- Verbalize acceptance of self in situation (e.g., chronic progressive disease, amputee, decreased independence, weight as is, effects of therapeutic regimen).
- Verbalize relief of anxiety and adaptation to actual/altered body image.
- Verbalize understanding of body changes.
- Recognize and incorporate body image change into self-concept in accurate manner without negating self-esteem.
- Seek information and actively pursue growth.
- Acknowledge self as an individual who has responsibility for self.
- Use adaptive devices/prosthesis appropriately.

Actions/Interventions

NURSING PRIORITY NO. 1. To assess causative/contributing factors:

- Discuss pathophysiology present and/or situation affecting the individual and refer to additional NDs as appropriate. For example, when alteration in body image is related to neurologic deficit (e.g., cerebrovascular accident—CVA), refer to ND Unilateral Neglect; in the presence of severe, ongoing pain, refer to Pain, chronic; or in loss of sexual desire/ability, refer to Sexual Dysfunction.
- Determine whether condition is permanent/no hope for resolution. (May be associated with other NDs, such as Self-Esteem [specify] or Attachment, risk for impaired parent/infant/child when child is affected.)
- Assess mental/physical influence of illness/condition on the client's emotional state (e.g., diseases of the endocrine system, use of steroid therapy, and so on).
- Evaluate level of client's knowledge of and anxiety related to situation. Observe emotional changes.
- Recognize behavior indicative of overconcern with body and its processes.
- Have client describe self, noting what is positive and what is negative. Be aware of how client believes others see self.
- Discuss meaning of loss/change to client. **A small (seemingly trivial) loss may have a big impact (such as the use of a urinary catheter or enema for continence). A change in function (such as immobility) may be more difficult for some to deal with than a change in appearance. Permanent facial scarring of child may be difficult for parents to accept.**
- Use developmentally appropriate communication techniques

for determining exact expression of body image in child (e.g., puppet play or constructive dialogue for toddler). **Developmental capacity must guide interaction to gain accurate information.**

- Note signs of grieving/indicators of severe or prolonged depression **to evaluate need for counseling and/or medications.**
- Determine ethnic background and cultural/religious perceptions and considerations.
- Identify social aspects of illness/disease (e.g., sexually transmitted diseases, sterility, chronic conditions).
- Observe interaction of client with SO(s). **Distortions in body image may be unconsciously reinforced by family members, and/or secondary gain issues may interfere with progress.**

NURSING PRIORITY NO. **2.** To determine coping abilities and skills:

- Assess client's current level of adaptation and progress.
- Listen to client's comments and responses to the situation. **Different situations are upsetting to different people, depending on individual coping skills and past experiences.**
- Note withdrawn behavior and the use of denial. **May be normal response to situation or may be indicative of mental illness (e.g., schizophrenia).** (Refer to ND Denial, ineffective.)
- Note use of addictive substances/alcohol; **may reflect dysfunctional coping.**
- Identify previously used coping strategies and effectiveness.
- Determine individual/family/community resources.

NURSING PRIORITY NO. **3.** To assist client and SO(s) to deal with/accept issues of self-concept related to body image:

- Establish therapeutic nurse-client relationship conveying an attitude of caring and developing a sense of trust.
- Visit client frequently and acknowledge the individual as someone who is worthwhile. **Provides opportunities for listening to concerns and questions.**
- Assist in correcting underlying problems **to promote optimal healing/adaptation.**
- Provide assistance with self-care needs/measures as necessary while promoting individual abilities/independence.
- Work with client's self-concept without moral judgments regarding client's efforts or progress (e.g., "You should be progressing faster; you're weak/lazy/not trying hard enough").
- Discuss concerns about fear of mutilation, prognosis, rejection when client facing surgery or potentially poor outcome of procedure/illness, **to address realities and provide emotional support.**
- Acknowledge and accept feelings of dependency, grief, and hostility.

- Encourage verbalization of and role-play anticipated **conflicts to enhance handling of potential situations.**
- Encourage client and SO(s) to communicate feelings to each other.
- Assume all individuals are sensitive to changes in appearance but avoid stereotyping.
- Alert staff to monitor own facial expressions and other nonverbal behaviors **because they need to convey acceptance and not revulsion when the client's appearance is affected.**
- Encourage family members to treat client normally and not as an invalid.
- Encourage client to look at/touch affected body part **to begin to incorporate changes into body image.**
- Allow client to use denial without participating (e.g., client may at first refuse to look at a colostomy; the nurse says "I am going to change your colostomy now" and proceeds with the task). **Provides individual time to adapt to situation.**
- Set limits on maladaptive behavior and assist client to identify positive behaviors **to aid in recovery.**
- Provide accurate information as desired/requested. Reinforce previously given information.
- Discuss the availability of prosthetics, reconstructive surgery, and physical/occupational therapy or other referrals as dictated by individual situation.
- Help client to select and use clothing/makeup **to minimize body changes and enhance appearance.**
- Discuss reasons for infectious isolation and procedures when used and make time to sit down and talk/listen to client while in the room **to decrease sense of isolation/loneliness.**

NURSING PRIORITY NO. 4. To promote wellness (Teaching/ Discharge Considerations):

- Begin counseling/other therapies (e.g., biofeedback/relaxation) as soon as possible **to provide early/ongoing sources of support.**
- Provide information at client's level of acceptance and in small pieces **to allow for easier assimilation.** Clarify misconceptions. Reinforce explanations given by other health team members.
- Include client in decision-making process and problemsolving activities.
- Assist client to incorporate therapeutic regimen into activi-ties of daily living (ADLs) (e.g., including specific exercises, housework activities). **Promotes continuation of program.**
- Identify/plan for alterations to home and work environment/activities **to accommodate individual needs and support independence.**

- Assist client in learning strategies for dealing with feelings/venting emotions.
- Offer positive reinforcement for efforts made (e.g., wearing makeup, using prosthetic device).
- Refer to appropriate support groups.

Documentation Focus

ASSESSMENT/REASSESSMENT

- Observations, presence of maladaptive behaviors, emotional changes, stage of grieving, level of independence.
- Physical wounds, dressings; use of life-support–type machine (e.g., ventilator, dialysis machine).
- Meaning of loss/change to client.
- Support systems available (e.g., SOs, friends, groups).

PLANNING

- Plan of care and who is involved in planning.
- Teaching plan.

IMPLEMENTATION/EVALUATION

- Client's response to interventions/teaching and actions performed.
- Attainment/progress toward desired outcome(s).
- Modifications of plan of care.

DISCHARGE PLANNING

- Long-term needs and who is responsible for actions.
- Specific referrals made (e.g., rehabilitation center, community resources).

SAMPLE NURSING OUTCOMES & INTERVENTIONS CLASSIFICATIONS (NOC/NIC)

NOC—Body Image
NIC—Body Image Enhancement

Body Temperature, risk for imbalanced

Taxonomy II: Safety/Protection—Class 6
Thermoregulation (00005)
[Diagnostic division: Safety]
Submitted 1986; Revised 2000

Definition: At risk for failure to maintain body temperature within normal range

Information that appears in brackets has been added by the authors to clarify and enhance the use of nursing diagnoses.

Risk Factors

Extremes of age, weight
Exposure to cold/cool or warm/hot environments
Dehydration
Inactivity or vigorous activity
Medications causing vasoconstriction/vasodilation, altered metabolic rate, sedation, [use or overdose of certain drugs or exposure to anesthesia]
Inappropriate clothing for environmental temperature
Illness or trauma affecting temperature regulation [e.g., infections, systemic or localized; neoplasms, tumors; collagen/vascular disease]

> NOTE: A risk diagnosis is not evidenced by signs and symptoms, as the problem has not occurred and nursing interventions are directed at prevention.

Desired Outcomes/Evaluation Criteria—Client Will:

- Maintain body temperature within normal range.
- Verbalize understanding of individual risk factors and appropriate interventions.
- Demonstrate behaviors for monitoring and maintaining appropriate body temperature.

Actions/Interventions

NURSING PRIORITY NO. 1. To identify causative/risk factors present:

- Determine if present illness/condition results from exposure to environmental factors, surgery, infection, trauma.
- Monitor laboratory values (**e.g., tests indicative of infection, drug screens**).
- Note client's age (e.g., premature neonate, young child, or aging individual), **as it can directly impact ability to maintain/regulate body temperature and respond to changes in environment.**
- Assess nutritional status.

NURSING PRIORITY NO. 2. To prevent occurrence of temperature alteration:

- Monitor/maintain comfortable ambient environment. Provide heating/cooling measures as indicated.
- Cover head with knit cap, place infant under radiant warmer or adequate blankets. **Heat loss in newborn/infants is greatest through head and by evaporation and convection.**
- Monitor core body temperature. (Tympanic temperature may be preferred, **as it is the most accurate noninvasive method.**)

- Restore/maintain core temperature within client's normal range. (Refer to NDs Hypothermia and Hyperthermia.)
- Refer at-risk persons to appropriate community resources (e.g., home care/social services, Foster Adult Care, housing agencies) **to provide assistance to meet individual needs.**

NURSING PRIORITY NO. **3**. To promote wellness (Teaching/Discharge Considerations):

- Review potential problem/individual risk factors with client/SO(s).
- Instruct in measures to protect from identified risk factors (e.g., too warm, too cold environment; improper medication regimen; drug overdose; inappropriate clothing/shelter; poor nutritional status).
- Review ways to prevent accidental alterations, such as induced hypothermia as a result of overzealous cooling to reduce fever or maintaining too warm an environment for client who has lost the ability to perspire.

Documentation Focus

ASSESSMENT/REASSESSMENT

- Identified individual causative/risk factors.
- Record of core temperature, initially and prn.
- Results of diagnostic studies/laboratory tests.

PLANNING

- Plan of care and who is involved in planning.
- Teaching plan, including best ambient temperature, and ways to prevent hypothermia or hyperthermia.

IMPLEMENTATION/EVALUATION

- Response to interventions/teaching and actions performed.
- Attainment/progress toward desired outcome(s).
- Modifications to plan of care.

DISCHARGE PLANNING

- Long-term needs and who is responsible for actions.
- Specific referrals made.

SAMPLE NURSING OUTCOMES & INTERVENTIONS CLASSIFICATIONS (NOC/NIC)

NOC—Risk Control
NIC—Temperature Regulation

Bowel Incontinence

Taxonomy II: Elimination—Class 2 Gastrointestinal
System (00014)
[Diagnostic Division: Elimination]
Submitted 1975; Nursing Diagnosis Extension and
Classification (NDEC) Revision 1998

Definition: Change in normal bowel habits characterized by involuntary passage of stool

Related Factors

Self-care deficit—toileting; impaired cognition; immobility; environ-
    mental factors (e.g., inaccessible bathroom)
Dietary habits; medications; laxative abuse
Stress
Colorectal lesions
Incomplete emptying of bowel; impaction; chronic diarrhea
General decline in muscle tone; abnormally high abdominal or intes-
    tinal pressure
Impaired reservoir capacity
Rectal sphincter abnormality; loss of rectal sphincter control;
    lower/upper motor nerve damage

Defining Characteristics

SUBJECTIVE

Recognizes rectal fullness but reports inability to expel formed stool
Urgency
Inability to delay defecation
Self-report of inability to feel rectal fullness

OBJECTIVE

Constant dribbling of soft stool
Fecal staining of clothing and/or bedding
Fecal odor
Red perianal skin
Inability to recognize/inattention to urge to defecate

Desired Outcomes/Evaluation
Criteria—Client Will:

- Verbalize understanding of causative/controlling factors.
- Identify individually appropriate interventions.
- Participate in therapeutic regimen to control incontinence.
- Establish/maintain as regular a pattern of bowel functioning
  as possible.

ACTIONS/INTERVENTIONS

NURSING PRIORITY NO. **1.** To assess causative/contributing
factors:

Information that appears in brackets has been added by the authors
to clarify and enhance the use of nursing diagnoses. **105**

- Identify pathophysiologic factors present (e.g., multiple sclerosis, acute/chronic cognitive impairment, spinal cord injury, stroke, ileus, ulcerative colitis).
- Note times/aspects of incontinent occurrence, preceding/precipitating events.
- Check for presence/absence of anal sphincter reflex or impaction, which may be contributing factors.
- Review medication regimen **for side effects/interactions.**
- Test stool for blood (guaiac) as appropriate.
- Palpate abdomen **for distention, masses, tenderness.**

NURSING PRIORITY NO. 2. To determine current pattern of elimination:

- Note stool characteristics (color, odor, consistency, amount, shape, and frequency). **Provides comparative baseline.**
- Encourage client or SO to record times at which incontinence occurs, **to note relationship to meals, activity, client's behavior.**
- Auscultate abdomen **for presence, location, and characteristics of bowel sounds.**

NURSING PRIORITY NO. 3. To promote control/management of incontinence:

- Assist in treatment of causative/contributing factors (e.g., as listed in the Related Factors and Defining Characteristics).
- Establish bowel program with regular time for defecation; use suppositories and/or digital stimulation when indicated. Maintain daily program initially. Progress to alternate days dependent on usual pattern/amount of stool.
- Take client to the bathroom/place on commode or bedpan at specified intervals, taking into consideration individual needs and incontinence patterns **to maximize success of program.**
- Encourage and instruct client/caregiver in providing diet high in bulk/fiber and adequate fluids (minimum of 2000 to 2400 mL/day). Encourage warm fluids after meals. Identify/eliminate problem foods **to avoid diarrhea/constipation, gas formation.**
- Give stool softeners/bulk formers as indicated/needed.
- Provide pericare **to avoid excoriation of the area.**
- Promote exercise program, as individually able, **to increase muscle tone/strength, including perineal muscles.**
- Provide incontinence aids/pads until control is obtained.
- Demonstrate techniques (e.g., contracting abdominal muscles, leaning forward on commode, manual compression) **to increase intra-abdominal pressure during defecation, and left to right abdominal massage to stimulate peristalsis.**

- Refer to ND Diarrhea if incontinence is due to uncontrolled diarrhea; ND Constipation if diarrhea is due to impaction.

NURSING PRIORITY NO. 4. To promote wellness (Teaching/Discharge Considerations):

- Review and encourage continuation of successful interventions as individually identified.
- Instruct in use of laxatives or stool softeners, if indicated, **to stimulate timed defecation.**
- Identify foods that promote bowel regularity.
- Provide emotional support to client and SO(s), especially when condition is long-term or chronic.
- Encourage scheduling of social activities within time frame of bowel program as indicated (e.g., avoid a 4-hour excursion if bowel program requires toileting every 3 hours and facilities will not be available) **to maximize social functioning and success of bowel program.**

Documentation Focus

ASSESSMENT/REASSESSMENT

- Current and previous pattern of elimination/physical findings, character of stool, actions tried.

PLANNING

- Plan of care and who is involved in planning.
- Teaching plan.

IMPLEMENTATION/EVALUATION

- Client's/caregiver's responses to interventions/teaching and actions performed.
- Changes in pattern of elimination, characteristics of stool.
- Attainment/progress toward desired outcome(s).
- Modifications to plan of care.

DISCHARGE PLANNING

- Identified long-term needs, noting who is responsible for each action.
- Specific bowel program at time of discharge.

SAMPLE NURSING OUTCOMES & INTERVENTIONS CLASSIFICATIONS (NOC/NIC)

NOC—Bowel Continence
NIC—Bowel Incontinence Care

Breastfeeding, effective [Learning Need]*

Taxonomy II: Role Relationships—Class 3 Role
Performance (00106)
[Diagnostic Division: Food/Fluid]
Submitted 1990

Definition: Mother-infant dyad/family exhibits
adequate proficiency and satisfaction with breastfeeding
process

Related Factors

Basic breastfeeding knowledge
Normal breast structure
Normal infant oral structure
Infant gestational age greater than 34 weeks
Support sources [available]
Maternal confidence

Defining Characteristics

SUBJECTIVE

Maternal verbalization of satisfaction with the breastfeeding process

OBJECTIVE

Mother able to position infant at breast to promote a successful
   latchon response
Infant is content after feedings
Regular and sustained suckling/swallowing at the breast [e.g., 8 to 10
   times/24 h]
Appropriate infant weight patterns for age
Effective mother/infant communication pattern (infant cues, maternal
   interpretation and response)
Signs and/or symptoms of oxytocin release (letdown or milk ejection
   reflex)
Adequate infant elimination patterns for age; [stools soft; more than 6
   wet diapers/day of unconcentrated urine]
Eagerness of infant to nurse

Desired Outcomes/Evaluation Criteria—Client Will:

• Verbalize understanding of breastfeeding techniques.
• Demonstrate effective techniques for breastfeeding.

---

*This is difficult to address, as the Related Factors and Defining
Characteristics are in fact the outcome/evaluation criteria that would
be desired. We believe that normal breastfeeding behaviors need to be
learned and supported, with interventions directed at learning activities for enhancement.

   Information that appears in brackets has been added by the authors
to clarify and enhance the use of nursing diagnoses.

- Demonstrate family involvement and support.
- Attend classes/read appropriate materials as necessary.

Actions/Interventions

NURSING PRIORITY NO. **1**. To assess individual learning needs:

- Assess mother's knowledge and previous experience with breastfeeding.
- Monitor effectiveness of current breastfeeding efforts.
- Determine support systems available to mother/family.

NURSING PRIORITY NO. **2**. To promote effective breastfeeding behaviors:

- Initiate breastfeeding within first hour after birth.
- Demonstrate how to support and position infant.
- Observe mother's return demonstration.
- Keep infant with mother **for unrestricted breastfeeding duration and frequency.**
- Encourage mother to drink at least 2000 mL of fluid per day or 8 oz every hour.
- Provide information as needed.

NURSING PRIORITY NO. **3**. To promote wellness (Teaching/Discharge Considerations):

- Provide for follow-up contact/home visit 48 hours after discharge; repeat visit as necessary **to provide support and assist with problem solving, if needed.**
- Recommend monitoring number of infant's wet diapers **(at least 6 wet diapers in 24 hours suggests adequate hydration).**
- Encourage mother/other family members to express feelings/concerns, and Active-listen **to determine nature of concerns.**
- Review techniques for expression and storage of breast milk **to help sustain breastfeeding activity.**
- Problem-solve return-to-work issues or periodic infant care requiring bottle feeding.
- Refer to support groups, such as La Leche League, as indicated.
- Refer to ND Breastfeeding, ineffective for more specific information as appropriate.

Documentation Focus

ASSESSMENT/REASSESSMENT

- Identified assessment factors (maternal and infant).
- Number of daily wet diapers and periodic weight.

PLANNING

- Plan of care/interventions and who is involved in the planning.
- Teaching plan.

IMPLEMENTATION/EVALUATION

- Mother's response to actions/teaching plan and actions performed.
- Effectiveness of infant's efforts to feed.
- Attainment/progress toward desired outcome(s).
- Modifications to plan of care.

DISCHARGE PLANNING

- Long-term needs/referrals and who is responsible for follow-up actions.

SAMPLE NURSING OUTCOMES & INTERVENTIONS CLASSIFICATIONS (NOC/NIC)

NOC—Breastfeeding Establishment: Maternal
NIC—Lactation Counseling

Breastfeeding, ineffective

Taxonomy II: Role Relationships—Class 3 Role
Performance (00104)
[Diagnostic Division: Food/Fluid]
Submitted 1988

Definition: Dissatisfaction or difficulty a mother, infant, or child experiences with the breastfeeding process

Related Factors

Prematurity; infant anomaly; poor infant sucking reflex
Infant receiving [numerous or repeated] supplemental feedings with artificial nipple
Maternal anxiety or ambivalence
Knowledge deficit
Previous history of breastfeeding failure
Interruption in breastfeeding
Nonsupportive partner/family
Maternal breast anomaly; previous breast surgery; [painful nipples/breast engorgement]

Defining Characteristics

SUBJECTIVE

Unsatisfactory breastfeeding process
Persistence of sore nipples beyond the first week of breastfeeding

---

Information that appears in brackets has been added by the authors to clarify and enhance the use of nursing diagnoses.

Insufficient emptying of each breast per feeding
Actual or perceived inadequate milk supply

OBJECTIVE

Observable signs of inadequate infant intake [decrease in number of
    wet diapers, inappropriate weight loss/or inadequate gain]
Nonsustained or insufficient opportunity for suckling at the breast;
    infant inability [failure] to attach onto maternal breast correctly
Infant arching and crying at the breast; resistant latching on
Infant exhibiting fussiness and crying within the first hour after
    breastfeeding; unresponsive to other comfort measures
No observable signs of oxytocin release

Desired Outcomes/Evaluation Criteria—Client Will:

- Verbalize understanding of causative/contributing factors.
- Demonstrate techniques to improve/enhance breastfeeding.
- Assume responsibility for effective breastfeeding.
- Achieve mutually satisfactory breastfeeding regimen with infant content after feedings and gaining weight appropriately.

Actions/Interventions

NURSING PRIORITY NO. 1. To identify maternal causative/
contributing factors:

- Assess client knowledge about breastfeeding and extent of instruction that has been given.
- Encourage discussion of current/previous breastfeeding experience(s).
- Note previous unsatisfactory experience (including self or others) **because it may be affecting current situation.**
- Do physical assessment, noting appearance of breasts/ nipples, marked asymmetry of breasts, obvious inverted or flat nipples, minimal or no breast enlargement during pregnancy.
- Determine whether lactation failure is primary (**i.e., maternal prolactin deficiency/serum prolactin levels, inadequate mammary gland tissue, breast surgery that has damaged the nipple, areola enervation-irremediable**) or secondary (**i.e., sore nipples, severe engorgement, plugged milk ducts, mastitis, inhibition of letdown reflex, maternal/infant separation with disruption of feedings-treatable**).
- Note history of pregnancy, labor and delivery (vaginal or cesarean section), other recent or current surgery; preexisting medical problems (e.g., diabetes, epilepsy, cardiac diseases, or presence of disabilities).
- Identify maternal support systems; presence and response of SO(s), extended family, friends.

- Ascertain mother's age, number of children at home, and need to return to work.
- Determine maternal feelings (e.g., fear/anxiety, ambivalence, depression).
- Ascertain cultural expectations/conflicts.

NURSING PRIORITY NO. 2. To assess infant causative/contributing factors:

- Determine suckling problems, as noted in Related Factors/Defining Characteristics.
- Note prematurity and/or infant anomaly (e.g., cleft palate).
- Review feeding schedule, **to note increased demand for feeding (at least 8 times/day, taking both breasts at each feeding for more than 15 minutes on each side) or use of supplements with artificial nipple.**
- Evaluate observable signs of inadequate infant intake (e.g., baby latches onto mother's nipples with sustained suckling but minimal audible swallowing/gulping noted, infant arching and crying at the breasts with resistance to latching on, decreased urinary output/frequency of stools, inadequate weight gain).
- Determine whether baby is content after feeding, or exhibits fussiness and crying within the first hour after breastfeeding, **suggesting unsatisfactory breastfeeding process.**
- Note any correlation between maternal ingestion of certain foods and "colicky" response of infant.

NURSING PRIORITY NO. 3. To assist mother to develop skills of adequate breastfeeding:

- Give emotional support to mother. Use 1:1 instruction with each feeding during hospital stay/clinic visit.
- Inform mother that some babies do not cry when they are hungry; instead some make "rooting" motions and suck their fingers.
- Recommend avoidance or overuse of supplemental feedings and pacifiers (unless specifically indicated) **that can lessen infant's desire to breastfeed.**
- Restrict use of breast shields (i.e., only temporarily to help draw the nipple out), then place baby directly on nipple.
- Demonstrate use of electric piston-type breast pump with bilateral collection chamber when necessary **to maintain or increase milk supply.**
- Encourage frequent rest periods, sharing household/child-care duties **to limit fatigue and facilitate relaxation at feeding times.**
- Suggest abstinence/restriction of tobacco, caffeine, alcohol, drugs, excess sugar **because they may affect milk production/letdown reflex or be passed on to the infant.**

- Promote early management of breastfeeding problems. For example:

Engorgement: Heat and/or cool applications to the breasts, massage from chest wall down to nipple; use synthetic oxytocin nasal spray **to enhance letdown reflex;** soothe "fussy baby" before latching on the breast, properly position baby on breast/nipple, alternate the side baby starts nursing on, nurse round-the-clock and/or pump with piston-type electric breast pump with bilateral collection chambers at least 8 to 12 times/day.

Sore nipples: Wear 100% cotton fabrics, do not use soap/alcohol/ drying agents on nipples, avoid use of nipple shields or nursing pads that contain plastic; cleanse and then air dry, use thin layers of lanolin (if mother/baby not sensitive to wool); provide exposure to sunlight/sunlamps with extreme caution; administer mild pain reliever as appropriate, apply ice before nursing; soak with warm water before attaching infant **to soften nipple and remove dried milk,** begin with least sore side or begin with hand expression **to establish letdown reflex,** properly position infant on breast/ nipple, and use a variety of nursing positions.

Clogged ducts: Use larger bra or extender to avoid pressure on site; use moist or dry heat, gently massage from above plug down to nipple; nurse infant, hand express, or pump after massage; nurse more often on affected side.

Inhibited letdown: Use relaxation techniques before nursing (e.g., maintain quiet atmosphere, assume position of comfort, massage, apply heat to breasts, have beverage available); develop a routine for nursing, concentrate on infant; administer synthetic oxytocin nasal spray as appropriate.

Mastitis: Promote bedrest (with infant) for several days; administer antibiotics; provide warm, moist heat before and during nursing; empty breasts completely, continuing to nurse baby at least 8 to 12 times/day, or pumping breasts for 24 hours; then resuming breast-feeding as appropriate.

NURSING PRIORITY NO. 4. To condition infant to breastfeed:

- Scent breast pad with breast milk and leave in bed with infant along with mother's photograph when separated from mother for medical purposes (e.g., prematurity).
- Increase skin-to-skin contact.
- Provide practice times at breast.
- Express small amounts of milk into baby's mouth.
- Have mother pump breast after feeding to enhance milk production.
- Use supplemental nutrition system cautiously when necessary.
- Identify special interventions for feeding in presence of cleft lip/palate.

NURSING PRIORITY NO. 5. To promote wellness (Teaching/ Discharge Considerations):

- Schedule follow-up visit with healthcare provider 48 hours after hospital discharge and 2 weeks after birth **for evaluation of milk intake/breastfeeding process.**

- Recommend monitoring number of infant's wet diapers (**at least 6 wet diapers in 24 hours suggests adequate hydration**).
- Weigh infant at least every third day as indicated and record (**to verify adequacy of nutritional intake**).
- Encourage spouse education and support when appropriate. Review mother's need for rest, relaxation, and time together and with other children as appropriate.
- Discuss importance of adequate nutrition/fluid intake, prenatal vitamins, or other vitamin/mineral supplements, such as vitamin C, as indicated.
- Address specific problems (e.g., suckling problems, prematurity/anomalies).
- Inform mother that return of menses within first 3 months after infant's birth may indicate inadequate prolactin levels.
- Refer to support groups (e.g., La Leche League, parenting support groups, stress reduction, or other community resources as indicated).
- Provide bibliotherapy for further information.

Documentation Focus

ASSESSMENT/REASSESSMENT

- Identified assessment factors, both maternal and infant (e.g., is engorgement present, is infant demonstrating adequate weight gain without supplementation).

PLANNING

- Plan of care/interventions and who is involved in planning.
- Teaching plan.

IMPLEMENTATION/EVALUATION

- Mother's/infant's responses to interventions/teaching and actions performed.
- Attainment/progress toward desired outcome(s).
- Modifications to plan of care.

DISCHARGE PLANNING

- Referrals that have been made and mother's choice of participation.

SAMPLE NURSING OUTCOMES & INTERVENTIONS CLASSIFICATIONS (NOC/NIC)

NOC—Knowledge Breastfeeding
NIC—Breastfeeding Assistance

Breastfeeding, interrupted

Taxonomy II: Role Relationships—Class 3 Role
Performance (00105)
[Diagnostic Division: Food/Fluid]
Submitted 1992

Definition: Break in the continuity of the breastfeeding process as a result of inability or inadvisability to put baby to breast for feeding

Related Factors

Maternal or infant illness
Prematurity
Maternal employment
Contraindications to breastfeeding (e.g., drugs, true breast milk jaundice)
Need to abruptly wean infant

Defining Characteristics

SUBJECTIVE

Infant does not receive nourishment at the breast for some or all of feedings
Maternal desire to maintain lactation and provide (or eventually provide) her breast milk for her infant's nutritional needs
Lack of knowledge regarding expression and storage of breast milk

OBJECTIVE

Separation of mother and infant

Desired Outcomes/Evaluation Criteria—Client Will:

- Identify and demonstrate techniques to sustain lactation until breastfeeding is reinitiated.
- Achieve mutually satisfactory feeding regimen with infant content after feedings and gaining weight appropriately.
- Achieve weaning and cessation of lactation if desired or necessary.

Actions/Interventions

NURSING PRIORITY NO. 1. To identify causative/contributing factors:

- Assess client knowledge and perceptions about breastfeeding and extent of instruction that has been given.
- Encourage discussion of current/previous breastfeeding experience(s).

Information that appears in brackets has been added by the authors to clarify and enhance the use of nursing diagnoses.

- Determine maternal responsibilities, routines, and scheduled activities (e.g., caretaking of siblings, employment in/out of home, work/school schedules of family members, ability to visit hospitalized infant).
- Note contraindications to breastfeeding (e.g., maternal illness, drug use); desire/need to wean infant.
- Ascertain cultural expectations/conflicts.

NURSING PRIORITY NO. 2. To assist mother to maintain or conclude breastfeeding as desired/required:
- Give emotional support to mother and accept decision regarding cessation/continuation of breastfeeding.
- Demonstrate use of manual and/or electric piston-type breast pump.
- Suggest abstinence/restriction of tobacco, caffeine, alcohol, drugs, excess sugar as appropriate when breastfeeding is reinitiated **because they may affect milk production/letdown reflex or be passed on to the infant**.
- Provide information (e.g., wearing a snug, well-fitting brassiere, avoiding stimulation, and using medication for discomfort **to support weaning process**).

NURSING PRIORITY NO. 3. To promote successful infant feeding:
- Review techniques for storage/use of expressed breast milk **to provide optimal nutrition and promote continuation of breastfeeding process**.
- Discuss proper use and choice of supplemental nutrition and alternate feeding method (e.g., bottle/syringe).
- Review safety precautions (e.g., proper flow of formula from nipple, frequency of burping, holding bottle instead of propping, formula preparation, and sterilization techniques).
- Determine if a routine visiting schedule or advance warning can be provided **so that infant will be hungry/ready to feed.**
- Provide privacy, calm surroundings when mother breastfeeds in hospital setting.
- Recommend/provide for infant sucking on a regular basis, especially if gavage feedings are part of the therapeutic regimen. Reinforces that feeding time is pleasurable and enhances digestion.

NURSING PRIORITY NO. 4. To promote wellness (Teaching/Discharge Considerations):
- Encourage mother to obtain adequate rest, maintain fluid and nutritional intake, and schedule breast pumping every 3 hours while awake as indicated **to sustain adequate milk production and breastfeeding process**.
- Identify other means of nurturing/strengthening infant attachment (e.g., comforting, consoling, play activities).
- Refer to support groups (e.g., La Leche League, Lact-Aid),

community resources (e.g., public health nurse, lactation specialist).
• Promote use of bibliotherapy for further information.

Documentation Focus

ASSESSMENT/REASSESSMENT

• Baseline findings maternal/infant factors.
• Number of wet diapers daily/periodic weight.

PLANNING

• Plan of care and who is involved in planning.
• Teaching plan.

IMPLEMENTATION/EVALUATION

• Maternal response to interventions/teaching and actions performed.
• Infant's response to feeding and method.
• Whether infant appears satisfied or still seems to be hungry.
• Attainment/progress toward desired outcome(s).
• Modifications to plan of care.

DISCHARGE PLANNING

• Referrals, plan for follow-up and who is responsible.
• Specific referrals made.

SAMPLE NURSING OUTCOMES & INTERVENTIONS CLASSIFICATIONS (NOC/NIC)

NOC—Breastfeeding Maintenance
NIC—Lactation Counseling

Breathing Pattern, ineffective

Taxonomy II: Activity/Rest—Class 4
Cardiovascular/Pulmonary Responses (00032)
[Diagnostic Division: Respiration]
Submitted 1980; Revised 1996, and Nursing Diagnosis
Extension and Classification (NDEC) 1998

Definition: Inspiration and/or expiration that does not provide adequate ventilation

Related Factors

Neuromuscular dysfunction; SCI; neurological immaturity
Musculoskeletal impairment; bony/chest wall deformity

Information that appears in brackets has been added by the authors to clarify and enhance the use of nursing diagnoses.

Anxiety

Pain

Perception/cognitive impairment

Decreased energy/fatigue; respiratory muscle fatigue

Body position; obesity

Hyperventilation; hypoventilation syndrome; [alteration of client's normal $O_2:CO_2$ ratio (e.g., O_2 therapy in COPD)]

Defining Characteristics

SUBJECTIVE

Shortness of breath

OBJECTIVE

Dyspnea; orthopnea

Respiratory rate:

Adults >14 yr: ≤11 or [>]24

Children 1 to 4 yr, <20 or >30

5 to 14 yr, <14 or >25

Infants [0 to 12 mo], <25 or >60

Depth of breathing:

    Adult tidal volume: 500 mL at rest

    Infant tidal volume: 6 to 8 mL/kg

Timing ratio; prolonged expiration phases; pursed-lip breathing

Decreased minute ventilation; vital capacity

Decreased inspiratory/expiratory pressure

Use of accessory muscles to breathe; assumption of three-point position

Altered chest excursion; [paradoxical breathing patterns]

Nasal flaring; [grunting]

Increased anterior-posterior diameter

Desired Outcomes/Evaluation Criteria—Client Will:

- Establish a normal/effective respiratory pattern.
- Be free of cyanosis and other signs/symptoms of hypoxia with ABGs within client's normal/acceptable range.
- Verbalize awareness of causative factors and initiate needed lifestyle changes.
- Demonstrate appropriate coping behaviors.

Actions/Interventions

NURSING PRIORITY NO. 1. To identify etiology/precipitating factors:

- Auscultate chest, noting presence/character of breath sounds, presence of secretions.
- Note rate and depth of respirations, type of breathing pattern: tachypnea, Cheyne-Stokes, other irregular patterns.

- Assist with necessary testing (e.g., lung volumes/flow studies, pulmonary function/sleep studies) **to diagnose presence/ severity of lung diseases.**
- Review chest x-rays as indicated **for severity of acute/chronic conditions.**
- Review laboratory data, for example, ABGs (degree of oxygenation, CO_2 retention); drug screens; and pulmonary function studies (vital capacity/tidal volume).
- Note emotional responses, for example, gasping, crying, tingling fingers. **(Hyperventilation may be a factor.)**
- Assess for concomitant pain/discomfort **that may restrict/ limit respiratory effort.**

NURSING PRIORITY NO. 2. To provide for relief of causative factors:

- Administer oxygen at lowest concentration indicated for underlying pulmonary condition, respiratory distress, or cyanosis.
- Suction airway as needed **to clear secretions.**
- Assist with bronchoscopy or chest tube insertion as indicated.
- Elevate HOB as appropriate **to promote physiologic/psychologic ease of maximal inspiration.**
- Encourage slower/deeper respirations, use of pursed-lip technique, and so on **to assist client in "taking control" of the situation.**
- Have client breathe into a paper bag **to correct hyperventilation.**
- Maintain calm attitude while dealing with client and SO(s) **to limit level of anxiety.**
- Assist client in the use of relaxation techniques.
- Deal with fear/anxiety that may be present. (Refer to NDs Fear and/or Anxiety.)
- Encourage position of comfort. Reposition client frequently if immobility is a factor.
- Splint rib cage during deep-breathing exercises/cough if indicated.
- Medicate with analgesics as appropriate **to promote deeper respiration and cough.** (Refer to ND Pain, acute or Pain, chronic.)
- Encourage ambulation as individually indicated.
- Avoid overeating/gas-forming foods; **may cause abdominal distention.**
- Provide use of adjuncts, such as incentive spirometer, **to facilitate deeper respiratory effort.**
- Supervise use of respirator/diaphragmatic stimulator, rocking bed, apnea monitor, and so forth **when neuromuscular impairment is present.**
- Maintain emergency equipment in readily accessible location

and include age/size appropriate ET/trach tubes (e.g., infant, child, adolescent, or adult).

NURSING PRIORITY NO. 3. To promote wellness (Teaching/Discharge Considerations):

- Review etiology and possible coping behaviors.
- Teach conscious control of respiratory rate as appropriate.
- Maximize respiratory effort with good posture and effective use of accessory muscles.
- Assist client to learn breathing exercises: diaphragmatic, abdominal breathing, inspiratory resistive, and pursed-lip as indicated.
- Recommend energy conservation techniques and pacing of activities.
- Encourage adequate rest periods between activities **to limit fatigue.**
- Discuss relationship of smoking to respiratory function.
- Encourage client/SO(s) to develop a plan for smoking cessation. Provide appropriate referrals.
- Instruct in proper use and safety concerns for home oxygen therapy as indicated.
- Make referral to support groups/contact with individuals who have encountered similar problems.

Documentation Focus

ASSESSMENT/REASSESSMENT

- Relevant history of problem.
- Respiratory pattern, breath sounds, use of accessory muscles.
- Laboratory values.
- Use of respiratory supports, ventilator settings, and so forth.

PLANNING

- Plan of care/interventions and who is involved in the planning.
- Teaching plan.

IMPLEMENTATION/EVALUATION

- Response to interventions/teaching, actions performed, and treatment regimen.
- Mastery of skills, level of independence.
- Attainment/progress toward desired outcome(s).
- Modifications to plan of care.

DISCHARGE PLANNING

- Long-term needs, including appropriate referrals and action taken, available resources.
- Specific referrals provided.

SAMPLE NURSING OUTCOMES
& INTERVENTIONS CLASSIFICATIONS (NOC/NIC)

NOC—Respiratory Status: Ventilation
NIC—Ventilation Assistances

Cardiac Output, decreased

Taxonomy II: Activity/Rest—Class 4
Cardiovascular/Pulmonary Responses (00029)
Submitted 1975; Revised 1996, 2000
[Diagnostic Division: Circulation]

Definition: Inadequate blood pumped by the heart to meet the metabolic demands of the body. [Note: In a hypermetabolic state, although cardiac output may be within normal range, it may still be inadequate to meet the needs of the body's tissues. Cardiac output and tissue perfusion are interrelated, although there are differences. When cardiac output is decreased, tissue perfusion problems will develop; however, tissue perfusion problems can exist without decreased cardiac output.]

Related Factors

Altered heart rate/rhythm, [conduction]
Altered stroke volume: altered preload [e.g., decreased venous return]; altered afterload [e.g., systemic vascular resistance]; altered contractility [e.g., ventricular-septal rupture, ventricular aneurysm, papillary muscle rupture, valvular disease]

Defining Characteristics

SUBJECTIVE

Altered Heart Rate/Rhythm: Palpitations
Altered Preload: Fatigue
Altered Afterload: Shortness of breath/dyspnea
Altered Contractility: Orthopnea/paroxysmal nocturnal dyspnea [PND]
Behavioral/Emotional: Anxiety

OBJECTIVE

Altered Heart Rate/Rhythm: [Dys]arrhythmias (tachycardia, bradycardia); EKG [ECG] changes
Altered Preload: Jugular vein distention (JVD); edema; weight gain;

Information that appears in brackets has been added by the authors to clarify and enhance the use of nursing diagnoses.

increased/decreased central venous pressure (CVP); increased/decreased pulmonary artery wedge pressure (PAWP); murmurs

Altered Afterload: Cold, clammy skin; skin [and mucous membrane] color changes [cyanosis, pallor]; prolonged capillary refill; decreased peripheral pulses; variations in blood pressure readings; increased/decreased systemic vascular resistance (SVR)/pulmonary vascular resistance (PVR); oliguria; [anuria]

Altered Contractility: Crackles; cough; cardiac output, 4 L/min; cardiac index, 2.5 L/min; decreased ejection fraction, stroke volume index (SVI), left ventricular stroke work index (LVSWI); S3 or S4 sounds [gallop rhythm]

Behavioral/Emotional: Restlessness

Desired Outcomes/Evaluation Criteria—Client Will:

- Display hemodynamic stability (e.g., blood pressure, cardiac output, renal perfusion/urinary output, peripheral pulses).
- Report/demonstrate decreased episodes of dyspnea, angina, and dysrhythmias.
- Demonstrate an increase in activity tolerance.
- Verbalize knowledge of the disease process, individual risk factors, and treatment plan.
- Participate in activities that reduce the workload of the heart (e.g., stress management or therapeutic medication regimen program, weight reduction, balanced activity/rest plan, proper use of supplemental oxygen, cessation of smoking).
- Identify signs of cardiac decompensation, alter activities, and seek help appropriately.

Actions/Interventions

NURSING PRIORITY NO. **1.** To identify causative/contributing factors:

- Review clients at risk as noted in Related Factors. Note: Individuals with brainstem trauma, spinal cord injuries at T7 or above, **may be at risk for altered cardiac output due to an uninhibited sympathetic response.** (Refer to ND Autonomic Dysreflexia, risk for.)
- Evaluate medication regimen; note drug use/abuse.
- Assess potential for/type of developing shock states: hematogenic, bacteremic, cardiogenic, vasogenic, and psychogenic.
- Review laboratory data (e.g., complete blood cell—CBC—count, electrolytes, ABGs, blood urea nitrogen/creatinine—BUN/Cr—cardiac enzymes, and cultures, such as blood/wound/secretions).

NURSING PRIORITY NO. **2.** To assess degree of debilitation:

- Determine baseline vital signs/hemodynamic parameters

including peripheral pulses. (**Provides opportunities to track changes.**)

- Review signs of impending failure/shock, noting vital signs, invasive hemodynamic parameters, breath sounds, heart tones, and urinary output. Note presence of pulsus paradoxus, **reflecting cardiac tamponade.**
- Review diagnostic studies (e.g., pharmacologic stress testing, ECG, scans, echocardiogram, heart catheterization).
- Note response to activity/procedures and time required to return to baseline vital signs.

NURSING PRIORITY NO. 3. To minimize/correct causative factors, maximize cardiac output:

ACUTE PHASE

- Position with HOB flat or keep trunk horizontal while raising legs 20 to 30 degrees in shock situation (contraindicated in congestive state, in which semi-Fowler's position is preferred).
- Monitor vital signs frequently **to note response to activities.**
- Perform periodic hemodynamic measurements as indicated (e.g., arterial, CVP, pulmonary, and left atrial pressures; cardiac output).
- Monitor cardiac rhythm continuously **to note effectiveness of medications and/or devices (e.g., implanted pacemaker/defibrillator).**
- Administer blood/fluid replacement, antibiotics, diuretics, inotropic drugs, antidysrhythmics, steroids, vasopressors, and/or dilators as indicated. Evaluate response **to determine therapeutic, adverse, or toxic effects of therapy.**
- Restrict or administer fluids (IV/PO) as indicated. Provide adequate fluid/free water, depending on client needs. Assess hourly or periodic urinary output, noting total fluid balance **to allow for timely alterations in therapeutic regimen.**
- Monitor rate of IV drugs closely, using infusion pumps as appropriate **to prevent bolus/overdose.**
- Administer supplemental oxygen as indicated **to increase oxygen available to tissues.**
- Promote adequate rest by decreasing stimuli, providing quiet environment. Schedule activities and assessments **to maximize sleep periods.**
- Assist with or perform self-care activities for client.
- Avoid the use of restraints whenever possible if client is confused. (**May increase agitation and increase the cardiac workload.**)
- Use sedation and analgesics as indicated with caution **to achieve desired effect without compromising hemodynamic readings.**
- Maintain patency of invasive intravascular monitoring and

infusion lines. Tape connections **to prevent air embolus and/or exsanguination.**
- Maintain aseptic technique during invasive procedures. Provide site care as indicated.
- Provide antipyretics/fever control actions as indicated.
- Weigh daily.
- Avoid activities, such as isometric exercises, rectal stimulation, vomiting, spasmodic coughing, **which may stimulate a Valsalva response.** Administer stool softener as indicated.
- Encourage client to breathe deeply in/out during activities that increase risk of Valsalva effect.
- Alter environment/bed linens **to maintain body temperature in near-normal range.**
- Provide psychologic support. Maintain calm attitude but admit concerns if questioned by the client. **Honesty can be reassuring when so much activity and "worry" are apparent to the client.**
- Provide information about testing procedures and client participation.
- Assist with special procedures as indicated (e.g., invasive line placement, intra-aortic—IA—balloon insertion, pericardiocentesis, cardioversion, pacemaker insertion).
- Explain dietary/fluid restrictions.
- Refer to ND Tissue Perfusion, ineffective.

NURSING PRIORITY NO. 4. To promote venous return:

POSTACUTE/CHRONIC PHASE

- Provide for adequate rest, positioning client for maximum comfort. Administer analgesics as appropriate.
- Encourage relaxation techniques **to reduce anxiety.**
- Elevate legs when in sitting position; apply abdominal binder if indicated, use tilt table as needed **to prevent orthostatic hypotension.**
- Give skin care, provide sheepskin or air/water/gel/foam mattress, and assist with frequent position changes **to avoid the development of pressure sores.**
- Elevate edematous extremities and avoid restrictive clothing. When support hose are used, be sure they are individually fitted and appropriately applied.
- Increase activity levels as permitted by individual condition.

NURSING PRIORITY NO. 5. To maintain adequate nutrition and fluid balance:

- Provide for diet restrictions (e.g., low-sodium, bland, soft, low-calorie/residue/fat diet, with frequent small feedings as indicated).

- Note reports of anorexia/nausea and withhold oral intake as indicated.
- Provide fluids as indicated (may have some restrictions; may need to consider electrolyte replacement/supplementation **to minimize dysrhythmias**).
- Monitor intake/output and calculate 24-hour fluid balance.

NURSING PRIORITY NO. 6. To promote wellness (Teaching/ Discharge Considerations):

- Note individual risk factors present (e.g., smoking, stress, obesity) and specify interventions for reduction of identified factors.
- Review specifics of drug regimen, diet, exercise/activity plan.
- Discuss significant signs/symptoms that need to be reported to healthcare provider (e.g., muscle cramps, headaches, dizziness, skin rashes) **that may be signs of drug toxicity and/or mineral loss, especially potassium.**
- Review "danger" signs requiring immediate physician notification (e.g., unrelieved or increased chest pain, dyspnea, edema).
- Encourage changing positions slowly, dangling legs before standing **to reduce risk of orthostatic hypotension.**
- Give information about positive signs of improvement, such as decreased edema, improved vital signs/circulation **to provide encouragement.**
- Teach home monitoring of weight, pulse, and/or blood pressure as appropriate **to detect change and allow for timely intervention.**
- Promote visits from family/SO(s) who provide positive input.
- Encourage relaxing environment, using relaxation techniques, massage therapy, soothing music, quiet activities.
- Teach stress management techniques as indicated, including appropriate exercise program.
- Identify resources for weight reduction, cessation of smoking, and so forth **to provide support for change.**
- Refer to NDs Activity Intolerance; Diversional Activity, deficient; Coping, ineffective and Coping, family: compromised; Sexual Dysfunction; Pain, acute/chronic; Nutrition, imbalanced; Fluid Volume, deficient/excess, as indicated.

Documentation Focus

ASSESSMENT/REASSESSMENT

- Baseline and subsequent findings and individual hemodynamic parameters, heart and breath sounds, ECG pattern, presence/strength of peripheral pulses, skin/tissue status, renal output, and mentation.

PLANNING

- Plan of care and who is involved in planning.
- Teaching plan.

IMPLEMENTATION/EVALUATION

- Client's responses to interventions/teaching and actions performed.
- Status and disposition at discharge.
- Attainment/progress toward desired outcome(s).
- Modifications to plan of care.

DISCHARGE PLANNING

- Discharge considerations and who will be responsible for carrying out individual actions.
- Long-term needs.
- Specific referrals made.

SAMPLE NURSING OUTCOMES & INTERVENTIONS CLASSIFICATIONS (NOC/NIC)

NOC—Cardiac Pump Effectiveness
NIC—Hemodynamic Regulations

Caregiver Role Strain

Taxonomy II: Role Relationships—Class 1 Caregiving Roles (00061)
[Diagnostic Division: Social Interaction]
Submitted 1992; Nursing Diagnosis Extension and Classification (NDEC) Revision 1998; 2000

Definition: Difficulty in performing caregiver role

Related Factors

CARE RECEIVER HEALTH STATUS

Illness severity/chronicity
Unpredictability of illness course; instability of care receiver's health
Increasing care needs and dependency
Problem behaviors; psychological or cognitive problems
Addiction or codependency of care receiver

CAREGIVING ACTIVITIES

Discharge of family member to home with significant care needs [e.g., premature birth/congenital defect]

Information that appears in brackets has been added by the authors to clarify and enhance the use of nursing diagnoses.

Unpredictability of care situation; 24-hour care responsibility; amount/complexity of activities
Ongoing changes in activities; years of caregiving

CAREGIVER HEALTH STATUS

Physical problems; psychological or cognitive problems
Inability to fulfill one's own or others' expectations; unrealistic expectations of self
Marginal coping patterns
Addiction or codependency

SOCIOECONOMIC

Competing role commitments
Alienation from family, friends, and coworkers; isolation from others
Insufficient recreation

CAREGIVER-CARE RECEIVER RELATIONSHIP

Unrealistic expectations of caregiver by care receiver
History of poor relationship
Mental status of elder inhibits conversation
Presence of abuse or violence

FAMILY PROCESSES

History of marginal family coping/dysfunction

RESOURCES

Inadequate physical environment for providing care (e.g., housing, temperature, safety)
Inadequate equipment for providing care; inadequate transportation
Insufficient finances
Inexperience with caregiving; insufficient time; physical energy; emotional strength; lack of support
Lack of caregiver privacy
Lack of knowledge about or difficulty accessing community resources; inadequate community services (e.g., respite care, recreational resources); assistance and support (formal and informal)
Caregiver is not developmentally ready for caregiver role

[Author's note: The presence of this problem may encompass other numerous problems/high-risk concerns, such as Diversional Activity, deficient; Sleep Pattern, disturbed; Fatigue; Anxiety; Coping, ineffective; Coping, compromised family and Coping, disabled family; Conflict, decisional; Denial, ineffective; Grieving, anticipatory; Hopelessness; Powerlessness; Spiritual Distress; Health Maintenance, ineffective; Home Maintenance, impaired; Sexuality Patterns, ineffective; Coping, readiness for enhanced family; Family Processes, interrupted; Social Isolation. Careful attention to data gathering will identify and clarify the client's specific needs, which can then be coordinated under this single diagnostic label.]

Defining Characteristics

SUBJECTIVE

CAREGIVING ACTIVITIES

Apprehension about possible institutionalization of care receiver, the future regarding care receiver's health and caregiver's ability to provide care, care receiver's care if caregiver becomes ill or dies

CAREGIVER HEALTH STATUS — PHYSICAL

Gastrointestinal (GI) upset (e.g., mild stomach cramps, vomiting, diarrhea, recurrent gastric ulcer episodes)
Weight change, rash, headaches, hypertension, cardiovascular disease, diabetes, fatigue

CAREGIVER HEALTH STATUS — EMOTIONAL

Feeling depressed; anger; stress; frustration; increased nervousness
Disturbed sleep
Lack of time to meet personal needs

CAREGIVER HEALTH STATUS — SOCIOECONOMIC

Changes in leisure activities; refuses career advancement

CAREGIVER-CARE RECEIVER RELATIONSHIP

Difficulty watching care receiver go through the illness
Grief/uncertainty regarding changed relationship with care receiver

FAMILY PROCESSES — CAREGIVING ACTIVITIES

Concern about family members

OBJECTIVE

CAREGIVING ACTIVITIES

Difficulty performing/completing required tasks
Preoccupation with care routine
Dysfunctional change in caregiving activities

CAREGIVER HEALTH STATUS — EMOTIONAL

Impatience; increased emotional lability; somatization
Impaired individual coping

CAREGIVER HEALTH STATUS — SOCIOECONOMIC

Low work productivity; withdraws from social life

FAMILY PROCESSES

Family conflict

Desired Outcomes/Evaluation Criteria — Caregiver Will:

- Identify resources within self to deal with situation.
- Provide opportunity for care receiver to deal with situation in own way.

- Express more realistic understanding and expectations of the care receiver.
- Demonstrate behavior/lifestyle changes to cope with and/or resolve problematic factors.
- Report improved general well-being, ability to deal with situation.

Actions/Interventions

NURSING PRIORITY NO. 1. To assess degree of impaired function:

- Inquire about/observe physical condition of care receiver and surroundings as appropriate.
- Assess caregiver's current state of functioning (e.g., hours of sleep, nutritional intake, personal appearance, demeanor).
- Determine use of prescription/over-the-counter (OTC) drugs, alcohol to deal with situation.
- Identify safety issues concerning caregiver and receiver.
- Assess current actions of caregiver and how they are received by care receiver (e.g., caregiver may be trying to be helpful but is not perceived as helpful; may be too protective or may have unrealistic expectations of care receiver). **May lead to misunderstanding and conflict.**
- Note choice/frequency of social involvement and recreational activities.
- Determine use/effectiveness of resources and support systems.

NURSING PRIORITY NO. 2. To identify the causative/contributing factors relating to the impairment:

- Note presence of high-risk situations (e.g., elderly client with total self-care dependence, or family with several small children with one child requiring extensive assistance due to physical condition/developmental delays). **May necessitate role reversal resulting in added stress or place excessive demands on parenting skills.**
- Determine current knowledge of the situation, noting misconceptions, lack of information. **May interfere with caregiver/care receiver's response to illness/condition.**
- Identify relationship of caregiver to care receiver (e.g., spouse/lover, parent/child, sibling, friend).
- Ascertain proximity of caregiver to care receiver.
- Note physical/mental condition, complexity of therapeutic regimen of care receiver.
- Determine caregiver's level of responsibility, involvement in and anticipated length of care.
- Ascertain developmental level/abilities and additional responsibilities of caregiver.

- Use assessment tool, such as Burden Interview, when appropriate, **to further determine caregiver's abilities.**
- Identify individual cultural factors and impact on caregiver. **Helps clarify expectations of caregiver/receiver, family, and community.**
- Note codependency needs/enabling behaviors of caregiver.
- Determine availability/use of support systems and resources.
- Identify presence/degree of conflict between caregiver/care receiver/family.
- Determine preillness/current behaviors that may be interfering with the care/recovery of the care receiver.

NURSING PRIORITY NO. 3. To assist caregiver to identify feelings and begin to deal with problems:

- Establish a therapeutic relationship, conveying empathy and unconditional positive regard.
- Acknowledge difficulty of the situation for the caregiver/family.
- Discuss caregiver's view of and concerns about situation.
- Encourage caregiver to acknowledge and express feelings. Discuss normalcy of the reactions without using false reassurance.
- Discuss caregiver's/family members' life goals, perceptions and expectations of self **to clarify unrealistic thinking and identify potential areas of flexibility or compromise.**
- Discuss impact of and ability to handle role changes necessitated by situation.

NURSING PRIORITY NO. 4. To enhance caregiver's ability to deal with current situation:

- Identify strengths of caregiver and care receiver.
- Discuss strategies to coordinate caregiving tasks and other responsibilities (e.g., employment, care of children/dependents, housekeeping activities).
- Facilitate family conference **to share information and develop plan for involvement in care activities as appropriate.**
- Identify classes and/or needed specialists (e.g., first aid/CPR classes, enterostomal/physical therapist).
- Determine need for/sources of additional resources (e.g., financial, legal, respite care).
- Provide information and/or demonstrate techniques for dealing with acting out/violent or disoriented behavior. **Enhances safety of caregiver and receiver.**
- Identify equipment needs/resources, adaptive aids **to enhance the independence and safety of the care receiver.**

- Provide contact person/case manager **to coordinate care, provide support, assist with problem solving.**

NURSING PRIORITY NO. 5. To promote wellness (Teaching/ Discharge Considerations):

- Assist caregiver to plan for changes that may be necessary (e.g., home care providers, eventual placement in long-term care facility).
- Discuss/demonstrate stress management techniques and importance of self-nurturing (e.g., pursuing self-development interests, personal needs, hobbies, and social activities).
- Encourage involvement in support group.
- Refer to classes/other therapies as indicated.
- Identify available 12-step program when indicated to provide tools **to deal with enabling/codependent behaviors that impair level of function.**
- Refer to counseling or psychotherapy as needed.
- Provide bibliotherapy of appropriate references **for self-paced learning** and encourage discussion of information.

Documentation Focus

ASSESSMENT/REASSESSMENT

- Assessment findings, functional level/degree of impairment, caregiver's understanding/perception of situation.
- Identified risk factors.

PLANNING

- Plan of care and individual responsibility for specific activities.
- Needed resources, including type and source of assistive devices/durable equipment.
- Teaching plan.

IMPLEMENTATION/EVALUATION

- Caregiver's/receiver's response to interventions/teaching and actions performed.
- Identification of inner resources, behavior/lifestyle changes to be made.
- Attainment/progress toward desired outcome(s).
- Modifications to plan of care.

DISCHARGE PLANNING

- Plan for continuation/follow-through of needed changes.
- Referrals for assistance/evaluation.

SAMPLE NURSING OUTCOMES
& INTERVENTIONS CLASSIFICATIONS (NOC/NIC)

NOC—Caregiver Lifestyle Disruption
NIC—Caregiver Support

Caregiver Role Strain, risk for

Taxonomy II: Role Relationships—Class 1 Caregiving
Roles (00062)
[Diagnostic Division: Social Interaction]
Submitted 1992

Definition: Caregiver is vulnerable for felt difficulty in
performing the family caregiver role

Risk Factors

Illness severity of the care receiver; psychological or cognitive prob-
lems in care receiver; addiction or codependency
Discharge of family member with significant home-care needs; prema-
ture birth/congenital defect
Unpredictable illness course or instability in the care receiver's health
Duration of caregiving required; inexperience with caregiving;
complexity/amount of caregiving tasks; caregiver's competing role
commitments
Caregiver health impairment
Caregiver is female/spouse
Caregiver not developmentally ready for caregiver role (e.g., a young
adult needing to provide care for middle-aged parent); developmental delay or retardation of the care receiver or caregiver
Presence of situational stressors that normally affect families (e.g.,
significant loss, disaster or crisis, economic vulnerability, major life
events [such as birth, hospitalization, leaving home, returning
home, marriage, divorce, change in employment, retirement, death])
Inadequate physical environment for providing care (e.g., housing,
transportation, community services, equipment)
Family/caregiver isolation
Lack of respite and recreation for caregiver
Marginal family adaptation or dysfunction prior to the caregiving situ-
ation
Marginal caregiver's coping patterns
Past history of poor relationship between caregiver and care receiver
Care receiver exhibits deviant, bizarre behavior
Presence of abuse or violence

> NOTE: A risk diagnosis is not evidenced by signs and symptoms, as
> the problem has not occurred and nursing interventions are
> directed at prevention.

Information that appears in brackets has been added by the authors
to clarify and enhance the use of nursing diagnoses.

Desired Outcomes/Evaluation Criteria—Caregiver Will:

- Identify individual risk factors and appropriate interventions.
- Demonstrate/initiate behaviors or lifestyle changes to prevent development of impaired function.
- Use available resources appropriately.
- Report satisfaction with current situation.

Actions/Interventions

NURSING PRIORITY NO. 1. To assess factors affecting current situation:

- Note presence of high-risk situations (e.g., elderly client with total self-care dependence or several small children with one child requiring extensive assistance due to physical condition/developmental delays). **May necessitate role reversal resulting in added stress or place excessive demands on parenting skills.**
- Identify relationship and proximity of caregiver to care receiver (e.g., spouse/lover, parent/child, friend).
- Note therapeutic regimen and physical/mental condition of care receiver.
- Determine caregiver's level of responsibility, involvement in and anticipated length of care.
- Ascertain developmental level/abilities and additional responsibilities of caregiver.
- Use assessment tool, such as Burden Interview, when appropriate, **to further determine caregiver's abilities.**
- Identify strengths/weaknesses of caregiver and care receiver.
- Verify safety of caregiver/receiver.
- Discuss caregiver's and care receiver's view of and concerns about situation.
- Determine available supports and resources currently used.
- Note any codependency needs of caregiver.

NURSING PRIORITY NO. 2. To enhance caregiver's ability to deal with current situation:

- Discuss strategies to coordinate care and other responsibilities (e.g., employment, care of children/dependents, housekeeping activities).
- Facilitate family conference as appropriate **to share information and develop plan for involvement in care activities.**
- Refer to classes and/or specialists (e.g., first aid/CPR classes, enterostomal/physical therapist) **for special training as indicated.**

- Identify additional resources to include financial, legal, respite care.
- Identify equipment needs/resources, adaptive aids **to enhance the independence and safety of the care receiver.**
- Identify contact person/case manager as needed **to coordinate care, provide support, and assist with problem solving.**
- Provide information and/or demonstrate techniques for dealing with acting out/violent or disoriented behavior.
- Assist caregiver to recognize codependent behaviors (i.e., doing things for others that others are able to do for themselves) and how these behaviors affect the situation.

NURSING PRIORITY NO. 3. To promote wellness (Teaching/Discharge Considerations):

- Stress importance of self-nurturing (e.g., pursuing self-development interests, personal needs, hobbies, and social activities) **to improve/maintain quality of life for caregiver.**
- Discuss/demonstrate stress-management techniques.
- Encourage involvement in specific support group(s).
- Provide bibliotherapy of appropriate references and encourage discussion of information.
- Assist caregiver to plan for changes that may become necessary for the care receiver (e.g., home care providers, eventual placement in long-term care facility).
- Refer to classes/therapists as indicated.
- Identify available 12-step program when indicated **to provide tools to deal with codependent behaviors that impair level of function.**
- Refer to counseling or psychotherapy as needed.

Documentation Focus

ASSESSMENT/REASSESSMENT

- Identified risk factors and caregiver perceptions of situation.
- Reactions of care receiver/family.

PLANNING

- Treatment plan and individual responsibility for specific activities.
- Teaching plan.

IMPLEMENTATION/EVALUATION

- Caregiver/receiver response to interventions/teaching and actions performed.
- Attainment/progress toward desired outcome(s).
- Modifications to plan of care.

- Long-term needs and who is responsible for actions to be taken.
- Specific referrals provided for assistance/evaluation.

SAMPLE NURSING OUTCOMES & INTERVENTIONS CLASSIFICATIONS (NOC/NIC)

NOC—Caregiving Endurance Potential
NIC—Caregiver Support

Communication, impaired verbal

Taxonomy II: Perception/Cognition—Class 5 Communication (00051)
[Diagnostic Division: Social Interaction]
Submitted 1983; Revised 1998 (by small group work 1996)

Definition: Decreased, delayed, or absent ability to receive, process, transmit, and use a system of symbols

Related Factors

Decrease in circulation to brain, brain tumor
Anatomic deficit (e.g., cleft palate, alteration of the neurovascular visual system, auditory system, or phonatory apparatus)
Difference related to developmental age
Physical barrier (tracheostomy, intubation)
Physiological conditions [e.g., dyspnea]; alteration of central nervous system (CNS); weakening of the musculoskeletal system
Psychological barriers (e.g., psychosis, lack of stimuli); emotional conditions [depression, panic, anger]; stress
Environmental barriers
Cultural difference
Lack of information
Side effects of medication
Alteration of self-esteem or self-concept
Altered perceptions
Absence of SOs

Defining Characteristics

SUBJECTIVE

[Reports of difficulty expressing self]

OBJECTIVE

Unable to speak dominant language
Speaks or verbalizes with difficulty

Information that appears in brackets has been added by the authors to clarify and enhance the use of nursing diagnoses.

Does not or cannot speak
Disorientation in the three spheres of time, space, person
Stuttering; slurring
Dyspnea
Difficulty forming words or sentences (e.g., aphonia, dyslalia, dysarthria)
Difficulty expressing thoughts verbally (e.g., aphasia, dysphasia, apraxia, dyslexia)
Inappropriate verbalization, [incessant, loose association of ideas; flight of ideas]
Difficulty in comprehending and maintaining the usual communicating pattern
Absence of eye contact or difficulty in selective attending; partial or total visual deficit
Inability or difficulty in use of facial or body expressions
Willful refusal to speak
[Inability to modulate speech]
[Message inappropriate to content]
[Use of nonverbal cues (e.g., pleading eyes, gestures, turning away)]
[Frustration, anger, hostility]

Desired Outcomes/Evaluation Criteria—Client Will:

- Verbalize or indicate an understanding of the communication difficulty and plans for ways of handling.
- Establish method of communication in which needs can be expressed.
- Participate in therapeutic communication (e.g., using silence, acceptance, restating reflecting, Active-listening, and I-messages).
- Demonstrate congruent verbal and nonverbal communication.
- Use resources appropriately.

Actions/Interventions

NURSING PRIORITY NO. 1. To assess causative/contributing factors:

- Review history for neurologic conditions **that could affect speech, such as CVA, tumor, multiple sclerosis, hearing loss, and so forth.** Note results of neurologic testing such as electroencephalogram (EEG), computed tomography (CT) scan.
- Note whether aphasia is motor (expressive: loss of images for articulated speech), sensory (receptive: unable to understand words and does not recognize the defect), conduction (slow comprehension, uses words inappropriately but knows the error), and/or global (total loss of ability to comprehend and speak). Evaluate the degree of impairment.
- Evaluate mental status, note presence of psychotic conditions

(e.g., manic-depressive, schizoid/affective behavior). Assess psychologic response to communication impairment, willingness to find alternate means of communication.

- Note presence of ET tube/tracheostomy or other physical blocks to speech (e.g., cleft palate, jaws wired).
- Assess environmental factors that may affect ability to communicate (e.g., room noise level).
- Determine primary language spoken and cultural factors.
- Assess style of speech (as outlined in Defining Characteristics).
- Note level of anxiety present; presence of angry, hostile behavior; frustration.
- Interview parent to determine child's developmental level of speech and language comprehension.
- Note parent's speech patterns and manner of communicating with child, including gestures.

NURSING PRIORITY NO. 2. To assist client to establish a means of communication to express needs, wants, ideas, and questions:

- Determine ability to read/write. Evaluate musculoskeletal states, including manual dexterity (e.g., ability to hold a pen and write).
- Obtain a translator/written translation or picture chart **when writing is not possible.**
- Facilitate hearing and vision examinations/obtaining necessary aids **when needed/desired for improving communication.** Assist client to learn to use and adjust to aids.
- Establish relationship with the client, listening carefully and attending to client's verbal/nonverbal expressions.
- Maintain eye contact, preferably at client's level. Be aware of cultural factors that may preclude eye contact (e.g., some Native-Americans).
- Keep communication simple, using all modes for accessing information: visual, auditory, and kinesthetic.
- Maintain a calm, unhurried manner. Provide sufficient time for client to respond. **Individuals with expressive aphasia may talk more easily when they are rested and relaxed and when they are talking to one person at a time.**
- Determine meaning of words used by the client and congruency of communication and nonverbal messages.
- Validate meaning of nonverbal communication; do not make assumptions, **because they may be wrong.** Be honest; if you do not understand, seek assistance from others.
- Individualize techniques using breathing for relaxation of the vocal cords, rote tasks (such as counting), and singing or melodic intonation to assist aphasic clients relearn speech.
- Anticipate needs until effective communication is reestablished.

Communication, impaired verbal

- Plan for alternative methods of communication (e.g., slate board, letter/picture board, hand/eye signals, typewriter/ computer) incorporating information about type of disability present.
- Identify previous solutions tried/used if situation is chronic or recurrent.
- Provide reality orientation by responding with simple, straightforward, honest statements.
- Provide environmental stimuli as needed **to maintain contact with reality;** or reduce stimuli **to lessen anxiety that may worsen problem.**
- Use confrontation skills, when appropriate, within an established nurse-client relationship **to clarify discrepancies between verbal and nonverbal cues.**

NURSING PRIORITY NO. 3. To promote wellness (Teaching/ Discharge Considerations):

- Review information about condition, prognosis, and treatment with client/SO(s). Reinforce that loss of speech does not imply loss of intelligence.
- Discuss individual methods of dealing with impairment.
- Recommend placing a tape recorder with a prerecorded emergency message near the telephone. Information to include: client's name, address, telephone number, type of airway, and that emergency assistance is immediately required.
- Use and assist client/SO(s) to learn therapeutic communication skills of acknowledgment, Active-listening, and I-messages. **Improves general communication skills.**
- Involve family/SO(s) in plan of care as much as possible. **Enhances participation and commitment to plan.**
- Refer to appropriate resources (e.g., speech therapist, group therapy, individual/family and/or psychiatric counseling).
- Refer to NDs Coping, ineffective; Coping, family: disabled (as indicated); Anxiety; Fear.

Documentation Focus

ASSESSMENT/REASSESSMENT

- Assessment findings/pertinent history information (i.e., physical/psychological/cultural concerns).
- Meaning of nonverbal cues, level of anxiety client exhibits.

PLANNING

- Plan of care and interventions (e.g., type of alternative communication/translator).
- Teaching plan.

IMPLEMENTATION/EVALUATION

- Response to interventions/teaching and actions performed.
- Attainment/progress toward desired outcome(s).
- Modifications to plan of care.

DISCHARGE PLANNING

- Discharge needs/referrals made, additional resources available.

SAMPLE NURSING OUTCOMES & INTERVENTIONS CLASSIFICATIONS (NOC/NIC)

NOC—Communication Ability
NIC—Communication Enhancement: Speech Deficit

Communication, readiness for enhanced

Taxonomy II: Perception/Cognition—Class 4 Cognition (00161)
[Diagnostic Division: Teaching/Learning]
Submitted 2002

Definition: A pattern of exchanging information and ideas with others that is sufficient for meeting one's needs and life goals and can be strengthened

Related Factors

To be developed

Defining Characteristics

SUBJECTIVE

Expresses willingness to enhance communication
Expresses thoughts and feelings
Expresses satisfaction with ability to share information and ideas with others

OBJECTIVE

Able to speak or write a language
Forms words, phrases, and language
Uses and interprets nonverbal cues appropriately

Desired Outcomes/Evaluation Criteria: Client/SO/Caregiver Will:

- Verbalize or indicate an understanding of the communication difficulty and ways of handling.

Information that appears in brackets has been added by the authors to clarify and enhance the use of nursing diagnoses.

- Be able to express information, thoughts, and feelings in a satisfactory manner.

Actions/Interventions

NURSING PRIORITY NO **1.** To assess how client is managing communication and potential difficulties:

- Ascertain circumstances that result in client's desire to improve communication. **Many factors are involved in communication, and identifying specific needs/expectations help in developing realistic goals and determining likelihood of success.**
- Evaluate mental status. **Disorientation and psychotic conditions may be affecting speech and the communication of thoughts, needs, and desires.**
- Determine client's developmental level of speech and language comprehension. **Provides baseline information for developing plan for improvement.**
- Determine ability to read/write. **Evaluating grasp of language as well as musculoskeletal states, including manual dexterity (e.g., ability to hold a pen and write), provides information about nature of client's situation. Educational plan can address language skills. Neuromuscular deficits will require individual program to correct.**
- Determine country of origin, dominant language, whether client is recent immigrant and what cultural, ethnic group client identifies as own. **Recent immigrant may identify with home country, and its people, language, beliefs, and health-care practices affecting desire to learn language and improve ability to interact in new country.**
- Ascertain if interpreter is needed/desired. **Law mandates that interpretation services be made available. Trained, professional interpreter who translates precisely and possesses a basic understanding of medical terminology and healthcare ethics is preferred to enhance client and provider satisfaction.**
- Determine comfort level in expression of feelings and concepts in nonproficient language. **Anxiety about language difficulty can interfere with ability to communicate effectively.**
- Note any physical barriers to effective communication (e.g., talking tracheostomy, wired jaws) or physiologic/neurologic conditions (e.g., severe shortness of breath, neuromuscular weakness, stroke, brain trauma, hearing impairment, cleft palate, facial trauma). **Client may be dealing with speech/language comprehension or have voice production problems (pitch, loudness, or quality), which call attention to voice rather than what speaker is saying. These barriers will**

need to be addressed to enable client to improve communication skills.

- Clarify meaning of words used by the client to describe important aspects of life and health/well-being (e.g., pain, sorrow, anxiety). **Words can easily be misinterpreted when sender and receiver have different ideas about their meanings. This can affect the way both client and caregiver communicate important concepts. Restating what one has heard can clarify whether an expressed statement has been understood or misinterpreted.**
- Evaluate level of anxiety, frustration, or fear; presence of angry, hostile behavior. **Emotional/psychiatric issues can affect communication and interfere with understanding.**
- Evaluate congruency of verbal and nonverbal messages. **It is estimated that 65% to 95% of communication is nonverbal, and communication is enhanced when verbal and nonverbal messages are congruent.**
- Determine lack of knowledge or misunderstanding of terms related to client's specific situation. **Indicators of need for additional information, clarification to help client improve ability to communicate.**
- Evaluate need/desire for pictures or written communications and instructions as part of treatment plan. **Alternative methods of communication can help client feel understood and promote feelings of satisfaction with interaction.**

NURSING PRIORITY NO. 2. To improve client's ability to communicate thoughts, needs, and ideas:

- Maintain a calm, unhurried manner. Provide sufficient time for client to respond. **An atmosphere in which client is free to speak without fear of criticism provides the opportunity to explore all the issues involved in making decisions to improve communication skills.**
- Pay attention to speaker. Be an active listener. **The use of Active-listening communicates acceptance and respect for the client, establishing trust and promoting openness and honest expression. It communicates a belief that the client is a capable and competent person.**
- Sit down, maintain eye contact, preferably at client's level, and spend time with the client. **Conveys message that the nurse has time and interest in communicating.**
- Observe body language, eye movements, and behavioral clues. **May reveal unspoken concerns, for example, when pain is present, client may react with tears, grimacing, stiff posture, turning away, and angry outbursts.**
- Help client identify and learn to avoid use of nontherapeutic communication. **These barriers are recognized as detriments to open communication and learning to avoid them**

maximizes the effectiveness of communication between client and others.

- Establish hand/eye signals if indicated. Neurologic impairments may allow client to understand language but not be able to speak and/or may have a physical barrier to writing.
- Obtain interpreter with language or signing abilities as needed. May be needed to enhance understanding of words, language concepts, or needs to promote accurate interpretation of communication.
- Provide pad and pencil, slate board, letter/picture board, if indicated. When client has physical impairments that interfere with spoken communication, alternate means can provide concepts that are understandable to both parties.
- Obtain/provide access to typewriter/computer. Use of these devices may be more helpful when impairment is long-standing or when client is used to using them.
- Respect client's cultural communication needs. Different cultures can dictate beliefs of what is normal or abnormal (i.e., in some cultures, eye-to-eye contact is considered disrespectful, impolite, or an invasion of privacy; silence and tone of voice has various meanings, and slang words can cause confusion).
- Provide glasses, hearing aids, dentures, electronic speech devices as needed. These devices maximize sensory perception and can improve understanding and enhance speech patterns.
- Reduce distractions and background noises (e.g., close the door, turn down the radio/TV). A distracting environment can interfere with communication, limiting attention to tasks and making speech and communication more difficult. Reducing noise can help both parties hear clearly, improving understanding.
- Associate words with objects using repetition and redundancy, point to objects, or demonstrate desired actions. Speaker's own body language can be used to enhance client's understanding when neurologic conditions result in difficulty understanding language.
- Use confrontation skills carefully when appropriate, within an established nurse-client relationship. Can be used to clarify discrepancies between verbal and nonverbal cues, enabling client to look at areas that may require change.

NURSING PRIORITY NO. 3. To promote optimum communication:

- Discuss with family/SO and other caregivers effective ways in which the client communicates. **Identifying positive aspects of current communication skills enables family members to learn and move forward in desire to enhance ways of interacting.**

- Encourage client and family use of successful techniques for communication, whether it is speech/language techniques or alternate modes of communicating. **Enhances family relationships and promotes self-esteem for all members as they are able to communicate clearly regardless of the problems which have interfered with ability to interact.**
- Reinforce client/SO(s) learning and use of therapeutic communication skills of acknowledgment, Active-listening, and I-messages. **Improves general communication skills, emphasizes acceptance, and conveys respect enabling family relationships to improve.**
- Refer to appropriate resources (e.g., speech therapist, language classes, individual/family and/or psychiatric counseling). **May need further assistance to overcome problems that are preventing family from reaching desired goal of enhanced communication.**

Documentation Focus

ASSESSMENT/REASSESSMENT

- Assessment findings/pertinent history information (i.e., physical/psychologic/cultural concerns).
- Meaning of nonverbal cues, level of anxiety client exhibits.

PLANNING

- Plan of care and interventions (e.g., type of alternative communication/translator).
- Teaching plan.

IMPLEMENTATION/EVALUATION

- Progress toward desired outcome(s).
- Modifications to plan of care.

DISCHARGE PLANNING

- Discharge needs/referrals made, additional resources available.

SAMPLE NURSING OUTCOMES & INTERVENTIONS CLASSIFICATIONS (NOC/NIC)

NOC—Communication Ability
NIC—Communication Enhancement [specify]

Conflict, decisional (specify)

Taxonomy II: Life Principles—Class 3 Value/Belief/Action
Congruence (00083)
[Diagnostic Division: Ego Integrity]
Submitted 1988

Definition: Uncertainty about course of action to be
taken when choice among competing actions involves
risk, loss, or challenge to personal life values

Related Factors

Unclear personal values/beliefs; perceived threat to value system
Lack of experience or interference with decision making
Lack of relevant information, multiple or divergent sources of infor-
    mation
Support system deficit
[Age, developmental state]
[Family system, sociocultural factors]
[Cognitive, emotional, behavioral level of functioning]

Defining Characteristics

SUBJECTIVE

Verbalized uncertainty about choices or of undesired consequences of
    alternative actions being considered
Verbalized feeling of distress or questioning personal values and beliefs
    while attempting a decision

OBJECTIVE

Vacillation between alternative choices; delayed decision making
Self-focusing
Physical signs of distress or tension (increased heart rate; increased
    muscle tension; restlessness; etc.)

Desired Outcomes/Evaluation
Criteria—Client Will:

- Verbalize awareness of positive and negative aspects of
  choices/alternative actions.
- Acknowledge/ventilate feelings of anxiety and distress associated with choice/related to making difficult decision.
- Identify personal values and beliefs concerning issues.
- Make decision(s) and express satisfaction with choices.
- Meet psychologic needs as evidenced by appropriate expression of feelings, identification of options, and use of
  resources.
- Display relaxed manner/calm demeanor, free of physical signs
  of distress.

Information that appears in brackets has been added by the authors
to clarify and enhance the use of nursing diagnoses.

Actions/Interventions

NURSING PRIORITY NO. **1.** To assess causative/contributing factors:

- Determine usual ability to manage own affairs. Clarify who has legal right to intervene on behalf of child (e.g., parent, other relative, or court appointed guardian/advocate). (**Family disruption/conflicts can complicate decision process.**)
- Note expressions of indecision, dependence on others, availability/involvement of support persons (e.g., lack of/conflicting advice). Ascertain dependency of other(s) on client and/or issues of codependency.
- Active-listen/identify reason for indecisiveness **to help client to clarify problem.**
- Determine effectiveness of current problem-solving techniques.
- Note presence/intensity of physical signs of anxiety (e.g., increased heart rate, muscle tension).
- Listen for expressions of inability to find meaning in life/reason for living, feelings of futility, or alienation from God and others around them. (Refer to ND Spiritual Distress as indicated.)

NURSING PRIORITY NO. **2.** To assist client to develop/effectively use problem-solving skills:

- Promote safe and hopeful environment, as needed, while client regains inner control.
- Encourage verbalization of conflicts/concerns.
- Accept verbal expressions of anger/guilt, setting limits on maladaptive behavior **to promote client safety.**
- Clarify and prioritize individual goals, noting where the subject of the "conflict" falls on this scale.
- Identify strengths and presence of positive coping skills (e.g., use of relaxation technique, willingness to express feelings).
- Identify positive aspects of this experience and assist client to view it as a learning opportunity **to develop new and creative solutions.**
- Correct misperceptions client may have and provide factual information. **Provides for better decision making.**
- Provide opportunities for client to make simple decisions regarding self-care and other daily activities. Accept choice not to do so. Advance complexity of choices as tolerated.
- Encourage child to make developmentally appropriate decisions concerning own care. **Fosters child's sense of self-worth, enhances ability to learn/exercise coping skills.**

- Discuss time considerations, setting time line for small steps and considering consequences related to not making/postponing specific decisions **to facilitate resolution of conflict.**
- Have client list some alternatives to present situation or decisions, using a brainstorming process. Include family in this activity as indicated (e.g., placement of parent in long-term care facility, use of intervention process with addicted member). Refer to NDs Family Processes, interrupted; Family Processes, dysfunctional: alcoholism; Coping, family: compromised.
- Practice use of problem-solving process with current situation/decision.
- Discuss/clarify spiritual concerns, accepting client's values in a nonjudgmental manner.

NURSING PRIORITY NO. **3.** To promote wellness (Teaching/Discharge Considerations):

- Promote opportunities for using conflict-resolution skills, identifying steps as client does each one.
- Provide positive feedback for efforts and progress noted. **Promotes continuation of efforts.**
- Encourage involvement of family/SO(s) as desired/available to provide support for the client.
- Support client for decisions made, especially if consequences are unexpected, difficult to cope with.
- Encourage attendance at stress reduction, assertiveness classes.
- Refer to other resources as necessary (e.g., clergy, psychiatric clinical nurse specialist/psychiatrist, family/marital therapist, addiction support groups).

Documentation Focus

ASSESSMENT/REASSESSMENT

- Assessment findings/behavioral responses, degree of impairment in lifestyle functioning.
- Individuals involved in the conflict.
- Personal values/beliefs.

PLANNING

- Plan of care/interventions and who is involved in the planning process.
- Teaching plan.

IMPLEMENTATION/EVALUATION

- Client's and involved individual's responses to interventions/teaching and actions performed.

- Ability to express feelings, identify options; use of resources.
- Attainment/progress toward desired outcome(s).
- Modifications to plan of care.

DISCHARGE PLANNING

- Long-term needs/referrals, actions to be taken, and who is responsible for doing.
- Specific referrals made.

SAMPLE NURSING OUTCOMES & INTERVENTIONS CLASSIFICATIONS (NOC/NIC)

NOC—Decision Making
NIC—Decision-Making Support

Confusion, acute

Taxonomy II: Perception/Cognition—Class 4 Cognition (00128)
[Diagnostic Division: Neurosensory]
Submitted 1994

Definition: Abrupt onset of a cluster of global, transient changes and disturbances in attention, cognition, psychomotor activity, level of consciousness, and/or sleep/wake cycle

Related Factors

Over 60 years of age
Dementia
Alcohol abuse, drug abuse
Delirium [including febrile epilepticum (following or instead of an epileptic attack), toxic and traumatic]
[Medication reaction/interaction; anesthesia/surgery; metabolic imbalances]
[Exacerbation of a chronic illness, hypoxemia]
[Severe pain]
[Sleep deprivation]

Defining Characteristics

SUBJECTIVE

Hallucinations [visual/auditory]
[Exaggerated emotional responses]

OBJECTIVE

Fluctuation in cognition
Fluctuation in sleep/wake cycle
Fluctuation in level of consciousness

Information that appears in brackets has been added by the authors to clarify and enhance the use of nursing diagnoses.

Fluctuation in psychomotor activity [tremors, body movement]

Increased agitation or restlessness

Misperceptions, [inappropriate responses]

Lack of motivation to initiate and/or follow through with goal-directed or purposeful behavior

Desired Outcomes/Evaluation Criteria—Client Will:

- Regain/maintain usual reality orientation and level of consciousness.
- Verbalize understanding of causative factors when known.
- Initiate lifestyle/behavior changes to prevent or minimize recurrence of problem.

Actions/Interventions

NURSING PRIORITY NO. 1. To assess causative/contributing factors:

- Identify factors present, including substance abuse, seizure history, recent ETC therapy, episodes of fever/pain, presence of acute infection (especially urinary tract infection in elderly client), exposure to toxic substances, traumatic events; change in environment, including unfamiliar noises, excessive visitors.
- Investigate possibility of drug withdrawal, exacerbation of psychiatric conditions (e.g., mood disorder, dissociative disorders, dementia).
- Evaluate vital signs **for signs of poor tissue perfusion (i.e., hypotension, tachycardia, tachypnea).**
- Determine current medications/drug use—especially anti-anxiety agents, barbiturates, lithium, methyldopa, disulfiram, cocaine, alcohol, amphetamines, hallucinogens, opiates (associated with high risk of confusion)—and schedule of use **as combinations increase risk of adverse reactions/interactions (e.g., cimetidine + antacid, digoxin + diuretics, antacid + propranolol).**
- Assess diet/nutritional status.
- Note presence of anxiety, fear, other physiologic reactions.
- Monitor laboratory values, noting hypoxemia, electrolyte imbalances, BUN/Cr, ammonia levels, serum glucose, signs of infection, and drug levels (including peak/trough as appropriate).
- Evaluate sleep/rest status, noting deprivation/oversleeping. Refer to ND Sleep Pattern, disturbed as appropriate.

NURSING PRIORITY NO. 2. To determine degree of impairment:

- Talk with SO(s) **to determine historic baseline, observed changes, and onset/recurrence of changes.**
- Evaluate extent of impairment in orientation, attention span,

ability to follow directions, send/receive communication, appropriateness of response.

- Note occurrence/timing of agitation, hallucinations, violent behaviors. (**"Sundown syndrome" may occur, with client oriented during daylight hours but confused during night.**)
- Determine threat to safety of client/others.

NURSING PRIORITY NO. 3. To maximize level of function, prevent further deterioration:

- Assist with treatment of underlying problem (e.g., drug intoxication/substance abuse, infectious process, hypoxemia, biochemical imbalances, nutritional deficits, pain management).
- Monitor/adjust medication regimen and note response. Eliminate nonessential drugs as appropriate.
- Orient client to surroundings, staff, necessary activities as needed. Present reality concisely and briefly. Avoid challenging illogical thinking—**defensive reactions may result.**
- Encourage family/SO(s) to participate in reorientation as well as providing ongoing input (e.g., current news and family happenings).
- Maintain calm environment and eliminate extraneous noise/**stimuli to prevent overstimulation.** Provide normal levels of essential sensory/tactile stimulation—include personal items/pictures, and so on.
- Encourage client to use vision/hearing aids when needed.
- Give simple directions. Allow sufficient time for client to respond, to communicate, to make decisions.
- Provide for safety needs (e.g., supervision, siderails, seizure precautions, placing call bell within reach, positioning needed items within reach/clearing traffic paths, ambulating with devices).
- Note behavior that may be indicative of potential for violence and take appropriate actions.
- Administer psychotropics cautiously **to control restlessness, agitation, hallucinations.**
- Avoid/limit use of restraints—**may worsen situation, increase likelihood of untoward complications.**
- Provide undisturbed rest periods. Administer short-acting, nonbenzodiazepine sleeping medication (e.g., Benadryl) at bedtime.

NURSING PRIORITY NO. 4. To promote wellness (Teaching/ Discharge Considerations):

- Explain reason for confusion, if known.
- Review drug regimen.
- Assist in identifying ongoing treatment needs.
- Stress importance of keeping vision/hearing aids in good

repair and necessity of periodic evaluation **to identify changing client needs.**

- Discuss situation with family and involve in planning **to meet identified needs.**
- Provide appropriate referrals (e.g., cognitive retraining, substance abuse support groups, medication monitoring program, Meals on Wheels, home health, and adult day care).

Documentation Focus

ASSESSMENT/REASSESSMENT

- Nature, duration, frequency of problem.
- Current and previous level of function, effect on independence/lifestyle (including safety concerns).

PLANNING

- Plan of care and who is involved in planning.
- Teaching plan.

IMPLEMENTATION/EVALUATION

- Response to interventions and actions performed.
- Attainment/progress toward desired outcomes.
- Modifications to plan of care.

DISCHARGE PLANNING

- Long-term needs and who is responsible for actions to be taken.
- Available resources and specific referrals.

SAMPLE NURSING OUTCOMES & INTERVENTIONS CLASSIFICATIONS (NOC/NIC)

NOC—Cognitive Ability
NIC—Delirium Management

Confusion, chronic

Taxonomy II: Perception/Cognition—Class 4 Cognition (00129)
[Diagnostic Division: Neurosensory]
Submitted 1994

Definition: Irreversible, long-standing, and/or progressive deterioration of intellect and personality characterized by decreased ability to interpret environmental stimuli; decreased capacity for intellectual thought processes; and manifested by disturbances of memory, orientation, and behavior

Information that appears in brackets has been added by the authors to clarify and enhance the use of nursing diagnoses.

Related Factors

Alzheimer's disease [dementia of the Alzheimer's type]
Korsakoff's psychosis
Multi-infarct dementia
Cerebral vascular accident
Head injury

Defining Characteristics

OBJECTIVE

Clinical evidence of organic impairment
Altered interpretation/response to stimuli
Progressive/long-standing cognitive impairment
No change in level of consciousness
Impaired socialization
Impaired memory (short-term, long-term)
Altered personality

Desired Outcome/Evaluation Criteria—Client Will:

• Remain safe and free from harm.

Family/SO Will:

• Verbalize understanding of disease process/prognosis and client's needs.
• Identify/participate in interventions to deal effectively with situation.
• Provide for maximal independence while meeting safety needs of client.

Actions/Interventions

NURSING PRIORITY NO. 1. To assess degree of impairment:

• Evaluate responses on diagnostic examinations (e.g., memory impairments, reality orientation, attention span, calculations).
• Test ability to receive and send effective communication.
• Note deterioration/changes in personal hygiene or behavior.
• Talk with SO(s) regarding baseline behaviors, length of time since onset/progression of problem, their perception of prognosis, and other pertinent information and concerns for client.
• Evaluate response to care providers/receptiveness to interventions.
• Determine anxiety level in relation to situation. Note behavior that may be indicative of potential for violence.

NURSING PRIORITY NO. 2. To prevent further deterioration/ maximize level of function:

- Provide calm environment, eliminate extraneous noise/ stimuli.
- Ascertain interventions previously used/tried and evaluate effectiveness.
- Avoid challenging illogical thinking **because defensive reactions may result.**
- Encourage family/SO(s) to provide ongoing orientation/ input to include current news and family happenings.
- Maintain reality-oriented relationship/environment (e.g., clocks, calendars, personal items, seasonal decorations). Encourage participation in resocialization groups.
- Allow client to reminisce, exist in own reality if not detrimental to well-being.
- Provide safety measures (e.g., close supervision, identification bracelet, medication lockup, lower temperature on hot water tank).

NURSING PRIORITY NO. 3. To assist SO(s) to develop coping strategies:

- Determine family resources, availability and willingness to participate in meeting client's needs.
- Identify appropriate community resources (e.g., Alzheimer's or brain injury support group, respite care) **to provide support and assist with problem solving.**
- Evaluate attention to own needs, including grieving process.
- Refer to ND Caregiver Role Strain, risk for.

NURSING PRIORITY NO. 4. To promote wellness (Teaching/ Discharge Considerations):

- Determine ongoing treatment needs and appropriate resources.
- Develop plan of care with family **to meet client's and SO's individual needs.**
- Provide appropriate referrals (e.g., Meals on Wheels, adult day care, home care agency, respite care).

Documentation Focus

ASSESSMENT/REASSESSMENT

- Individual findings, including current level of function and rate of anticipated changes.

PLANNING

- Plan of care and who is involved in planning.

IMPLEMENTATION/EVALUATION

- Response to interventions and actions performed.
- Attainment/progress toward desired outcomes.
- Modifications to plan of care.

DISCHARGE PLANNING

- Long-term needs/referrals and who is responsible for actions to be taken.
- Available resources, specific referrals made.

SAMPLE NURSING OUTCOMES & INTERVENTIONS CLASSIFICATIONS (NOC/NIC)

NOC—Cognitive Ability
NIC—Dementia Management

Constipation

Taxonomy II: Elimination—Class 2 Gastrointestinal
System (00011)
[Diagnostic Division: Elimination]
Submitted 1975; Nursing Diagnosis Extension and
Classification (NDEC) Revision 1998

Definition: Decrease in normal frequency of defecation
accompanied by difficult or incomplete passage of stool
and/or passage of excessively hard, dry stool

Related Factors

FUNCTIONALS

Irregular defecation habits; inadequate toileting (e.g., timeliness, positioning for defecation, privacy)
Insufficient physical activity; abdominal muscle weakness
Recent environmental changes
Habitual denial/ignoring of urge to defecate

PSYCHOLOGICAL

Emotional stress; depression; mental confusion

PHARMACOLOGICAL

Antilipemic agents; laxative overdose; calcium carbonate; aluminum-containing antacids; nonsteroidal anti-inflammatory agents; opiates; anticholinergics; diuretics; iron salts; phenothiazides; sedatives; sympathomimetics; bismuth salts; antidepressants; calcium channel blockers

---

Information that appears in brackets has been added by the authors to clarify and enhance the use of nursing diagnoses.

MECHANICAL

Hemorrhoids; pregnancy; obesity

Rectal abscess or ulcer, anal fissures, prolapse; anal strictures; rectocele

Prostate enlargement; postsurgical obstruction

Neurological impairment; megacolon (Hirschsprung's disease); tumors

Electrolyte imbalance

PHYSIOLOGICAL

Poor eating habits; change in usual foods and eating patterns; insufficient fiber intake; insufficient fluid intake, dehydration

Inadequate dentition or oral hygiene

Decreased motility of gastrointestinal tract

Defining Characteristics

SUBJECTIVE

Change in bowel pattern; unable to pass stool; decreased frequency; decreased volume of stool

Change in usual foods and eating patterns; increased abdominal pressure; feeling of rectal fullness or pressure

Abdominal pain; pain with defecation; nausea and/or vomiting; headache; indigestion; generalized fatigue

OBJECTIVE

Dry, hard, formed stool

Straining with defecation

Hypoactive or hyperactive bowel sounds; change in abdominal growling (borborygmi)

Distended abdomen; abdominal tenderness with or without palpable muscle resistance

Percussed abdominal dullness

Presence of soft pastelike stool in rectum; oozing liquid stool; bright red blood with stool; dark or black or tarry stool

Severe flatus; anorexia

Atypical presentations in older adults (e.g., change in mental status, urinary incontinence, unexplained falls, elevated body temperature)

Desired Outcomes/Evaluation Criteria—Client Will:

- Establish/regain normal pattern of bowel functioning.
- Verbalize understanding of etiology and appropriate interventions/solutions for individual situation.
- Demonstrate behaviors or lifestyle changes to prevent recurrence of problem.
- Participate in bowel program as indicated.

Actions/Interventions

NURSING PRIORITY NO. 1. To identify causative/contributing factors:

- Review daily dietary regimen. Note oral/dental health **that can impact intake.**
- Determine fluid intake, **to note deficits.**
- Evaluate medication/drug usage and note interactions or side effects (e.g., narcotics, antacids, chemotherapy, iron, contrast media such as barium, steroids).
- Note energy/activity level and exercise pattern.
- Identify areas of stress (e.g., personal relationships, occupational factors, financial problems).
- Determine access to bathroom, privacy, and ability to perform self-care activities.
- Investigate reports of pain with defecation. Inspect perianal area for hemorrhoids, fissures, skin breakdown, or other abnormal findings.
- Discuss laxative/enema use. Note signs/reports of laxative abuse.
- Review medical/surgical history (e.g., metabolic or endocrine disorders, pregnancy, prior surgery, megacolon).
- Palpate abdomen **for presence of distention, masses.**
- Check for presence of fecal impaction as indicated.
- Assist with medical workup **for identification of other possible causative factors.**

NURSING PRIORITY NO. 2. To determine usual pattern of elimination:

- Discuss usual elimination pattern and problem.
- Note factors that usually stimulate bowel activity and any interferences present.

NURSING PRIORITY NO. 3. To assess current pattern of elimination:

- Note color, odor, consistency, amount, and frequency of stool. **Provides a baseline for comparison, promotes recognition of changes.**
- Ascertain duration of current problem and degree of concern (e.g., long-standing condition that client has "lived with" or a postsurgical event that causes great distress) **as client's response may be inappropriate in relation to severity of condition.**
- Auscultate abdomen for presence, location, and characteristics of bowel sounds **reflecting bowel activity.**
- Note laxative/enema use.
- Review current fluid/dietary intake.

NURSING PRIORITY NO. 4. To facilitate return to usual/acceptable pattern of elimination:

- Instruct in/encourage balanced fiber and bulk in **diet to improve consistency of stool and facilitate passage through colon.**

- Promote adequate fluid intake, including high-fiber fruit juices; suggest drinking warm, stimulating fluids (e.g., decaffeinated coffee, hot water, tea) **to promote moist/soft stool.**
- Encourage activity/exercise within limits of individual ability **to stimulate contractions of the intestines.**
- Provide privacy and routinely scheduled time for defecation (bathroom or commode preferable to bedpan).
- Encourage/support treatment of underlying medical cause where appropriate (e.g., thyroid treatment) **to improve body function, including the bowel.**
- Administer stool softeners, mild stimulants, or bulk-forming agents as ordered, and/or routinely when appropriate (e.g., client receiving opiates, decreased level of activity/immobility).
- Apply lubricant/anesthetic ointment to anus if needed.
- Administer enemas; digitally remove impacted stool.
- Provide sitz bath after stools **for soothing effect to rectal area.**
- Establish bowel program to include glycerin suppositories and digital stimulation as appropriate **when long-term or permanent bowel dysfunction is present.**

NURSING PRIORITY NO. **5.** To promote wellness (Teaching/Discharge Considerations):

- Discuss physiology and acceptable variations in elimination.
- Provide information about relationship of diet, exercise, fluid, and appropriate use of laxatives as indicated.
- Discuss rationale for and encourage continuation of successful interventions.
- Encourage client to maintain elimination diary if appropriate **to facilitate monitoring of long-term problem.**
- Identify specific actions to be taken if problem recurs **to promote timely intervention, enhancing client's independence.**

Documentation Focus

ASSESSMENT/REASSESSMENT

- Usual and current bowel pattern, duration of the problem, and individual contributing factors.
- Characteristics of stool.
- Underlying dynamics.

PLANNING

- Plan of care/interventions and changes in lifestyle that are necessary to correct individual situation, and who is involved in planning.
- Teaching plan.

IMPLEMENTATION/EVALUATION

- Responses to interventions/teaching and actions performed.
- Change in bowel pattern, character of stool.
- Attainment/progress toward desired outcomes.
- Modifications to plan of care.

DISCHARGE PLANNING

- Individual long-term needs, noting who is responsible for actions to be taken.
- Recommendations for follow-up care.
- Specific referrals made.

SAMPLE NURSING OUTCOMES & INTERVENTIONS CLASSIFICATIONS (NOC/NIC)

NOC—Bowel Elimination
NIC—Constipation/Impaction Management

Constipation, perceived

Taxonomy II: Elimination—Class 2 Gastrointestinal System (00012)
[Diagnostic Division: Elimination]
Submitted 1988

Definition: Self-diagnosis of constipation and abuse of laxatives, enemas, and suppositories to ensure a daily bowel movement

Related Factors

Cultural/family health beliefs
Faulty appraisal, [long-term expectations/habits]
Impaired thought processes

Defining Characteristics

SUBJECTIVE

Expectation of a daily bowel movement with the resulting overuse of laxatives, enemas, and suppositories
Expected passage of stool at same time every day

Desired Outcomes/Evaluation Criteria—Client Will:

- Verbalize understanding of physiology of bowel function.
- Identify acceptable interventions to promote adequate bowel function.

Information that appears in brackets has been added by the authors to clarify and enhance the use of nursing diagnoses.

- Decrease reliance on laxatives/enemas.
- Establish individually appropriate pattern of elimination.

Actions/Interventions

NURSING PRIORITY NO. **1.** To identify factors affecting individual beliefs:

- Determine client's understanding of a "normal" bowel pattern.
- Compare with client's current bowel functioning.
- Identify interventions used by client to correct perceived problem.

NURSING PRIORITY NO. **2.** To promote wellness (Teaching/Discharge Considerations):

- Discuss physiology and acceptable variations in elimination.
- Identify detrimental effects of drug/enema use.
- Review relationship of diet/exercise to bowel elimination.
- Provide support by Active-listening and discussing client's concerns/fears.
- Encourage use of stress-reduction activities/refocusing of attention while client works to establish individually appropriate pattern.

Documentation Focus

ASSESSMENT/REASSESSMENT

- Assessment findings/client's perceptions of the problem.
- Current bowel pattern, stool characteristics.

PLANNING

- Plan of care/interventions and who is involved in the planning.
- Teaching plan.

IMPLEMENTATION/EVALUATION

- Client's responses to interventions/teaching and actions performed.
- Changes in bowel pattern, character of stool.
- Attainment/progress toward desired outcome(s).
- Modifications to plan of care.

DISCHARGE PLANNING

- Referral for follow-up care.

SAMPLE NURSING OUTCOMES
& INTERVENTIONS CLASSIFICATIONS (NOC/NIC)

NOC—Health Beliefs
NIC—Bowel Management

Constipation, risk for

Taxonomy II: Elimination—Class 2 Gastrointestinal
System (00015)
[Diagnostic Division: Elimination]
Nursing Diagnosis Extension and Classification (NDEC)
Submission 1998

Definition: At risk for a decrease in normal frequency
of defecation accompanied by difficult or incomplete
passage of stool and/or passage of excessively hard, dry
stool

Risk Factors

FUNCTIONAL

Irregular defecation habits; inadequate toileting (e.g., timeliness, posi-
tioning for defecation, privacy)
Insufficient physical activity; abdominal muscle weakness
Recent environmental changes
Habitual denial/ignoring of urge to defecate

PSYCHOLOGICAL

Emotional stress; depression; mental confusion

PHYSIOLOGICAL

Change in usual foods and eating patterns; insufficient fiber/fluid
intake, dehydration; poor eating habits
Inadequate dentition or oral hygiene
Decreased motility of gastrointestinal tract

PHARMACOLOGICAL

Phenothiazides; nonsteroidal anti-inflammatory agents; sedatives;
aluminum-containing antacids; laxative overuse; iron salts; anticholinergics; antidepressants; anticonvulsants; antilipemic agents;
calcium channel blockers; calcium carbonate; diuretics; sympathomimetics; opiates; bismuth salts

MECHANICAL

Hemorrhoids; pregnancy; obesity
Rectal abscess or ulcer; anal stricture; anal fissures; prolapse; rectocele
Prostate enlargement; postsurgical obstruction

Information that appears in brackets has been added by the authors
to clarify and enhance the use of nursing diagnoses.

Neurological impairment; megacolon (Hirschsprung's disease); tumors
Electrolyte imbalance

> NOTE: A risk diagnosis is not evidenced by signs and symptoms, as the problem has not occurred and nursing interventions are directed at prevention.

Desired Outcomes/Evaluation Criteria—Client Will:

- Maintain usual pattern of bowel functioning.
- Verbalize understanding of risk factors and appropriate interventions/solutions related to individual situation.
- Demonstrate behaviors or lifestyle changes to prevent developing problem.

Actions/Interventions

NURSING PRIORITY NO. 1. To identify individual risk factors/ needs:

- Auscultate abdomen for presence, location, and characteristics of bowel sounds **reflecting bowel activity.**
- Discuss usual elimination pattern and use of laxatives.
- Ascertain client's beliefs and practices about bowel elimination, such as "must have a bowel movement every day or I need an enema."
- Determine current situation and possible impact on bowel function (e.g., surgery, use of medications affecting intestinal function, advanced age, weakness, depression, and other risk factors as listed previously).
- Evaluate current dietary and fluid intake and implications for effect on bowel function.
- Review medications (new and chronic use) **for impact on/effects of changes in bowel function.**

NURSING PRIORITY NO. 2. To facilitate normal bowel function:

- Instruct in/encourage balanced fiber and bulk in diet **to improve consistency of stool and facilitate passage through the colon.**
- Promote adequate fluid intake, including water and high-fiber fruit juices; suggest drinking warm, stimulating fluids (e.g., decaffeinated coffee, hot water, tea) **to promote moist/soft stool.**
- Encourage activity/exercise within limits of individual ability **to stimulate contractions of the intestines.**
- Provide privacy and routinely scheduled time for defecation (bathroom or commode preferable to bedpan).

- Administer routine stool softeners, mild stimulants, or bulk-forming agents prn and/or routinely when appropriate (e.g., client taking pain medications, especially opiates, or who is inactive, immobile, or unconscious).
- Ascertain frequency, color, consistency, amount of stools. **Provides a baseline for comparison, promotes recognition of changes.**

NURSING PRIORITY NO. 3. To promote wellness (Teaching/Discharge Considerations):

- Discuss physiology and acceptable variations in elimination. **May help reduce concerns/anxiety about situation.**
- Review individual risk factors/potential problems and specific interventions.
- Review appropriate use of medications.
- Encourage client to maintain elimination diary if appropriate **to help monitor bowel pattern.**
- Refer to NDs Constipation; Constipation, perceived.

Documentation Focus

ASSESSMENT/REASSESSMENT

- Current bowel pattern, characteristics of stool, medications.

PLANNING

- Plan of care and who is involved in planning.
- Teaching plan.

IMPLEMENTATION/EVALUATION

- Responses to interventions/teaching and actions performed.
- Attainment/progress toward desired outcomes.
- Modifications to plan of care.

DISCHARGE PLANNING

- Individual long-term needs, noting who is responsible for actions to be taken.
- Specific referrals made.

SAMPLE NURSING OUTCOMES & INTERVENTIONS CLASSIFICATIONS (NOC/NIC)

NOC—Bowel Elimination
NIC—Constipation/Impaction Management

Coping, community: ineffective

Taxonomy II: Coping/Stress Tolerance—Class 2 Coping
Responses (00077)
[Diagnostic Division: Social Interaction]
Submitted 1994; Nursing Diagnosis Extension and
Classification (NDEC) Revision 1998

Definition: Pattern of community activities (for adaptation and problem solving) that is unsatisfactory for meeting the demands or needs of the community

Related Factors

Deficits in social support services and resources
Inadequate resources for problem solving
Ineffective or nonexistent community systems (e.g., lack of emergency medical system, transportation system, or disaster planning systems)
Natural or human-made disasters

Defining Characteristics

SUBJECTIVE

Community does not meet its own expectations
Expressed vulnerability; community powerlessness
Stressors perceived as excessive

OBJECTIVE

Deficits of community participation
Excessive community conflicts
High illness rates
Increased social problems (e.g., homicide, vandalism, arson, terrorism, robbery, infanticide, abuse, divorce, unemployment, poverty, militance, mental illness)

Desired Outcomes/Evaluation Criteria—Community Will:

- Recognize negative and positive factors affecting community's ability to meet its own demands or needs.
- Identify alternatives to inappropriate activities for adaptation/problem solving.
- Report a measurable increase in necessary/desired activities to improve community functioning.

Actions/Interventions

NURSING PRIORITY NO. 1. To identify causative or precipitating factors:

- Evaluate community activities **as related to meeting collective needs within the community itself and between the community and the larger society.**

Information that appears in brackets has been added by the authors to clarify and enhance the use of nursing diagnoses.

- Note community reports of community functioning, including areas of weakness or conflict.
- Identify effects of Related Factors on community activities.
- Determine availability and use of resources.
- Identify unmet demands or needs of the community.

NURSING PRIORITY NO. 2. To assist the community to reactivate/develop skills to deal with needs:
- Determine community strengths.
- Identify and prioritize community goals.
- Encourage community members/groups to engage in problem-solving activities.
- Develop a plan jointly with community **to deal with deficits in support to meet identified goals.**

NURSING PRIORITY NO. 3. To promote wellness as related to community health:
- Create plans managing interactions within the community itself and between the community and the larger society **to meet collective needs.**
- Assist the community to form partnerships within the community and between the community and the larger society. **Promotes long-term development of the community to deal with current and future problems.**
- Provide channels for dissemination of information to the community as a whole, for example, print media; radio/television reports and community bulletin boards; speakers' bureau; reports to committees, councils, advisory boards on file and accessible to the public.
- Make information available in different modalities and geared to differing educational levels/cultures of the community.
- Seek out and evaluate underserved populations.

Documentation Focus

ASSESSMENT/REASSESSMENT

- Assessment findings, including perception of community members regarding problems.

PLANNING

- Plan of care and who is involved in planning.
- Teaching plan.

IMPLEMENTATION/EVALUATION

- Response of community entities to plan/interventions and actions performed.
- Attainment/progress toward desired outcome(s).
- Modifications to plan of care.

DISCHARGE PLANNING

• Long-range plans and who is responsible for actions to be taken.

SAMPLE NURSING OUTCOMES & INTERVENTIONS CLASSIFICATIONS (NOC/NIC)

NOC—Community Health Status
NIC—Community Health Development

Coping, community: readiness for enhanced

Taxonomy II: Coping/Stress Tolerance—Class 2 Coping Responses (00076)
[Diagnostic Division: Social Interaction]
Submitted 1994

Definition: Pattern of community activities for adaptation and problem solving that is satisfactory for meeting the demands or needs of the community but can be improved for management of current and future problems/stressors

Related Factors

Social supports available
Resources available for problem solving
Community has a sense of power to manage stressors

Defining Characteristics

SUBJECTIVE

Agreement that community is responsible for stress management

OBJECTIVE

Deficits in one or more characteristics that indicate effective coping
Active planning by community for predicted stressors
Active problem solving by community when faced with issues
Positive communication among community members
Positive communication between community/aggregates and larger community
Programs available for recreation and relaxation
Resources sufficient for managing stressors

Desired Outcomes/Evaluation Criteria—Community Will:

• Identify positive and negative factors affecting management of current and future problems/stressors.

Information that appears in brackets has been added by the authors to clarify and enhance the use of nursing diagnoses.

- Have an established plan in place to deal with problems/stressors.
- Describe management of deficits in characteristics that indicate effective coping.
- Report a measurable increase in ability to deal with problems/stressors.

Actions/Interventions

NURSING PRIORITY NO. 1. To determine existence of and deficits or weaknesses in management of current and future problems/stressors:

- Review community plan for dealing with problems/stressors.
- Assess effects of Related Factors on management of problems/stressors.
- Determine community's strengths and weaknesses.
- Identify limitations in current pattern of community activities that can be improved through adaptation and problem solving.
- Evaluate community activities as related to management of problems/stressors within the community itself and between the community and the larger society.

NURSING PRIORITY NO. 2. To assist the community in adaptation and problem solving for management of current and future needs/stressors:

- Define and discuss current needs and anticipated or projected concerns. **Agreement on scope/parameters of needs is essential for effective planning.**
- Prioritize goals **to facilitate accomplishment.**
- Identify available resources (e.g., persons, groups, financial, governmental, as well as other communities).
- Make a joint plan with the community to deal with adaptation and problem solving **for management of problems/stressors.**
- Seek out and involve underserved/at-risk groups within the community. **Supports communication and commitment of community as a whole.**

NURSING PRIORITY NO. 3. To promote well-being of community:

- Assist the community to form partnerships within the community and between the community and the larger society **to promote long-term developmental growth of the community.**
- Support development of plans for maintaining these interactions.
- Establish mechanism for self-monitoring of community needs and evaluation of efforts. **Facilitates proactive rather than reactive responses by the community.**

- Use multiple formats, for example, TV, radio, print media, billboards and computer bulletin boards, speakers' bureau, reports to community leaders/groups on file and accessible to the public, **to keep community informed regarding plans, needs, outcomes.**

Documentation Focus

ASSESSMENT/REASSESSMENT

- Assessment findings and community's perception of situation.
- Identified areas of concern, community strengths/weaknesses.

PLANNING

- Plan of care and who is involved and responsible for each action.
- Teaching plan.

IMPLEMENTATION/EVALUATION

- Response of community entities to the actions performed.
- Attainment/progress toward desired outcomes.
- Modifications to plan of care.

DISCHARGE PLANNING

- Short-range and long-range plans to deal with current, anticipated, and potential needs and who is responsible for follow-through.
- Specific referrals made, coalitions formed.

SAMPLE NURSING OUTCOMES & INTERVENTIONS CLASSIFICATIONS (NOC/NIC)

NOC—Community Competence
NIC—Program Development

Coping, defensive

Taxonomy II: Coping/Stress Tolerance—Class 2 Coping
Responses (00071)
[Diagnostic Division: Ego Integrity]
Submitted 1988

Definition: Repeated projection of falsely positive self-evaluation based on a self-protective pattern that defends against underlying perceived threats to positive self-regard

Information that appears in brackets has been added by the authors to clarify and enhance the use of nursing diagnoses.

Related Factors

To be developed
[Refer to ND Coping, ineffective]

Defining Characteristics

SUBJECTIVE

Denial of obvious problems/weaknesses
Projection of blame/responsibility
Hypersensitive to slight/criticism
Grandiosity
Rationalizes failures
[Refuses or rejects assistance]

OBJECTIVE

Superior attitude toward others
Difficulty establishing/maintaining relationships, [avoidance of intimacy]
Hostile laughter or ridicule of others, [aggressive behavior]
Difficulty in reality testing perceptions
Lack of follow-through or participation in treatment or therapy
[Attention-seeking behavior]

Desired Outcomes/Evaluation Criteria—Client Will:

- Verbalize understanding of own problems/stressors.
- Identify areas of concern/problems.
- Demonstrate acceptance of responsibility for own actions, successes, and failures.
- Participate in treatment program/therapy.
- Maintain involvement in relationships.

Actions/Interventions

- Refer to ND Coping, ineffective for additional interventions.

NURSING PRIORITY NO. 1. To determine degree of impairment:

- Assess ability to comprehend current situation, developmental level of functioning.
- Determine level of anxiety and effectiveness of current coping mechanisms.
- Determine coping mechanisms used (e.g., projection, avoidance, rationalization) and purpose of coping strategy (e.g., may mask low self-esteem) **to note how these behaviors affect current situation.**
- Assist client to identify/consider need to address problem differently.
- Describe all aspects of the problem using therapeutic communication skills, such as Active-listening.

- Observe interactions with others **to note difficulties/ability to establish satisfactory relationships.**
- Note expressions of grandiosity in the face of contrary evidence (e.g., "I'm going to buy a new car" when the individual has no job or available finances).

NURSING PRIORITY NO. 2. To assist client to deal with current situation:

- Provide explanation of the rules of the treatment setting and consequences of lack of cooperation.
- Set limits on manipulative behavior; be consistent in enforcing consequences when rules are broken and limits tested.
- Develop therapeutic relationship to enable client **to test new behaviors in a safe environment.** Use positive, nonjudgmental approach and "I" language **to promote sense of self-esteem.**
- Encourage control in all situations possible, include client in decisions, and planning **to preserve autonomy.**
- Acknowledge individual strengths and incorporate awareness of personal assets/strengths in plan.
- Convey attitude of acceptance and respect (unconditional positive regard) **to avoid threatening client's self-concept, preserve existing self-esteem.**
- Encourage identification and expression of feelings.
- Provide healthy outlets for release of hostile feelings (e.g., punching bags, pounding boards). Involve in outdoor recreation program when available.
- Provide opportunities for client to interact with others in a positive manner, **promoting self-esteem.**
- Assist client with problem-solving process. Identify and discuss responses to situation, maladaptive coping skills. Suggest alternative responses to situation **to help client select more adaptive strategies for coping.**
- Use confrontation judiciously **to help client begin to identify defense mechanisms (e.g., denial/projection) that are hindering development of satisfying relationships.**

NURSING PRIORITY NO. 3. To promote wellness (Teaching/Discharge Considerations):

- Encourage client to learn relaxation techniques, use of guided imagery, and positive affirmation of self **in order to incorporate and practice new behaviors.**
- Promote involvement in activities/classes where client can practice new skills and develop new relationships.
- Refer to additional resources (e.g., substance rehabilitation, family/marital therapy) as indicated.

Documentation Focus

ASSESSMENT/REASSESSMENT

- Assessment findings/presenting behaviors.
- Client perception of the present situation and usual coping methods/degree of impairment.

PLANNING

- Plan of care and interventions and who is involved in development of the plan.
- Teaching plan.

IMPLEMENTATION/EVALUATION

- Response to interventions/teaching and actions performed.
- Attainment/progress toward desired outcome(s).
- Modifications to plan of care.

DISCHARGE PLANNING

- Referrals and follow-up program.

SAMPLE NURSING OUTCOMES & INTERVENTIONS CLASSIFICATIONS (NOC/NIC)

NOC—Self-Esteem
NIC—Self-Awareness Enhancement

Coping, family: compromised

Taxonomy II: Coping/Stress Tolerance—Class 2 Coping Responses (00074)
[Diagnostic Division: Social Interaction]
Submitted 1980; Revised 1996

Definition: Usually supportive primary person (family member or close friend [SO]) provides insufficient, ineffective, or compromised support, comfort, assistance, or encouragement that may be needed by the client to manage or master adaptive tasks related to his/her health challenge

Related Factors

Inadequate or incorrect information or understanding by a primary person
Temporary preoccupation by a significant person who is trying to manage emotional conflicts and personal suffering and is unable to perceive or act effectively in regard to client's needs
Temporary family disorganization and role changes
Other situational or developmental crises or situations the significant person may be facing

Information that appears in brackets has been added by the authors to clarify and enhance the use of nursing diagnoses.

Little support provided by client, in turn, for primary person

Prolonged disease or disability progression that exhausts the supportive capacity of SO(s)

[Unrealistic expectations of client/SO(s) or each other]

[Lack of mutual decision-making skills]

[Diverse coalitions of family members]

Defining Characteristics

SUBJECTIVE

Client expresses or confirms a concern or complaint about SO's response to his or her health problem

SO describes preoccupation with personal reaction (e.g., fear, anticipatory grief, guilt, anxiety) to client's illness/disability or other situational or developmental crises

SO describes or confirms an inadequate understanding or knowledge base that interferes with effective assistive or supportive behaviors

OBJECTIVE

SO attempts assistive or supportive behaviors with less-than-satisfactory results

SO withdraws or enters into limited or temporary personal communication with the client at the time of need

SO displays protective behavior disproportionate (too little or too much) to the client's abilities or need for autonomy

[SO displays sudden outbursts of emotions/shows emotional lability or interferes with necessary nursing/medical interventions]

Desired Outcomes/Evaluation Criteria—Family Will:

- Identify/verbalize resources within themselves to deal with the situation.
- Interact appropriately with the client, providing support and assistance as indicated.
- Provide opportunity for client to deal with situation in own way.
- Verbalize knowledge and understanding of illness/disability/disease.
- Express feelings honestly.
- Identify need for outside support and seek such.

Actions/Interventions

NURSING PRIORITY NO. 1. To assess causative/contributing factors:

- Identify underlying situation(s) that may contribute to the inability of family to provide needed assistance to the client. **Circumstances may have preceded the illness and now have a significant effect (e.g., client had a heart attack during sexual activity, mate is afraid of repeating).**

- Note the length of illness, such as cancer, multiple sclerosis, and/or other long-term situations that may exist.
- Assess information available to and understood by the family/SO(s).
- Discuss family perceptions of situation. **Expectations of client and family members may/may not be realistic.**
- Identify role of the client in family and how illness has changed the family organization.
- Note other factors besides the client's illness that are affecting abilities of family members **to provide needed support.**

NURSING PRIORITY NO. **2.** To assist family to reactivate/develop skills to deal with current situation:

- Listen to client's/SO's comments, remarks, and expression of concern(s). Note nonverbal behaviors and/or responses and congruency.
- Encourage family members to verbalize feelings openly/ clearly.
- Discuss underlying reasons for behaviors with family **to help them understand and accept/deal with client behaviors.**
- Assist the family and client to understand "who owns the problem" and who is responsible for resolution. Avoid placing blame or guilt.
- Encourage client and family to develop problem-solving skills **to deal with the situation.**

NURSING PRIORITY NO. **3.** To promote wellness (Teaching/ Discharge Considerations):

- Provide information for family/SO(s) about specific illness/condition.
- Involve client and family in planning care as often as possible. **Enhances commitment to plan.**
- Promote assistance of family in providing client care as appropriate. **Identifies ways of demonstrating support while maintaining client's independence (e.g., providing favorite foods, engaging in diversional activities).**
- Refer to appropriate resources for assistance as indicated (e.g., counseling, psychotherapy, financial, spiritual).
- Refer to NDs Fear; Anxiety/Anxiety, death; Coping, ineffective; Coping, family: readiness for enhanced; Coping, family: disabled; Grieving, anticipatory as appropriate.

Documentation Focus

ASSESSMENT/REASSESSMENT

- Assessment findings, including current/past coping behaviors, emotional response to situation/stressors, support systems available.

- Plan of care, who is involved in planning and areas of responsibility.
- Teaching plan.

IMPLEMENTATION/EVALUATION

- Responses of family members/client to interventions/teaching and actions performed.
- Attainment/progress toward desired outcome(s).
- Modifications to plan of care.

DISCHARGE PLANNING

- Long-range plan and who is responsible for actions.
- Specific referrals made.

SAMPLE NURSING OUTCOMES
& INTERVENTIONS CLASSIFICATION (NOC/NIC)

NOC—Family Coping
NIC—Family Involvement Promotion

Coping, family: disabled

Taxonomy II: Coping/Stress Tolerance—Class 2 Coping Responses (00073)
[Diagnostic Division: Social Interaction]
Submitted 1980; Revised 1996

Definition: Behavior of SO (family member or other primary person) that disables his/her capacities and the client's capacity to effectively address tasks essential to either person's adaptation to the health challenge

Related Factors

Significant person with chronically unexpressed feelings of guilt, anxiety, hostility, despair, and so forth
Dissonant discrepancy of coping styles for dealing with adaptive tasks by the significant person and client or among significant people
Highly ambivalent family relationships
Arbitrary handling of a family's resistance to treatment that tends to solidify defensiveness as it fails to deal adequately with underlying anxiety
[High-risk family situations, such as single or adolescent parent, abusive relationship, substance abuse, acute/chronic disabilities, member with terminal illness]

Information that appears in brackets has been added by the authors to clarify and enhance the use of nursing diagnoses.

Defining Characteristics

[Expresses despair regarding family reactions/lack of involvement]

Intolerance, rejection, abandonment, desertion
Psychosomaticism
Agitation, depression, aggression, hostility
Taking on illness signs of client
Neglectful relationships with other family members
Carrying on usual routines disregarding client's needs
Neglectful care of the client in regard to basic human needs and/or
    illness treatment
Distortion of reality regarding the client's health problem, including
    extreme denial about its existence or severity
Decisions and actions by family that are detrimental to economic or
    social well-being
Impaired restructuring of a meaningful life for self, impaired individu-
    alization, prolonged overconcern for client
Client's development of helpless, inactive dependence

Desired Outcomes/Evaluation
Criteria—Family Will:

- Verbalize more realistic understanding and expectations of
  the client.
- Visit/contact client regularly.
- Participate positively in care of client, within limits of family's
  abilities and client's needs.
- Express feelings and expectations openly and honestly as
  appropriate.

Actions/Interventions

NURSING PRIORITY NO. 1. To assess causative/contributing
factors:

- Ascertain preillness behaviors/interactions of the family.
  Provides comparative baseline.
- Identify current behaviors of the family members (e.g., withdrawal—not visiting, brief visits, and/or ignoring client when
  visiting; anger and hostility toward client and others; ways of
  touching between family members, expressions of guilt).
- Discuss family perceptions of situation. **Expectations of client
  and family members may/may not be realistic.**
- Note other factors that may be stressful for the family (e.g.,
  financial difficulties or lack of community support, as when
  illness occurs when out of town). **Provides opportunity for
  appropriate referrals.**

- Determine readiness of family members to be involved with care of the client.

NURSING PRIORITY NO. 2. To provide assistance to enable family to deal with the current situation:

- Establish rapport with family members who are available. **Promotes therapeutic relationship and support for problem-solving solutions.**
- Acknowledge difficulty of the situation for the family. **Reduces blaming/guilt feelings.**
- Active-listen concerns, note both overconcern/lack of concern, which may interfere with ability to resolve situation.
- Allow free expression of feelings, including frustration, anger, hostility, and hopelessness. Place limits on acting-out/inappropriate behaviors **to minimize risk of violent behavior.**
- Give accurate information to SO(s) from the beginning.
- Be liaison between family and healthcare providers **to provide explanations and clarification of treatment plan.**
- Provide brief, simple explanations about use and alarms when equipment (such as a ventilator) is involved. Identify appropriate professional(s) **for continued support/problem solving.**
- Provide time for private interaction between client/family.
- Include SO(s) in the plan of care; provide instruction **to assist them to learn necessary skills to help client.**
- Accompany family when they visit **to be available for questions, concerns, and support.**
- Assist SO(s) to initiate therapeutic communication with client.
- Refer client to protective services as necessitated by risk of physical harm. **Removing client from home enhances individual safety and may reduce stress on family to allow opportunity for therapeutic intervention.**

NURSING PRIORITY NO. 3. To promote wellness (Teaching/Discharge Considerations):

- Assist family to identify coping skills being used and how these skills are/are not helping them deal with situation.
- Answer family's questions patiently and honestly. Reinforce information provided by other providers.
- Reframe negative expressions into positive whenever possible. **(A positive frame contributes to supportive interactions and can lead to better outcomes.)**
- Respect family needs for withdrawal and intervene judiciously. **Situation may be overwhelming and time away can be beneficial to continued participation.**
- Encourage family to deal with the situation in small increments rather than the whole picture.

- Assist the family to identify familiar things that would be helpful to the client (e.g., a family picture on the wall) **to reinforce/maintain orientation.**
- Refer family to appropriate resources as needed (e.g., family therapy, financial counseling, spiritual advisor).
- Refer to ND Grieving, anticipatory as appropriate.

Documentation Focus

ASSESSMENT/REASSESSMENT

- Assessment findings, current/past behaviors, including family members who are directly involved and support systems available.
- Emotional response(s) to situation/stressors.

PLANNING

- Plan of care/interventions and who is involved in planning.
- Teaching plan.

IMPLEMENTATION/EVALUATION

- Responses of individuals to interventions/teaching and actions performed.
- Attainment/progress toward desired outcome(s).
- Modifications to plan of care.

DISCHARGE PLANNING

- Ongoing needs/resources/other follow-up recommendations and who is responsible for actions.
- Specific referrals made.

SAMPLE NURSING OUTCOMES & INTERVENTIONS CLASSIFICATIONS (NOC/NIC)

NOC—Family Normalization
NIC—Family Therapy

Coping, family: readiness for enhanced

Taxonomy II: Coping/Stress Tolerance—Class 2 Coping Responses (00075)
[Diagnostic Division: Social Interaction]
Submitted 1980
Definition: Effective managing of adaptive tasks by family member involved with the client's health challenge, who now exhibits desire and readiness for enhanced health and growth in regard to self and in relation to the client

Information that appears in brackets has been added by the authors to clarify and enhance the use of nursing diagnoses.

Related Factors

Needs sufficiently gratified and adaptive tasks effectively addressed to enable goals of self-actualization to surface
[Developmental stage, situational crises/supports]

Defining Characteristics

SUBJECTIVE

Family member attempting to describe growth impact of crisis on his or her own values, priorities, goals, or relationships
Individual expressing interest in making contact on a one-to-one basis or on a mutual-aid group basis with another person who has experienced a similar situation

OBJECTIVE

Family member moving in direction of health-promoting and enriching lifestyle that supports and monitors maturational processes, audits and negotiates treatment programs, and generally chooses experiences that optimize wellness

Desired Outcomes/Evaluation Criteria—Family Will:

- Express willingness to look at own role in the family's growth.
- Verbalize desire to undertake tasks leading to change.
- Report feelings of self-confidence and satisfaction with progress being made.

Actions/Interventions

NURSING PRIORITY NO. 1. To assess situation and adaptive skills being used by the family members:

- Determine individual situation and stage of growth family is experiencing/demonstrating.
- Observe communication patterns of family. Listen to family's expressions of hope, planning, effect on relationships/life.
- Note expressions, such as "Life has more meaning for me since this has occurred," **to identify changes in values.**

NURSING PRIORITY NO. 2. To assist family to develop/strengthen potential for growth:

- Provide time to talk with family **to discuss their view of the situation.**
- Establish a relationship with family/client **to foster growth.**
- Provide a role model with which the family may identify.

- Discuss importance of open communication and of not having secrets.
- Demonstrate techniques, such as Active-listening, I-messages, and problem solving, **to facilitate effective communication.**

NURSING PRIORITY NO. 3. To promote wellness (Teaching/ Discharge Considerations):

- Assist family to support the client in meeting own needs within ability and/or constraints of the illness/situation.
- Provide experiences for the family **to help them learn ways of assisting/supporting client.**
- Identify other clients/groups with similar conditions and assist client/family to make contact (groups such as Reach for Recovery, CanSurmount, Al-Anon, etc.). **Provides ongoing support for sharing common experiences, problem solving, and learning new behaviors.**
- Assist family members to learn new, effective ways of dealing with feelings/reactions.

Documentation Focus

ASSESSMENT/REASSESSMENT

- Adaptive skills being used, stage of growth.
- Family communication patterns.

PLANNING

- Plan of care/interventions and who is involved in planning.
- Teaching plan.

IMPLEMENTATION/EVALUATION

- Client's/family's responses to interventions/teaching and actions performed.
- Attainment/progress toward desired outcome(s).
- Modifications to plan of care.

DISCHARGE PLANNING

- Identified needs/referrals for follow-up care, support systems.
- Specific referrals made.

SAMPLE NURSING OUTCOMES & INTERVENTIONS CLASSIFICATIONS (NOC/NIC)

NOC—Family Participation in Professional Care
NIC—Normalization Promotion

Coping, ineffective

Taxonomy II: Coping/Stress Tolerance—Class 2 Coping
Responses (00069)
[Diagnostic Division: Ego Integrity]
Submitted 1978; Nursing Diagnosis Extension and
Classification (NDEC) Revision 1998

Definition: Inability to form a valid appraisal of the
stressors, inadequate choices of practiced responses,
and/or inability to use available resources

Related Factors

Situational/maturational crises
High degree of threat
Inadequate opportunity to prepare for stressor; disturbance in pattern
of appraisal of threat
Inadequate level of confidence in ability to cope/perception of control;
uncertainty
Inadequate resources available; inadequate social support created by
characteristics of relationships
Disturbance in pattern of tension release; inability to conserve adap-
tive energies
Gender differences in coping strategies
[Work overload, no vacations, too many deadlines; little or no exercise]
[Impairment of nervous system; cognitive/sensory/perceptual impair-
ment, memory loss]
[Severe/chronic pain]

Defining Characteristics

SUBJECTIVE

Verbalization of inability to cope or inability to ask for help
Sleep disturbance; fatigue
Abuse of chemical agents
[Reports of muscular/emotional tension, lack of appetite]

OBJECTIVE

Lack of goal-directed behavior/resolution of problem, including
inability to attend to and difficulty with organizing information;
[lack of assertive behavior]
Use of forms of coping that impede adaptive behavior [including
inappropriate use of defense mechanisms, verbal manipulation]
Inadequate problem solving
Inability to meet role expectations/basic needs
Decreased use of social supports
Poor concentration
Change in usual communication patterns
High illness rate [including high blood pressure, ulcers, irritable bowel,
frequent headaches/neckaches]

Information that appears in brackets has been added by the authors
to clarify and enhance the use of nursing diagnoses.

Risk taking

Destructive behavior toward self or others [including overeating, excessive smoking/drinking, overuse of prescribed/OTC medications, illicit drug use]

[Behavioral changes (e.g., impatience, frustration, irritability, discouragement)]

Desired Outcomes/Evaluation Criteria—Client Will:

- Assess the current situation accurately.
- Identify ineffective coping behaviors and consequences.
- Verbalize awareness of own coping abilities.
- Verbalize feelings congruent with behavior.
- Meet psychologic needs as evidenced by appropriate expression of feelings, identification of options, and use of resources.

Actions/Interventions

NURSING PRIORITY NO. 1. To determine degree of impairment:
- Evaluate ability to understand events, provide realistic appraisal of situation.
- Identify developmental level of functioning. (**People tend to regress to a lower developmental stage during illness/crisis.**)
- Assess current functional capacity and note how it is affecting the individual's coping ability.
- Determine alcohol intake, drug use, smoking habits, sleeping and eating patterns.
- Ascertain impact of illness on sexual needs/relationship.
- Assess level of anxiety and coping on an ongoing basis.
- Note speech and communication patterns.
- Observe and describe behavior in objective terms. Validate observations.

NURSING PRIORITY NO. 2. To assess coping abilities and skills:
- Ascertain client's understanding of current situation and its impact.
- Active-listen and identify client's perceptions of what is happening.
- Evaluate client's decision-making ability.
- Determine previous methods of dealing with life problems **to identify successful techniques that can be used in current situation.**

NURSING PRIORITY NO. 3. To assist client to deal with current situation:
- Call client by name. Ascertain how client prefers to be addressed. **Using client's name enhances sense of self and promotes individuality/self-esteem.**

- Encourage communication with staff/SO(s).
- Use reality orientation (e.g., clocks, calendars, bulletin boards) and make frequent references to time, place as indicated. Place needed/familiar objects within sight for visual cues.
- Provide for continuity of care with same personnel taking care of the client as often as possible.
- Explain disease process/procedures/events in a simple, concise manner. Devote time for listening; **may help client to express emotions, grasp situation, and feel more in control.**
- Provide for a quiet environment/position equipment out of view as much as possible **when anxiety is increased by noisy surroundings.**
- Schedule activities so periods of rest alternate with nursing care. Increase activity slowly.
- Assist client in use of diversion, recreation, relaxation techniques.
- Stress positive body responses to medical conditions but do not negate the seriousness of the situation (e.g., stable blood pressure during gastric bleed or improved body posture in depressed client).
- Encourage client to try new coping behaviors and gradually master situation.
- Confront client when behavior is inappropriate, pointing out difference between words and actions. **Provides external locus of control, enhancing safety.**
- Assist in dealing with change in concept of body image as appropriate. (Refer to ND Body Image, disturbed.)

NURSING PRIORITY NO. 4. To provide for meeting psychologic needs:

- Treat the client with courtesy and respect. Converse at client's level, providing meaningful conversation while performing care. (**Enhances therapeutic relationship.**) Take advantage of teachable moments.
- Allow client to react in own way without judgment by staff. Provide support and diversion as indicated.
- Encourage verbalization of fears and anxieties and expression of feelings of denial, depression, and anger. Let the client know that these are normal reactions.
- Provide opportunity for expression of sexual concerns.
- Help client to set limits on acting-out behaviors and learn ways to express emotions in an acceptable manner. (**Promotes internal locus of control.**)

NURSING PRIORITY NO. 5. To promote wellness (Teaching/Discharge Considerations):

- Give updated/additional information needed about events,

cause (if known), and potential course of illness as soon as possible. **Knowledge helps reduce anxiety/fear, allows client to deal with reality.**

- Provide and encourage an atmosphere of realistic hope.
- Give information about purposes and side effects of medications/treatments.
- Stress importance of follow-up care.
- Encourage and support client in evaluating lifestyle, occupation, and leisure activities.
- Assess effects of stressors (e.g., family, social, work environment, or nursing/healthcare management) and ways to deal with them.
- Provide for gradual implementation and continuation of necessary behavior/lifestyle changes. **Enhances commitment to plan.**
- Discuss/review anticipated procedures and client concerns, as well as postoperative expectations when surgery is recommended.
- Refer to outside resources and/or professional therapy as indicated/ordered.
- Determine need/desire for religious representative/spiritual counselor and arrange for visit.
- Provide information, privacy, or consultation as indicated for sexual concerns.
- Refer to other NDs as indicated (e.g., Pain; Anxiety; Communication, impaired verbal; Violence, [actual/] risk for other-directed and Violence, [actual/] risk for self-directed).

Documentation Focus

ASSESSMENT/REASSESSMENT

- Baseline findings, degree of impairment, and client's perceptions of situation.
- Coping abilities and previous ways of dealing with life problems.

PLANNING

- Plan of care/interventions and who is involved in planning.
- Teaching plan.

IMPLEMENTATION/EVALUATION

- Client's responses to interventions/teaching and actions performed.
- Medication dose, time, and client's response.
- Attainment/progress toward desired outcome(s).
- Modifications to plan of care.

- Long-term needs and actions to be taken.
- Support systems available, specific referrals made, and who is responsible for actions to be taken.

SAMPLE NURSING OUTCOMES & INTERVENTIONS CLASSIFICATIONS (NOC/NIC)

NOC—Coping
NIC—Coping Enhancement

Coping, readiness for enhanced

Taxonomy II: Coping/Stress Tolerance—Class 2 Coping Responses (00158)
[Diagnostic Divisions: Ego Integrity]
Submitted 2002

Definition: A pattern of cognitive and behavioral efforts to manage demands that is sufficient for well-being and can be strengthened

Related Factors

To be developed

Defining Characteristics

SUBJECTIVE

Defines stressors as manageable
Seeks social support; knowledge of new strategies
Acknowledges power
Is aware of possible environmental changes

OBJECTIVE

Uses a broad range of problem-oriented strategies; spiritual resources

Desired Outcomes/Evaluation Criteria—Client Will:

- Assess current situation accurately.
- Identify effective coping behaviors currently being used.
- Verbalize feelings congruent with behavior.
- Meet psychologic needs as evidenced by appropriate expression of feelings, identification of options, and use of resources.

Information that appears in brackets has been added by the authors to clarify and enhance the use of nursing diagnoses.

Actions/Interventions

NURSING PRIORITY NO. 1. To determine needs and desire for improvement:

- Evaluate ability to understand events, provide realistic appraisal of situation. **Provides information about client's perception, cognitive ability, and whether the client is aware of the facts of the situation. This is essential for planning care.**
- Determine stressors that are currently affecting client. **Accurate identification of situation that client is dealing with provides information for planning interventions to enhance coping abilities.**
- Identify social supports available to client. **Available support systems, such as family and friends, can provide client with ability to handle current stressful events and often "talking it out" with an empathic listener will help client move forward to enhance coping skills.**
- Review coping strategies client is aware of and using. **The desire to improve one's coping ability is based on an awareness of the current status of the stressful situation.**
- Determine alcohol intake, other drug use, smoking habits, sleeping and eating patterns. **Use of these substances impairs ability to deal with anxiety and affects ability to cope with life's stressors. Identification of impaired sleeping and eating patterns provides clues to need for change.**
- Assess level of anxiety and coping on an ongoing basis. **Provides information for baseline to develop plan of care to improve coping abilities.**
- Note speech and communication patterns. **Assesses ability to understand and provides information necessary to help client make progress in desire to enhance coping abilities.**
- Evaluate client's decision-making ability. **Understanding client's ability provides a starting point for developing plan and determining what information client needs to develop more effective coping skills.**

NURSING PRIORITY NO. 2. To assist client to develop enhanced coping skills:

- Active-listen and identify client's perceptions of current status. **Reflecting client's statements and thoughts can provide a forum for understanding perceptions in relation to reality for planning care and determining accuracy of interventions needed.**
- Determine previous methods of dealing with life problems. **Enables client to identify successful techniques used in the past promoting feelings of confidence in own ability.**

- Discuss desire to improve ability to manage stressors of life. **Understanding motivation behind decision to seek new information to enhance life will help client know what is needed to learn new skills of coping.**
- Discuss understanding of concept of knowing what can and cannot be changed. **Acceptance of reality that some things cannot be changed allows client to focus energies on dealing with things that can be changed.**

NURSING PRIORITY NO. 3. To promote optimum wellness:

- Discuss predisposing factors related to any individual's response to stress. **Understanding that genetic influences, past experiences, and existing conditions determine whether a person's response is adaptive or maladaptive will give client a base on which to continue to learn what is needed to improve life.**
- Assist client to develop a stress management program. **An individualized program of relaxation, meditation, involvement with caring for others/pets will enhance coping skills and strengthen client's ability to manage challenging situations.**
- Help client develop problem-solving skills. **Learning the process for problem solving will promote successful resolution of potentially stressful situations that arise.**
- Encourage involvement in activities of interest, such as exercise/sports, music, and art. **Individuals must decide for themselves what coping strategies are adaptive for them. Most people find enjoyment and relaxation in these kinds of activities.**
- Discuss possibility of doing volunteer work in an area of the client's choosing. **Many people report satisfaction in helping others and client may find pleasure in such involvement.**
- Refer to classes and/or reading material as appropriate. **May be helpful to further learning and pursuing goal of enhanced coping ability.**

Documentation Focus

ASSESSMENT/REASSESSMENT

- Baseline information, client's perception of need.
- Coping abilities and previous ways of dealing with life problems.

PLANNING

- Plan of care/interventions and who is involved in planning.
- Teaching plan.

IMPLEMENTATION/EVALUATION

- Client's responses to interventions/teaching and actions performed.
- Attainment/progress toward desired outcome(s).
- Modifications to plan of care.

DISCHARGE PLANNING

- Long-term needs and actions to be taken.
- Support systems available, specific referrals made, and who is responsible for actions to be taken.

SAMPLE NURSING OUTCOMES & INTERVENTIONS CLASSIFICATIONS (NOC/NIC)

NOC—Coping
NIC—Coping Enhancement

Death Syndrome, risk for sudden infant

Taxonomy II: Safety/Protection—Class 2 Physical Injury (00156)
[Diagnostic Division: Safety]
Submitted 2002

Definition: Presence of risk factors for sudden death of an infant under 1 year of age [Sudden Infant Death Syndrome (SIDS) is the sudden death of an infant under 1 year of age, which remains unexplained after a thorough case investigation, including performance of a complete autopsy, examination of the death scene, and review of the clinical history. SIDS is a subset of Sudden Unexpected Death in Infancy (SUDI) that is the sudden and unexpected death of an infant due to natural or unnatural causes.]

Risk Factors

MODIFIABLE

Delayed or nonattendance of prenatal care
Infants placed to sleep in the prone or side-lying position
Soft underlayment/loose articles in the sleep environment
Infant overheating/overwrapping
Prenatal and postnatal smoke exposure

POTENTIALLY MODIFIABLE

Young maternal age
Low birth weight; prematurity

Information that appears in brackets has been added by the authors to clarify and enhance the use of nursing diagnoses.

NONMODIFIABLE

Male gender
Ethnicity (e.g., African-American, Native-American race of mother)
Seasonality of SIDS deaths (higher in winter and fall months)
SIDS mortality peaks between infant aged 2 to 4 months

NOTE: A risk diagnosis is not evidenced by signs and symptoms, as the problem has not occurred and nursing interventions are directed at prevention.

Desired Outcomes/Evaluation Criteria—Client Will:

• Verbalize knowledge of modifiable factors that can be addressed.
• Make changes in environment to prevent death occurring from other factors.
• Follow medically recommended prenatal and postnatal care.

Actions/Interventions

NURSING PRIORITY NO. 1. To assess causative/contributing factors:

• Identify individual risk factors pertaining to situation. **Determines modifiable or potentially modifiable factors that can be addressed and treated. SIDS is the most common cause of death between 2 weeks and 1 year of age, with peak incidence occurring between the 2nd and 4th month.**
• Determine ethnicity, cultural background of family. **Although distribution is worldwide, African-American babies are twice as likely to die of SIDS and American-Indian babies are nearly three times more likely to die than white babies.**
• Note whether mother smoked during pregnancy or is currently smoking. **Smoking is known to negatively affect the fetus prenatally as well as after birth. Some reports indicate an increased risk of SIDS in babies of smoking mothers.**
• Assess extent of prenatal care and extent to which mother followed recommended care measures. **Prenatal care is important for all pregnancies to afford the optimal opportunity for all infants to have a healthy start to life.**
• Note use of alcohol or other drugs/medications during and after pregnancy **that may have a negative impact on the developing fetus. Enables management to minimize any damaging effects. (Note: Infants of American-Indian mothers who drank any amount of alcohol 3 months before conception through the first trimester had six times the risk of SIDS as those whose mothers did not drink.)**

NURSING PRIORITY NO. 2. To promote use of activities to mini-mize risk of SIDS:

- Recommend that baby be placed on his or her back to sleep, both at nighttime and naptime. **Research shows that fewer babies die of SIDS when they sleep on their backs.**
- Advise all caregivers of the infant regarding the importance of maintaining correct sleep position. **Anyone who will have responsibility for the care of the child during sleep needs to be reminded of the importance of the back sleep position.**
- Encourage parents to schedule awake tummy time with infant. **This activity promotes strengthening of back and neck muscles while parents are close and baby is not sleeping.**
- Encourage early and medically recommended prenatal care and continue with well-baby checkups and immunizations after birth. Include information about signs of premature labor and actions to be taken to avoid problems if possible. **Prematurity presents many problems for the newborn and keeping babies healthy prevents problems that could put the infant at risk for SIDS. Immunizing infants prevents many illnesses that can also be life threatening.**
- Encourage breastfeeding, if possible. Recommend sitting up in chair when nursing at night. **Breastfeeding has many advantages, immunological, nutritional, and psychosocial promoting a healthy infant. Although this does not preclude the occurrence of SIDS, healthy babies are less prone to many illnesses/problems. The risk of the mother falling asleep while feeding infant in bed with resultant accidental suffoca-tion has been shown to be of concern.**
- Discuss issues of bedsharing and the concerns regarding sudden and unexpected infant deaths from accidental entrap-ment under a sleeping adult or suffocation by becoming wedged in a couch or cushioned chair. **Bedsharing or putting infant to sleep in an unsafe situation results in dangerous sleep environments that place infants at substantial risk for SUDI or SIDS.**
- Note cultural beliefs about bedsharing. **Bedsharing is more common among breastfed infants and mothers who are young, unmarried, low income, or from a minority group. Additional study is needed to better understand bedsharing practices and its associated risks and benefits.**

NURSING PRIORITY NO. 3. To promote wellness (Teaching/Discharge Considerations):

- Discuss known facts about SIDS with parents. **Corrects misconceptions and helps reduce level of anxiety.**
- Avoid overdressing or overheating infants during sleep. **Infants dressed in two or more layers of clothes as they**

slept had six times the risk of SIDS as those dressed in fewer layers.
- Place the baby on a firm mattress in an approved crib. Avoiding soft mattresses, sofas, cushions, waterbeds, other soft surfaces, while not known to prevent SIDS, will minimize chance of suffocation/SUDI.
- Remove fluffy and loose bedding from sleep area making sure baby's head and face are not covered during sleep. Minimizes possibility of suffocation.
- Discuss the use of apnea monitors. Apnea monitors are not recommended to prevent SIDS but may be used to monitor other medical problems.
- Discourage frequent checking of the infant. This will not prevent the occurrence of SIDS and frequent checking only tires the parents and creates an atmosphere of tension and anxiety.
- Recommend public health nurse visit new mothers at least once or twice following discharge. Researchers found that American-Indian infants whose mothers received such visits were 80% less likely to die from SIDS than those who were never visited.
- Refer parents to local SIDS programs and encourage consultation with healthcare provider if baby shows any signs of illness or behaviors that concern them. Can provide information and support for risk reduction and correction of treatable problems. Healthcare providers will deal with illnesses, and so forth.

Documentation Focus

ASSESSMENT/REASSESSMENT

- Baseline findings, degree of parental anxiety/concern.

PLANNING

- Plan of care/interventions and who is involved in planning.
- Teaching plan.

IMPLEMENTATION/EVALUATION

- Parent's responses to interventions/teaching and actions performed.
- Attainment/progress toward desired outcome(s).
- Modifications to plan of care.

DISCHARGE PLANNING

- Long-term needs and actions to be taken.
- Support systems available, specific referrals made, and who is responsible for actions to be taken.

NOC—Risk Detection
NIC—Risk Identification

Denial, ineffective

Taxonomy II: Coping/Stress Tolerance—Class 2 Coping
Responses (00072)
[Diagnostic Division: Ego Integrity]
Submitted 1988

Definition: Conscious or unconscious attempt to
disavow the knowledge or meaning of an event to
reduce anxiety/fear, but leading to the detriment of
health

Related Factors

To be developed
[Personal vulnerability; unmet self-needs]
[Presence of overwhelming anxiety-producing feelings/situation; real-
ity factors that are consciously intolerable]
[Fear of consequences, negative past experiences]
[Learned response patterns, e.g., avoidance]
[Cultural factors, personal/family value systems]

Defining Characteristics

SUBJECTIVE

Minimizes symptoms; displaces source of symptoms to other organs
Unable to admit impact of disease on life pattern
Displaces fear of impact of the condition
Does not admit fear of death or invalidism

OBJECTIVE

Delays seeking or refuses healthcare attention to the detriment of
health
Does not perceive personal relevance of symptoms or danger
Makes dismissive gestures or comments when speaking of distressing
events
Displays inappropriate affect
Uses home remedies (self-treatment) to relieve symptoms

Desired Outcomes/Evaluation
Criteria—Client Will:

- Acknowledge reality of situation/illness.
- Express realistic concern/feelings about symptoms/illness.

Information that appears in brackets has been added by the authors
to clarify and enhance the use of nursing diagnoses.

- Seek appropriate assistance for presenting problem.
- Display appropriate affect.

Actions/Interventions

NURSING PRIORITY NO. 1. To assess causative/contributing factors:

- Identify situational crisis/problem and client's perception of the situation.
- Determine stage and degree of denial.
- Compare client's description of symptoms/conditions to reality of clinical picture.
- Note client's comments about impact of illness/problem on lifestyle.

NURSING PRIORITY NO. 2. To assist client to deal appropriately with situation:

- Develop trusting nurse-client relationship. Use therapeutic communication skills of Active-listening and I-messages.
- Provide safe, nonthreatening environment.
- Encourage expressions of feelings, accepting client's view of the situation without confrontation. Set limits on maladaptive behavior **to promote safety.**
- Present accurate information as appropriate, without insisting that the client accept what has been presented. **Avoids confrontation, which may further entrench client in denial.**
- Discuss client's behaviors in relation to illness (e.g., diabetes, alcoholism) and point out the results of these behaviors.
- Encourage client to talk with SO(s)/friends. **May clarify concerns and reduce isolation and withdrawal.**
- Involve in group sessions **so client can hear other views of reality and test own perceptions.**
- Avoid agreeing with inaccurate statements/perceptions **to prevent perpetuating false reality.**
- Provide positive feedback for constructive moves toward independence **to promote repetition of behavior.**

NURSING PRIORITY NO. 3. To promote wellness (Teaching/Discharge Considerations):

- Provide written information about illness/situation **for client and family to refer to as they consider options.**
- Involve family members/SO(s) in long-range planning for meeting individual needs.
- Refer to appropriate community resources (e.g., Diabetes Association, Multiple Sclerosis Society, Alcoholics Anonymous) **to help client with long-term adjustment.**
- Refer to ND Coping, ineffective.

Documentation Focus

ASSESSMENT/REASSESSMENT

- Assessment findings, degree of personal vulnerability/denial.
- Impact of illness/problem on lifestyle.

PLANNING

- Plan of care and who is involved in the planning.
- Teaching plan.

IMPLEMENTATION/EVALUATION

- Client's response to interventions/teaching and actions performed.
- Use of resources.
- Attainment/progress toward desired outcome(s).
- Modifications to plan of care.

DISCHARGE PLANNING

- Long-term needs and who is responsible for actions taken.
- Specific referrals made.

SAMPLE NURSING OUTCOMES & INTERVENTIONS CLASSIFICATIONS (NOC/NIC)

NOC—Acceptance: Health Status
NIC—Anxiety Reduction

Dentition, impaired

Taxonomy II: Safety/Protection—Class 2 Physical Injury (00048)
[Diagnostic Division: Food/Fluid]
Nursing Diagnosis Extension and Classification (NDEC) Submission 1998

Definition: Disruption in tooth development/eruption patterns or structural integrity of individual teeth

Related Factors

Dietary habits; nutritional deficits
Selected prescription medications; chronic use of tobacco, coffee or tea, red wine
Ineffective oral hygiene, sensitivity to heat or cold; chronic vomiting
Lack of knowledge regarding dental health; excessive use of abrasive cleaning agents/intake of fluorides
Barriers to self-care; access or economic barriers to professional care
Genetic predisposition; premature loss of primary teeth; bruxism
[Traumatic injury/surgical intervention]

Information that appears in brackets has been added by the authors to clarify and enhance the use of nursing diagnoses.

Defining Characteristics

SUBJECTIVE

Toothache

OBJECTIVE

Halitosis

Tooth enamel discoloration; erosion of enamel; excessive plaque

Worn down or abraded teeth; crown or root caries; tooth fracture(s); loose teeth; missing teeth or complete absence

Premature loss of primary teeth; incomplete eruption for age (may be primary or permanent teeth)

Excessive calculus

Malocclusion or tooth misalignment; asymmetrical facial expression

Desired Outcomes/Evaluation Criteria—Client Will:

- Display healthy gums, mucous membranes and teeth in good repair.
- Report adequate nutritional/fluid intake.
- Verbalize and demonstrate effective dental hygiene skills.
- Follow through on referrals for appropriate dental care.

Action/Interventions

NURSING PRIORITY NO. 1. To assess causative/contributing factors:

- Note presence/absence of teeth and/or dentures and ascertain its significance in terms of nutritional needs and aesthetics.
- Evaluate current status of dental hygiene and oral health.
- Document presence of factors affecting dentition (e.g., chronic use of tobacco, coffee, tea; bulimia/chronic vomiting; abscesses, tumors, braces, bruxism/chronic grinding of teeth) **to evaluate for possible interventions and/or treatment needs.**
- Note current factors impacting dental health (e.g., presence of ET intubation, facial fractures, chemotherapy) **that require special mouth care activities.**

NURSING PRIORITY NO. 2. To treat/manage dental care needs:

- Administer saline rinses, diluted alcohol-free mouthwashes.
- Provide gentle gum massage with soft toothbrush.
- Assist with/encourage brushing and flossing **when client is unable to do self-care.**
- Provide appropriate diet for optimal nutrition, considering client's ability to chew (e.g., liquids or soft foods).
- Increase fluids as needed **to enhance hydration and general well-being of oral mucous membranes.**
- Reposition ET tubes and airway adjuncts routinely, carefully

padding/protecting teeth/prosthetics. Suction with care when indicated.

- Avoid thermal stimuli when teeth are sensitive. Recommend use of specific toothpaste designed **to reduce sensitivity of teeth.**
- Document (photo) facial injuries before treatment **to provide "pictorial baseline" for future comparison/evaluation.**
- Maintain good jaw/facial alignment when fractures are present.
- Administer antibiotics as needed **to treat oral/gum infections.**
- Recommend use of analgesics and topical analgesics as needed **when dental pain is present.**
- Administer antibiotic therapy prior to dental procedures in susceptible individuals (e.g., prosthetic heart valve clients) and/or ascertain that bleeding disorders or coagulation deficits are not present **to prevent excess bleeding.**
- Refer to appropriate care providers (e.g., dental hygienists, dentists, oral surgeons, etc.).

NURSING PRIORITY NO. **3.** To promote wellness (Teaching/Discharge Considerations):

- Instruct client/caregiver in home-care interventions **to treat condition and/or prevent further complications.**
- Review resources that are needed for the client to perform adequate dental hygiene care (e.g., toothbrush/paste, clean water, referral to dental care providers, access to financial assistance, personal care assistant).
- Encourage cessation of tobacco, especially smokeless, enrolling in smoking-cessation classes.
- Discuss advisability of dental checkup and/or care prior to instituting chemotherapy or radiation **to minimize oral/dental/tissue damage.**

Documentation Focus

ASSESSMENT/REASSESSMENT

- Individual findings, including individual factors influencing dentition problems.
- Baseline photos/description of oral cavity/structures.

PLANNING

- Plan of care and who is involved in planning.
- Teaching plan.

IMPLEMENTATION/EVALUATION

- Responses to interventions/teaching and actions performed.
- Attainment/progress toward desired outcome(s).
- Modifications to plan of care.

DISCHARGE PLANNING

- Individual long-term needs, noting who is responsible for actions to be taken.
- Specific referrals made.

SAMPLE NURSING OUTCOMES
& INTERVENTIONS CLASSIFICATIONS (NOC/NIC)

NOC—Knowledge: Health
NIC—Oral Health Maintenance

Development, risk for delayed

Taxonomy II: Growth/Development—Class 2
Development (00112)
[Diagnostic Division: Teaching/Learning]
Nursing Diagnosis Extension and Classification (NDEC)
Submission 1998

Definition: At risk for delay of 25% or more in one or more of the areas of social or self-regulatory behavior, or cognitive, language, gross or fine motor skills

Risk Factors

PRENATAL

Maternal age <15 or >35 years
Unplanned or unwanted pregnancy; lack of, late, or poor prenatal care
Inadequate nutrition; poverty; illiteracy
Genetic or endocrine disorders; infections; substance abuse

INDIVIDUAL

Prematurity; congenital or genetic disorders
Vision/hearing impairment or frequent otitis media
Failure to thrive, inadequate nutrition; chronic illness
Brain damage (e.g., hemorrhage in postnatal period, shaken baby, abuse, accident); seizures
Positive drug screening test; substance abuse
Lead poisoning; chemotherapy; radiation therapy
Foster or adopted child
Behavior disorders
Technology dependent
Natural disaster

ENVIRONMENTAL

Poverty
Violence

Information that appears in brackets has been added by the authors to clarify and enhance the use of nursing diagnoses.

Mental retardation or severe learning disability
Abuse
Mental illness

> NOTE: A risk diagnosis is not evidenced by signs and symptoms, as the problem has not occurred and nursing interventions are directed at prevention.

Desired Outcomes/Evaluation Criteria—Client Will:

- Perform motor, social, self-regulatory behavior, cognitive and language skills appropriate for age within scope of present capabilities.

Caregiver Will

- Verbalize understanding of age-appropriate development/expectations
- Identify individual risk factors for developmental delay/deviation and plan(s) for prevention.

Actions/Interventions

NURSING PRIORITY NO. 1. To assess causative/contributing factors:

- Identify condition(s) that could contribute to developmental deviations; for example, prematurity, extremes of maternal age, substance abuse, brain injury/damage, chronic severe illness, mental illness, poverty, shaken baby syndrome, abuse, violence, failure to thrive, inadequate nutrition, (and/or others) as listed in Risk Factors.
- Ascertain nature of caregiver-required activities and abilities to perform needed activities.
- Note severity/pervasiveness of situation (e.g., potential for long-term stress leading to abuse/neglect versus situational disruption during period of crisis or transition).
- Evaluate environment in which long-term care will be provided.

NURSING PRIORITY NO. 2. To assist in preventing and/or limiting developmental delays:

- Avoid blame when discussing contributing factors. **Blame engenders negative feelings and does nothing to contribute to solution of the situation.**
- Note chronological age **to help determine developmental expectations.**
- Review expected skills/activities using authoritative text (e.g., Gesell, Musen/Congor) or assessment tools (e.g.,

Drawa-Person, Denver Developmental Screening Test, Bender's Visual Motor Gestalt test). **Provides guide for comparative measurement as child/individual progresses.**

- Consult professional resources (e.g., occupational/rehabilitation/speech therapists, special-education teacher, job counselor) **to formulate plan and address specific individual needs.**
- Encourage setting of short-term realistic goals for achieving developmental potential. **Small incremental steps are often easier to deal with.**
- Identify equipment needs (e.g., adaptive/growth-stimulating computer programs, communication devices).

NURSING PRIORITY NO. **3.** To promote wellness (Teaching/Discharge Considerations):

- Provide information regarding normal development, as appropriate, including pertinent reference materials.
- Encourage attendance at appropriate educational programs (e.g., parenting classes, infant stimulation sessions, seminars on life stresses, aging process).
- Identify available community resources as appropriate (e.g., early-intervention programs, seniors' activity/support groups, gifted and talented programs, sheltered workshop, crippled children's services, medical equipment/supplier). **Provides additional assistance to support family efforts in treatment program.**

Documentation Focus

ASSESSMENT/REASSESSMENT

- Assessment findings/individual needs including developmental level.
- Caregiver's understanding of situation and individual role.

PLANNING

- Plan of care and who is involved in the planning.
- Teaching plan.

IMPLEMENTATION/EVALUATION

- Client's response to interventions/teaching and actions performed.
- Caregiver response to teaching.
- Attainment/progress toward desired outcome(s).
- Modifications to plan of care.

DISCHARGE PLANNING

- Identified long-range needs and who is responsible for actions to be taken.

- Specific referrals made, sources for assistive devices, educational tools.

SAMPLE NURSING OUTCOMES & INTERVENTIONS CLASSIFICATIONS (NOC/NIC)

NOC—Child Development: [specify age]
NIC—Developmental Enhancement: Child

Diarrhea

Taxonomy II: Elimination—Class 2 Gastrointestinal System (0013)
[Diagnostic Division: Elimination]
Submitted 1975; Nursing Diagnosis Extension and Classification (NDEC) Revision 1998

Definition: Passage of loose, unformed stools

Related Factors

PSYCHOLOGICAL

High stress levels and anxiety

SITUATIONAL

Laxative/alcohol abuse; toxins; contaminants
Adverse effects of medications; radiation
Tube feedings
Travel

PHYSIOLOGICAL

Inflammation; irritation
Infectious processes; parasites
Malabsorption

Defining Characteristics

SUBJECTIVE

Abdominal pain
Urgency, cramping

OBJECTIVE

Hyperactive bowel sounds
At least three loose liquid stools per day

Desired Outcomes/Evaluation Criteria—Client Will:

- Reestablish and maintain normal pattern of bowel functioning.

Information that appears in brackets has been added by the authors to clarify and enhance the use of nursing diagnoses.

- Verbalize understanding of causative factors and rationale for treatment regimen.
- Demonstrate appropriate behavior to assist with resolution of causative factors (e.g., proper food preparation or avoidance of irritating foods).

Actions/Interventions

NURSING PRIORITY NO. 1. To assess causative factors/etiology:

- Ascertain onset and pattern of diarrhea, noting whether acute or chronic.
- Observe and record frequency, characteristics, amount, time of day, and precipitating factors related to occurrence of diarrhea.
- Note reports of pain associated with episodes.
- Auscultate abdomen **for presence, location, and characteristics of bowel sounds.**
- Observe for presence of associated factors, such as fever/chills, abdominal pain/cramping, emotional upset, physical exertion, and so forth.
- Evaluate diet history and note nutritional/fluid and electrolyte status.
- Review medications, noting side effects, possible interactions; note new prescriptions—particularly antibiotics, **which often cause changes in bowel habits, especially in children.**
- Determine recent exposure to different/foreign environments, change in drinking water/food intake, similar illness of others **that may help identify causative environmental factors.**
- Note history of recent gastrointestinal surgery; concurrent/ chronic illnesses/treatment; food/drug allergies, lactose intolerance.
- Review results of laboratory testing on stool specimens (for fat, blood, infections, etc.).
- Assess for fecal impaction **that may be accompanied by diarrhea.**

NURSING PRIORITY NO. 2. To eliminate causative factors:

- Restrict solid food intake as indicated **to allow for bowel rest/reduced intestinal workload.**
- Provide for changes in dietary intake **to avoid foods/substances that precipitate diarrhea.**
- Limit caffeine and high-fiber foods; avoid milk and fruits as appropriate.
- Adjust strength/rate of enteral tube feedings; change formula as indicated **when diarrhea is associated with tube feedings.**
- Recommend change in drug therapy as appropriate (e.g., choice of antacid).

- Promote the use of relaxation techniques (e.g., progressive relaxation exercise, visualization techniques) **to decrease stress/anxiety.**

NURSING PRIORITY NO. 3. To maintain hydration/electrolyte balance:

- Assess baseline hydration, note presence of postural hypotension, tachycardia, skin hydration/turgor, and condition of mucous membranes.
- Weigh infant's diapers **to determine amount of output and fluid replacement needs.**
- Review laboratory work for abnormalities.
- Administer antidiarrheal medications as indicated **to decrease gastrointestinal motility and minimize fluid losses.**
- Encourage oral intake of fluids containing electrolytes, such as juices, bouillon, or commercial preparations as appropriate.
- Administer enteral and IV fluids as indicated.

NURSING PRIORITY NO. 4. To maintain skin integrity:

- Assist as needed with pericare after each bowel movement.
- Provide prompt diaper change and gentle cleansing, because skin breakdown can occur quickly when diarrhea occurs.
- Apply lotion/ointment skin barrier as needed.
- Provide dry linen as necessary.
- Expose perineum/buttocks to air/use heat lamp if needed to keep area dry.
- Refer to ND Skin Integrity, impaired.

NURSING PRIORITY NO. 5. To promote return to normal bowel functioning:

- Increase oral fluid intake and return to normal diet as tolerated.
- Encourage intake of nonirritating liquids.
- Discuss possible change in infant formula. **Diarrhea may be result of/aggravated by intolerance to specific formula.**
- Recommend products such as natural fiber, plain natural yogurt, Lactinex **to restore normal bowel flora.**
- Give medications as ordered **to treat infectious process, decrease motility, and/or absorb water.**

NURSING PRIORITY NO. 6. To promote wellness (Teaching/ Discharge Considerations):

- Review causative factors and appropriate interventions **to prevent recurrence.**
- Evaluate and identify individual stress factors and coping behaviors.
- Review food preparation, emphasizing adequate cooking time and proper refrigeration/storage **to prevent bacterial growth/ contamination.**

- Discuss possibility of dehydration and the importance of fluid replacement.
- Respond to call for assistance promptly.
- Place bedpan in bed with client (if desired) or commode chair near bed **to provide quick access/reduce need to wait for assistance of others.**
- Provide privacy and psychologic support as necessary.
- Discuss use of incontinence pads **to protect bedding/furniture, depending on the severity of the problem.**

Documentation Focus

ASSESSMENT/REASSESSMENT

- Assessment findings, including characteristics/pattern of elimination.

PLANNING

- Plan of care and who is involved in planning.
- Teaching plan.

IMPLEMENTATION/EVALUATION

- Client's response to treatment/teaching and actions performed.
- Attainment/progress toward desired outcome(s).
- Modifications to plan of care.

DISCHARGE PLANNING

- Recommendations for follow-up care.

SAMPLE NURSING OUTCOMES & INTERVENTIONS CLASSIFICATIONS (NOC/NIC)

NOC—Bowel Elimination
NIC—Diarrhea Management

Disuse Syndrome, risk for

Taxonomy II: Activity/Rest—Class 2 Activity/Exercise (00040)
[Diagnostic Division: Activity/Rest]
Submitted 1988

Definition: At risk for deterioration of body systems as the result of prescribed or unavoidable musculoskeletal inactivity

Information that appears in brackets has been added by the authors to clarify and enhance the use of nursing diagnoses.

> NOTE: NANDA-identified complications from immobility can include pressure ulcers, constipation, stasis of pulmonary secretions, thrombosis, urinary tract infection/retention, decreased strength/endurance, orthostatic hypotension, decreased range of joint motion, disorientation, disturbed body image, and powerlessness.

Risk Factors

Severe pain, [chronic pain]
Paralysis, [other neuromuscular impairment]
Mechanical or prescribed immobilization
Altered level of consciousness
[Chronic physical or mental illness]

> NOTE: A risk diagnosis is not evidenced by signs and symptoms, as the problem has not occurred and nursing interventions are directed at prevention.

Desired Outcomes/Evaluation Criteria—Client Will:

- Display intact skin/tissues or achieve timely wound healing.
- Maintain/reestablish effective elimination patterns.
- Be free of signs/symptoms of infectious processes.
- Demonstrate adequate peripheral perfusion with stable vital signs, skin warm and dry, palpable peripheral pulses.
- Maintain usual reality orientation.
- Maintain/regain optimal level of cognitive, neurosensory, and musculoskeletal functioning.
- Express sense of control over the present situation and potential outcome.
- Recognize and incorporate change into self-concept in accurate manner without negative self-esteem.

Actions/Interventions

NURSING PRIORITY NO. 1. To evaluate probability of developing complications:

- Identify specific and potential concerns, including client's age, use of wheelchair, restraints. (**Ageist perspective of care provider may result in reluctance to engage in early mobilization of older client.**)
- Ascertain availability and use of support systems.
- Determine if client's condition is acute/short-term or whether it may be a long-term/permanent condition.
- Evaluate client's/family's understanding and ability to manage care for long period.

NURSING PRIORITY NO. 2. To identify individually appropriate preventive/corrective interventions:

SKIN

- Monitor skin over bony prominences.
- Reposition frequently as individually indicated **to relieve pressure.**
- Provide skin care daily and prn, drying well and using gentle massage and lotion to stimulate circulation.
- Initiate use of pressure-reducing devices (e.g., egg-crate/gel/water/air mattress or cushions).
- Review nutritional status and monitor nutritional intake.
- Provide/reinforce teaching regarding dietary needs, position changes, cleanliness.
- Refer to ND Skin or Tissue Integrity.

ELIMINATION

- Encourage balanced diet, including fruits and vegetables high in fiber and with adequate fluids **for optimal stool consistency and to facilitate passage through colon.** Include 8 oz/day of cranberry juice cocktail **to reduce risk of urinary infections.**
- Maximize mobility at earliest opportunity, using assistive devices as individually appropriate.
- Evaluate need for stool softeners, bulk-forming laxatives.
- Implement consistent bowel management/bladder training programs as indicated.
- Monitor urinary output/characteristics. Observe for signs of infection.
- Refer to NDs Constipation; Diarrhea; Bowel Incontinence; Urinary Elimination, impaired; Urinary Retention.

RESPIRATION

- Monitor breath sounds and characteristics of secretions **for early detection of complications** (e.g., pneumonia).
- Reposition, cough, deep-breathe on a regular schedule **to facilitate clearing of secretions/prevent atelectasis.**
- Suction as indicated **to clear airways.**
- Encourage use of incentive spirometry.
- Demonstrate techniques/assist with postural drainage.
- Assist with/instruct family and caregivers in quad coughing techniques/diaphragmatic weight training **to maximize ventilation in presence of spinal cord injury (SCI).**
- Discourage smoking. Involve in smoking-cessation program as indicated.
- Refer to NDs Airway Clearance/Breathing Pattern, ineffective.

VASCULAR (TISSUE PERFUSION)

- Determine core and skin temperature. Investigate development of cyanosis, changes in mentation **to identify changes in oxygenation status.**
- Routinely evaluate circulation/nerve function of affected body parts. Note changes in temperature, color, sensation, and movement.
- Institute peripheral vascular support measures (e.g., elastic hose, Ace wraps, sequential compression devices—SCDs) **to enhance venous return.**
- Monitor blood pressure before, during, and after activity— sitting, standing, and lying if possible **to ascertain response to/tolerance of activity.**
- Assist with position changes as needed. Raise head gradually. Institute use of tilt table where appropriate. **Injury may occur as a result of orthostatic hypotension.**
- Maintain proper body position; avoid use of constricting garments/restraints **to prevent vascular congestion.**
- Refer to NDs Tissue Perfusion, ineffective; Peripheral Neurovascular Dysfunction, risk for.

MUSCULOSKELETAL (MOBILITY/RANGE OF MOTION, STRENGTH/ENDURANCE)

- Perform range-of-motion (ROM) exercises and involve client in active exercises with physical/occupational therapy (e.g., muscle strengthening).
- Maximize involvement in self-care.
- Pace activities as possible to increase strength/endurance.
- Apply functional positioning splints as appropriate.
- Evaluate role of pain in mobility problem.
- Implement pain management program as individually indicated.
- Limit/monitor closely the use of restraints and immobilize client as little as possible. Remove restraints periodically and assist with ROM exercises.
- Refer to NDs Activity Intolerance; Mobility, impaired physical; Pain, acute; Pain, chronic.

SENSORY-PERCEPTION

- Orient client as necessary to time, place, person, and so forth. Provide cues for orientation (e.g., clock, calendar).
- Provide appropriate level of environmental stimulation (e.g., music, TV/radio, clock, calendar, personal possessions, visitors).
- Encourage participation in recreational/diversional activities and regular exercise program (as tolerated).

- Suggest use of sleep aids/usual presleep rituals to promote normal sleep/rest.
- Refer to NDs Sensory Perception, disturbed; Sleep Pattern, disturbed; Social Isolation; Diversional Activity, deficient.

SELF-ESTEEM, POWERLESSNESS

- Explain/review all care procedures.
- Provide for/assist with mutual goal setting, involving SO(s). Promotes sense of control and enhances commitment to goals.
- Provide consistency in caregivers whenever possible.
- Ascertain that client can communicate needs adequately (e.g., call light, writing tablet, picture/letter board, interpreter).
- Encourage verbalization of feelings/questions.
- Refer to NDs Powerlessness; Communication, impaired verbal; Self-Esteem [specify]; Role Performance, ineffective.

BODY IMAGE

- Orient to body changes through verbal description, written information; encourage looking at and discussing changes to promote acceptance.
- Promote interactions with peers and normalization of activities within individual abilities.
- Refer to NDs Body Image, disturbed; Self-Esteem, situational low; Social Isolation; Personal Identity, disturbed.

NURSING PRIORITY NO. 3. To promote wellness (Teaching/Discharge Considerations):

- Provide/review information about individual needs/areas of concern.
- Encourage involvement in regular exercise program, including isometric/isotonic activities, active or assistive ROM to limit consequences of disuse and maximize level of function.
- Review signs/symptoms requiring medical evaluation/follow-up to promote timely interventions.
- Identify community support services (e.g., financial, home maintenance, respite care, transportation).
- Refer to appropriate rehabilitation/home-care resources.
- Note sources for assistive devices/necessary equipment.

Documentation Focus

ASSESSMENT/REASSESSMENT

- Assessment findings, noting individual areas of concern, functional level, degree of independence, support systems/available resources.

PLANNING

- Plan of care and who is involved in planning.
- Teaching plan.

IMPLEMENTATION/EVALUATION

- Client's response to interventions/teaching and actions performed.
- Changes in level of functioning.
- Attainment/progress toward desired outcome(s).
- Modifications to plan of care.

DISCHARGE PLANNING

- Long-term needs and who is responsible for actions to be taken.
- Specific referrals made, resources for specific equipment needs.

SAMPLE NURSING OUTCOMES & INTERVENTIONS CLASSIFICATIONS (NOC/NIC)

NOC—Immobility Consequences: Physiological
NIC—Energy Management

Diversional Activity, deficient

Taxonomy II: Activity/Rest—Class 2 Activity/Exercise
(00097)
[Diagnostic Division: Activity/Rest]
Submitted 1980

Definition: Decreased stimulation from (or interest or engagement in) recreational or leisure activities [Note: Internal/external factors may or may not be beyond the individual's control.]

Related Factors

Environmental lack of diversional activity as in long-term hospitalization; frequent, lengthy treatments, [home-bound]
[Physical limitations, bedridden, fatigue, pain]
[Situational, developmental problem, lack of sources]
[Psychological condition, such as depression]

Defining Characteristics

SUBJECTIVE

Client's statement regarding the following:
Boredom; wish there were something to do, to read, and so on

Information that appears in brackets has been added by the authors to clarify and enhance the use of nursing diagnoses.

Usual hobbies cannot be undertaken in hospital [home or other care setting]

[Changes in abilities/physical limitations]

OBJECTIVE

[Flat affect; disinterest, inattentiveness]
[Restlessness; crying]
[Lethargy; withdrawal]
[Hostility]
[Overeating or lack of interest in eating; weight loss or gain]

Desired Outcomes/Evaluation Criteria—Client Will:

- Recognize own psychologic response (e.g., hopelessness and helplessness, anger, depression) and initiate appropriate coping actions.
- Engage in satisfying activities within personal limitations.

Actions/Interventions

NURSING PRIORITY NO. 1. To assess precipitating/etiologic factors:

- Validate reality of environmental deprivation.
- Note impact of disability/illness on lifestyle. Compare with previous/normal activity level.
- Determine ability to participate/interest in activities that are available. **Presence of depression, problems of mobility, protective isolation, or sensory deprivation may interfere with desired activity.**

NURSING PRIORITY NO. 2. To motivate and stimulate client involvement in solutions:

- Acknowledge reality of situation and feelings of the client **to establish therapeutic relationship.**
- Review history of activity/hobby preferences and possible modifications.
- Institute appropriate actions to deal with concomitant conditions, such as depression, immobility, and so forth.
- Provide for physical as well as mental diversional activities.
- Encourage mix of desired activities/stimuli (e.g., music; news program; educational presentations—TV/tapes, reading materials or "living" books; visitors; games; crafts; and hobbies interspersed with rest/quiet periods as appropriate). **Activities need to be personally meaningful for client to derive the most enjoyment.**
- Participate in decisions about timing and spacing of lengthy treatments to promote relaxation/reduce sense of boredom.
- Encourage client to assist in scheduling required and optional activity choices. For example, client may want to watch

favorite TV show at bathtime; if bath can be rescheduled later, **client's sense of control is enhanced.**

- Refrain from making changes in schedule without discussing with client. **It is important for staff to be responsible in making and following through on commitments to client.**
- Provide change of scenery (indoors and outdoors where possible).
- Identify requirements for mobility (wheelchair/walker/van/ volunteers, and the like).
- Provide for periodic changes in the personal environment when the client is confined. Use the individual's input in creating the changes (e.g., seasonal bulletin boards, color changes, rearranging furniture, pictures).
- Suggest activities, such as bird feeders/baths for bird-watching, a garden in a window box/terrarium, or a fish bowl/ aquarium, **to stimulate observation as well as involvement and participation in activity, such as identification of birds, choice of seeds, and so forth.**
- Accept hostile expressions while limiting aggressive acting-out behavior. (**Permission to express feelings of anger, hopelessness allows for beginning resolution. However, destructive behavior is counterproductive to self-esteem and problem solving.**)
- Involve occupational therapist as appropriate **to help identify and procure assistive devices and/or gear specific activities to individual situation.**

NURSING PRIORITY NO. 3. To promote wellness (Teaching/ Discharge Considerations):

- Explore options for useful activities using the person's strengths/abilities.
- Make appropriate referrals to available support groups, hobby clubs, service organizations.
- Refer to NDs Powerlessness; Social Isolation.

Documentation Focus

ASSESSMENT/REASSESSMENT

- Specific assessment findings, including blocks to desired activities.
- Individual choices for activities.

PLANNING

- Plan of care/interventions and who is involved in planning.

IMPLEMENTATION/EVALUATION

- Client's responses to interventions/teaching and actions performed.

- Attainment/progress toward desired outcome(s).
- Modifications to plan of care.

DISCHARGE PLANNING

- Long-term needs and who is responsible for actions to be taken.
- Referrals/community resources.

SAMPLE NURSING OUTCOMES & INTERVENTIONS CLASSIFICATIONS (NOC/NIC)

NOC—Leisure Participation
NIC—Recreation Therapy

Energy Field, disturbed

Taxonomy II: Activity/Rest—Class 3 Energy Balance
(00050)
[Diagnostic Division: Ego Integrity]
Submitted 1994

Definition: Disruption of the flow of energy [aura] surrounding a person's being that results in a disharmony of the body, mind, and/or spirit

Related Factors

To be developed
[Block in energy field]
[Depression]
[Increased state anxiety]
[Impaired immune system]
[Pain]

Defining Characteristics

OBJECTIVE

Temperature change (warmth/coolness)
Visual changes (image/color)
Disruption of the field (vacant/hold/spike/bulge)
Movement (wave/spike/tingling/dense/flowing)
Sounds (tone/words)

Desired Outcomes/Evaluation Criteria—Client Will:

- Acknowledge feelings of anxiety and distress.
- Verbalize sense of relaxation/well-being.
- Display reduction in severity/frequency of symptoms.

Information that appears in brackets has been added by the authors to clarify and enhance the use of nursing diagnoses.

Actions/Interventions

NURSING PRIORITY NO. 1. To determine causative/contributing factors:

- Develop therapeutic nurse-client relationship, initially accepting role of healer/guide as client desires.
- Provide opportunity for client to talk about illness, concerns, past history, emotional state, or other relevant information. Note body gestures, tone of voice, words chosen to express feelings/issues.
- Determine client's motivation/desire for treatment.
- Note use of medications, other drug use (e.g., alcohol).
- Use testing as indicated, such as the State-Trait Anxiety Inventory (STAI) or the Affect Balance Scale, **to provide measures of the client's anxiety.**

NURSING PRIORITY NO. 2. To evaluate energy field:

- Place client in sitting or supine position with legs/arms uncrossed. Place pillows or other supports **to enhance comfort and relaxation.**
- Center self physically and psychologically **to quiet mind and turn attention to the healing intent.**
- Move hands slowly over the client at level of 2 to 3 inches above skin **to assess state of energy field and flow of energy within the system.**
- Identify areas of imbalance or obstruction in the field (i.e., areas of asymmetry; feelings of heat/cold, tingling, congestion or pressure).

NURSING PRIORITY NO. 3. To provide therapeutic intervention:

- Explain the process of Therapeutic Touch (TT) and answer questions as indicated **to prevent unrealistic expectation. Fundamental focus of TT is on healing and wholeness, not curing signs/symptoms of disease.**
- Discuss findings of evaluation with client.
- Assist client with exercises **to promote "centering" and increase potential to self-heal, enhance comfort, reduce anxiety.**
- Perform unruffling process, keeping hands 2 to 3 inches from client's body **to dissipate impediments to free flow of energy within the system and between nurse and client.**
- Focus on areas of disturbance identified, holding hands over or on skin, and/or place one hand in back of body with other hand in front, **allows client's body to pull/repattern energy as needed**. At the same time, concentrate on the intent to help the client heal.
- Shorten duration of treatment as appropriate. **Children and elderly individuals are generally more sensitive to therapeutic intervention.**

- Make coaching suggestions in a soft voice **for enhancing feelings of relaxation** (e.g., pleasant images/other visualizations, deep breathing).
- Use hands-on massage/apply pressure to acupressure points as appropriate during process.
- Pay attention to changes in energy sensations as session progresses. Stop when the energy field is symmetric and there is a change to feelings of peaceful calm.
- Hold client's feet for a few minutes at end of session **to assist in "grounding" the body energy.**
- Provide client time for a period of peaceful rest following procedure.

NURSING PRIORITY NO. **4.** To promote wellness (Teaching/Discharge Considerations):

- Allow period of client dependency, as appropriate, **for client to strengthen own inner resources.**
- Encourage ongoing practice of the therapeutic process.
- Instruct in use of stress-reduction activities (e.g., centering/meditation, relaxation exercises) **to promote harmony between mind-body-spirit.**
- Discuss importance of integrating techniques into daily activity plan **for sustaining/enhancing sense of well-being.**
- Have client practice each step and demonstrate the complete TT process following the session as client displays readiness to assume responsibilities for self-healing.
- Promote attendance at a support group **where members can help each other practice and learn the techniques of TT.**
- Refer to other resources as identified (e.g., psychotherapy, clergy, medical treatment of disease processes, hospice) **for the individual to address total well-being/facilitate peaceful death.**

Documentation Focus

ASSESSMENT/REASSESSMENT

- Assessment findings, including characteristics and differences in the energy field.
- Client's perception of problem/need for treatment.

PLANNING

- Plan of care and who is involved in planning.
- Teaching plan.

IMPLEMENTATION/EVALUATION

- Changes in energy field.
- Client's response to interventions/teaching and actions performed.

- Attainment/progress toward desired outcomes.
- Modifications to plan of care.

DISCHARGE PLANNING

- Long-term needs and who is responsible for actions to be taken.
- Specific referrals made.

SAMPLE NURSING OUTCOMES
& INTERVENTIONS CLASSIFICATIONS (NOC/NIC)

NOC—Well-Being
NIC—Therapeutic Touch

Environmental Interpretation Syndrome, impaired

Taxonomy II: Perception/Cognition—Class 2 Orientation (00127)
[Diagnostic Division: Safety]
Submitted 1994

Definition: Consistent lack of orientation to person, place, time, or circumstances over more than 3 to 6 months, necessitating a protective environment

Related Factors

Dementia (Alzheimer's disease, multi-infarct dementia, Pick's disease, AIDS dementia)
Parkinson's disease
Huntington's disease
Depression
Alcoholism

Defining Characteristics

SUBJECTIVE

[Loss of occupation or social functioning from memory decline]

OBJECTIVE

Consistent disorientation in known and unknown environments
Chronic confusional states
Inability to follow simple directions, instructions
Inability to reason; to concentrate; slow in responding to questions
Loss of occupation or social functioning from memory decline

Information that appears in brackets has been added by the authors to clarify and enhance the use of nursing diagnoses.

Desired Outcomes/Evaluation Criteria—Client Will:

- Be free of harm.

Caregiver Will:

- Identify individual client safety concerns/needs.
- Modify activities/environment to provide for safety.

Actions/Interventions

NURSING PRIORITY NO. 1. To assess causative/precipitating factors:

- Discuss history and progression of condition. Note length of time since onset, future expectations, and incidents of injury/accidents.
- Review client's behavioral changes with SO(s) to note difficulties/problems, as well as additional impairments (e.g., decreased agility, reduced ROM of joints, loss of balance, decline in visual acuity).
- Identify potential environmental dangers and client's level of awareness (if any) of threat.
- Review results of cognitive screening tests.

NURSING PRIORITY NO. 2. To provide/promote safe environment:

- Provide consistent caregivers as much as possible.
- Include SO(s)/caregivers in planning process. **Enhances commitment to plan.**
- Identify previous/usual patterns for activities, such as sleeping, eating, self-care, and so on to include in plan of care.
- Promote and structure activities and rest periods.
- Limit number of decisions/choices client needs to make at one time **to conserve emotional energy.**
- Keep communication/questions simple. Use concrete terms.
- Limit number of visitors client interacts with at one time.
- Provide simple orientation measures, such as one-number calendar, holiday lights, and so on.
- Provide for safety/protection against hazards, such as to lock doors to unprotected areas/stairwells, discourage/supervise smoking, monitor ADLs (e.g., use of stove/sharp knives, choice of clothing in relation to environment/season), lock up medications/poisonous substances.
- Distract/redirect client's attention when behavior is agitated or dangerous.

- Use symbols instead of words when hearing/other impaired **to improve communication.**
- Use identity tags in clothes/belongings, bracelet/necklace **to provide identification if client wanders away/gets lost.**
- Incorporate information from results of cognitive testing into care planning.
- Refer to NDs Trauma, risk for; Confusion, chronic.

NURSING PRIORITY NO. **3.** To assist caregiver to deal with situation:

- Determine family's ability to care for client at home on an ongoing basis relative to individual responsibilities and availability.
- Discuss need for time for self away from client. (Refer to ND Caregiver Role Strain.)

NURSING PRIORITY NO. **4.** To promote wellness (Teaching/Discharge Considerations):

- Provide specific information about disease process/prognosis and client's particular needs.
- Discuss need for/appropriateness of genetic counseling for family members.
- Promote/plan for continuing care as appropriate. Identify resources for respite care needs.
- Refer to appropriate outside resources, such as adult day care, homemaker services, support groups. **Provides assistance, promotes problem solving.**

Documentation Focus

ASSESSMENT/REASSESSMENT

- Assessment findings, including degree of impairment.

PLANNING

- Plan of care and who is involved in planning.
- Teaching plan.

IMPLEMENTATION/EVALUATION

- Response to treatment plan/interventions and actions performed.
- Attainment/progress toward desired outcomes.
- Modifications to plan of care.

DISCHARGE PLANNING

- Long-range needs, who is responsible for actions to be taken.
- Specific referrals made.

SAMPLE NURSING OUTCOMES & INTERVENTIONS CLASSIFICATIONS (NOC/NIC)

NOC—Cognitive Ability
NIC—Reality Orientation

Failure to Thrive, adult

Taxonomy II: Growth/Development—Class 1 Growth
(00101)
[Diagnostic Division: Food/Fluid]
Submitted 1998

Definition: Progressive functional deterioration of a physical and cognitive nature. The individual's ability to live with multisystem diseases, cope with ensuing problems, and manage his or her care are remarkably diminished

Related Factors

Depression; apathy
Fatigue
[Major disease/degenerative condition]
[Aging process]

Defining Characteristics

SUBJECTIVE

States does not have an appetite, not hungry, or "I don't want to eat"
Expresses loss of interest in pleasurable outlets, such as food, sex, work, friends, family, hobbies, or entertainment
Difficulty performing simple self-care tasks
Altered mood state—expresses feelings of sadness, being low in spirit
Verbalizes desire for death

OBJECTIVE

Inadequate nutritional intake—eating less than body requirements; consumption of minimal to no food at most meals (i.e., consumes less than 75% of normal requirements); anorexia—does not eat meals when offered
Weight loss (decreased body mass from baseline weight)—5% unintentional weight loss in 1 month, 10% unintentional weight loss in 6 months
Physical decline (decline in bodily function)—evidence of fatigue, dehydration, incontinence of bowel and bladder
Cognitive decline (decline in mental processing)—as evidenced by problems with responding appropriately to environmental stimuli; demonstrates difficulty in reasoning, decision making, judgment, memory, concentration; decreased perception

---

Information that appears in brackets has been added by the authors to clarify and enhance the use of nursing diagnoses.

Apathy as evidenced by lack of observable feeling or emotion in terms of normal ADLs and environment

Decreased participation in ADLs that the older person once enjoyed; self-care deficit—no longer looks after or takes charge of physical cleanliness or appearance; neglects home environment and/or financial responsibilities

Decreased social skills/social withdrawal—noticeable decrease from usual past behavior in attempts to form or participate in cooperative and interdependent relationships (e.g., decreased verbal communication with staff, family, friends)

Frequent exacerbations of chronic health problems, such as pneumonia or urinary tract infections (UTIs)

Desired Outcomes/Evaluation Criteria—Client Will:

- Acknowledge presence of factors affecting well-being.
- Identify corrective/adaptive measures for individual situation.
- Demonstrate behaviors/lifestyle changes necessary to promote improved status.

Actions/Interventions

NURSING PRIORITY NO. **1.** To identify causative/contributing factors:

- Assess client's perception of factors leading to present condition, noting onset, duration, presence/absence of physical complaints, social withdrawal.
- Review with client previous and current life situations, including role changes, losses, and so on **to identify stressors affecting current situation.**
- Determine presence of malnutrition and factors contributing to failure to eat (e.g., chronic nausea, loss of appetite, no access to food or cooking, poorly fitting dentures, financial problems).
- Determine client's cognitive and perceptual status and effect on self-care ability.
- Evaluate level of adaptive behavior, knowledge, and skills about health maintenance, environment, and safety.
- Ascertain safety and effectiveness of home environment, persons providing care, and potential for/presence of neglectful/abusive situations.

NURSING PRIORITY NO. **2.** To assess degree of impairment:

- Perform physical and/or psychosocial assessment **to determine the extent of limitations affecting ability to thrive.**
- Active-listen client's/caregiver's perception of problem.
- Survey past and present availability/use of support systems.

NURSING PRIORITY NO. **3.** To assist client to achieve/maintain general well-being:

- Develop plan of action with client/caregiver to meet immediate needs (physical safety, hygiene, nutrition, emotional support) and assist in implementation of plan.
- Explore previously used successful coping skills and application to current situation. Refine/develop new strategies as appropriate.
- Assist client to develop goals for dealing with life/illness situation. Involve SO in long-range planning. **Promotes commitment to goals and plan, maximizing outcomes.**

NURSING PRIORITY NO. **4.** To promote wellness (Teaching/Discharge Considerations):

- Refer to other resources (e.g., social worker, occupational therapy, home care, assistive care, placement services, spiritual advisor). **Enhances coping, assists with problem solving, and may reduce risks to client and caregiver.**
- Promote socialization within individual limitations. **Provides additional stimulation, reduces sense of isolation.**
- Help client find a reason for living or begin to deal with end-of-life issues and provide support for grieving. **Enhances sense of control.**

Documentation Focus

ASSESSMENT/REASSESSMENT

- Individual findings, including current weight, dietary pattern, perceptions of self, food and eating, motivation for loss, support/feedback from SO(s).
- Ability to perform ADLs/participate in care, meet own needs.

PLANNING

- Plan of care/interventions and who is involved in planning.
- Teaching plan.

IMPLEMENTATION/EVALUATION

- Responses to interventions and actions performed, general well-being, weekly weight.
- Attainment/progress toward desired outcome(s).
- Modifications to plan of care.

DISCHARGE PLANNING

- Long-term needs and who is responsible for actions to be taken.
- Community resources/support groups.
- Specific referrals made.

SAMPLE NURSING OUTCOMES
& INTERVENTIONS CLASSIFICATIONS (NOC/NIC)

NOC—Will to Live
NIC—Mood Management

Falls, risk for

Taxonomy II: Safety/Protection—Class 2 Physical Injury
(00155)
[Diagnostic Division: Safety]
Submitted 2000

Definition: Increased susceptibility to falling that may
cause physical harm

Risk Factors

ADULTS

History of falls
Wheelchair use; use of assistive devices (e.g., walker, cane)
Age 65 or over; female (if elderly)
Lives alone
Lower limb prosthesis

PHYSIOLOGICAL

Presence of acute illness; postoperative conditions
Visual/hearing difficulties
Arthritis
Orthostatic hypotension; faintness when turning or extending
    neck
Sleeplessness
Anemias; vascular disease
Endoplasms (i.e., fatigue/limited mobility)
Urgency and/or incontinence; diarrhea
Postprandial blood sugar changes
Impaired physical mobility; foot problems; decreased lower extremity
    strength
Impaired balance; difficulty with gait; proprioceptive deficits (e.g.,
    unilateral neglect)
Neuropathy

COGNITIVE

Diminished mental status (e.g., confusion, delirium, dementia,
    impaired reality testing)
Medications; antihypertensive agents; ACE inhibitors; diuretics;
    tricyclic antidepressants; antianxiety agents; hypnotics or tranquil-
    izers
Alcohol use; narcotics

Information that appears in brackets has been added by the authors
to clarify and enhance the use of nursing diagnoses.

ENVIRONMENT

Restraints
Weather conditions (e.g., wet floors/ice)
Cluttered environment; throw/scatter rugs; no antislip material in bath and/or shower
Unfamiliar, dimly lit room

CHILDREN

2 years of age; male gender when <1 year of age
Lack of gate on stairs; window guards; auto restraints
Unattended infant on bed/changing table/sofa; bed located near window
Lack of parental supervision

NOTE: A risk diagnosis is not evidenced by signs and symptoms, as the problem has not occurred and nursing interventions are directed at prevention.

Desired Outcomes/Evaluation Criteria—Client/Caregivers Will:

- Verbalize understanding of individual risk factors that contribute to possibility of falls and take steps to correct situation(s).
- Demonstrate behaviors, lifestyle changes to reduce risk factors and protect self from injury.
- Modify environment as indicated to enhance safety.
- Be free of injury.

Actions/Interventions

NURSING PRIORITY NO. 1. To evaluate source/degree of risk:

- Note age and sex (child, young adult, elderly women are at greater risk).
- Evaluate developmental level, decision-making ability, level of cognition and competence. **Infants, young children, and elderly are at greatest risk because of developmental issues and weakness. Individuals with physical injuries or cognitive impairments are also at risk for falls caused by immobility, use of assistive aids, environmental hazards, or inability to recognize danger.**
- Assess muscle strength, gross and fine motor coordination. Note individual's general health status, determining what physical factors may affect safety, such as use of oxygen, chronic or debilitating conditions.
- Evaluate client's cognitive status. **Affects ability to perceive own limitations and risk for falling.**

- Assess mood, coping abilities, personality styles. **Individual's temperament, typical behavior, stressors and level of self-esteem can affect attitude toward safety issues, resulting in carelessness or increased risk-taking without consideration of consequences.**
- Ascertain knowledge of safety needs/injury prevention and motivation to prevent injury. **Client/caregivers may not be aware of proper precautions or may not have the knowledge, desire, or resources to attend to safety issues in all settings.**
- Note socioeconomic status/availability and use of resources in other circumstances. Can affect current coping abilities.

NURSING PRIORITY NO. 2. To assist client/caregiver to reduce or correct individual risk factors:

- Provide information regarding client's disease/condition(s) that may result in increased risk of falls.
- Identify needed interventions and safety devices **to promote safe environment and individual safety.**
- Review consequences of previously determined risk factors (e.g., falls caused by failure to make provisions for impairments caused by physical, cognitive, or environmental factors).
- Review medication regimen and how it affects client. Instruct in monitoring of effects/side effects. **Use of pain medications may contribute to weakness and confusion; multiple medications and combinations of medications affecting blood pressure or cardiac function may contribute to dizziness or loss of balance.**
- Discuss importance of monitoring conditions that contribute to occurrence of injury (e.g., fatigue, objects that block traffic patterns, lack of sufficient light, attempting tasks that are too difficult for present level of functioning, lack of ability to contact someone when help is needed).
- Determine caregiver's expectations of children, cognitively impaired and/or elderly family members and compare with actual abilities. **Reality of client's abilities and needs may be different than perception or desires of caregivers.**
- Discuss need for and sources of supervision (e.g., babysitters, before- and after-school programs, elderly day care, personal companions, etc.).
- Plan for home visit when appropriate. Determine that home safety issues are addressed, including supervision, access to emergency assistance, and client's ability to manage self care in the home. **May be needed to adequately determine client's needs and available resources.**
- Refer to physical or occupational therapist as appropriate.

May require exercises to improve strength or mobility, improve/relearn ambulation, or identify and obtain appropriate assistive devices for mobility, bathroom safety, or home modification.

NURSING PRIORITY NO. **3**. To promote wellness (Teaching/ Discharge Considerations):

- Refer to other resources as indicated. **Client/caregivers may need financial assistance, home modifications, referrals for counseling, homecare, sources for safety equipment, or placement in extended care facility.**
- Provide written resources **for later review/reinforcement of learning.**
- Promote education geared to increasing individual's awareness of safety measures and available resources.
- Promote community awareness about the problems of design of buildings, equipment, transportation, and workplace accidents that contribute to falls.
- Connect client/family with community resources, neighbors, friends to assist elderly/handicapped individuals in providing such things as structural maintenance, clearing of snow, gravel or ice from walks and steps, and so on.

Documentation Focus

ASSESSMENT/REASSESSMENT

- Individual risk factors noting current physical findings (e.g., bruises, cuts, anemia, and use of alcohol, drugs and prescription medications).
- Client's/caregiver's understanding of individual risks/safety concerns.

PLANNING

- Plan of care and who is involved in planning.
- Teaching plan.

IMPLEMENTATION/EVALUATION

- Individual responses to interventions/teaching and actions performed.
- Specific actions and changes that are made.
- Attainment/progress toward desired outcomes.
- Modifications to plan of care.

DISCHARGE PLANNING

- Long-range plans for discharge needs, lifestyle, home setting and community changes, and who is responsible for actions to be taken.
- Specific referrals made.

SAMPLE NURSING OUTCOMES & INTERVENTIONS CLASSIFICATIONS (NOC/NIC)

NOC—Safety Behavior: Fall Prevention
NIC—Fall Prevention

Family Processes, dysfunctional: alcoholism

Taxonomy II: Role Relationships—Class 2 Family Relationships (00063)
[Diagnostic Division: Social Interaction]
Submitted 1994

Definition: Psychosocial, spiritual, and physiological functions of the family unit are chronically disorganized, which leads to conflict, denial of problems, resistance to change, ineffective problem solving, and a series of self-perpetuating crises

Related Factors

Abuse of alcohol; resistance to treatment
Family history of alcoholism
Inadequate coping skills; addictive personality; lack of problem-solving skills
Biochemical influences; genetic predisposition

Defining Characteristics

SUBJECTIVE

Feelings
Anxiety/tension/distress; decreased self-esteem/worthlessness; lingering resentment
Anger/suppressed rage; frustration; shame/embarrassment; hurt; unhappiness; guilt
Emotional isolation/loneliness; powerlessness; insecurity; hopelessness; rejection
Responsibility for alcoholic's behavior; vulnerability; mistrust
Depression; hostility; fear; confusion; dissatisfaction; loss; repressed emotions
Being different from other people; misunderstood
Emotional control by others; being unloved; lack of identity
Abandonment; confused love and pity; moodiness; failure
Roles and Relationships
Family denial; deterioration in family relationships/disturbed family dynamics; ineffective spouse communication/marital problems; intimacy dysfunction
Altered role function/disruption of family roles; inconsistent parenting/low perception of parental support; chronic family problems

Information that appears in brackets has been added by the authors to clarify and enhance the use of nursing diagnoses.

Lack of skills necessary for relationships; lack of cohesiveness; disrupted family rituals

Family unable to meet security needs of its members

Pattern of rejection; economic problems; neglected obligations

OBJECTIVE

Roles and Relationships

Closed communication systems

Triangulating family relationships; reduced ability of family members to relate to each other for mutual growth and maturation

Family does not demonstrate respect for individuality and autonomy of its members

Behaviors

Expression of anger inappropriately; difficulty with intimate relationships; impaired communication; ineffective problem-solving skills; inability to meet emotional needs of its members; manipulation; dependency; criticizing; broken promises; rationalization/denial of problems

Refusal to get help/inability to accept and receive help appropriately; blaming

Loss of control of drinking; enabling to maintain drinking [substance use]; alcohol [substance] abuse; inadequate understanding or knowledge of alcoholism [substance abuse]

Inability to meet spiritual needs of its members

Inability to express or accept wide range of feelings; orientation toward tension relief rather than achievement of goals; escalating conflict

Lying; contradictory, paradoxical communication; lack of dealing with conflict; harsh self-judgment; isolation; difficulty having fun; self-blaming; unresolved grief

Controlling communication/power struggles; seeking approval and affirmation

Lack of reliability; disturbances in academic performance in children; disturbances in concentration; chaos; failure to accomplish current or past developmental tasks/difficulty with life-cycle transitions

Verbal abuse of spouse or parent; agitation; diminished physical contact

Family special occasions are alcohol-centered; nicotine addiction; inability to adapt to change; immaturity; stress-related physical illnesses; inability to deal with traumatic experiences constructively; substance abuse other than alcohol

Desired Outcomes/Evaluation Criteria—Family Will:

- Verbalize understanding of dynamics of codependence.
- Participate in individual/family treatment programs.
- Identify ineffective coping behaviors/consequences.
- Demonstrate/plan for necessary lifestyle changes.
- Take action to change self-destructive behaviors/alter behaviors that contribute to client's drinking/substance use.

Actions/Interventions

NURSING PRIORITY NO. 1. To assess contributing factors/underlying problem(s):

- Assess current level of functioning of family members.
- Ascertain family's understanding of current situation; note results of previous involvement in treatment.
- Review family history, explore roles of family members and circumstances involving substance use.
- Determine history of accidents/violent behaviors within family and safety issues.
- Discuss current/past methods of coping.
- Determine extent of enabling behaviors being evidenced by family members.
- Identify sabotage behaviors of family members. **Issues of secondary gain (conscious or unconscious) may impede recovery.**
- Note presence/extent of behaviors of family, client, and self that might be "too helpful," such as frequent requests for help, excuses for not following through on agreed-on behaviors, feelings of anger/irritation with others. **Enabling behaviors can complicate acceptance and resolution of problem.**

NURSING PRIORITY NO. 2. To assist family to change destructive behaviors:

- Mutually agree on behaviors/responsibilities for nurse and client. **Maximizes understanding of what is expected.**
- Confront and examine denial and sabotage behaviors used by family members. **Helps individuals move beyond blocks to recovery.**
- Discuss use of anger, rationalization, and/or projection and ways in which these interfere with problem resolution.
- Encourage family to deal with anger **to prevent escalation to violence.** Problem-solve concerns.
- Determine family strengths, areas for growth, individual/family successes.
- Remain nonjudgmental in approach to family members and to member who uses alcohol/drugs.
- Provide information regarding effects of addiction on mood/personality of the involved person. **Helps family members understand and cope with negative behaviors without being judgmental or reacting angrily.**
- Distinguish between destructive aspects of enabling behavior and genuine motivation to aid the user.
- Identify use of manipulative behaviors and discuss ways to avoid/prevent these situations.

NURSING PRIORITY NO. **3**. To promote wellness (Teaching/Discharge Considerations):

- Provide factual information to client/family about the effects of addictive behaviors on the family and what to expect after discharge.
- Provide information about enabling behavior, addictive disease characteristics for both user and nonuser who is codependent.
- Discuss importance of restructuring life activities, work/leisure relationships. **Previous lifestyle/relationships supported substance use requiring change to prevent relapse.**
- Encourage family to refocus celebrations excluding alcohol use **to reduce risk of relapse.**
- Provide support for family members; encourage participation in group work.
- Encourage involvement with/refer to self-help groups, Al-Anon, AlaTeen, Narcotics Anonymous, family therapy groups **to provide ongoing support and assist with problem solving.**
- Provide bibliotherapy as appropriate.
- In addition, refer to NDs Family Processes, interrupted; Coping, family: compromised/disabled as appropriate.

Documentation Focus

ASSESSMENT/REASSESSMENT

- Assessment findings, including history of substance(s) that have been used and family risk factors/safety concerns.
- Family composition and involvement.
- Results of prior treatment involvement.

PLANNING

- Plan of care and who is involved in planning.
- Teaching plan.

IMPLEMENTATION/EVALUATION

- Responses of family members to treatment/teaching and actions performed.
- Attainment/progress toward desired outcome(s).
- Modifications to plan of care.

DISCHARGE PLANNING

- Long-term needs, who is responsible for actions to be taken.
- Specific referrals made.

SAMPLE NURSING OUTCOMES
& INTERVENTIONS CLASSIFICATIONS (NOC/NIC)

NOC—Family Environment: Internal
NIC—Substance Use Treatment

Family Processes, interrupted

Taxonomy II: Role Relationships—Class 2 Family
Relationships (00060)
[Diagnostic Division: Social Interactions]
Submitted 1982; Nursing Diagnosis Extension and
Classification (NDEC) Revision 1998

Definition: Change in family relationships and/or functioning

Related Factors

Situational transition and/or crises [e.g., economic, change in roles,
    illness, trauma, disabling/expensive treatments]
Developmental transition and/or crises [e.g., loss or gain of a family
    member, adolescence, leaving home for college]
Shift in health status of a family member
Family roles shift; power shift of family members
Modification in family finances, family social status
Informal or formal interaction with community

Defining Characteristics

SUBJECTIVE

Changes in: power alliances; satisfaction with family; expressions of
    conflict within family; effectiveness in completing assigned tasks;
    stress-reduction behaviors; expressions of conflict with and/or isola-
    tion from community resources; somatic complaints
[Family expresses confusion about what to do; verbalizes they are
    having difficulty responding to change]

OBJECTIVE

Changes in: assigned tasks; participation in problem solving/decision
    making; communication patterns; mutual support; availability for
    emotional support/affective responsiveness and intimacy; patterns
    and rituals

Desired Outcomes/Evaluation
Criteria—Family Will:

- Express feelings freely and appropriately.
- Demonstrate individual involvement in problem-solving

Information that appears in brackets has been added by the authors
to clarify and enhance the use of nursing diagnoses.

processes directed at appropriate solutions for the situation/
crisis.
- Direct energies in a purposeful manner to plan for resolution
of the crisis.
- Verbalize understanding of illness/trauma, treatment regimen, and prognosis.
- Encourage and allow member who is ill to handle situation in
own way, progressing toward independence.

Actions/Interventions

NURSING PRIORITY NO. 1. To assess individual situation for
causative/contributing factors:

- Determine pathophysiology, illness/trauma, developmental
crisis present.
- Identify family developmental stage (e.g., marriage, birth of a
child, children leaving home).
- Note components of family: parent(s), children, male/female,
extended family available.
- Observe patterns of communication in this family. Are feelings expressed? Freely? Who talks to whom? Who makes
decisions? For whom? Who visits? When? What is the interaction between family members? (**Not only identifies weak-
ness/areas of concern to be addressed but also strengths that
can be used for resolution of problem.**)
- Assess boundaries of family members. Do members share
family identity and have little sense of individuality? Do they
seem emotionally distant, not connected with one another?
- Ascertain role expectations of family members. Who is the ill
member (e.g., nurturer, provider)? How does the illness affect
the roles of others?
- Determine "Family Rules." For example, adult concerns
(finances, illness, etc.) are kept from the children.
- Identify parenting skills and expectations.
- Note energy direction. Are efforts at resolution/problem solving purposeful or scattered?
- Listen for expressions of despair/helplessness (e.g., "I don't
know what to do") **to note degree of distress.**
- Note cultural and/or religious factors **that may affect percep-
tions/expectations of family members.**
- Assess support systems available outside of the family.

NURSING PRIORITY NO. 2. To assist family to deal with situa-
tion/crisis:

- Deal with family members in warm, caring, respectful way.
- Acknowledge difficulties and realities of the situation.
**Reinforces that some degree of conflict is to be expected and
can be used to promote growth.**

- Encourage expressions of anger. Avoid taking them personally. **Maintains boundaries between nurse and family.**
- Stress importance of continuous, open dialogue between family members **to facilitate ongoing problem solving.**
- Provide information as necessary, verbal and written. Reinforce as necessary.
- Assist family to identify and encourage their use of previously successful coping behaviors.
- Recommend contact by family members on a regular, frequent basis.
- Arrange for/encourage family participation in multidisciplinary team conference/group therapy as appropriate.
- Involve family in social support and community activities of their interest and choice.

NURSING PRIORITY NO. 3. To promote wellness (Teaching/ Discharge Considerations):

- Encourage use of stress-management techniques (e.g., appropriate expression of feelings, relaxation exercises).
- Provide educational materials and information **to assist family members in resolution of current crisis.**
- Refer to classes (e.g., Parent Effectiveness, specific disease/ disability support groups, self-help groups, clergy, psychologic counseling/family therapy) as indicated.
- Assist family to identify situations that may lead to fear/anxiety. (Refer to NDs Fear; Anxiety.)
- Involve family in planning for future and mutual goal setting. **Promotes commitment to goals/continuation of plan.**
- Identify community agencies (e.g., Meals on Wheels, visiting nurse, trauma support group, American Cancer Society, Veterans Administration) for both immediate and long-term support.

Documentation Focus

ASSESSMENT/REASSESSMENT

- Assessment findings, including family composition, developmental stage of family, and role expectations.
- Family communication patterns.

PLANNING

- Plan of care/interventions and who is involved in planning.
- Teaching plan.

IMPLEMENTATION/EVALUATION

- Each individual's response to interventions/teaching and actions performed.

- Attainment/progress toward desired outcome(s).
- Modifications to plan of care.

DISCHARGE PLANNING

- Long-range needs, noting who is responsible for actions to be taken.
- Specific referrals made.

SAMPLE NURSING OUTCOMES & INTERVENTIONS CLASSIFICATIONS (NOC/NIC)

NOC—Family Functioning
NIC—Family Process Maintenance

Family Processes, readiness for enhanced

Taxonomy II: Role Relationships—Class 2 Family Relationships (00159)
[Diagnostic Division: Social Interaction]
Submitted 2002

Definition: A pattern of family functioning that is sufficient to support the well-being of family members and can be strengthened

Defining Characteristics

SUBJECTIVE

Expresses willingness to enhance family dynamics
Communication is adequate
Relationships are generally positive; interdependent with community;
    family tasks are accomplished
Energy level of family supports activities of daily living
Family adapts to change

OBJECTIVE

Family functioning meets physical, social, and psychological needs of
    family members
Activities support the safety and growth of family members
Family roles are flexible and appropriate for developmental
    stages
Respect for family members is evident
Boundaries of family members are maintained
Family resilience is efficient
Balance exists between autonomy and cohesiveness

Information that appears in brackets has been added by the authors to clarify and enhance the use of nursing diagnoses.

Desired Outcomes/Evaluation Criteria—Client Will:

- Express feelings freely and appropriately.
- Verbalize understanding of desire for enhanced family dynamics.
- Demonstrate individual involvement in problem solving to improve family communications.
- Acknowledge awareness of boundaries of family members.

Actions/Interventions

NURSING PRIORITY NO. **1**. To determine current status of family:

- Assess family composition: parent(s), children, male/female, extended family. **Many family forms exist in society today, such as biological, nuclear, single-parent, stepfamily, communal, and same-sex couple or family. A better way to determine a family may be to determine the attribute of affection, strong emotional ties, a sense of belonging, and durability of membership.**
- Note participating members of family: parent(s), children, male/female, extended family. **Identifies members of family who need to be directly involved and taken into consideration in developing plan of care to improve family functioning.**
- Note stage of family development (e.g., single, young adult, newly married, family with young children, family with adolescents, grown children, later life). **Tasks may vary greatly among cultural groups, and this information provides a framework for developing plan to enhance family processes.**
- Observe patterns of communication in the family. Are feelings expressed: Freely? Who talks to whom? Who makes decisions? For Whom? Who visits? When? What is the interaction between family members? **Not only identifies weakness/areas of concern to be addressed but also strengths that can be used for planning improvement in family communication.**
- Assess boundaries of family members. Do members share family identity and have little sense of individuality? Do they seem emotionally connected with one another? **Individuals need to respect one another and boundaries need to be clear so family members are free to be responsible for themselves.**
- Identify 'family rules' that are accepted in the family. **Families interact in certain ways over time and develop patterns of behavior that are accepted as the way 'we behave' in this**

family. 'Functional families' rules are constructive and promote the needs of all family members.

● Note energy direction. Efforts at problem solving and resolution of different opinions may be purposeful or may be scattered and ineffective.

● Determine cultural and/or religious factors influencing family interactions. Expectations related to socioeconomic beliefs may be different in various cultures, for instance, traditional views of marriage and family life may be strongly influenced by Roman Catholicism in Italian-American and Latino-American families. In some cultures the father is considered the authority figure and the mother is the homemaker. These beliefs may be functional or dysfunctional in any given family and may even change with stressors/circumstances (e.g., financial, loss/gain of a family member, personal growth).

NURSING PRIORITY NO. 2. To assist the family to improve interactions:

● Establish nurse-family relationship. Promotes a warm, caring atmosphere in which family members can share thoughts, ideas, and feelings openly and nonjudgmentally.

● Acknowledge realities, and possible difficulties, of individual situation. Reinforces that some degree of conflict is to be expected in family interactions that can be used to promote growth.

● Stress importance of continuous, open dialogue between family members. Facilitates ongoing expression of open, honest feelings and opinions and effective problem solving.

● Assist family to identify and encourage use of previously successful coping behaviors. Promotes recognition of previous successes and confidence in own abilities to learn and improve family interactions.

● Acknowledge differences among family members with open dialogue about how these differences have occurred. Conveys an acceptance of these differences among individuals and helps to look at how they can be used to strengthen the family.

● Identify effective parenting skills already being used and suggest new ways of handling difficult behaviors. Allows individual family members to realize that some of what has been done already has been helpful and encourages them to learn new skills to manage family interactions in a more effective manner.

NURSING PRIORITY NO. 3. To promote optimum well-being:

● Discuss and encourage use and participation in stress-management techniques. **Relaxation exercises, visualization, and similar skills can be useful for promoting reduction of anxiety and ability to manage stress that occurs in their lives.**

- Encourage participation in learning role-reversal activities. **Helps individuals to gain insight and understanding of other person's feelings and point of view.**
- Involve family members in setting goals and planning for the future. **When individuals are involved in the decision making, they are more committed to carrying through a plan to enhance family interactions as life goes on.**
- Provide educational materials and information. **Enhances learning to assist in developing positive relationships among family members.**
- Assist family members to identify situations that may create problems and lead to fear/anxiety. **Thinking ahead can help individuals anticipate helpful actions to prevent conflict and untoward consequences.**
- Refer to classes/support groups as appropriate. **Family Effectiveness, self-help, psychology, religious affiliations can provide new information to assist family members to learn and apply to enhancing family interactions.**

Documentation Focus

ASSESSMENT/REASSESSMENT

- Assessment findings, including family composition, developmental stage of family, and role expectations.
- Family communication patterns.

PLANNING

- Plan of care/interventions and who is involved in planning.
- Educational plan.

IMPLEMENTATION/EVALUATION

- Each individual's response to interventions/teaching and actions performed.
- Attainment/progress toward desired outcome(s).
- Modifications to lifestyle/treatment plan.

DISCHARGE PLANNING

- Long-range needs, noting who is responsible for actions to be taken.
- Specific referrals made.

SAMPLE NURSING OUTCOMES
& INTERVENTIONS CLASSIFICATION (NOC/NIC)

NOC—Family Functioning
NIC—Family Process Maintenance

Fatigue

Taxonomy II: Activity/Rest—Class 3 Energy Balance
(00093)
[Diagnostic Division: Activity/Rest]
Submitted 1988; Nursing Diagnosis Extension and
Classification (NDEC) Revision 1998

Definition: An overwhelming sustained sense of
exhaustion and decreased capacity for physical and
mental work at usual level

Related Factors

PSYCHOLOGICAL

Stress; anxiety; boring lifestyle; depression

ENVIRONMENTAL

Noise; lights; humidity; temperature

SITUATIONAL

Occupation; negative life events

PHYSIOLOGICAL

Increased physical exertion; sleep deprivation
Pregnancy; disease states; malnutrition; anemia
Poor physical condition
[Altered body chemistry (e.g., medications, drug withdrawal,
chemotherapy)]

Defining Characteristics

SUBJECTIVE

Verbalization of an unremitting and overwhelming lack of energy;
inability to maintain usual routines/level of physical activity
Perceived need for additional energy to accomplish routine tasks;
increase in rest requirements
Tired; inability to restore energy even after sleep
Feelings of guilt for not keeping up with responsibilities
Compromised libido
Increase in physical complaints

Information that appears in brackets has been added by the authors
to clarify and enhance the use of nursing diagnoses.

OBJECTIVE

Lethargic or listless; drowsy
Compromised concentration
Disinterest in surroundings/introspection
Decreased performance, [accident-prone]

Fatigue

Desired Outcomes/Evaluation Criteria—Client Will:

- Report improved sense of energy.
- Identify basis of fatigue and individual areas of control.
- Perform ADLs and participate in desired activities at level of ability.
- Participate in recommended treatment program.

Actions/Interventions

NURSING PRIORITY NO. 1. To assess causative/contributing factors:

- Review medication regimen/use (e.g., beta blockers with fatigue as a side effect, cancer chemotherapy).
- Identify presence of physical and/or psychological disease states (e.g., multiple sclerosis, lupus, chronic pain, hepatitis, AIDS, major depressive disorder, anxiety states).
- Note stage of disease process, nutrition state, fluid balance.
- Determine ability to participate in activities/level of mobility.
- Assess presence/degree of sleep disturbances.
- Note lifestyle changes, expanded responsibilities/demands of others, job-related conflicts.
- Assess psychologic and personality factors that may affect reports of fatigue level.
- Note client's belief about what is causing the fatigue and what relieves it.
- Evaluate aspect of "learned helplessness" that may be manifested by giving up. **Can perpetuate a cycle of fatigue, impaired functioning, and increased anxiety and fatigue.**

NURSING PRIORITY NO. 2. To determine degree of fatigue/impact on life:

- Use a scale, such as Piper Fatigue Self-Report or Nail's General Fatigue Scale, as appropriate. **Can help determine manifestation, intensity, duration, and emotional meaning of fatigue.**
- Note daily energy patterns (i.e., peaks/valleys). **Helpful in determining pattern/timing of activity.**
- Discuss lifestyle changes/limitations imposed by fatigue state.
- Interview parent/care provider regarding specific changes

NURSING DIAGNOSES IN ALPHABETICAL ORDER **233**

observed in child/elder. (**These individuals may not be able to verbalize feelings or relate meaningful information.**)
- Review availability and current use of support systems/ resources.
- Evaluate need for individual assistance/assistive devices.
- Measure physiologic response to activity (e.g., changes in blood pressure or heart/respiratory rate).

NURSING PRIORITY NO. 3. To assist client to cope with fatigue and manage within individual limits of ability:

- Accept reality of client reports of fatigue and do not underestimate effect on quality of life the client experiences (**e.g., clients with MS are prone to more frequent/severe fatigue following minimal energy expenditure and require longer recovery period; post-polio clients often display a cumulative effect if they fail to pace themselves and rest when early signs of fatigue are encountered**).
- Establish realistic activity goals with client. **Enhances commitment to promoting optimal outcomes.**
- Plan care to allow individually adequate rest periods. Schedule activities for periods when client has the most energy **to maximize participation.**
- Involve client/SO(s) in schedule planning.
- Encourage client to do whatever possible (e.g., self-care, sit up in chair, walk). Increase activity level as tolerated.
- Instruct in methods to conserve energy (e.g., sit instead of stand during activities/shower; plan steps of activity before beginning so that all needed materials are at hand).
- Assist with self-care needs; keep bed in low position and travelways clear of furniture, assist with ambulation as indicated.
- Provide environment conducive to relief of fatigue. **Temperature and level of humidity are known to affect exhaustion (especially in clients with MS).**
- Provide diversional activities. Avoid overstimulation/understimulation (cognitive and sensory). **Impaired concentration can limit ability to block competing stimuli/distractions.**
- Discuss routines to promote restful sleep. (Refer to ND Sleep Pattern, disturbed.)
- Instruct in stress-management skills of visualization, relaxation, and biofeedback when appropriate.
- Refer to physical/occupational therapy for programmed daily exercises and activities **to maintain/increase strength and muscle tone and to enhance sense of well-being.**

NURSING PRIORITY NO. 4. To promote wellness (Teaching/ Discharge Considerations):

- Discuss therapy regimen relating to individual causative

factors (e.g., physical and/or psychological illnesses) and help client/SO(s) to understand relationship of fatigue to illness.

- Assist client/SO(s) to develop plan for activity and exercise within individual ability. Stress necessity of allowing sufficient time to finish activities.
- Instruct client in ways to monitor responses to activity and significant signs/symptoms **that indicate the need to alter activity level.**
- Promote overall health measures (e.g., nutrition, adequate fluid intake, appropriate vitamin/iron supplementation).
- Provide supplemental oxygen as indicated. **Presence of anemia/hypoxemia reduces oxygen available for cellular uptake and contributes to fatigue.**
- Encourage client to develop assertiveness skills, prioritizing goals/activities, learning to say "No." Discuss burnout syndrome when appropriate and actions client can take to change individual situation.
- Assist client to identify appropriate coping behaviors. **Promotes sense of control and improves self-esteem.**
- Identify support groups/community resources.
- Refer to counseling/psychotherapy as indicated.
- Obtain resources to assist with routine needs (e.g., Meals on Wheels, homemaker/housekeeper services, yard care).

Documentation Focus

ASSESSMENT/REASSESSMENT

- Manifestations of fatigue and other assessment findings.
- Degree of impairment/effect on lifestyle.
- Expectations of client/SO relative to individual abilities/ specific condition.

PLANNING

- Plan of care/interventions and who is involved in the planning.
- Teaching plan.

IMPLEMENTATION/EVALUATION

- Client's response to interventions/teaching and actions performed.
- Attainment/progress toward desired outcome(s).
- Modifications to plan of care.

DISCHARGE PLANNING

- Discharge needs/plan, actions to be taken, and who is responsible.
- Specific referrals made.

SAMPLE NURSING OUTCOMES
& INTERVENTIONS CLASSIFICATIONS (NOC/NIC)

NOC—Endurance
NIC—Energy Management

Fear [specify focus]

Taxonomy II: Coping/Stress Tolerance—Class 2 Coping
Responses (00148)
[Diagnostic Division: Ego Integrity]
Submitted 1980; Revised 2000

Definition: Response to perceived threat [real or imag-
ined] that is consciously recognized as a danger

Related Factors

Natural/innate origin (e.g., sudden noise, height, pain, loss of physical
   support); innate releasers (neurotransmitters); phobic stimulus
Learned response (e.g., conditioning, modeling from identification
   with others)
Unfamiliarity with environmental experiences
Separation from support system in potentially stressful situation (e.g.,
   hospitalization, hospital procedures [/treatments])
Language barrier; sensory impairment

Defining Characteristics

SUBJECTIVE

Cognitive: Identifies object of fear; stimulus believed to be a threat
Physiological: Anorexia, nausea, fatigue, dry mouth, [palpitations]
Apprehension; excitement; being scared; alarm; panic; terror; dread
Decreased self-assurance
Increased tension; jitteriness

OBJECTIVE

Cognitive: Diminished productivity, learning ability, problem solving
Behaviors: Increased alertness; avoidance[/flight] or attack behaviors;
   impulsiveness; narrowed focus on "it" (e.g., the focus of the fear)
Physiological: Increased pulse; vomiting; diarrhea; muscle tightness;
   increased respiratory rate and shortness of breath; increased systolic
   blood pressure; pallor; increased perspiration; pupil dilation

Desired Outcomes/Evaluation
Criteria—Client Will:

• Acknowledge and discuss fears, recognizing healthy versus
   unhealthy fears.

   Information that appears in brackets has been added by the authors
to clarify and enhance the use of nursing diagnoses.

- Verbalize accurate knowledge of/sense of safety related to current situation.
- Demonstrate understanding through use of effective coping behaviors (e.g., problem solving) and resources.
- Display appropriate range of feelings and lessened fear.

Actions/Interventions

NURSING PRIORITY NO. 1. To assess degree of fear and reality of threat perceived by the client:

- Ascertain client/SO(s) perception of what is occurring and how this affects life.
- Note degree of incapacitation (e.g., "frozen with fear," inability to engage in necessary activities).
- Compare verbal/nonverbal responses **to note congruencies or misperceptions of situation.**
- Be alert to signs of denial/depression.
- Identify sensory deficits that may be present, such as hearing impairment. Affects sensory reception and interpretation.
- Note degree of concentration, focus of attention.
- Investigate client's reports of subjective experiences (may be delusions/hallucinations).
- Be alert to and evaluate potential for violence.
- Measure vital signs/physiologic responses to situation.
- Assess family dynamics. (Refer to other NDs, such as Family Processes, interrupted; Coping, family: readiness for enhanced; Coping, family: compromised/disabled; Anxiety.)

NURSING PRIORITY NO. 2. To assist client/SO(s) in dealing with fear/situation:

- Stay with the client or make arrangements to have someone else be there. **Sense of abandonment can exacerbate fear.**
- Listen to, Active-listen client concerns.
- Provide information in verbal and written form. Speak in simple sentences and concrete terms. **Facilitates understanding and retention of information.**
- Acknowledge normalcy of fear, pain, despair, and give "permission" to express feelings appropriately/freely.
- Provide opportunity for questions and answer honestly. **Enhances sense of trust and nurse-client relationship.**
- Present objective information when available and allow client to use it freely. Avoid arguing about client's perceptions of the situation. **Limits conflicts when fear response may impair rational thinking.**
- Promote client control where possible and help client identify and accept those things over which control is not possible. **(Strengthens internal locus of control.)**

- Encourage contact with a peer who has successfully dealt with a similarly fearful situation. **Provides a role model, and client is more likely to believe others who have had similar experience(s).**

NURSING PRIORITY NO. 3. To assist client in learning to use own responses for problem solving:

- Acknowledge usefulness of fear for taking care of self.
- Identify client's responsibility for the solutions. (Reinforce that the nurse will be available for help.) **Enhances sense of control.**
- Determine internal/external resources for help (e.g., awareness/use of effective coping skills in the past; SOs who are available for support).
- Explain procedures within level of client's ability to understand and handle. (Be aware of how much information client wants **to prevent confusion/overload.**)
- Explain relationship between disease and symptoms if appropriate.
- Review use of antianxiety medications and reinforce use as prescribed.

NURSING PRIORITY NO. 4. To promote wellness (Teaching/ Discharge Considerations):

- Support planning for dealing with reality.
- Assist client to learn relaxation/visualization and guided imagery skills.
- Encourage and assist client to develop exercise program (within limits of ability). **Provides a healthy outlet for energy generated by feelings and promotes relaxation.**
- Provide for/deal with sensory deficits in appropriate manner (e.g., speak clearly and distinctly, use touch carefully as indicated by situation).
- Refer to support groups, community agencies/organizations as indicated. **Provides ongoing assistance for individual needs.**

Documentation Focus

ASSESSMENT/REASSESSMENT

- Assessment findings, noting individual factors contributing to current situation.
- Manifestations of fear.

PLANNING

- Plan of care and who is involved in the planning.
- Teaching plan.

IMPLEMENTATION/EVALUATION

- Client's responses to treatment plan/interventions and actions performed.
- Attainment/progress toward desired outcome(s).
- Modifications to plan of care.

DISCHARGE PLANNING

- Long-term needs and who is responsible for actions to be taken.
- Specific referrals made.

SAMPLE NURSING OUTCOMES & INTERVENTIONS CLASSIFICATIONS (NOC/NIC)

NOC—Anxiety Control
NIC—Anxiety Reduction

Fluid Balance, readiness for enhanced

Taxonomy II: Nutrition—Class 5 Hydration (00160)
[Diagnostic Division: Food/Fluid]
Submitted 2002

Definition: A pattern of equilibrium between fluid volume and chemical composition of body fluids that is sufficient for meeting physical needs and can be strengthened

Related Factors

To be developed

Defining Characteristics

SUBJECTIVE

Expresses willingness to enhance fluid balance
No excessive thirst

OBJECTIVE

Stable weight
Moist mucous membranes
Food and fluid intake adequate for daily needs
Straw-colored urine with specific gravity within normal limits
Good tissue turgor
Urine output appropriate for intake
No evidence of edema or dehydration

Information that appears in brackets has been added by the authors to clarify and enhance the use of nursing diagnoses.

Desired Outcome/Evaluation Criteria—Client Will:

- Maintain fluid volume at a functional level as indicated by adequate urinary output, stable vital signs, moist mucous membranes, good skin turgor.
- Demonstrate behaviors to monitor fluid balance.
- Be free of thirst.
- Be free of evidence of fluid overload (e.g., absence of edema and adventitious lung sounds).

Actions/Interventions

NURSING PRIORITY NO. **1.** To determine potential for fluid imbalance and ways that client is managing:

- Note presence of medical diagnoses with potential for fluid imbalance: (1) diagnoses/disease processes that may lead to deficits (e.g., diuretic therapy, hyperglycemia; ulcerative colitis, COPD, burns, cirrhosis of the liver, vomiting, diarrhea, hemorrhage; hot/humid climate, prolonged exercise; getting overheated/fever; diuretic effect of caffeine/alcohol); or (2) fluid excess (e.g., renal failure, cardiac failure, stroke, cerebral lesions, renal/adrenal insufficiency, psychogenic polydipsia, acute stress, surgical/anesthetic procedures, excessive or rapid infusion of IV fluids). **Body fluid balance is regulated by intake (food and fluid), output (kidney, gastrointestinal tract, skin, and lungs), and regulatory hormonal mechanisms. Balance is maintained within relatively narrow margin and can be easily disrupted by multiple factors.**
- Determine potential effects of age and developmental stage. **Elderly individuals have less body water than younger adults, decreased thirst response, and reduced effectiveness of compensatory mechanisms (e.g., kidneys are less efficient in conserving sodium and water). Infants and children have a relatively higher percentage of total body water and metabolic rate and are sometimes less able than adults to control their fluid intake.**
- Evaluate environmental factors that could impact fluid balance. **Persons with impaired mobility, diminished vision, or confined to bed cannot as easily meet their own needs and may be reluctant to ask for assistance. Persons whose work environment is restrictive or outside may also have greater challenges in meeting fluid needs.**
- Assess vital signs (e.g., temperature, blood pressure, heart rate), skin/mucous membrane moisture, and urine output. Weigh as indicated. **Predictors of fluid balance that should be in client's usual range in a healthy state.**

NURSING PRIORITY NO. **2.** To prevent occurrence of imbalance:

- Monitor I/O (e.g., frequency of voids/diaper changes) as appropriate, being aware of insensible losses (e.g., hot environment, use of oxygen/permanent tracheostomy) and "hidden sources" of intake (e.g., foods high in water content) **to ensure accurate picture of fluid status.**
- Weigh client and compare with recent weight history. **Provides baseline for future monitoring.**
- Establish and review with client individual fluid needs/replacement schedule. **Active participation in planning for own needs enhances likelihood of adhering to plan.**
- Encourage regular oral intake (e.g., fluids between meals, additional fluids during hot weather or when exercising) **to maximize intake and maintain fluid balance.**
- Distribute fluids over 24-hour period in presence of fluid restriction. **Prevents peaks/valleys in fluid level and associated thirst.**
- Administer/discuss judicious use of medications as indicated (e.g., antiemetics, antidiarrheals, antipyretics, and diuretics). **Medications may be indicated to prevent fluid imbalance if individual becomes sick.**

NURSING PRIORITY NO. **3.** To promote optimum wellness:

- Discuss client's individual conditions/factors that could cause occurrence of fluid imbalance as individually appropriate (such as prevention of hyperglycemic episodes) **so that client/SO can take corrective action.**
- Identify and instruct in ways to meet specific fluid needs (e.g., client could carry water bottle when going to sports events or measure specific 24-hour fluid portions if restrictions apply) **to manage fluid intake over time.**
- Recommend restriction of caffeine, alcohol as indicated. **Prevents untoward diuretic effect and possible dehydration.**
- Instruct client/SO(s) in how to measure and record I/O if needed for home management. **Provides means of monitoring status and adjusting therapy to meet changing needs.**
- Establish regular schedule for weighing. **To help monitor changes in fluid status.**
- Identify actions (if any) client may take to correct imbalance. **Encourages responsibility for self-care.**
- Review any dietary needs/restrictions and safe substitutes for salt as appropriate. **Helps prevent fluid retention/edema formation.**
- Review/instruct in medication regimen and administration and discuss potential for interactions/side effects that could disrupt fluid balance.

- Instruct in signs and symptoms indicating need for immediate/further evaluation and follow-up **to prevent complications and/or allow for early intervention.**

Documentation Focus

ASSESSMENT/REASSESSMENT

- Individual findings, including factors affecting ability to manage (regulate) body fluids.
- I/O, fluid balance, changes in weight, and vital signs.
- Results of diagnostic testing/laboratory studies.

PLANNING

- Plan of care and who is involved in the planning.
- Teaching plan.

IMPLEMENTATION/EVALUATION

- Client's responses to treatment/teaching and actions performed.
- Attainment/progress toward desired outcome(s).
- Modifications to plan of care.

DISCHARGE PLANNING

- Long-term needs, noting who is responsible for actions to be taken.
- Specific referrals made.

SAMPLE NURSING OUTCOMES & INTERVENTIONS CLASSIFICATIONS (NOC/NIC)

NOC—Fluid Balance
NIC   Fluid Monitoring

[Fluid Volume, deficient hyper/hypotonic]

NOTE: NANDA has restricted Fluid Volume, deficient to address only isotonic dehydration. For client needs related to dehydration associated with alterations in sodium, the authors have provided this second diagnostic category.
[Diagnostic Division: Food/Fluid]

Definition: [Decreased intravascular, interstitial, and/or intracellular fluid. This refers to dehydration with changes in sodium.]

Information that appears in brackets has been added by the authors to clarify and enhance the use of nursing diagnoses.

Related Factors

[Hypertonic dehydration: uncontrolled diabetes mellitus/insipidus, HHNC, increased intake of hypertonic fluids/IV therapy, inability to respond to thirst reflex/inadequate free water supplementation (high-osmolarity enteral feeding formulas), renal insufficiency/ failure]

[Hypotonic dehydration: chronic illness/malnutrition, excessive use of hypotonic IV solutions (e.g., D5W), renal insufficiency]

Defining Characteristics

SUBJECTIVE

[Reports of fatigue, nervousness, exhaustion]
[Thirst]

OBJECTIVE

[Increased urine output, dilute urine (initially) and/or decreased output/oliguria]
[Weight loss]
[Decreased venous filling]
[Hypotension (postural)]
[Increased pulse rate; decreased pulse volume and pressure]
[Decreased skin turgor]
[Change in mental status (e.g., confusion)]
[Increased body temperature]
[Dry skin/mucous membranes]
[Hemoconcentration; altered serum sodium]

Desired Outcomes/Evaluation Criteria—Client Will:

- Maintain fluid volume at a functional level as evidenced by individually adequate urinary output, stable vital signs, moist mucous membranes, good skin turgor.
- Verbalize understanding of causative factors and purpose of individual therapeutic interventions and medications.
- Demonstrate behaviors to monitor and correct deficit as indicated when condition is chronic.

Actions/Interventions

NURSING PRIORITY NO. 1. To assess causative/precipitating factors:

- Note possible medical diagnoses/disease processes that may lead to deficits (e.g., chronic renal failure with loss of sodium, diuretic therapy, increased respiratory losses secondary to acidosis, hyperglycemia).
- Determine effects of age. **(For example, elderly individuals often have a decreased thirst reflex and may not be aware of additional water needs.)**
- Evaluate nutritional status, noting current intake, weight

changes, problems with oral intake, use of supplements/tube feedings. Measure subcutaneous fat/muscle mass.

NURSING PRIORITY NO. 2. To evaluate degree of fluid deficit:

- Assess vital signs; note strength of peripheral pulses.
- Measure blood pressure (lying/sitting/standing) when possible and monitor invasive hemodynamic parameters as indicated (e.g., CVP, PAP/PCWP).
- Note presence of physical signs (e.g., dry mucous membranes, poor skin turgor, delayed capillary refill).
- Observe urinary output, color, and measure amount and specific gravity.
- Review laboratory data (e.g., Hb/Hct, electrolytes, total protein/albumin).

NURSING PRIORITY NO. 3. To correct/replace fluid losses to reverse pathophysiologic mechanisms:

- Establish 24-hour replacement needs and routes to be used (e.g., IV/PO). **Prevents peaks/valleys in fluid level.**
- Note client preferences concerning fluids and foods with high fluid content.
- Provide nutritious diet via appropriate route; give adequate free water with enteral feedings.
- Administer IV fluids as appropriate.
- Maintain accurate intake and output (I/O), calculate 24-hour fluid balance, and weigh daily.

NURSING PRIORITY NO. 4. To promote comfort and safety:

- Bathe less frequently using mild cleanser/soap and provide optimal skin care with suitable emollients **to maintain skin integrity and prevent excessive dryness.**
- Provide frequent oral care, eye care **to prevent injury from dryness.**
- Change position frequently.
- Provide for safety measures when client is confused.
- Replace electrolytes as ordered.
- Administer medications (e.g., insulin, antidiuretic hormone—ADH, vasopressin—Pitressin therapy) as indicated by contributing disease process.
- Correct acidosis (e.g., administration of sodium bicarbonate or changes in mechanical ventilation as appropriate).

NURSING PRIORITY NO. 5. To promote wellness (Teaching/Discharge Considerations):

- Discuss factors related to occurrence of deficit as individually appropriate.
- Identify and instruct in ways to meet specific nutritional needs.
- Instruct client/SO(s) in how to measure and record I/O.
- Identify actions (if any) client may take to correct deficiencies.

- Review/instruct in medication regimen and administration and interactions/side effects.
- Instruct in signs and symptoms indicating need for immediate/further evaluation and follow-up.

Documentation Focus

ASSESSMENT/REASSESSMENT

- Individual findings, including factors affecting ability to manage (regulate) body fluids and degree of deficit.
- I/O, fluid balance, changes in weight, urine specific gravity, and vital signs.
- Results of diagnostic testing/laboratory studies.

PLANNING

- Plan of care and who is involved in the planning.
- Teaching plan.

IMPLEMENTATION/EVALUATION

- Client's responses to treatment/teaching and actions performed.
- Attainment/progress toward desired outcome(s).
- Modifications to plan of care.

DISCHARGE PLANNING

- Long-term needs, noting who is responsible for actions to be taken.
- Specific referrals made.

SAMPLE NURSING OUTCOMES & INTERVENTIONS CLASSIFICATIONS (NOC/NIC)

NOC—Fluid Balance
NIC—Fluid/Electrolyte Management

Fluid Volume, deficient [isotonic]

NOTE: This diagnosis has been structured to address isotonic dehydration (hypovolemia) excluding states in which changes in sodium occur. For client needs related to dehydration associated with alterations in sodium, refer to Fluid Volume, deficient [hyper/hypotonic].

Taxonomy II: Nutrition—Class 5 Hydration (00027)
[Diagnostic Division: Food/Fluid]
Submitted 1978; Revised 1996

Definition: Decreased intravascular, interstitial, and/or intracellular fluid. This refers to dehydration, water loss alone without change in sodium

Information that appears in brackets has been added by the authors to clarify and enhance the use of nursing diagnoses.

Related Factors

Active fluid volume loss [e.g., hemorrhage, gastric intubation, diarrhea, wounds; abdominal cancer; burns, fistulas, ascites (third spacing); use of hyperosmotic radiopaque contrast agents]

Failure of regulatory mechanisms [e.g., fever/thermoregulatory response, renal tubule damage]

Defining Characteristics

SUBJECTIVE

Thirst
Weakness

OBJECTIVE

Decreased urine output; increased urine concentration
Decreased venous filling; decreased pulse volume/pressure
Sudden weight loss (except in third spacing)
Decreased BP; increased pulse rate/body temperature
Decreased skin/tongue turgor; dry skin/mucous membranes
Change in mental state
Elevated Hct

Desired Outcomes/Evaluation Criteria—Client Will:

- Maintain fluid volume at a functional level as evidenced by individually adequate urinary output with normal specific gravity, stable vital signs, moist mucous membranes, good skin turgor and prompt capillary refill, resolution of edema (e.g., ascites).
- Verbalize understanding of causative factors and purpose of individual therapeutic interventions and medications.
- Demonstrate behaviors to monitor and correct deficit as indicated.

Actions/Interventions

NURSING PRIORITY NO. 1. To assess causative/precipitating factors:

- Note possible diagnoses that may create a fluid volume deficit (e.g., ulcerative colitis, burns, cirrhosis of the liver, abdominal cancer); other factors, such as laryngectomy/tracheostomy tubes, drainage from wounds/fistulas or suction devices; water deprivation/fluid restrictions; decreased level of consciousness; vomiting, hemorrhage, dialysis; hot/humid climate, prolonged exercise; increased metabolic rate secondary to fever; increased caffeine/alcohol.
- Determine effects of age. (**Elderly individuals are at higher risk because of decreasing response/effectiveness of compensatory mechanisms [e.g., kidneys are less efficient in conserv-**

ing sodium and water]. Infants and children have a relatively high percentage of total body water, are sensitive to loss, and are less able to control their fluid intake.)

NURSING PRIORITY NO. 2. To evaluate degree of fluid deficit:

- Estimate traumatic/procedural fluid losses and note possible routes of insensible fluid losses.
- Assess vital signs; note strength of peripheral pulses.
- Note physical signs of dehydration (e.g., concentrated urine, dry mucous membranes, delayed capillary refill, poor skin turgor, confusion).
- Determine customary and current weight.
- Measure abdominal girth when ascites or third spacing of fluid occurs. Assess for peripheral edema formation.
- Review laboratory data (e.g., Hb/Hct, electrolytes, total protein/albumin, BUN/Cr).

NURSING PRIORITY NO. 3. To correct/replace losses to reverse pathophysiologic mechanisms:

- Stop blood loss (e.g., gastric lavage with room-temperature or cool saline solution, drug administration, prepare for surgical intervention).
- Establish 24-hour fluid replacement needs and routes to be used. **Prevents peaks/valleys in fluid level.**
- Note client preferences regarding fluids and foods with high fluid content.
- Keep fluids within client's reach and encourage frequent intake as appropriate.
- Administer IV fluids as indicated. Replace blood products/plasma expanders as ordered.
- Control humidity and ambient air temperature as appropriate, especially when major burns are present, or increase/decrease in presence of fever. Reduce bedding/clothes, provide tepid sponge bath. Assist with hypothermia when ordered **to reduce high fever and elevated metabolic rate.** (Refer to ND Hyperthermia.)
- Maintain accurate I/O and weigh daily. Monitor urine specific gravity.
- Monitor vital signs (lying/sitting/standing) and invasive hemodynamic parameters as indicated (e.g., CVP, PAP/PCWP).

NURSING PRIORITY NO. 4. To promote comfort and safety:

- Change position frequently.
- Bathe every other day, provide optimal skin care with emollients.
- Provide frequent oral care as well as eye care **to prevent injury from dryness.**

- Change dressings frequently/use adjunct appliances as indicated for draining wounds **to protect skin and monitor losses.**
- Provide for safety measures when client is confused.
- Administer medications (e.g., **antiemetics or antidiarrheals to limit gastric/intestinal losses; antipyretics to reduce fever**).
- Refer to ND Diarrhea.

NURSING PRIORITY NO. 5. To promote wellness (Teaching/Discharge Considerations):

- Discuss factors related to occurrence of dehydration.
- Assist client/SO(s) to learn to measure own I/O.
- Identify actions client may take to correct deficiencies.
- Recommend restriction of caffeine, alcohol as indicated.
- Review medications and interactions/side effects.
- Note signs/symptoms indicating need for emergent/further evaluation and follow-up.

Documentation Focus

ASSESSMENT/REASSESSMENT

- Assessment findings, including degree of deficit and current sources of fluid intake.
- I/O, fluid balance, changes in weight/edema, urine specific gravity, and vital signs.

PLANNING

- Plan of care and who is involved in planning.
- Teaching plan.

IMPLEMENTATION/EVALUATION

- Client's responses to interventions/teaching and actions performed.
- Attainment/progress toward desired outcome(s).
- Modifications to plan of care.

DISCHARGE PLANNING

- Long-term needs, plan for correction, and who is responsible for actions to be taken.
- Specific referrals made.

SAMPLE NURSING OUTCOMES & INTERVENTIONS CLASSIFICATIONS (NOC/NIC)

NOC—Hydration
NIC—Hypovolemia Management

Taxonomy II: Nutrition—Class 5 Hydration (00026)
[Diagnostic division: Food/Fluid]
Submitted 1982; Revised 1996

Definition: Increased isotonic fluid retention

Related Factors

Compromised regulatory mechanism [e.g., syndrome of inappropriate
antidiuretic hormone—SIADH—or decreased plasma proteins as
found in conditions such as malnutrition, draining fistulas, burns,
organ failure]
Excess fluid intake
Excess sodium intake
[Drug therapies, such as chlorpropamide, tolbutamide, vincristine,
triptylines, carbamazepine]

Defining Characteristics

SUBJECTIVE

Shortness of breath, orthopnea
Anxiety

OBJECTIVE

Edema, may progress to anasarca; weight gain over short period of
time
Intake exceeds output; oliguria
Abnormal breath sounds (rales or crackles), changes in respiratory
pattern, dyspnea
Increased CVP; jugular vein distention; positive hepatojugular reflex
S3 heart sound
Pulmonary congestion, pleural effusion, pulmonary artery pressure
changes; BP changes
Change in mental status; restlessness
Specific gravity changes
Decreased Hb/Hct, azotemia, altered electrolytes

Desired Outcomes/Evaluation Criteria—Client Will:

• Stabilize fluid volume as evidenced by balanced I/O, vital
signs within client's normal limits, stable weight, and free of
signs of edema.
• Verbalize understanding of individual dietary/fluid restrictions.
• Demonstrate behaviors to monitor fluid status and reduce
recurrence of fluid excess.
• List signs that require further evaluation.

Information that appears in brackets has been added by the authors
to clarify and enhance the use of nursing diagnoses.

Actions/Interventions

NURSING PRIORITY NO. **1.** To assess causative/precipitating factors:

- Be aware of risk factors (e.g., cardiac failure, cerebral lesions, renal/adrenal insufficiency, psychogenic polydipsia, acute stress, surgical/anesthetic procedures, excessive or rapid infusion of IV fluids, decrease or loss of serum proteins).
- Note amount/rate of fluid intake from all sources: PO, IV, ventilator, and so forth.
- Review intake of sodium (dietary, drug, IV) and protein.

NURSING PRIORITY NO. **2.** To evaluate degree of excess:

- Compare current weight with admission and/or previously stated weight.
- Measure vital signs and invasive hemodynamic parameters (e.g., CVP, PAP/PCWP) if available.
- Auscultate breath sounds **for presence of crackles/congestion.**
- Record occurrence of dyspnea (exertional, nocturnal, and so on).
- Auscultate heart tones for S3, **ventricular gallop.**
- Assess for presence of neck vein distention/hepatojugular reflux.
- Note presence of edema (puffy eyelids, dependent swelling ankles/feet if ambulatory or up in chair; sacrum and posterior thighs when recumbent), anasarca.
- Measure abdominal **girth for changes that may indicate increasing fluid retention/edema.**
- Note patterns and amount of urination (e.g., nocturia, oliguria).
- Evaluate mentation **for confusion, personality changes.**
- Assess neuromuscular reflexes.
- Assess appetite; note presence of nausea/vomiting.
- Observe skin and mucous membranes (**prone to decubitus/ ulceration**).
- Note fever (**at increased risk of infection**).
- Review laboratory data (e.g., BUN/Cr, Hb/Hct, serum albumin, proteins, and electrolytes; urine specific gravity/osmolality/sodium excretion) and chest x-ray.

NURSING PRIORITY NO. **3.** To promote mobilization/elimination of excess fluid:

- Restrict sodium and fluid intake as indicated.
- Record I/O accurately; calculate fluid balance (plus/minus).
- Set an appropriate rate of fluid intake/infusion throughout 24-hour period **to prevent peaks/valleys in fluid level.**
- Weigh daily or on a regular schedule as indicated. **Provides a comparative baseline.**

- Administer medications (e.g., diuretics, cardiotonics, steroid replacement, plasma or albumin volume expanders).
- Evaluate edematous extremities, change position frequently **to reduce tissue pressure and risk of skin breakdown.**
- Place in semi-Fowler's position as appropriate **to facilitate movement of diaphragm improving respiratory effort.**
- Promote early mobility.
- Provide quiet environment, limiting external stimuli.
- Use safety precautions if confused/debilitated.
- Assist with procedures as indicated (e.g., thoracentesis, dialysis).

NURSING PRIORITY NO. 4. To maintain integrity of skin and oral mucous membranes:

- Refer to NDs Skin Integrity, impaired/risk for impaired and Oral Mucous Membrane, impaired.

NURSING PRIORITY NO. 5. To promote wellness (Teaching/ Discharge Considerations):

- Review dietary restrictions and safe substitutes for salt (e.g., lemon juice or spices, such as oregano).
- Discuss importance of fluid restrictions and "hidden sources" of intake (such as foods high in water content).
- Instruct client/family in use of voiding record, I/O.
- Consult dietitian as needed.
- Suggest interventions, such as frequent oral care, chewing gum/hard candy, use of lip balm, **to reduce discomforts of fluid restrictions.**
- Review drug regimen/side effects.
- Stress need for mobility and/or frequent position changes **to prevent stasis and reduce risk of tissue injury.**
- Identify "danger" signs requiring notification of healthcare provider **to ensure timely evaluation/intervention.**

Documentation Focus

ASSESSMENT/REASSESSMENT

- Assessment findings, noting existing conditions contributing to and degree of fluid retention (vital signs, amount, presence and location of edema, and weight changes).
- I/O, fluid balance.

PLANNING

- Plan of care and who is involved in the planning.
- Teaching plan.

IMPLEMENTATION/EVALUATION

- Response to interventions/teaching and actions performed.

- Attainment/progress toward desired outcome(s).
- Modifications to plan of care.

DISCHARGE PLANNING

- Long-range needs, noting who is responsible for actions to be taken.

SAMPLE NURSING OUTCOMES & INTERVENTIONS CLASSIFICATIONS (NOC/NIC)

NOC—Fluid Balance
NIC—Hypervolemia Management

Fluid Volume, risk for deficient

Taxonomy II: Nutrition—Class 5 Hydration (00028)
[Diagnostic Division: Food/Fluid]
Submitted 1978

Definition: At risk for experiencing vascular, cellular, or intracellular dehydration

Risk Factors

Extremes of age and weight
Loss of fluid through abnormal routes (e.g., indwelling tubes)
Knowledge deficiency related to fluid volume
Factors influencing fluid needs (e.g., hypermetabolic states)
Medications (e.g., diuretics)
Excessive losses through normal routes (e.g., diarrhea)
Deviations affecting access, intake, or absorption of fluids (e.g., physical immobility)

NOTE: A risk diagnosis is not evidenced by signs and symptoms, as the problem has not occurred and nursing interventions are directed at prevention.

Desired Outcomes/Evaluation Criteria—Client Will:

- Identify individual risk factors and appropriate interventions.
- Demonstrate behaviors or lifestyle changes to prevent development of fluid volume deficit.

Actions/Interventions

NURSING PRIORITY NO. 1. To assess causative/contributing factors:

- Note client's age, level of consciousness/mentation.

Information that appears in brackets has been added by the authors to clarify and enhance the use of nursing diagnoses.

- Assess other etiologic factors present (e.g., availability of fluids, mobility, presence of fever).

NURSING PRIORITY NO. 2. To prevent occurrence of deficit:

- Weigh client and compare with recent weight history.
- Establish individual fluid needs/replacement schedule.
- Encourage oral intake (e.g., offer fluids between meals, provide water with drinking straw) **to maximize intake.**
- Provide supplemental fluids (tube feed, IV) as indicated. Distribute fluids over 24-hour period. **Prevents peaks/valleys in fluid level.**
- Monitor I/O balance being aware of insensible losses **to ensure accurate picture of fluid status.**
- Perform serial weights **to note trends.**
- Note changes in vital signs (e.g., orthostatic hypotension, tachycardia, fever).
- Assess skin turgor/oral mucous membranes.
- Review laboratory data (e.g., Hb/Hct, electrolytes, BUN/Cr).
- Administer medications as indicated (e.g., antiemetics, antidiarrheals, antipyretics).

NURSING PRIORITY NO. 3. To promote wellness (Teaching/Discharge Considerations):

- Discuss individual risk factors/potential problems and specific interventions.
- Review appropriate use of medication.
- Encourage client to maintain diary of food/fluid intake; number and amount of voidings and stools, and so forth.
- Refer to NDs [Fluid Volume, deficient hyper/hypotonic] or [isotonic].

Documentation Focus

ASSESSMENT/REASSESSMENT

- Individual findings, including individual factors influencing fluid needs/requirements.
- Baseline weight, vital signs.
- Specific client preferences for fluids.

PLANNING

- Plan of care and who is involved in planning.
- Teaching plan.

IMPLEMENTATION/EVALUATION

- Responses to interventions/teaching and actions performed.
- Attainment/progress toward desired outcome(s).
- Modifications to plan of care.

DISCHARGE PLANNING

* Individual long-term needs, noting who is responsible for actions to be taken.
* Specific referrals made.

SAMPLE NURSING OUTCOMES & INTERVENTIONS CLASSIFICATIONS (NOC/NIC)

NOC—Fluid Balance
NIC—Fluid Monitoring

Fluid Volume, risk for imbalanced

Taxonomy II: Nutrition—Class 5 Hydration (00025)
[Diagnostic Division: Food/Fluid]
Submitted 1998

Definition: At risk for a decrease, an increase, or a rapid shift from one to the other of intravascular, interstitial, and/or intracellular fluid. This refers to body fluid loss, gain, or both

Risk Factors

Scheduled for major invasive procedures
[Rapid/sustained loss, (e.g., hemorrhage, burns, fistulas)]
[Rapid fluid replacement]
Other risk factors to be determined

> NOTE: A risk diagnosis is not evidenced by signs and symptoms, as the problem has not occurred and nursing interventions are directed at prevention.

Desired Outcomes/Evaluation Criteria—Client Will:

* Demonstrate adequate fluid balance as evidenced by stable vital signs, palpable pulses/good quality, normal skin turgor, moist mucous membranes; individual appropriate urinary output; lack of excessive weight fluctuation (loss/gain), and no edema present.

Actions/Interventions

NURSING PRIORITY NO. **1.** To determine causative/contributing factors:

* Note potential sources of fluid loss/intake; presence of conditions, such as diabetes insipidus, hyperosmolar nonketotic

---

Information that appears in brackets has been added by the authors to clarify and enhance the use of nursing diagnoses.

syndrome; need for major invasive procedures, medications (e.g., diuretics); use of IV fluids and delivery device, administration of total parenteral nutrition (TPN).

- Note client's age, current level of hydration, and mentation. **Provides information regarding ability to tolerate fluctuations in fluid level and risk for creating or failing to respond to problem (e.g., confused client may have inadequate intake, disconnect tubings, or readjust IV flow rate).**

NURSING PRIORITY NO. 2. To prevent fluctuations/imbalances in fluid levels:

- Measure and record I/O. Monitor urine output (hourly as needed), noting amount, color, time of day, diuresis.
- Note presence of vomiting, liquid stool; inspect dressing(s), drainage devices **to include losses in output calculations.**
- Calculate fluid balance (intake > output or output > intake).
- Auscultate BP, calculate pulse pressure. (**PP widens before systolic BP drops in response to fluid loss.**)
- Monitor BP responses to activities (e.g., **BP/heart and respiratory rate often increases when either fluid deficit or excess is present**).
- Weigh daily or as indicated and evaluate changes **as they relate to fluid status.**
- Assess for clinical signs of dehydration (hypotension, dry skin/mucous membranes, delayed capillary refill) or fluid excess (e.g., peripheral/dependent edema, adventitious breath sounds, distended neck veins).
- Note increased lethargy, hypotension, muscle cramping. (**Electrolyte imbalances may be present.**)
- Review laboratory data, chest x-ray **to determine changes indicative of electrolyte and/or fluid imbalance.**
- Establish fluid oral intake, incorporating beverage preferences when possible.
- Maintain fluid/sodium restrictions when needed.
- Administer IV fluids as prescribed using infusion pumps **to promote fluid management.**
- Tape tubing connections longitudinally **to reduce risk of disconnection and loss of fluids.**
- Administer diuretics, antiemetics, as prescribed.
- Assist with rotating tourniquet phlebotomy, dialysis, or ultra-filtration **to correct fluid overload situation.**

NURSING PRIORITY NO. 3. To promote wellness (Teaching/ Discharge Considerations):

- Discuss individual risk factors/potential problems and specific interventions.
- Instruct client/SO in how to measure and record I/O as appropriate.

- Review/instruct in medication/TPN regimen.
- Identify signs and symptoms indicating need for prompt evaluation/follow-up.

Documentation Focus

ASSESSMENT/REASSESSMENT

- Individual findings, including individual factors influencing fluid needs/requirements.
- Baseline weight, vital signs.
- Specific client preferences for fluids.

PLANNING

- Plan of care and who is involved in planning.
- Teaching plan.

IMPLEMENTATION/EVALUATION

- Responses to interventions/teaching and actions performed.
- Attainment/progress toward desired outcome(s).
- Modifications to plan of care.

DISCHARGE PLANNING

- Individual long-term needs, noting who is responsible for actions to be taken.
- Specific referrals made.

SAMPLE NURSING OUTCOMES
& INTERVENTIONS CLASSIFICATIONS (NOC/NIC)

NOC—Fluid Balance
NIC—Fluid Monitoring

Gas Exchange, impaired

Taxonomy II: Elimination—Class 4 Pulmonary System (00030)
[Diagnostic Division: Respiration]
Submitted 1980; Revised 1996, Nursing Diagnosis Extension and Classification (NDEC) Revision 1998

Definition: Excess or deficit in oxygenation and/or carbon dioxide elimination at the alveoli-capillary membrane [This may be an entity of its own but also may be an end result of other pathology with an interrelatedness between airway clearance and/or breathing pattern problems.]

Information that appears in brackets has been added by the authors to clarify and enhance the use of nursing diagnoses.

Related Factors

Ventilation perfusion imbalance [as in the following: altered blood flow (e.g., pulmonary embolus, increased vascular resistance), vasospasm, heart failure, hypovolemic shock]

Alveolar-capillary membrane changes (e.g., acute respiratory distress syndrome); chronic conditions, such as restrictive/obstructive lung disease, pneumoconiosis, respiratory depressant drugs, brain injury, asbestosis/silicosis

[Altered oxygen supply (e.g., altitude sickness)]

[Altered oxygen-carrying capacity of blood (e.g., sickle cell/other anemia, carbon monoxide poisoning)]

Defining Characteristics

SUBJECTIVE

Dyspnea
Visual disturbances
Headache upon awakening
[Sense of impending doom]

OBJECTIVE

Confusion; [decreased mental acuity]
Restlessness; irritability; [agitation]
Somnolence; [lethargy]
Abnormal ABGs/arterial pH; hypoxia/hypoxemia; hypercapnia; hypercarbia; decreased carbon dioxide
Cyanosis (in neonates only); abnormal skin color (pale, dusky)
Abnormal rate, rhythm, depth of breathing; nasal flaring
Tachycardia [development of dysrhythmias]
Diaphoresis
[Polycythemia]

Desired Outcomes/Evaluation Criteria—Client Will:

- Demonstrate improved ventilation and adequate oxygenation of tissues by ABGs within client's normal limits and absence of symptoms of respiratory distress (as noted in Defining Characteristics).
- Verbalize understanding of causative factors and appropriate interventions.
- Participate in treatment regimen (e.g., breathing exercises, effective coughing, use of oxygen) within level of ability/situation.

Actions/Interventions

NURSING PRIORITY NO. 1. To assess causative/contributing factors:

- Note presence of factors listed in Related Factors. Refer to

NDs Airway Clearance, ineffective and Breathing Pattern, ineffective as appropriate.

NURSING PRIORITY NO. 2. To evaluate degree of compromise:

- Note respiratory rate, depth; use of accessory muscles, pursed-lip breathing; note areas of pallor/cyanosis; for example, peripheral (nailbeds) versus central (circumoral) or general duskiness.
- Auscultate breath sounds, note areas of decreased/adventitious breath sounds as well as fremitus.
- Assess level of consciousness and mentation changes. Note somnolence, restlessness, reports of headache on arising.
- Monitor vital signs and cardiac rhythm.
- Evaluate pulse oximetry to determine oxygenation; evaluate vital capacity **to assess respiratory insufficiency.**
- Review pertinent laboratory data (e.g., ABGs, CBC); chest x-rays.
- Assess energy level and activity tolerance.
- Note effect of illness on self-esteem/body image.

NURSING PRIORITY NO. 3. To correct/improve existing deficiencies:

- Elevate head of bed/position client appropriately, provide airway adjuncts and suction as indicated **to maintain airway.**
- Encourage frequent position changes and deep-breathing/coughing exercises. Use incentive spirometer, chest physiotherapy, IPPB, and so forth as indicated. **Promotes optimal chest expansion and drainage of secretions.**
- Provide supplemental oxygen at lowest concentration indicated by laboratory results and client symptoms/situation.
- Monitor for carbon dioxide narcosis (e.g., change in level of consciousness, changes in O_2 and CO_2 blood gas levels, flushing, decreased respiratory rate, headaches), **which may occur in clients receiving long-term oxygen therapy.**
- Maintain adequate I/O **for mobilization of secretions** but avoid fluid overload.
- Use sedation judiciously **to avoid depressant effects on respiratory functioning.**
- Ensure availability of proper emergency equipment, including ET/trach set and suction catheters appropriate for age and size of infant/child/adult. Avoid use of face mask in elderly emaciated client.
- Encourage adequate rest and limit activities to within client tolerance. Promote calm/restful environment. **Helps limit oxygen needs/consumption.**
- Provide psychologic support, listening to questions/concerns.

- Administer medications as indicated (e.g., corticosteroids, antibiotics, bronchodilators, expectorants, heparin) **to treat underlying conditions.**
- Monitor therapeutic and adverse effects as well as interactions of drug therapy.
- Minimize blood loss from procedures (e.g., tests, hemodialysis).
- Assist with procedures as individually indicated (e.g., transfusion, phlebotomy, bronchoscopy) **to improve respiratory function/oxygen-carrying capacity.**
- Monitor/adjust ventilator settings (e.g., Fio_2, tidal volume, inspiratory/expiratory ratio, sigh, positive end-expiratory pressure—PEEP) as indicated when mechanical support is being used.
- Keep environment allergen/pollutant free **to reduce irritant effect on airways.**

NURSING PRIORITY NO. **4.** To promote wellness (Teaching/Discharge Considerations):

- Review risk factors, particularly environmental/employment-related **to promote prevention/management of risk.**
- Discuss implications of smoking related to the illness/condition.
- Encourage client and SO(s) to stop smoking, attend cessation programs as necessary **to improve lung function.**
- Discuss reasons for allergy testing when indicated. Review individual drug regimen and ways of dealing with side effects.
- Instruct in the use of relaxation, stress-reduction techniques as appropriate.
- Reinforce need for adequate rest, while encouraging activity within client's limitations.
- Review oxygen-conserving techniques (e.g., sitting instead of standing to perform tasks, eating small meals; performing slower, purposeful movements).
- Review job description/work activities **to identify need for job modifications/vocational rehabilitation.**
- Discuss home oxygen therapy and safety measures as indicated when home oxygen implemented.
- Identify specific supplier for supplemental oxygen/necessary respiratory devices, as well as other individually appropriate resources, such as home-care agencies, Meals on Wheels, and so on, **to facilitate independence.**

Documentation Focus

ASSESSMENT/REASSESSMENT

- Assessment findings, including respiratory rate, character of breath sounds; frequency, amount, and appearance of

secretions; presence of cyanosis, laboratory findings, and mentation level.
- Conditions that may interfere with oxygen supply.

PLANNING

- Plan of care/interventions and who is involved in the planning.
- Ventilator settings, liters of supplemental oxygen.
- Teaching plan.

IMPLEMENTATION/EVALUATION

- Client's responses to treatment/teaching and actions performed.
- Attainment/progress toward desired outcome(s).
- Modifications to plan of care.

DISCHARGE PLANNING

- Long-range needs, identifying who is responsible for actions to be taken.
- Community resources for equipment/supplies postdischarge.
- Specific referrals made.

SAMPLE NURSING OUTCOMES & INTERVENTIONS CLASSIFICATIONS (NOC/NIC)

NOC—Respiratory Status: Gas Exchange
NIC—Respiratory Monitoring

Grieving, anticipatory

Taxonomy II: Coping/Stress Tolerance—Class 2 Coping Responses (00136)
[Diagnostic Division: Ego Integrity]
Submitted 1980; Revised 1996

Definition: Intellectual and emotional responses and behaviors by which individuals, families, communities work through the process of modifying self-concept based on the perception of potential loss [Note: May be a healthy response requiring interventions of support and information giving.]

Related Factors

To be developed
[Perceived potential loss of SO, physiological/psychosocial well-being (body part/function, social role), lifestyle/personal possessions]

Information that appears in brackets has been added by the authors to clarify and enhance the use of nursing diagnoses.

Defining Characteristics

SUBJECTIVE

Sorrow, guilt, anger, [choked feelings]

Denial of potential loss; denial of the significance of the loss

Expression of distress at potential loss, [ambivalence, sense of unreality]; bargaining

Alteration in activity level; sleep/dream patterns; eating habits; libido

OBJECTIVE

Potential loss of significant object (e.g., people, job, status, home, ideals, part and processes of the body)

Altered communication patterns

Difficulty taking on new or different roles

Resolution of grief prior to the reality of loss

[Altered affect]

[Crying]

[Social isolation, withdrawal]

Desired Outcomes/Evaluation Criteria—Client Will:

- Identify and express feelings (e.g., sadness, guilt, fear) freely/effectively.
- Acknowledge impact/effect of the grieving process (e.g., physical problems of eating, sleeping) and seek appropriate help.
- Look toward/plan for future, one day at a time.

Actions/Interventions

NURSING PRIORITY NO. 1. To assess causative/contributing factors:

- Determine client's perception of anticipated loss and meaning to him or her. "What are your concerns?" "What are your fears? Your greatest fear?" "How do you see this affecting you/your lifestyle?"
- Ascertain response of family/SO(s) to client's situation/concerns.

NURSING PRIORITY NO. 2. To determine current response to anticipated loss:

- Note emotional responses, such as withdrawal, angry behavior, crying.
- Observe client's body language and check out meaning with the client. Note congruency with verbalizations.
- Note cultural factors/expectations that may impact client's responses **to assess how the client is responding to the situation.**
- Identify problems with eating, activity level, sexual desire, role performance (e.g., work, parenting).
- Note family communication/interaction patterns.

• Determine use/availability of community resources/support groups.

NURSING PRIORITY NO. **3.** To assist client to deal with situation:

• Provide open environment and trusting relationship. **Promotes a free discussion of feelings and concerns.**

• Use therapeutic communication skills of Active-listening, silence, acknowledgment. Respect client desire/request not to talk.

• Provide puppets or play therapy for toddlers/young children. **(May help express grief and deal with loss.)**

• Permit appropriate expressions of anger, fear. Note hostility toward/feelings of abandonment by spiritual power. (Refer to appropriate NDs, e.g., Spiritual Distress.)

• Provide information about normalcy of individual grief reaction.

• Be honest when answering questions, providing information. **Enhances sense of trust and nurse-client relationship.**

• Provide assurance to child that cause for situation is not client's own doing, bearing in mind age and developmental level. **May lessen sense of guilt and affirm there is no need to assign blame to any family member.**

• Provide hope within parameters of individual situation. Do not give false reassurance.

• Review past life experiences/previous loss(es), role changes, and coping skills, noting strengths/successes. **Useful in dealing with current situation and problem solving existing needs.**

• Discuss control issues, such as what is in the power of the individual to change and what is beyond control. **Recognition of these factors helps client focus energy for maximal benefit/outcome.**

• Incorporate family/SO(s) in problem solving. **Encourages family to support/assist client to deal with situation while meeting needs of family members.**

• Determine client's status and role in family (e.g., parent, sibling, child, and address loss of family member role).

• Instruct in use of visualization and relaxation techniques.

• Use sedatives/tranquilizers with caution. **May retard passage through the grief process.**

NURSING PRIORITY NO. **4.** To promote wellness (Teaching/Discharge Considerations):

• Give information that feelings are OK and are to be expressed appropriately. **Expression of feelings can facilitate the grieving process, but destructive behavior can be damaging.**

• Encourage continuation of usual activities/schedule and involvement in appropriate exercise program.

• Identify/promote family and social support systems.

- Discuss and assist with planning for future/funeral as appropriate.
- Refer to additional resources, such as pastoral care, counseling/psychotherapy, community/organized support groups as indicated for both client and family/SO, **to meet ongoing needs and facilitate grief work.**

Documentation Focus

ASSESSMENT/REASSESSMENT

- Assessment findings, including client's perception of anticipated loss and signs/symptoms that are being exhibited.
- Responses of family/SO(s).
- Availability/use of resources.

PLANNING

- Plan of care and who is involved in planning.
- Teaching plan.

IMPLEMENTATION/EVALUATION

- Client's response to interventions/teaching and actions performed.
- Attainment/progress toward desired outcome(s).
- Modifications to plan of care.

DISCHARGE PLANNING

- Long-range needs and who is responsible for actions to be taken.
- Specific referrals made.

SAMPLE NURSING OUTCOMES & INTERVENTIONS CLASSIFICATIONS (NOC/NIC)

NOC—Grief Resolution
NIC—Grief Work Facilitation

Grieving, dysfunctional

Taxonomy II: Coping/Stress Tolerance—Class 2 Coping Responses (00135)
[Diagnostic Division: Ego Integrity]
Submitted 1980; Revised 1996

Definition: Extended, unsuccessful use of intellectual and emotional responses by which individuals, families, and communities attempt to work through the process of modifying self-concept based on the perception of loss

Information that appears in brackets has been added by the authors to clarify and enhance the use of nursing diagnoses.

Related Factors

Actual or perceived object loss (e.g., people, possessions, job, status, home, ideals, parts and processes of the body [e.g., amputation, paralysis, chronic/terminal illness])

[Thwarted grieving response to a loss, lack of resolution of previous grieving response]

[Absence of anticipatory grieving]

Defining Characteristics

SUBJECTIVE

Expression of distress at loss; denial of loss

Expression of guilt; anger; sadness; unresolved issues; [hopelessness]

Idealization of lost object (e.g., people, possessions, job, status, home, ideals, parts and processes of the body)

Reliving of past experiences with little or no reduction (diminishment) of intensity of the grief

Alterations in eating habits, sleep/dream patterns, activity level, libido, concentration and/or pursuit of tasks

OBJECTIVE

Onset or exacerbation of somatic or psychosomatic responses

Crying; labile affect

Difficulty in expressing loss

Prolonged interference with life functioning; developmental regression

Repetitive use of ineffectual behaviors associated with attempts to reinvest in relationships

[Withdrawal; isolation]

Desired Outcomes/Evaluation
Criteria—Client Will:

- Acknowledge presence/impact of dysfunctional situation.
- Demonstrate progress in dealing with stages of grief at own pace.
- Participate in work and self-care/ADLs as able.
- Verbalize a sense of progress toward resolution of the grief and hope for the future.

Actions/Interventions

NURSING PRIORITY NO. 1. To assess causative/contributing factors:

- Identify loss that is present. Look for cues of sadness (e.g., sighing, faraway look, unkempt appearance, inattention to conversation).
- Identify stage of grief being expressed: denial, isolation, anger, bargaining, depression, acceptance.
- Determine level of functioning, ability to care for self.

- Note availability/use of support systems and community resources.
- Be aware of avoidance behaviors (e.g., anger, withdrawal, long periods of sleeping, or refusing to interact with family).
- Identify cultural factors and ways individual has dealt with previous loss(es) **to determine how the individual is expressing self.**
- Ascertain response of family/SO(s) to client's situation. Assess needs of SO(s).
- Refer to ND Grieving, anticipatory as appropriate.

NURSING PRIORITY NO. 2. To assist client to deal appropriately with loss:

- Encourage verbalization without confrontation about realities. **Helpful in beginning resolution and acceptance.**
- Encourage client to talk about what the client chooses and do not try to force the client to "face the facts."
- Active-listen feelings and be available for support/assistance. Speak in soft, caring voice.
- Encourage expression of anger/fear and anxiety. Refer to appropriate NDs.
- Permit verbalization of anger with acknowledgment of feelings and setting of limits regarding destructive behavior. **(Enhances client safety and promotes resolution of grief process).**
- Acknowledge reality of feelings of guilt/blame, including hostility toward spiritual power. (Refer to ND Spiritual Distress.) Assist client to take steps toward resolution.
- Respect the client's needs and wishes for quiet, privacy, talking, or silence.
- Give "permission" to be at this point when the client is depressed.
- Provide comfort and availability as well as caring for physical needs.
- Reinforce use of previously effective coping skills. Instruct in/encourage use of visualization and relaxation techniques.
- Assist SOs to cope with client's response and include age-specific interventions. **(Family/SOs may not be dysfunctional but may be intolerant.)**
- Include family/SO(s) in setting realistic goals for meeting needs of family members.

NURSING PRIORITY NO. 3. To promote wellness (Teaching/Discharge Considerations):

- Discuss with client healthy ways of dealing with difficult situations.
- Have client identify familial, religious, and cultural factors

that have meaning for him or her. **May help bring loss into perspective and promote grief resolution.**

- Encourage involvement in usual activities, exercise, and socialization within limits of physical ability, and psychologic state.
- Discuss and assist with planning for future/funeral as appropriate.
- Refer to other resources (e.g., pastoral care, counseling, psychotherapy, organized support groups). **Provides additional help when needed to resolve situation/continue grief work.**

Documentation Focus

ASSESSMENT/REASSESSMENT

- Assessment findings, including meaning of loss to the client, current stage of the grieving process, and responses of family/SO(s).
- Availability/use of resources.

PLANNING

- Plan of care and who is involved in the planning.
- Teaching plan.

IMPLEMENTATION/EVALUATION

- Client's response to interventions/teaching and actions performed.
- Attainment/progress toward desired outcome(s).
- Modifications to plan of care.

DISCHARGE PLANNING

- Long-term needs and who is responsible for actions to be taken.
- Specific referrals made.

SAMPLE NURSING OUTCOMES & INTERVENTIONS CLASSIFICATIONS (NOC/NIC)

NOC—Grief Resolution
NIC—Grief Work Facilitation

Growth and Development, delayed

Taxonomy II: Growth/Development—Class 2
Development (00111)
[Diagnostic Division: Teaching/Learning]
Submitted 1986

Definition: Deviations from age-group norms

Information that appears in brackets has been added by the authors to clarify and enhance the use of nursing diagnoses.

Related Factors

Inadequate caretaking, [physical/emotional neglect or abuse]
Indifference, inconsistent responsiveness, multiple caretakers
Separation from SO(s)
Environmental and stimulation deficiencies
Effects of physical disability [handicapping condition]
Prescribed dependence [insufficient expectations for self-care]
[Physical/emotional illness (chronic, traumatic), (e.g., chronic inflam-
    matory disease, pituitary tumors, impaired nutrition/ metabolism,
    greater-than-normal energy requirements, prolonged/painful treat-
    ments, prolonged/repeated hospitalizations)]
[Sexual abuse]
[Substance use/abuse]

Defining Characteristics

SUBJECTIVE

Inability to perform self-care or self-control activities appropriate
    for age

OBJECTIVE

Delay or difficulty in performing skills (motor, social, or expressive)
    typical of age group; [loss of previously acquired skills]
Altered physical growth
Flat affect, listlessness, decreased responses
[Sleep disturbances, negative mood/response]

Desired Outcomes/Evaluation
Criteria—Client Will:

- Perform motor, social, and/or expressive skills typical of age
  group within scope of present capabilities.
- Perform self-care and self-control activities appropriate
  for age.
- Demonstrate weight/growth stabilization or progress toward
  age-appropriate size.

Parents/Caregivers Will:

- Verbalize understanding of growth/developmental delay/
  deviation and plan(s) for intervention.

Actions/Interventions

NURSING PRIORITY NO. 1. To assess causative/contributing
factors:

- Determine existing condition(s) contributing to growth/
  developmental deviation, such as limited intellectual capacity,

physical disabilities, chronic illness, tumors, genetic anomalies, substance use/abuse, multiple birth (e.g., twins)/minimal length of time between pregnancies.

- Determine nature of parenting/caretaking activities (e.g., inadequate, inconsistent, unrealistic/insufficient expectations; lack of stimulation, limit setting, responsiveness).
- Note severity/pervasiveness of situation (e.g., long-term physical/emotional abuse versus situational disruption or inadequate assistance during period of crisis or transition).
- Assess significant stressful events, losses, separation, and environmental changes (e.g., abandonment, divorce; death of parent/sibling; aging; unemployment, new job; moves; new baby/sibling, marriage, new stepparent).
- Active-listen concerns about body size, ability to perform competitively (e.g., sports, body building).
- Determine use of drugs, **which may affect body growth.**
- Evaluate hospital/institutional environment for adequate stimulation, diversional or play activities.

NURSING PRIORITY NO. 2. To determine degree of deviation from growth/developmental norms:

- Note chronological age, familial factors, including body build/stature, **to determine individual expectations.**
- Carefully record height/weight over time **to determine trends.**
- Note findings of psychologic evaluation of client and family. (**Extreme emotional deprivation may retard physical growth by hypothalamic inhibition of growth hormone, as in failure to thrive or dwarfism.**)
- Identify present developmental age/stage. Note reported losses in functional level/evidence of precocious development. **Provides comparative baseline.**
- Review expected skills/activities, using authoritative text (e.g., Gesell, Musen/Congor) or assessment tools (e.g., Draw-a-Person, Denver Developmental Screening Test, Bender's Visual Motor Gestalt Test).
- Note degree of individual deviation, multiple skills affected (e.g., speech, motor activity, socialization versus one area of difficulty, such as toileting).
- Note whether difficulty is temporary or permanent (e.g., setback or delay versus irreversible condition, such as brain damage, stroke, Alzheimer's disease).
- Investigate sexual acting-out behaviors inappropriate for age. **May indicate sexual abuse.**

NURSING PRIORITY NO. 3. To correct/minimize growth deviations and associated complications:

- Review medication regimen given to stimulate/suppress growth as appropriate, or possibly to shrink tumor when present.
- Stress necessity of not stopping medications without approval of healthcare provider.
- Prepare for surgical interventions/radiation therapy **to treat tumor.**
- Discuss appropriateness and potential complications of bone-lengthening procedures.
- Discuss consequences of substance use/abuse.
- Include nutritionist and other specialists (e.g., physical/occupational therapists) in developing plan of care.
- Monitor growth periodically. **Aids in evaluating effectiveness of interventions/promotes early identification of need for additional actions.**

NURSING PRIORITY NO. 4. To assist client (and/or caregivers) to prevent, minimize, or overcome delay/regressed development:

- Consult appropriate professional resources (e.g., occupational/rehabilitation/speech therapists, special-education teacher, job counselor) **to address specific individual needs.**
- Encourage recognition that deviation/behavior is appropriate for a specific age level (e.g., 14-year-old is functioning at level of 6-year-old or 16-year-old is not displaying pubertal changes). **Promotes acceptance of client as presented and helps shape expectations reflecting actual situation.**
- Avoid blame when discussing contributing factors.
- Maintain positive, hopeful attitude. Support self-actualizing nature of the individual and attempts to maintain or return to optimal level of self-control or self-care activities.
- Refer family/client for counseling/psychotherapy **to deal with issues of abuse/neglect.**
- Encourage setting of short-term, realistic goals for achieving developmental potential.
- Involve client in opportunities to practice new behaviors (e.g., role-play, group activities). **Strengthens learning process.**
- Identify equipment needs (e.g., adaptive/growth-stimulating computer programs, communication devices).
- Evaluate progress on continual basis **to increase complexity of tasks/goals as indicated.**
- Provide positive feedback for efforts/successes and adaptation while minimizing failures. **Encourages continuation of efforts, improving outcome.**

- Assist client/caregivers to accept and adjust to irreversible developmental deviations (e.g., Down syndrome is not currently correctable).
- Provide support for caregiver during transitional crises (e.g., residential schooling, institutionalization).

NURSING PRIORITY NO. 5. To promote wellness (Teaching/ Discharge Considerations):

- Provide information regarding normal growth and development process as appropriate. Suggest genetic counseling for family/client dependent on causative factors.
- Determine reasonable expectations for individual without restricting potential (i.e., set realistic goals that, if met, can be advanced). **Promotes continued personal growth.**
- Discuss appropriateness of appearance, grooming, touching, language, and other associated developmental issues. Refer to ND Self-Care deficit [specify].
- Recommend involvement in regular exercise/sport medicine program **to enhance muscle tone/strength and appropriate body building.**
- Discuss actions to take to avoid preventable complications (e.g., periodic laboratory studies **to monitor hormone levels/nutritional status**).
- Recommend wearing medical alert bracelet when taking replacement hormones.
- Encourage attendance at appropriate educational programs (e.g., parenting classes, infant stimulation sessions, seminars on life stresses, aging process).
- Provide pertinent reference materials and pamphlets. **Enhances learning at own pace.**
- Discuss community responsibilities (e.g., services required to be provided to school-age child). Include social worker/ special-education team in process of **planning for meeting educational, physical, psychological, and monitoring needs of child.**
- Identify community resources as appropriate: public health programs, such as Women, Infants, and Children (WIC); nutritionist; substance abuse programs; early-intervention programs; seniors' activity/support groups; gifted and talented programs; Sheltered Workshop; crippled children's services; medical equipment/supplier. **Provides additional assistance to support family efforts in treatment program.**
- Evaluate/refer to social services **to determine safety of client and consideration of placement in foster care.**
- Refer to the NDs Parenting, impaired; Family Processes, interrupted.

Documentation Focus

ASSESSMENT/REASSESSMENT

- Assessment findings/individual needs, including current growth status/trends and developmental level/evidence of regression.
- Caregiver's understanding of situation and individual role.
- Safety of individual/need for placement.

PLANNING

- Plan of care and who is involved in the planning.
- Teaching plan.

IMPLEMENTATION/EVALUATION

- Client's responses to interventions/teaching and actions performed.
- Caregiver response to teaching.
- Attainment/progress toward desired outcome(s).
- Modifications to plan of care.

DISCHARGE PLANNING

- Identified long-range needs and who is responsible for actions to be taken.
- Specific referrals made; sources for assistive devices, educational tools.

SAMPLE NURSING OUTCOMES & INTERVENTIONS CLASSIFICATIONS (NOC/NIC)

NOC—Child Development: [specify age group]
NIC—Developmental Enhancement: Child

Growth, risk for disproportionate

Taxonomy II: Growth/Development—Class 1 Growth (00113)
[Diagnostic Division: Teaching/Learning]
Nursing Diagnosis Extension and Classification (NDEC)
Submission 1998

Definition: At risk for growth above the 97th percentile or below the 3rd percentile for age, crossing two percentile channels; disproportionate growth

Risk Factors

PRENATAL

Maternal nutrition; multiple gestation
Substance use/abuse; teratogen exposure

Information that appears in brackets has been added by the authors to clarify and enhance the use of nursing diagnoses.

Congenital/genetic disorders [e.g., dysfunction of endocrine gland, tumors]

INDIVIDUAL

Organic (e.g., pituitary tumors) and inorganic factors
Prematurity
Malnutrition; caregiver and/or individual maladaptive feeding behaviors; insatiable appetite; anorexia; [impaired metabolism, greater-than-normal energy requirements]
Infection; chronic illness [e.g., chronic inflammatory diseases]
Substance [use]/abuse [including anabolic steroids]

ENVIRONMENTAL

Deprivation; poverty
Violence; natural disasters
Teratogen; lead poisoning

CAREGIVER

Abuse
Mental illness/retardation, severe learning disability

NOTE: A risk diagnosis is not evidenced by signs and symptoms, as the problem has not occurred and nursing interventions are directed at prevention.

Desired Outcomes/Evaluation Criteria—Client Will:

* Receive appropriate nutrition as indicated by individual needs.
* Demonstrate weight/growth stabilizing or progress toward age-appropriate size.
* Participate in plan of care as appropriate for age/ability.

Caregiver Will:

* Verbalize understanding of growth delay/deviation and plans for intervention.

Actions/Interventions

NURSING PRIORITY NO. 1. To assess causative/contributing factors:

* Determine factors/condition(s) existing that could contribute to growth deviation as listed in Risk Factors, including familial history of pituitary tumors, Marfan's syndrome, genetic anomalies, and so forth.

- Identify nature and effectiveness of parenting/caregiving activities (e.g., inadequate, inconsistent, unrealistic/insufficient expectations; lack of stimulation, limit setting, responsiveness).
- Note severity/pervasiveness of situation (e.g., individual/ showing effects of long-term physical/emotional abuse/ neglect versus individual experiencing recent-onset situational disruption or inadequate resources during period of crisis or transition).
- Assess significant stressful events, losses, separation and environmental changes (e.g., abandonment, divorce, death of parent/sibling, aging, move).
- Assess cognition, awareness, orientation, behavior (e.g., withdrawal/aggression) reaction to environment and stimuli.
- Active-listen concerns about body size, ability to perform competitively (e.g., sports, body building) **to ascertain the potential for use of anabolic steroids/other drugs.**

NURSING PRIORITY NO. 2. To prevent/limit deviation from growth norms:

- Note chronological age, familial factors (body build/stature) **to determine growth expectations.** Note reported losses/ alterations in functional level. **Provides comparative baseline.**
- Identify present growth age/stage. Review expectations for current height/weight percentiles and degree of deviation.
- Investigate increase in height/weight especially exceeding 3 standard deviations (SDs) above the mean in prepubertal clients. Note presence of headache and other neurologic changes. (**May indicate gigantism due to pituitary tumor.**)
- Note reports of progressive increase in hat/glove/ring/shoe size in adults, especially after age 40. **Elongation of facial features, hands, and feet suggests acromegaly.**
- Review results of x-rays to determine bone age/extent of bone and soft-tissue overgrowth, laboratory studies **to measure hormone levels,** and diagnostic scans **to identify pathology.**
- Assist with therapy to treat/correct underlying conditions (e.g., Crohn's disease, cardiac problems, or renal disease); endocrine problems (e.g., hypothyroidism, type 1 diabetes mellitus, growth hormone abnormalities); genetic/intrauterine growth retardation; infant feeding problems, nutritional deficits. Refer to ND Nutrition, imbalanced [specify].
- Include nutritionist and other specialists (e.g., physical/occupational therapist) in developing plan of care.

- Determine need for medications (e.g., appetite stimulants or antidepressants, growth hormones, etc.).
- Discuss consequences of substance use/abuse.
- Monitor growth periodically. **Aids in evaluating effectiveness of interventions/promotes early identification of need for additional actions.**

NURSING PRIORITY NO. **3**. To promote wellness (Teaching/Discharge Considerations):

- Provide information regarding normal growth as appropriate, including pertinent reference materials.
- Discuss appropriateness of appearance, grooming, touching, language, and other associated developmental issues. Refer to NDs Growth and Development, delayed and Self-Care deficit [specify].
- Recommend involvement in regular exercise/sports medicine **program to enhance muscle tone/strength and appropriate body building.**
- Discuss actions to take to prevent/avoid preventable complications.
- Identify available community resources as appropriate (e.g., public health programs, such as WIC; medical equipment supplies; nutritionists; substance abuse programs; specialists in endocrine problems/genetics).

Documentation Focus

ASSESSMENT/REASSESSMENT

- Assessment findings/individual needs, including current growth status, and trends.
- Caregiver's understanding of situation and individual role.

PLANNING

- Plan of care and who is involved in the planning.
- Teaching plan.

IMPLEMENTATION/EVALUATION

- Client's responses to interventions/teaching and actions performed.
- Caregiver response to teaching.
- Attainment/progress toward desired outcome(s).
- Modifications to plan of care.

DISCHARGE PLANNING

- Identified long-range needs and who is responsible for actions to be taken.
- Specific referrals made, sources for assistive devices, educational tools.

SAMPLE NURSING OUTCOMES & INTERVENTIONS CLASSIFICATIONS (NOC/NIC)

NOC—Child Development: [specify age group]
NIC—Nutritional Monitoring

Health Maintenance, ineffective

Taxonomy II: Health Promotion—Class 2 Health
Management (00099)
[Diagnostic Division: Safety]
Submitted 1982

Definition: Inability to identify, manage, and/or seek
out help to maintain health [This diagnosis contains
components of other NDs. We recommend subsuming
health maintenance interventions under the "basic"
nursing diagnosis when a single causative factor is identified (e.g., Knowledge, deficient [Specify]; Therapeutic
Regimen Management: ineffective; Confusion, chronic;
Communication, impaired verbal; Thought Process,
disturbed; Coping, ineffective; Coping, family: compromised; Growth and Development, delayed).]

Related Factors

Lack of or significant alteration in communication skills (written,
verbal, and/or gestural)
Unachieved developmental tasks
Lack of ability to make deliberate and thoughtful judgments
Perceptual or cognitive impairment (complete or partial lack of gross
and/or fine motor skills)
Ineffective individual coping; dysfunctional grieving; disabling spiri-
tual distress
Ineffective family coping
Lack of material resource; [lack of psychosocial supports]

Defining Characteristics

SUBJECTIVE

Expressed interest in improving health behaviors
Reported lack of equipment, financial and/or other resources; impair-
ment of personal support systems
Reported inability to take the responsibility for meeting basic health
practices in any or all functional pattern areas
[Reported compulsive behaviors]

OBJECTIVE

Demonstrated lack of knowledge regarding basic health practices
Observed inability to take the responsibility for meeting basic health

---

Information that appears in brackets has been added by the authors
to clarify and enhance the use of nursing diagnoses.

practices in any or all functional pattern areas; history of lack of health-seeking behavior

Demonstrated lack of adaptive behaviors to internal/external environmental changes

Observed impairment of personal support system; lack of equipment, financial and/or other resources

[Observed compulsive behaviors]

Desired Outcomes/Evaluation Criteria—Client Will:

- Identify necessary health maintenance activities.
- Verbalize understanding of factors contributing to current situation.
- Assume responsibility for own healthcare needs within level of ability.
- Adopt lifestyle changes supporting individual healthcare goals.

SO/Caregiver Will:

- Verbalize ability to cope adequately with existing situation, provide support/monitoring as indicated.

Actions/Interventions

NURSING PRIORITY NO. 1. To assess causative/contributing factors:

- Determine level of dependence/independence and type/presence of developmental disabilities. **May range from complete dependence (dysfunctional) to partial or relative independence.**
- Assess communication skills/ability/need for interpreter.
- Note whether impairment is a progressive illness/long-term health problem, exacerbation or complication of chronic illness. **May require more intensive/long-lasting intervention.**
- Evaluate for substance use/abuse (e.g., alcohol, narcotics).
- Note desire/level of ability to meet health maintenance needs, as well as self-care ADLs.
- Note setting where client lives (e.g., long-term care facility, homebound, or homeless).
- Ascertain recent changes in lifestyle (e.g., man whose wife dies and he has no skills for taking care of his own/family's health needs).
- Determine level of adaptive behavior, knowledge, and skills about health maintenance, environment, and safety.
- Evaluate environment **to note individual adaptation needs (e.g., supplemental humidity, air purifier, change in heating system).**

- Note client's use of professional services and resources (e.g., appropriate or inappropriate/nonexistent).

NURSING PRIORITY NO. **2**. To assist client/caregiver(s) to maintain and manage desired health practices:

- Develop plan with client/SO(s) for self-care. **Allows for incorporating existing disabilities, adapting, and organizing care as necessary.**
- Provide time to listen to concerns of client/SO(s).
- Provide anticipatory guidance **to maintain and manage effective health practices during periods of wellness and identify ways client can adapt when progressive illness/long-term health problems occur.**
- Encourage socialization and personal involvement **to prevent regression.**
- Provide for communication and coordination between the healthcare facility team and community healthcare providers **to provide continuation of care.**
- Involve comprehensive specialty health teams when available/indicated (e.g., pulmonary, psychiatric, enterostomal, IV therapy, nutritional support, substance-abuse counselors).
- Monitor adherence to prescribed medical regimen **to alter the care plan as needed.**

NURSING PRIORITY NO. **3**. To promote wellness (Teaching/Discharge Considerations):

- Provide information about individual healthcare needs.
- Limit amount of information presented at one time, especially when dealing with elderly client. Present new material through self-paced instruction when possible. **Allows client time to process and store new information.**
- Help client/SO(s) develop healthcare goals. Provide a written copy to those involved in planning process **for future reference/revision as appropriate.**
- Assist client/SO(s) to develop stress management skills.
- Identify ways to adapt exercise program **to meet client's changing needs/abilities and environmental concerns.**
- Identify signs and symptoms requiring further evaluation and follow-up.
- Make referral as needed for community support services (e.g., homemaker/home attendant, Meals on Wheels, skilled nursing care, Well-Baby Clinic, senior citizen healthcare activities).
- Refer to social services as indicated **for assistance with financial, housing, or legal concerns (e.g., conservatorship).**
- Refer to support groups as appropriate (e.g., senior citizens, Red Cross, Alcoholics/Narcotics Anonymous).
- Arrange for hospice service for client with terminal illness.

Documentation Focus

ASSESSMENT/REASSESSMENT

- Assessment findings, including individual abilities; family involvement, and support factors/availability of resources.

PLANNING

- Plan of care and who is involved in planning.
- Teaching plan.

IMPLEMENTATION/EVALUATION

- Responses of client/SO(s) to plan/interventions/teaching and actions performed.
- Attainment/progress toward desired outcome(s).
- Modifications to plan of care.

DISCHARGE PLANNING

- Long-range needs and who is responsible for actions to be taken.
- Specific referrals made.

SAMPLE NURSING OUTCOMES & INTERVENTIONS CLASSIFICATIONS (NOC/NIC)

NOC—Health Promoting Behavior
NIC—Health System Guidance

Health-Seeking Behaviors (specify)

Taxonomy II: Health Promotion—Class 2 Health Management (00084)
[Diagnostic Division: Teaching/Learning]
Submitted 1988

Definition: Active seeking (by a person in stable health) of ways to alter personal health habits and/or the environment to move toward a higher level of health [Note: Stable health is defined as achievement of age-appropriate illness-prevention measures; client reports good or excellent health, and signs and symptoms of disease, if present, are controlled.]

Related Factors

To be developed
[Situational/maturational occurrence precipitating concern about current health status]

Information that appears in brackets has been added by the authors to clarify and enhance the use of nursing diagnoses.

Defining Characteristics

SUBJECTIVE

Expressed desire to seek a higher level of wellness
Expressed desire for increased control of health practice
Expression of concern about current environmental conditions on
    health status
Stated unfamiliarity with wellness community resources
[Expressed desire to modify codependent behaviors]

OBJECTIVE

Observed desire to seek a higher level of wellness
Observed desire for increased control of health practice
Demonstrated or observed lack of knowledge in health promo-
    tion behaviors, unfamiliarity with wellness community
    resources

Desired Outcomes/Evaluation Criteria—Client Will:

- Express desire to change specific habit/lifestyle patterns to achieve/maintain optimal health.
- Participate in planning for change.
- Seek community resources to assist with desired change.

Actions/Interventions

NURSING PRIORITY NO. **1.** To assess specific concerns/habits/
issues client desires to change:

- Discuss concerns with client and Active-listen **to identify underlying issues (e.g., physical and/or emotional stressors; and/or external factors, such as environmental pollutants or other hazards).**
- Review knowledge base and note coping skills that have been used previously to change behavior/habits.
- Use testing as indicated and review results with client/SO(s) **to help with development of plan of action.**
- Identify behaviors associated with health habits/poor health practices and measures may need to change.

NURSING PRIORITY NO. **2.** To assist client to develop plan for
improving health:

- Explore with client/SO(s) areas of health over which each individual has control.
- Problem-solve options for change. **Helps identify actions to be taken to achieve desired improvement.**
- Provide information about conditions/health risk factors or concerns in written and audiovisual forms as appropriate. **Use of multiple modalities enhances acquisition/retention of information.**

- Discuss assertive behaviors and provide opportunity for client to practice new behaviors.
- Use therapeutic communication skills **to provide support for desired changes.**

NURSING PRIORITY NO. 3. To promote wellness (Teaching/Discharge Considerations):

- Acknowledge client's strengths in present health management and build on in planning for future.
- Encourage use of relaxation skills, medication, visualization, and guided imagery **to assist in management of stress.**
- Instruct in individually appropriate wellness behaviors (e.g., breast self-examination, immunizations, regular medical and dental examinations, healthy diet, exercise program).
- Identify and refer child/family member to health resources for immunizations, basic health services, and to learn health promotion/monitoring skills (e.g., monitoring hydration, measuring fever). **May facilitate long-term attention to health issues.**
- Refer to community resources (e.g., dietitian/weight control program, smoking cessation groups, Alcoholics Anonymous, codependency support groups, assertiveness training/Parent Effectiveness classes, clinical nurse specialists/psychiatrists) **to address specific concerns.**

Documentation Focus

ASSESSMENT/REASSESSMENT

- Assessment findings, including individual concerns/risk factors.
- Client's request for change.

PLANNING

- Plan of care and who is involved in planning.
- Teaching plan.

IMPLEMENTATION/EVALUATION

- Responses to wellness plan, interventions/teaching, and actions performed.
- Attainment/progress toward desired outcome(s).
- Modifications to plan of care.

DISCHARGE PLANNING

- Long-range needs and who is responsible for actions to be taken.
- Specific referrals.

SAMPLE NURSING OUTCOMES
& INTERVENTIONS CLASSIFICATIONS (NOC/NIC)

NOC—Health Seeking Behavior
NIC—Self-Modification Assistance

Home Maintenance, impaired

Taxonomy II: Health Promotion—Class 2 Health
Management (00098)
[Diagnostic Division: Safety]
Submitted 1980

Definition: Inability to independently maintain a safe
growth-promoting immediate environment

Related Factors

Individual/family member disease or injury
Insufficient family organization or planning
Insufficient finances
Impaired cognitive or emotional functioning
Lack of role modeling
Unfamiliarity with neighborhood resources
Lack of knowledge
Inadequate support systems

Defining Characteristics

SUBJECTIVE

Household members express difficulty in maintaining their home in a
comfortable [safe] fashion
Household requests assistance with home maintenance
Household members describe outstanding debts or financial crises

OBJECTIVE

Accumulation of dirt, food, or hygienic wastes
Unwashed or unavailable cooking equipment, clothes, or linen
Overtaxed family members (e.g., exhausted, anxious)
Repeated hygienic disorders, infestations, or infections
Disorderly surroundings; offensive odors
Inappropriate household temperature
Lack of necessary equipment or aids
Presence of vermin or rodents

Desired Outcomes/Evaluation
Criteria—Client/Caregiver Will:

• Identify individual factors related to difficulty in maintaining
a safe environment.

Information that appears in brackets has been added by the authors
to clarify and enhance the use of nursing diagnoses.

- Verbalize plan to eliminate health and safety hazards.
- Adopt behaviors reflecting lifestyle changes to create and sustain a healthy/growth-promoting environment.
- Demonstrate appropriate, effective use of resources.

Actions/Interventions

NURSING PRIORITY NO. **1.** To assess causative/contributing factors:

- Determine reason for and degree of disability.
- Assess level of cognitive/emotional/physical functioning.
- Identify lack of knowledge/misinformation.
- Discuss home environment **to determine ability to care for self and to identify potential health and safety hazards.**
- Identify support systems available to client/SO(s).
- Determine financial resources to meet needs of individual situation.

NURSING PRIORITY NO. **2.** To help client/SO(s) to create/maintain a safe, growth-promoting environment:

- Coordinate planning with multidisciplinary team.
- Arrange for home visit/evaluation as needed.
- Assist client/SO(s) to develop plan for maintaining a clean, healthful environment (e.g., sharing of household tasks/repairs between family members, contract services, exterminators, trash removal).
- Assist client/SO(s) to identify and acquire necessary equipment (e.g., lifts, commode chair, safety grab bars, cleaning supplies) **to meet individual needs.**
- Identify resources available for appropriate assistance (e.g., visiting nurse, budget counseling, homemaker, Meals on Wheels, physical/occupational therapy, social services).
- Identify options for financial assistance.

NURSING PRIORITY NO. **3.** To promote wellness (Teaching/Discharge Considerations):

- Identify environmental hazards **that may negatively affect health.** Discuss long-term plan for taking care of environmental needs.
- Provide information necessary for the individual situation.
- Plan opportunities for family members/caregivers to have respite from care of client. **Prevents burnout/role strain.**
- Identify community resources and support systems (e.g., extended family, neighbors).
- Refer to NDs Knowledge, deficient (specify); Self-Care Deficit [specify]; Coping, ineffective; Coping, family: compromised; Injury, risk for.

Documentation Focus

ASSESSMENT/REASSESSMENT

- Assessment findings include individual/environmental factors, presence and use of support systems.

PLANNING

- Plan of care and who is involved in planning; support systems and community resources identified.
- Teaching plan.

IMPLEMENTATION/EVALUATION

- Client's/SO's responses to interventions/teaching and actions performed.
- Attainment/progress toward desired outcome(s).
- Modifications to plan of care.

DISCHARGE PLANNING

- Long-term needs and who is responsible for actions to be taken.
- Specific referrals made, equipment needs/resources.

SAMPLE NURSING OUTCOMES & INTERVENTIONS CLASSIFICATIONS (NOC/NIC)

NOC—Self-Care: Instrumental Activities of Daily Living (IADL)
NIC—Home Maintenance Assistance

Hopelessness

Taxonomy II: Self-Perception—Class 1 Self-Concept (00124)
[Diagnostic Division: Ego Integrity]
Submitted 1986

Definition: Subjective state in which an individual sees limited or no alternatives or personal choices available and is unable to mobilize energy on own behalf

Related Factors

Prolonged activity restriction creating isolation
Failing or deteriorating physiological condition
Long-term stress; abandonment
Lost belief in transcendent values/God

Information that appears in brackets has been added by the authors to clarify and enhance the use of nursing diagnoses.

Defining Characteristics

SUBJECTIVE

Verbal cues (despondent content, "I can't," sighing); [believes things will not change/problems will always be there]

OBJECTIVE

Passivity, decreased verbalization
Decreased affect
Lack of initiative
Decreased response to stimuli, [depressed cognitive functions, problems with decisions, thought processes; regression]
Turning away from speaker; closing eyes; shrugging in response to speaker
Decreased appetite, increased/decreased sleep
Lack of involvement in care/passively allowing care
[Withdrawal from environs]
[Lack of involvement/interest in SOs (children, spouse)]
[Angry outbursts]

Desired Outcomes/Evaluation Criteria—Client Will:

- Recognize and verbalize feelings.
- Identify and use coping mechanisms to counteract feelings of hopelessness.
- Involve self in and control (within limits of the individual situation) own self-care and ADLs.
- Set progressive short-term goals to develop/foster/sustain behavioral changes/outlook.
- Participate in diversional activities of own choice.

Actions/Interventions

NURSING PRIORITY NO. **1.** To identify causative/contributing factors:

- Review familial/social history and physiologic history for problems, such as history of poor coping abilities, disorder of familial relating patterns, emotional problems, language/cultural barriers (**leading to feelings of isolation**), recent or long-term illness of client or family member, multiple social and/or physiologic traumas to individual or family members.
- Note current familial/social/physical situation of client (e.g., newly diagnosed with chronic/terminal disease, language/cultural barriers, lack of support system, recent job loss, loss of spiritual/religious faith, recent multiple traumas).
- Determine coping behaviors and defense mechanisms displayed.

NURSING PRIORITY NO. 2. To assess level of hopelessness:

- Note behaviors indicative of hopelessness. (Refer to Defining Characteristics.)
- Determine coping behaviors previously used and client's perception of effectiveness then and now.
- Evaluate/discuss use of defense mechanisms (useful or not), such as increased sleeping, use of drugs, illness behaviors, eating disorders, denial, forgetfulness, daydreaming, ineffectual organizational efforts, exploiting own goal setting, regression.

NURSING PRIORITY NO. 3. To assist client to identify feelings and to begin to cope with problems as perceived by the client:

- Establish a therapeutic/facilitative relationship showing positive regard for the client. **Client may then feel safe to disclose feelings and feel understood and listened to.**
- Explain all tests/procedures thoroughly. Involve client in planning schedule for care. Answer questions truthfully. **Enhances trust and therapeutic relationship.**
- Encourage client to verbalize and explore feelings and perceptions (e.g., anger, helplessness, powerlessness, confusion, despondency, isolation, grief).
- Provide opportunity for children to "play out" feelings (e.g., puppets or art for preschooler, peer discussions for adolescents). **Provides insight into perceptions and may give direction for coping strategies.**
- Express hope to client and encourage SO(s) and other health-team members to do so. **Client may not identify positives in own situation.**
- Assist client to identify short-term goals. Encourage activities to achieve goals, and facilitate contingency planning. **Promotes dealing with situation in manageable steps, enhancing chances for success and sense of control.**
- Discuss current options and list actions that may be taken to gain some control of situation. Correct misconceptions expressed by the client.
- Endeavor to prevent situations that might lead to feelings of isolation or lack of control in client's perception.
- Promote client control in establishing time, place, and frequency of therapy sessions. Involve family members in the therapy situation as appropriate.
- Help client recognize areas in which he or she has control versus those that are not within his or her control.
- Encourage risk taking in situations in which the client can succeed.
- Help client begin to develop coping mechanisms that can be learned and used effectively **to counteract hopelessness.**

- Encourage structured/controlled increase in physical activity. **Enhances sense of well-being.**
- Demonstrate and encourage use of relaxation exercises, guided imagery.

NURSING PRIORITY NO. **4.** To promote wellness (Teaching/Discharge Considerations):

- Provide positive feedback for actions taken to deal with and overcome feelings of hopelessness. **Encourages continuation of desired behaviors.**
- Assist client/family to become aware of factors/situations leading to feelings of hopelessness. **Provides opportunity to avoid/modify situation.**
- Discuss initial signs of hopelessness (e.g., procrastination, increasing need for sleep, decreased physical activity, and withdrawal from social/familial activities).
- Facilitate client's incorporation of personal loss. **Enhances grief work and promotes resolution of feelings.**
- Encourage client/family to develop support systems in the immediate community.
- Help client to become aware of, nurture, and expand spiritual self. (Refer to ND Spiritual Distress.)
- Introduce the client into a support group before the individual therapy is terminated **for continuation of therapeutic process.**
- Refer to other resources for assistance as indicated (e.g., clinical nurse specialist, psychiatrist, social services, spiritual advisor).

Documentation Focus

ASSESSMENT/REASSESSMENT

- Assessment findings, including degree of impairment, use of coping skills, and support systems.

PLANNING

- Plan of care and who is involved in planning.
- Teaching plan.

IMPLEMENTATION/EVALUATION

- Responses to interventions/teaching and actions performed.
- Attainment/progress toward desired outcome(s).
- Modifications to plan of care.

DISCHARGE PLANNING

- Identified long-range needs/client's goals for change and who is responsible for actions to be taken.
- Specific referrals made.

SAMPLE NURSING OUTCOMES & INTERVENTIONS CLASSIFICATIONS (NOC/NIC)

NOC—Depression Control
NIC—Hope Instillation

Hyperthermia

Taxonomy II: Safety/Protection—Class 6
Thermoregulation (00007)
[Diagnostic Division: Safety]
Submitted 1986

Definition: Body temperature elevated above normal range

Related Factors

Exposure to hot environment; inappropriate clothing
Vigorous activity; dehydration
Inability or decreased ability to perspire
Medications or anesthesia
Increased metabolic rate; illness or trauma

Defining Characteristics

SUBJECTIVE

[Headache]

OBJECTIVE

Increase in body temperature above normal range
Flushed skin; warm to touch
Increased respiratory rate, tachycardia; [unstable BP]
Seizures or convulsions; [muscle rigidity/fasciculations]
[Confusion]

Desired Outcomes/Evaluation Criteria—Client Will:

- Maintain core temperature within normal range.
- Be free of complications such as irreversible brain/neurologic damage, and acute renal failure.
- Identify underlying cause/contributing factors and importance of treatment, as well as signs/symptoms requiring further evaluation or intervention.
- Demonstrate behaviors to monitor and promote normothermia.
- Be free of seizure activity.

Information that appears in brackets has been added by the authors to clarify and enhance the use of nursing diagnoses.

Actions/Interventions

NURSING PRIORITY NO. **1.** To assess causative/contributing factors:

- Identify underlying cause (e.g., excessive heat production such as hyperthyroid state, malignant hyperpyrexia; impaired heat dissipation such as heatstroke, dehydration; autonomic dysfunction as occurs with spinal cord transection; hypothalamic dysfunction, such as CNS infection, brain lesions, drug overdose; infection).
- Note chronological and developmental age of client. **Children are more susceptible to heatstroke, elderly or impaired individuals may not be able to recognize and/or act on symptoms of hyperthermia.**

NURSING PRIORITY NO. **2.** To evaluate effects/degree of hyperthermia:

- Monitor core temperature. **Note:** Rectal and tympanic temperatures most closely approximate core temperature; however, abdominal temperature monitoring may be done in the premature neonate.
- Assess neurologic response, noting level of consciousness and orientation, reaction to stimuli, reaction of pupils, presence of posturing or seizures.
- Monitor BP and invasive hemodynamic parameters if available (e.g., mean arterial pressure—MAP, CVP, PAP, PCWP). **Central hypertension or peripheral/postural hypotension can occur.**
- Monitor heart rate and rhythm. **Dysrhythmias and ECG changes are common due to electrolyte imbalance, dehydration, specific action of catecholamines, and direct effects of hyperthermia on blood and cardiac tissue.**
- Monitor respirations. **Hyperventilation may initially be present, but ventilatory effort may eventually be impaired by seizures, hypermetabolic state (shock and acidosis).**
- Auscultate breath sounds, noting adventitious sounds such as crackles (rales).
- Monitor/record all sources of fluid loss such as urine (**oliguria and/or renal failure may occur due to hypotension, dehydration, shock, and tissue necrosis**), vomiting and diarrhea, wounds/fistulas, and insensible losses (**potentiates fluid and electrolyte losses**).
- Note presence/absence of sweating as body attempts to increase heat loss by evaporation, conduction, and diffusion. **Evaporation is decreased by environmental factors of high humidity and high ambient temperature as well as body factors producing loss of ability to sweat or sweat gland**

dysfunction (e.g., spinal cord transection, cystic fibrosis, dehydration, vasoconstriction).

- Monitor laboratory studies such as ABGs, electrolytes, cardiac and liver enzymes (**may reveal tissue degeneration**); glucose; urinalysis (**myoglobinuria, proteinuria, and hemoglobinuria can occur as products of tissue necrosis**); and coagulation profile (**for presence of disseminated intravascular coagulation—DIC**).

NURSING PRIORITY NO. 3. To assist with measures to reduce body temperature/restore normal body/organ function:

- Administer antipyretics, orally/rectally (e.g., aspirin, acetaminophen), as ordered.
- Promote surface cooling by means of undressing (**heat loss by radiation and conduction**); cool environment and/or fans (**heat loss by convection**); cool/tepid sponge baths or immersion (**heat loss by evaporation and conduction**); local ice packs, especially in groin and axillae (**areas of high blood flow**); and/or use of hypothermia blanket. (**Note:** In pediatric clients, tepid water is preferred. **Alcohol sponges are no longer used because they can increase peripheral vascular constriction and CNS depression; cold-water sponges/immersion can increase shivering, producing heat.**) In presence of malignant hyperthermia, lavage of body cavities with cold water may be used **to promote core cooling**.
- Administer medications (e.g., chlorpromazine or diazepam) as ordered **to control shivering and seizures**.
- Wrap extremities with bath towels when hypothermia blanket is used **to minimize shivering**.
- Turn off hypothermia blanket when core temperature is within 1° to 3° of desired temperature **to allow for downward drift**.
- Promote client safety (e.g., maintain patent airway, padded siderails, skin protection from cold such as when hypothermia blanket is used, observation of equipment safety measures).
- Provide supplemental oxygen **to offset increased oxygen demands and consumption**.
- Administer medications as indicated **to treat underlying cause,** such as antibiotics (**for infection**), dantrolene (**for malignant hyperthermia**), beta blockers (**for thyroid storm**).
- Administer replacement fluids and electrolytes **to support circulating volume and tissue perfusion**.
- Maintain bedrest **to reduce metabolic demands/oxygen consumption**.
- Provide high-calorie diet, tube feedings, or parenteral nutrition **to meet increased metabolic demands**.

NURSING PRIORITY NO. **4.** To promote wellness (Teaching/Discharge Considerations):

- Review specific cause such as underlying disease process (thyroid storm); environmental factors (heatstroke); reaction to anesthesia (malignant hyperthermia).
- Identify those factors that client can control (if any), such as correction of underlying disease process (e.g., thyroid control medication); ways to protect oneself from excessive exposure to environmental heat (e.g., proper clothing, restriction of activity, scheduling outings during cooler part of day); and understanding of family traits (**e.g., malignant hyperthermia reaction to anesthesia is often familial**).
- Discuss importance of adequate fluid intake **to prevent dehydration.**
- Review signs/symptoms of hyperthermia (e.g., flushed skin, increased body temperature, increased respiratory/heart rate). **Indicates need for prompt intervention.**
- Recommend avoidance of hot tubs/saunas as appropriate (**e.g., clients with cardiac conditions, pregnancy that may affect fetal development or increase cardiac workload**).

Documentation Focus

ASSESSMENT/REASSESSMENT

- Temperature and other assessment findings, including vital signs and state of mentation.

PLANNING

- Plan of care/interventions and who is involved in the planning.
- Teaching plan.

IMPLEMENTATION/EVALUATION

- Responses to interventions/teaching and actions performed.
- Attainment/progress toward desired outcome(s).
- Modifications to plan of care.

DISCHARGE PLANNING

- Referrals that are made, those responsible for actions to be taken.

SAMPLE NURSING OUTCOMES & INTERVENTIONS CLASSIFICATIONS (NOC/NIC)

NOC—Thermoregulation
NIC—Temperature Regulation

Hypothermia

Taxonomy II: Safety/Protection—Class 6
Thermoregulation (00006)
[Diagnostic Division: Safety]
Submitted 1986; Revised 1988

Definition: Body temperature below normal range

Related Factors

Exposure to cool or cold environment [prolonged exposure, e.g., homeless, immersion in cold water/near-drowning, induced hypothermia/cardiopulmonary bypass]
Inadequate clothing
Evaporation from skin in cool environment
Inability or decreased ability to shiver
Aging [or very young]
[Debilitating] illness or trauma, damage to hypothalamus
Malnutrition; decreased metabolic rate, inactivity
Consumption of alcohol; medications[/drug overdose] causing vasodilation

Defining Characteristics

OBJECTIVE

Reduction in body temperature below normal range
Shivering; piloerection
Cool skin
Pallor
Slow capillary refill; cyanotic nailbeds
Hypertension; tachycardia
[Core temperature 95°F/35°C: increased respirations, poor judgment, shivering]
[Core temperature 95°F to 93.2°F/35°C to 34°C: bradycardia or tachycardia, myocardial irritability/dysrhythmias, muscle rigidity, shivering, lethargic/confused, decreased coordination]
[Core temperature 93.2°F to 86°F/34°C to 30°C: hypoventilation, bradycardia, generalized rigidity, metabolic acidosis, coma]
[Core temperature below 86°F/30°C: no apparent vital signs, heart rate unresponsive to drug therapy, comatose, cyanotic, dilated pupils, apneic, areflexic, no shivering (appears dead)]

Desired Outcomes/Evaluation Criteria—Client Will:

- Display core temperature within normal range.
- Be free of complications, such as cardiac failure, respiratory infection/failure, thromboembolic phenomena.
- Identify underlying cause/contributing factors that are within client control.

Information that appears in brackets has been added by the authors to clarify and enhance the use of nursing diagnoses.

- Verbalize understanding of specific interventions to prevent hypothermia.
- Demonstrate behaviors to monitor and promote normo-thermia.

Actions/Interventions

NURSING PRIORITY NO. **1**. To assess causative/contributing factors:

- Note underlying cause (e.g., exposure to cold weather, cold-water immersion, preparation for surgery, open wounds/exposed viscera, multiple rapid transfusions of banked blood, treatment for hyperthermia).
- Note contributing factors: age of client (e.g., premature neonate, child, elderly person); concurrent/coexisting medical problems (e.g., brainstem injury, near-drowning, sepsis, hypothyroidism, alcohol intoxication); nutrition status; living condition/relationship status (e.g., aged/cognitive impaired client living alone).

NURSING PRIORITY NO. **2**. To prevent further decrease in body temperature:

- Remove wet clothing. Prevent pooling of antiseptic/irrigating solutions under client in operating room.
- Wrap in warm blankets, extra clothing; cover skin areas outside of operative field.
- Avoid use of heat lamps or hot water bottles. (**Surface rewarming can result in rewarming shock due to surface vasodilation.**)
- Provide warm liquids if client can swallow.
- Warm blood transfusions as appropriate.
- Prevent drafts in room.

NURSING PRIORITY NO. **3**. To evaluate effects of hypothermia:

- Measure core temperature with low register thermometer (measuring below 94°F/34°C).
- Assess respiratory effort (**rate and tidal volume are reduced when metabolic rate decreases and respiratory acidosis occurs**).
- Auscultate lungs, noting adventitious sounds (**pulmonary edema, respiratory infection, and pulmonary embolus are possible complications of hypothermia**).
- Monitor heart rate and rhythm. **Cold stress reduces pacemaker function, and bradycardia (unresponsive to atropine), atrial fibrillation, atrioventricular blocks, and ventricular tachycardia can occur. Ventricular fibrillation occurs most frequently when core temperature is 82°F/28°C or below.**
- Monitor BP, noting hypotension. **Can occur due to vasocon-**

striction, and shunting of fluids as a result of cold injury effect on capillary permeability.

- Measure urine output (**oliguria/renal failure can occur due to low flow state and/or following hypothermic osmotic diuresis**).
- Note CNS effects (e.g., mood changes, sluggish thinking, amnesia, complete obtundation); and peripheral CNS effects (e.g., paralysis—87.7°F/31°C, dilated pupils—below 86°F/30°C, flat EEG—68°F/20°C).
- Monitor laboratory studies such as ABGs (**respiratory and metabolic acidosis**); electrolytes; CBC (**increased hematocrit, decreased white blood cell count**); cardiac enzymes (**myocardial infarct may occur owing to electrolyte imbalance, cold stress catecholamine release, hypoxia, or acidosis**); coagulation profile; glucose; pharmacological profile (**for possible cumulative drug effects**).

NURSING PRIORITY NO. 4. To restore normal body temperature/organ function:

- Assist with measures to normalize core temperature, such as warmed IV solutions and warm solution lavage of body cavities (gastric, peritoneal, bladder) or cardiopulmonary bypass if indicated.
- Rewarm no faster than 1° to 2°/h **to avoid sudden vasodilation, increased metabolic demands on heart, and hypotension (rewarming shock).**
- Assist with surface warming by means of warmed blankets, warm environment/radiant heater, electronic warming devices. Cover head/neck and thorax, leaving extremities uncovered as appropriate **to maintain peripheral vasoconstriction. Note:** Do not institute surface rewarming prior to core rewarming in severe hypothermia (**causes after drop of temperature by shunting cold blood back to heart in addition to rewarming shock as a result of surface vasodilation**).
- Protect skin/tissues by repositioning, applying lotion/lubricants, and avoiding direct contact with heating appliance/blanket. (**Impaired circulation can result in severe tissue damage.**)
- Keep client quiet; handle gently **to reduce potential for fibrillation in cold heart.**
- Provide CPR as necessary, with compressions initially at one-half normal heart rate (**severe hypothermia causes slowed conduction, and cold heart may be unresponsive to medications, pacing, and defibrillation**).
- Maintain patent airway. Assist with intubation if indicated.
- Provide heated, humidified oxygen when used.
- Turn off warming blanket when temperature is within 1° to 3° of desired temperature **to avoid hyperthermia situation.**

- Administer IV fluids with caution **to prevent overload as the vascular bed expands** (cold heart is slow to compensate for increased volume).
- Avoid vigorous drug therapy (**as rewarming occurs, organ function returns, correcting endocrine abnormalities, and tissues become more receptive to the effects of drugs previously administered**). **Note:** Iloprost IV may help control blood viscosity—**enhancing circulation and reducing risk of gangrene.**
- Immerse hands/feet in warm water/apply warm soaks once body temperature is stabilized. Place sterile cotton between digits and wrap hands/feet with a bulky gauze wrap.
- Perform range-of-motion exercises, provide support hose, reposition, do coughing/deep-breathing exercises, avoid restrictive clothing/restraints **to reduce circulatory stasis.**
- Provide well-balanced, high-calorie diet/feedings **to replenish glycogen stores and nutritional balance.**

NURSING PRIORITY NO. 5. To promote wellness (Teaching/Discharge Considerations):

- Inform client/SO(s) of procedures being used to rewarm client.
- Review specific cause of hypothermia.
- Discuss signs/symptoms of early hypothermia (e.g., changes in mentation, somnolence, impaired coordination, slurred speech) **to facilitate recognition of problem and timely intervention.**
- Identify factors that client can control (if any), such as protection from environment, potential risk for future hypersensitivity to cold, and so forth.

Documentation Focus

ASSESSMENT/REASSESSMENT

- Findings, noting degree of system involvement, respiratory rate, ECG pattern, capillary refill, and level of mentation.
- Graph temperature.

PLANNING

- Plan of care and who is involved in planning.
- Teaching plan.

IMPLEMENTATION/EVALUATION

- Responses to interventions/teaching, actions performed.
- Attainment/progress toward desired outcome(s).
- Modifications to plan of care.

DISCHARGE PLANNING

- Long-term needs, identifying who is responsible for each action.

SAMPLE NURSING OUTCOMES & INTERVENTIONS CLASSIFICATIONS (NOC/NIC)

NOC—Thermoregulation
NIC—Hypothermia Treatment

Infant Behavior, disorganized

Taxonomy II: Coping/Stress Tolerance—Class 3
Neurobehavioral Stress (00116)
[Diagnostic Division: Neurosensory]
Submitted 1994; Nursing Diagnosis Extension and
Classification (NDEC) Revision 1998

Definition: Disintegrated physiological and neurobe-havioral responses to the environment

Related Factors

PRENATAL

Congenital or genetic disorders; teratogenic exposure; [exposure to drugs]

POSTNATAL

Prematurity; oral/motor problems; feeding intolerance; malnutrition
Invasive/painful procedures; pain

INDIVIDUAL

Gestational/postconceptual age; immature neurological system
Illness; [infection]; [hypoxia/birth asphyxia]

ENVIRONMENTAL

Physical environment inappropriateness
Sensory inappropriateness/overstimulation/deprivation
[Lack of containment/boundaries]

CAREGIVER

Cue misreading/cue knowledge deficit
Environmental stimulation contribution

Information that appears in brackets has been added by the authors to clarify and enhance the use of nursing diagnoses.

Defining Characteristics

OBJECTIVE

Regulatory Problems
Inability to inhibit [e.g., "locking in"—inability to look away from stimulus]; irritability

State-Organization System
Active-awake (fussy, worried gaze); quiet-awake (staring, gaze aversion)
Diffuse/unclear sleep, state-oscillation
Irritable or panicky crying

Attention-Interaction System
Abnormal response to sensory stimuli (e.g., difficult to soothe, inability to sustain alert status)

Motor System
Increased, decreased, or limp tone
Finger splay, fisting or hands to face; hyperextension of arms and legs
Tremors, startles, twitches; jittery, jerky, uncoordinated movement
Altered primitive reflexes

Physiological
Bradycardia, tachycardia, or arrhythmias; bradypnea, tachypnea, apnea
Pale, cyanotic, mottled, or flushed color
"Time-out signals" (e.g., gaze, grasp, hiccough, cough, sneeze, sigh, slack jaw, open mouth, tongue thrust)
Oximeter desaturation
Feeding intolerances (aspiration or emesis)

Desired Outcomes/Evaluation Criteria—Infant Will:

- Exhibit organized behaviors that allow the achievement of optimal potential for growth and development as evidenced by modulation of physiologic, motor, state, and attentional-interactive functioning.

Parent/Caregiver Will:

- Recognize individual infant cues.
- Identify appropriate responses (including environmental modifications) to infant's cues.
- Verbalize readiness to assume caregiving independently.

Actions/Interventions

NURSING PRIORITY NO. 1. To assess causative/contributing factors:

- Determine infant's chronological and developmental age; note length of gestation.
- Observe for cues suggesting presence of situations that may result in pain/discomfort.
- Determine adequacy of physiological support.

- Evaluate level/appropriateness of environmental stimuli.
- Ascertain parents' understanding of infant's needs/abilities.
- Listen to parent's concerns about their capabilities to meet infant's needs.

NURSING PRIORITY NO. 2. To assist parents in providing co-regulation to the infant:

- Provide a calm, nurturant physical and emotional environment.
- Encourage parents to hold infant, including skin-to-skin contact as appropriate.
- Model gentle handling of baby and appropriate responses to infant behavior. **Provides cues to parent.**
- Support and encourage parents to be with infant and participate actively in all aspects of care. **Situation may be overwhelming and support may enhance coping.**
- Discuss infant growth/development, pointing out current status and progressive expectations as appropriate. **Augments parents' knowledge of co-regulation.**
- Incorporate the parents' observations and suggestions into plan of care. **Demonstrates valuing of parents' input and encourages continued involvement.**

NURSING PRIORITY NO. 3. To deliver cares within the infant's stress threshold:

- Provide a consistent caregiver. **Facilitates recognition of infant cues/changes in behavior.**
- Identify infant's individual self-regulatory behaviors, e.g., sucking, mouthing; grasp, hand-to-mouth, face behaviors; foot clasp, brace; limb flexion, trunk tuck; boundary seeking.
- Support hands to mouth and face; offer pacifier or non-nutritive sucking at the breast with gavage feedings. **Provides opportunities for infant to suck.**
- Avoid aversive oral stimulation, such as routine oral suctioning; suction ET tube only when clinically indicated.
- Use oxy-hood large enough to cover the infant's chest so arms will be inside the hood. **Allows for hand-to-mouth activities during this therapy.**
- Provide opportunities for infant to grasp.
- Provide boundaries and/or containment during all activities. Use swaddling, nesting, bunting, caregiver's hands as indicated.
- Allow adequate time/opportunities to hold infant. Handle infant very gently, move infant smoothly, slowly and contained, avoiding sudden/abrupt movements.
- Maintain normal alignment, position infant with limbs softly flexed, shoulders and hips adducted slightly. Use appropriate-sized diapers.

- Evaluate chest for adequate expansion, placing rolls under trunk if prone position indicated.
- Avoid restraints, including at IV sites. If IV board is necessary, secure to limb positioned in normal alignment.
- Provide a sheepskin, egg-crate mattress, water bed, and/or gel pillow/mattress for infant who does not tolerate frequent position changes. **Minimizes tissue pressure, lessens risk of tissue injury.**
- Visually assess color, respirations, activity, invasive lines without disturbing infant. Assess with "hands on" every 4 hours as indicated and prn. **Allows for undisturbed rest/quiet periods.**
- Schedule daily activities, time for rest, and organization of sleep/wake states to maximize tolerance of infant. Defer routine care when infant in quiet sleep.
- Provide care with baby in sidelying position. Begin by talking softly to the baby, then placing hands in containing hold on baby, **allows baby to prepare.** Proceed with least-invasive manipulations first.
- Respond promptly to infant's agitation or restlessness. Provide "time out" when infant shows early cues of overstimulation. Comfort and support the infant after stressful interventions.
- Remain at infant's bedside for several minutes after procedures/**caregiving to monitor infant's response and provide necessary support.**
- Administer analgesics as individually appropriate.

NURSING PRIORITY NO. 4. To modify the environment to provide appropriate stimulation:

- Introduce stimulation as a single mode and assess individual tolerance.

LIGHT/VISION

- Reduce lighting perceived by infant; introduce diurnal lighting (and activity) when infant achieves physiologic stability. (Day light levels of 20 to 30 candles and night light levels of less than 10 candles are suggested.) Change light levels gradually **to allow infant time to adjust.**
- Protect the infant's eyes from bright illumination during examinations/procedures, as well as from indirect sources such as neighboring phototherapy treatments, **to prevent retinal damage.**
- Deliver phototherapy (when required) with Biliblanket devices if available (**alleviates need for eye patches**).
- Provide caregiver face (preferably parent's) as visual stimulus when infant shows readiness (awake, attentive).

SOUND

- Identify sources of noise in environment and eliminate or reduce (e.g., speak in a low voice, reduce volume on alarms/telephones to safe but not excessive volume, pad metal trash can lids, open paper packages, such as IV tubing and suction catheters, slowly and at a distance from bedside, conduct rounds/report away from bedside, place soft/thick fabric such as blanket rolls and toys near infant's head **to absorb sound**).
- Keep all incubator portholes closed, closing with two **hands to avoid loud snap with closure and associated startle response.**
- Do not play musical toys or tape players inside incubator.
- Avoid placing items on top of incubator; if necessary to do so, pad surface well.
- Conduct regular decibel checks of interior noise level in incubator (recommended not to exceed 60 dB).
- Provide auditory stimulation **to console, support infant before and through handling or to reinforce restfulness.**

OLFACTORY

- Be cautious in exposing infant to strong odors (such as alcohol, Betadine, perfumes), **as olfactory capability of the infant is very sensitive.**
- Place a cloth or gauze pad scented with milk near the infant's face during gavage feeding. **Enhances association of milk with act of feeding/gastric fullness.**
- Invite parents to leave a handkerchief that they have scented by wearing close to their body near infant. **Strengthens infant recognition of parents.**

VESTIBULAR

- Move and handle the infant slowly and gently. Do not restrict spontaneous movement.
- Provide vestibular stimulation **to console, stabilize breathing/heart rate, or enhance growth.** Use a water bed (with or without oscillation), a motorized/moving bed or cradle, or rocking in the arms of a caregiver.

GUSTATORY

- Dip pacifier in milk and offer to infant for sucking and tasting during gavage feeding.

TACTILE

- Maintain skin integrity and monitor closely. Limit frequency of invasive procedures.

- Minimize use of chemicals on skin (e.g., alcohol, Betadine, solvents) and remove afterward with warm water **because skin is very sensitive/fragile.**
- Limit use of tape and adhesives directly on skin. Use DuoDerm under tape **to prevent dermal injury.**
- Touch infant with a firm containing touch, avoid light stroking. Provide a sheepskin, soft linen. **Note: Tactile experience is the primary sensory mode of the infant.**
- Encourage frequent parental holding of infant (including skin-to-skin). Supplement activity with extended family, staff, volunteers.

NURSING PRIORITY NO. 5. To promote wellness (Teaching/Discharge Considerations):

- Evaluate home environment **to identify appropriate modifications.**
- Identify community resources (e.g., early stimulation program, qualified child-care facilities/respite care, visiting nurse, home-care support, specialty organizations).
- Determine sources for equipment/therapy needs.
- Refer to support/therapy groups as indicated **to provide role models, facilitate adjustment to new roles/responsibilities, and enhance coping.**
- Provide contact number as appropriate (e.g., primary nurse) **to support adjustment to home setting.**
- Refer to additional NDs such as Attachment, risk for impaired parent/infant/child; Coping, family: compromised/disabled/readiness for enhanced; Growth and Development, delayed; Caregiver Role Strain, risk for.

Documentation Focus

ASSESSMENT/REASSESSMENT

- Findings, including infant's cues of stress, self-regulation, and readiness for stimulation; chronological/developmental age.
- Parent's concerns, level of knowledge.

PLANNING

- Plan of care and who is involved in the planning.
- Teaching plan.

IMPLEMENTATION/EVALUATION

- Infant's responses to interventions/actions performed.
- Parents' participation and response to interactions/teaching.
- Attainment/progress toward desired outcome(s).
- Modifications of plan of care.

DISCHARGE PLANNING

- Long-term needs and who is responsible for actions to be taken.
- Specific referrals made.

SAMPLE NURSING OUTCOMES & INTERVENTIONS CLASSIFICATIONS (NOC/NIC)

NOC—Neurological Status
NIC—Environmental Management

Infant Behavior, readiness for enhanced organized

Taxonomy II: Coping/Stress Tolerance—Class 3
Neurobehavioral (00117)
[Diagnostic Division: Neurosensory]
Submitted 1994

Definition: A pattern of modulation of the physiological and behavioral systems of functioning (i.e., autonomic, motor, state-organizational, self-regulators, and attentional-interactional systems) in an infant that is satisfactory but that can be improved resulting in higher levels of integration in response to environmental stimuli

Related Factors

Prematurity
Pain

Defining Characteristics

OBJECTIVE

Stable physiological measures
Definite sleep-wake states
Use of some self-regulatory behaviors
Response to visual/auditory stimuli

Desired Outcomes/Evaluation Criteria—Infant Will:

- Continue to modulate physiological and behavioral systems of functioning.
- Achieve higher levels of integration in response to environmental stimuli.

Information that appears in brackets has been added by the authors to clarify and enhance the use of nursing diagnoses.

Parent/Caregiver Will:

- Identify cues reflecting infant's stress threshold and current status.
- Develop/modify responses (including environment) to promote infant adaptation and development.

Actions/Interventions

NURSING PRIORITY NO. 1. To assess infant status and parental skill level:

- Determine infant's chronological and developmental age; note length of gestation.
- Identify infant's individual self-regulatory behaviors: suck, mouth; grasp, hand-to-mouth, face behaviors; foot clasp, brace; limb flexion, trunk tuck; boundary seeking.
- Observe for cues suggesting presence of situations that may result in pain/discomfort.
- Evaluate level/appropriateness of environmental stimuli.
- Ascertain parents' understanding of infant's needs/abilities.
- Listen to parents' perceptions of their capabilities to promote infant's development.

NURSING PRIORITY NO. 2. To assist parents to enhance infant's integration:

- Review infant growth/development, pointing out current status and progressive expectations. Identify cues reflecting infant stress.
- Discuss possible modifications of environmental stimuli/ activity schedule, sleep and pain control needs.
- Incorporate parents' observations and suggestions into plan of care. **Demonstrates valuing of parents' input and enhances sense of ability to deal with situation.**

NURSING PRIORITY NO. 3. To promote wellness (Teaching/ Learning Considerations):

- Identify community resources (e.g., visiting nurse, home care support, child care).
- Refer to support group/individual role model **to facilitate adjustment to new roles/responsibilities.**
- Refer to additional NDs, for example, Coping, family: readiness for enhanced.

Documentation Focus

ASSESSMENT/REASSESSMENT

- Findings, including infant's self-regulation and readiness for stimulation; chronological/developmental age.
- Parents' concerns, level of knowledge.

- Plan of care and who is involved in the planning.
- Teaching plan.

PLANNING

- Plan of care and who is involved in the planning.
- Teaching plan.

IMPLEMENTATION/EVALUATION

- Infant's responses to interventions/actions performed.
- Parents' participation and response to interactions/teaching.
- Attainment/progress toward desired outcome(s).
- Modifications of plan of care.

DISCHARGE PLANNING

- Long-term needs and who is responsible for actions to be taken.
- Specific referrals made.

SAMPLE NURSING OUTCOMES & INTERVENTIONS CLASSIFICATIONS (NOC/NIC)

NOC—Neurological Status
NIC—Developmental Care

Infant Behavior, risk for disorganized

Taxonomy II: Coping/Stress Tolerance—Class 3
Neurobehavioral Stress (00115)
[Diagnostic Division: Neurosensory]
Submitted 1994

Definition: Risk for alteration in integration and modulation of the physiological and behavioral systems of functioning (i.e., autonomic, motor, state, organizational, self-regulatory, and attentional-interactional systems)

Risk Factors

Pain
Oral/motor problems
Environmental overstimulation
Lack of containment/boundaries
Invasive/painful procedures
Prematurity; [immaturity of the CNS; genetic problems that alter neurological and/or physiological functioning, conditions resulting in hypoxia and/or birth asphyxia]
[Malnutrition; infection; drug addiction]
[Environmental events or conditions, such as separation from parents, exposure to loud noise, excessive handling, bright lights]

Information that appears in brackets has been added by the authors to clarify and enhance the use of nursing diagnoses.

> NOTE: A risk diagnosis is not evidenced by signs and symptoms, as the problem has not occurred and nursing interventions are directed at prevention.

Desired Outcomes/Evaluation Criteria—Infant Will:

- Exhibit organized behaviors that allow the achievement of optimal potential for growth and development as evidenced by modulation of physiologic, motor, state, and attentional-interactive functioning.

Parent/Caregiver Will:

- Identify cues reflecting infant's stress threshold and current status.
- Develop/modify responses (including environment) to promote infant adaptation and development.
- Verbalize readiness to assume caregiving independently. Refer to ND Infant Behavior, disorganized for Actions/ Interventions and Documentation Focus.

SAMPLE NURSING OUTCOMES & INTERVENTIONS CLASSIFICATIONS (NOC/NIC)

NOC—Neurological Status
NIC—Environmental Management

Infant Feeding Pattern, ineffective

Taxonomy II: Nutrition—Class 1 Ingestion (00107)
[Diagnostic Division: Food/Fluid]
Submitted 1992

Definition: Impaired ability to suck or coordinate the suck-swallow response

Related Factors

Prematurity
Neurological impairment/delay
Oral hypersensitivity
Prolonged NPO
Anatomic abnormality

Defining Characteristics

SUBJECTIVE

[Caregiver reports infant is unable to initiate or sustain an effective suck]

Information that appears in brackets has been added by the authors to clarify and enhance the use of nursing diagnoses.

OBJECTIVE

Inability to initiate or sustain an effective suck
Inability to coordinate sucking, swallowing, and breathing

Desired Outcomes/Evaluation Criteria—Client Will:

- Display adequate output as measured by sufficient number of wet diapers daily.
- Demonstrate appropriate weight gain.
- Be free of aspiration.

Actions/Interventions

NURSING PRIORITY NO. **1.** To identify contributing factors/degree of impaired function:

- Assess developmental age, structural abnormalities (e.g., cleft lip/palate), mechanical barriers (e.g., ET tube, ventilator).
- Determine level of consciousness, neurologic damage, seizure activity, presence of pain.
- Note type/scheduling of medications. (**May cause sedative effect/impair feeding activity.**)
- Compare birth and current weight/length measurements.
- Assess signs of stress when feeding (e.g., tachypnea, cyanosis, fatigue/lethargy).
- Note presence of behaviors indicating continued hunger after feeding.

NURSING PRIORITY NO. **2.** To promote adequate infant intake:

- Determine appropriate method for feeding (e.g., special nipple/feeding device, gavage/enteral tube feeding) and choice of formula/breast milk to meet infant needs.
- Demonstrate techniques/procedures for feeding. Note proper positioning of infant, "latching-on" techniques, rate of delivery of feeding, frequency of burping.
- Monitor caregiver's efforts. Provide feedback and assistance as indicated. **Enhances learning, encourages continuation of efforts.**
- Refer mother to lactation specialist for assistance and support in dealing with unresolved issues (e.g., teaching infant to suck).
- Emphasize importance of calm/relaxed environment during feeding.
- Adjust frequency and amount of feeding according to infant's response. **Prevents stress associated with under/over-feeding.**

- Advance diet, adding solids or thickening agent as appropriate for age and infant needs.
- Alternate feeding techniques (e.g., nipple and gavage) according to infant's ability and level of fatigue.
- Alter medication/feeding schedules as indicated **to minimize sedative effects.**

NURSING PRIORITY NO. **3.** To promote wellness (Teaching/Discharge Considerations):

- Instruct caregiver in techniques to prevent/alleviate aspiration.
- Discuss anticipated growth and development goals for infant, corresponding caloric needs.
- Suggest monitoring infant's weight and nutrient intake periodically.
- Recommend participation in classes as indicated (e.g., first aid, infant CPR).

Documentation Focus

ASSESSMENT/REASSESSMENT

- Type and route of feeding, interferences to feeding and reactions.
- Infant's measurements.

PLANNING

- Plan of care/interventions and who is involved in planning.
- Teaching plan.

IMPLEMENTATION/EVALUATION

- Infant's response to interventions (e.g., amount of intake, weight gain, response to feeding) and actions performed.
- Caregiver's involvement in infant care, participation in activities, response to teaching.
- Attainment of/progress toward desired outcome(s).
- Modifications to plan of care.

DISCHARGE PLANNING

- Long-term needs/referrals and who is responsible for follow-up actions.

SAMPLE NURSING OUTCOMES & INTERVENTIONS CLASSIFICATIONS (NOC/NIC)

NOC—Swallowing Status: Oral Phase
NIC—Nutritional Monitoring

Infection, risk for

Taxonomy II: Safety/Protection—Class 1 Infection
(00004)
[Diagnostic Division: Safety]
Submitted 1986

Definition: At increased risk for being invaded by pathogenic organisms

Risk Factors

Inadequate primary defenses (broken skin, traumatized tissue, decrease in ciliary action, stasis of body fluids, change in pH secretions, altered peristalsis)

Inadequate secondary defenses (e.g., decreased hemoglobin, leukopenia, suppressed inflammatory response) and immunosuppression

Inadequate acquired immunity; tissue destruction and increased environmental exposure; invasive procedures

Chronic disease, malnutrition, trauma

Pharmaceutical agents [including antibiotic therapy]

Rupture of amniotic membranes

Insufficient knowledge to avoid exposure to pathogens

> NOTE: A risk diagnosis is not evidenced by signs and symptoms, as the problem has not occurred and nursing interventions are directed at prevention.

Desired Outcomes/Evaluation Criteria—Client Will:

- Verbalize understanding of individual causative/risk factor(s).
- Identify interventions to prevent/reduce risk of infection.
- Demonstrate techniques, lifestyle changes to promote safe environment.
- Achieve timely wound healing; be free of purulent drainage or erythema; be afebrile.

Actions/Interventions

NURSING PRIORITY NO. 1. To assess causative/contributing factors:

- Note risk factors for occurrence of infection (e.g., compromised host, skin integrity, environmental exposure).
- Observe for localized signs of infection at insertion sites of invasive lines, sutures, surgical incisions/wounds.
- Assess and document skin conditions around insertions of pins, wires, and tongs, noting inflammation and drainage.
- Note signs and symptoms of sepsis (systemic infection): fever, chills, diaphoresis, altered level of consciousness, positive blood cultures.

Information that appears in brackets has been added by the authors to clarify and enhance the use of nursing diagnoses.

- Obtain appropriate tissue/fluid specimens for observation and culture/sensitivities testing.

NURSING PRIORITY NO. **2.** To reduce/correct existing risk factors:

- Stress proper handwashing techniques by all caregivers between therapies/clients. **A first-line defense against nosocomial infections/cross-contamination.**
- Monitor visitors/caregivers **to prevent exposure of client.**
- Provide for isolation as indicated (e.g., wound/skin, reverse). **Reduces risk of cross-contamination.**
- Perform/instruct in preoperative body shower/scrubs when indicated (e.g., orthopedic, plastic surgery).
- Maintain sterile technique for invasive procedures (e.g., IV, urinary catheter, pulmonary suctioning).
- Cleanse incisions/insertion sites daily and prn with povidone-iodine or other appropriate solution.
- Change dressings as needed/indicated.
- Separate touching surfaces when skin is excoriated, such as in herpes zoster. Use gloves when caring for open lesions to minimize autoinoculation/transmission of viral diseases (e.g., herpes simplex virus, hepatitis, AIDS).
- Cover dressings/casts with plastic when using bedpan **to prevent contamination when wound is in perineal/pelvic region.**
- Encourage early ambulation, deep breathing, coughing, position change **for mobilization of respiratory secretions.**
- Monitor/assist with use of adjuncts (e.g., respiratory aids such as incentive spirometry) **to prevent pneumonia.**
- Maintain adequate hydration, stand/sit to void, and catheterize if necessary **to avoid bladder distention.**
- Provide regular catheter/perineal care. **Reduces risk of ascending UTI.**
- Assist with medical procedures (e.g., wound/joint aspiration, incision and drainage of abscess, bronchoscopy) as indicated.
- Administer/monitor medication regimen (e.g., antimicrobials, drip infusion into osteomyelitis, subeschar clysis, topical antibiotics) and note client's response **to determine effectiveness of therapy/presence of side effects.**
- Administer prophylactic antibiotics and immunizations as indicated.

NURSING PRIORITY NO. **3.** To promote wellness (Teaching/Discharge Considerations):

- Review individual nutritional needs, appropriate exercise program, and need for rest.
- Instruct client/SO(s) in techniques to protect the integrity of skin, care for lesions, and prevention of spread of infection.

- Emphasize necessity of taking antibiotics as directed (e.g., dosage and length of therapy). **Premature discontinuation of treatment when client begins to feel well may result in return of infection.**
- Discuss importance of not taking antibiotics/using "leftover" drugs unless specifically instructed by healthcare provider. **Inappropriate use can lead to development of drug-resistant strains/secondary infections.**
- Discuss the role of smoking in respiratory infections.
- Promote safer-sex practices and report sexual contacts of infected individuals **to prevent the spread of sexually transmitted disease.**
- Involve in community education programs geared **to increasing awareness of spread/prevention of communicable diseases.**
- Promote childhood immunization program. Encourage adults to update immunizations as appropriate.
- Include information in preoperative teaching about ways to reduce potential for postoperative infection (e.g., respiratory measures to prevent pneumonia, wound/dressing care, avoidance of others with infection).
- Review use of prophylactic antibiotics if appropriate (e.g., prior to dental work for clients with history of rheumatic fever).
- Identify resources available to the individual (e.g., substance abuse/rehabilitation or needle exchange program as appropriate; available/free condoms, etc.).
- Refer to NDs Disuse Syndrome, risk for; Home Maintenance, impaired; Health Maintenance, ineffective.

Documentation Focus

ASSESSMENT/REASSESSMENT

- Individual risk factors that are present including recent/current antibiotic therapy.
- Wound and/or insertion sites, character of drainage/body secretions.
- Signs/symptoms of infectious process

PLANNING

- Plan of care/interventions and who is involved in planning.
- Teaching plan.

IMPLEMENTATION/EVALUATION

- Responses to interventions/teaching and actions performed.
- Attainment/progress toward desired outcome(s).
- Modifications to plan of care.

DISCHARGE PLANNING

- Discharge needs/referrals and who is responsible for actions to be taken.
- Specific referrals made.

SAMPLE NURSING OUTCOMES & INTERVENTIONS CLASSIFICATIONS (NOC/NIC)

NOC—Immune Status
NIC—Infection Protection

Injury, risk for

Taxonomy II: Safety/Protection—Class 2 Physical Injury (00035)
[Diagnostic Division: Safety]
Submitted 1978

Definition: At risk of injury as a result of environmental conditions interacting with the individual's adaptive and defensive resources

Risk Factors

INTERNAL

Biochemical, regulatory function (e.g., sensory disfunction)
Integrative or effector dysfunction; tissue hypoxia; immune/autoimmune dysfunction; malnutrition; abnormal blood profile (e.g., leukocytosis/leukopenia, altered clotting factors, thrombocytopenia, sickle cell, thalassemia, decreased hemoglobin)
Physical (e.g., broken skin, altered mobility); developmental age (physiological, psychosocial)
Psychological (affective, orientation)

EXTERNAL

Biological (e.g., immunization level of community, microorganism)
Chemical (e.g., pollutants, poisons, drugs, pharmaceutical agents, alcohol, caffeine, nicotine, preservatives, cosmetics, dyes); nutrients (e.g., vitamins, food types)
Physical (e.g., design, structure, and arrangement of community, building, and/or equipment), mode of transport or transportation
People/provider (e.g., nosocomial agent, staffing patterns; cognitive, affective, and psychomotor factors)

NOTE: A risk diagnosis is not evidenced by signs and symptoms, as the problem has not occurred and nursing interventions are directed at prevention.

Information that appears in brackets has been added by the authors to clarify and enhance the use of nursing diagnoses.

Desired Outcomes/Evaluation Criteria—Client/Caregivers Will:

- Verbalize understanding of individual factors that contribute to possibility of injury and take steps to correct situation(s).
- Demonstrate behaviors, lifestyle changes to reduce risk factors and protect self from injury.
- Modify environment as indicated to enhance safety.
- Be free of injury.

Actions/Interventions

In reviewing this ND, it is apparent there is much overlap with other diagnoses. We have chosen to present generalized interventions. Although there are commonalities to injury situations, we suggest that the reader refer to other primary diagnoses as indicated, such as Poisoning, Suffocation, Trauma, and Falls, risk for; Wandering; Mobility, impaired (specify); Thought Processes, disturbed; Confusion, acute or chronic; Sensory Perception, disturbed; Home Maintenance, ineffective; Nutrition: imbalanced, less than body requirements; Skin Integrity, impaired/risk for impaired; Gas Exchange, impaired; Tissue Perfusion, ineffective; Cardiac Output, decreased; Infection, risk for; Violence, risk for other-directed/self-directed; Parenting, impaired/risk for impaired.

NURSING PRIORITY NO. **1.** To evaluate degree/source of risk inherent in the individual situation:

- Note age and sex (**children, young adults, elderly persons, and men are at greater risk**).
- Evaluate developmental level, decision-making ability, level of cognition and competence.
- Assess mood, coping abilities, personality styles (e.g., temperament, aggression, impulsive behavior, level of self-esteem) **that may result in carelessness/increased risk-taking without consideration of consequences.**
- Evaluate individual's response to violence in surroundings (e.g., neighborhood, TV, peer group). **May enhance disregard for own/others' safety.**
- Ascertain knowledge of safety needs/injury prevention and motivation to prevent injury in home, community, and work setting.
- Determine potential for abusive behavior by family members/SO(s)/peers.
- Note socioeconomic status/availability and use of resources.
- Assess muscle strength, gross and fine motor coordination.
- Observe for signs of injury and age (e.g., old/new bruises, history of fractures, frequent absences from school/work).

NURSING PRIORITY NO. **2.** To assist client/caregiver to reduce or correct individual risk factors:

- Provide information regarding disease/condition(s) that may result in increased risk of injury (e.g., osteoporosis).
- Identify interventions/safety devices **to promote safe physical environment and individual safety.** Refer to physical or occupational therapist as appropriate.
- Review consequences of previously determined risk factors (e.g., increase in oral cancer among teenagers using smokeless tobacco; occurrence of spontaneous abortion, fetal alcohol syndrome/neonatal addiction in prenatal women using tobacco, alcohol, and other drugs).
- Demonstrate/encourage use of techniques to reduce/manage stress and vent emotions, such as anger, hostility.
- Discuss importance of self-monitoring of conditions/emotions that can contribute to occurrence of injury (e.g., fatigue, anger, irritability).
- Encourage participation in self-help programs, such as assertiveness training, positive self-image **to enhance self-esteem/sense of self-worth.**
- Review expectations caregivers have of children, cognitively impaired, and/or elderly family members.
- Discuss need for and sources of supervision (e.g., before- and after-school programs, elderly day care).
- Discuss concerns about child care, discipline practices.

NURSING PRIORITY NO. **3.** To promote wellness (Teaching/Discharge Considerations):

- Refer to other resources as indicated (e.g., counseling/psychotherapy, budget counseling, parenting classes).
- Provide bibliotherapy/written resources **for later review and self-paced learning.**
- Promote community education programs geared to increasing awareness of safety measures and resources available to the individual.
- Promote community awareness about the problems of design of buildings, equipment, transportation, and workplace practices that contribute to accidents.
- Identify community resources/neighbors/friends to assist elderly/handicapped individuals in providing such things as structural maintenance, snow and ice removal from walks and steps, and so forth.

Documentation Focus

ASSESSMENT/REASSESSMENT

- Individual risk factors, noting current physical findings (e.g., bruises, cuts).

- Client's/caregiver's understanding of individual risks/safety concerns.

PLANNING

- Plan of care and who is involved in planning.
- Teaching plan.

IMPLEMENTATION/EVALUATION

- Individual responses to interventions/teaching and actions performed.
- Specific actions and changes that are made.
- Attainment/progress toward desired outcome(s).
- Modifications to plan of care.

DISCHARGE PLANNING

- Long-range plans for discharge needs, lifestyle and community changes, and who is responsible for actions to be taken.
- Specific referrals made.

SAMPLE NURSING OUTCOMES & INTERVENTIONS CLASSIFICATIONS (NOC/NIC)

NOC—Safety Behavior: Personal
NIC—Surveillance: Safety

Injury, risk for perioperative positioning

Taxonomy II: Safety/Protection—Class 2 Physical Injury (00087)
[Diagnostic Division: Safety]
Submitted 1994

Definition: At risk for injury as a result of the environmental conditions found in the perioperative setting

Risk Factors

Disorientation; sensory/perceptual disturbances due to anesthesia
Immobilization, muscle weakness; [preexisting musculoskeletal conditions]
Obesity; emaciation; edema
[Elderly]

NOTE: A risk diagnosis is not evidenced by signs and symptoms, as the problem has not occurred and nursing interventions are directed at prevention.

Information that appears in brackets has been added by the authors to clarify and enhance the use of nursing diagnoses.

Desired Outcomes/Evaluation Criteria—Client Will:

- Be free of injury related to perioperative disorientation.
- Be free of untoward skin and tissue injury or changes lasting beyond 24 to 48 hours postprocedure.
- Report resolution of localized numbness, tingling, or changes in sensation related to positioning within 24 to 48 hours as appropriate.

Actions/Interventions

NURSING PRIORITY NO. **1.** To identify individual risk factors/needs:

- Note anticipated length of procedure and customary position to increase awareness of potential complications (e.g., supine position may cause low back pain and skin pressure at heels/elbows/sacrum; lateral chest position can cause shoulder and neck pain plus eye and ear injury on the client's downside).
- Review client's history, noting age, weight/height, nutritional status, physical limitations/preexisting conditions. May affect choice of position and skin/tissue integrity during surgery (e.g., elderly person with no subcutaneous padding, arthritis; thoracic outlet/cubital tunnel syndrome, diabetes, obesity, presence of abdominal stoma, peripheral vascular disease, level of hydration, temperature of extremities).
- Assess the individual's responses to preoperative sedation/medication, noting level of sedation and/or adverse effects (e.g., drop in BP) and report to surgeon as indicated.
- Evaluate environmental conditions/safety issues surrounding the sedated client (e.g., client holding area, siderails up on bed/cart, someone with the client, etc.).

NURSING PRIORITY NO. **2.** To position client to provide protection for anatomic structures and to prevent client injury:

- Lock cart/bed in place, provide body and limb support for client during transfers, using adequate numbers of personnel.
- Place safety strap strategically to secure client for specific procedure. Avoid pressure on extremities when securing straps.
- Maintain body alignment as much as possible, using pillows, padding, safety straps to secure position.
- Protect body from contact with metal parts of the operating table, which could produce burns.
- Position extremities to facilitate periodic evaluation of safety, circulation, nerve pressure, and body alignment, especially when moving table attachments.

- Apply and reposition padding of pressure points of bony prominences (e.g., arms, ankles) and neurovascular pressure points (e.g., breasts, knees) **to maintain position of safety.**
- Place legs in stirrups simultaneously, adjusting stirrup height to client's legs, maintaining symmetrical position (when lithotomy position used). Pad popliteal space as indicated.
- Check peripheral pulses and skin color/temperature periodically **to monitor circulation.**
- Reposition slowly at transfer and in bed (especially halothane-anesthetized client) **to prevent severe drop in BP, dizziness, or unsafe transfer.**
- Protect airway and facilitate respiratory effort following extubation.
- Determine specific position reflecting procedure guidelines (e.g., head of bed elevated following spinal anesthesia, turn to unoperated side following pneumonectomy).

NURSING PRIORITY NO. **3.** To promote wellness (Teaching/Discharge Considerations):

- Provide perioperative teaching relative to client safety issues including not crossing legs during procedures performed under local or light anesthesia; postoperative needs/limitations, and signs/symptoms requiring medical evaluation.
- Inform client and postoperative caregivers of expected/transient reactions (such as low backache, localized numbness, and reddening or skin indentations, all of which should disappear in 24 hours).
- Assist with therapies/nursing actions including skin care measures, application of elastic stockings, early mobilization **to promote skin and tissue integrity.**
- Encourage/assist with frequent range-of-motion exercises, especially when joint stiffness occurs.
- Identify potential hazards in the surgical suite and implement corrections as appropriate.
- Refer to appropriate resources as needed.

Documentation Focus

ASSESSMENT/REASSESSMENT

- Findings, including individual risk factors for problems in the perioperative setting/need to modify routine activities or positions.
- Periodic evaluation of monitoring activities.

PLANNING

- Plan of care and who is involved in planning.
- Teaching plan.

IMPLEMENTATION/EVALUATION

• Response to interventions and actions performed.
• Attainment/progress toward desired outcome(s).
• Modifications to plan of care.

DISCHARGE PLANNING

• Long-term needs and who is responsible for actions to be taken.

SAMPLE NURSING OUTCOMES & INTERVENTIONS CLASSIFICATIONS (NOC/NIC)

NOC—Risk Control
NIC—Positioning: Intraoperative

Intracranial Adaptive Capacity, decreased

Taxonomy II: Coping/Stress Tolerance—Class 3
Neurobehavioral Stress (00049)
[Diagnostic Division: Circulation]
Submitted 1994

Definition: Intracranial fluid dynamic mechanisms that normally compensate for increases in intracranial volume are compromised, resulting in repeated disproportionate increases in intracranial pressure (ICP) in response to a variety of noxious and non-noxious stimuli

Related Factors

Brain injuries
Sustained increase in ICP equals 10 to 15 mm Hg
Decreased cerebral perfusion pressure ≤50 to 60 mm Hg
Systemic hypotension with intracranial hypertension

Defining Characteristics

OBJECTIVE

Repeated increases in ICP of greater than 10 mm Hg for more than 5 minutes following a variety of external stimuli
Disproportionate increase in ICP following single environmental or nursing maneuver stimulus
Elevated P2 ICP waveform
Volume pressure response test variation (volume-pressure ratio 2, pressure-volume index <10)
Baseline ICP equal to or greater than 10 mm Hg
Wide amplitude ICP waveform

Information that appears in brackets has been added by the authors to clarify and enhance the use of nursing diagnoses.

[Altered level of consciousness—coma]
[Changes in vital signs, cardiac rhythm]

Desired Outcomes/Evaluation Criteria—Client Will:

- Demonstrate stable ICP as evidenced by normalization of pressure waveforms/response to stimuli.
- Display improved neurologic signs.

Actions/Interventions

NURSING PRIORITY NO. 1. To assess causative/contributing factors:

- Determine factors related to individual situation (e.g., cause of coma)
- Monitor/document changes in ICP waveform and corresponding event (e.g., suctioning, position change, monitor alarms, family visit) **to alter care appropriately.**

NURSING PRIORITY NO. 2. To note degree of impairment:

- Assess eye opening and position/movement, pupils (size, shape, equality, light reactivity), and consciousness/mental status.
- Note purposeful and nonpurposeful motor response (posturing, etc.), comparing right/left sides.
- Test for presence/absence of reflexes (e.g., blink, cough, gag, Babinski's reflex), nuchal rigidity.
- Monitor vital signs and cardiac rhythm before/during/after activity. **Helps determine parameters for "safe" activity.**

NURSING PRIORITY NO. 3. To minimize/correct causative factors/maximize perfusion:

- Elevate head of bed (HOB) 15 to 45 degrees (30 degrees for child), as individually appropriate.
- Maintain head/neck in neutral position, support with small towel rolls or pillows **to maximize venous return.** Avoid placing head on large pillow or causing hip flexion of 90 degrees or more.
- Decrease extraneous stimuli/provide comfort measures (e.g., quiet environment, soft voice, tapes of familiar voices played through earphones, back massage, gentle touch as tolerated) **to reduce CNS stimulation and promote relaxation.**
- Limit painful procedures (e.g., venipunctures, redundant neurologic evaluations) to those that are absolutely necessary.
- Provide rest periods between care activities and limit duration of procedures. Lower lighting/noise level, schedule and limit activities **to provide restful environment and promote regular sleep patterns (i.e., day/night pattern).**

- Limit/prevent activities that increase intrathoracic/abdominal pressures (e.g., coughing, vomiting, straining at stool). Avoid/limit use of restraints. **These factors markedly increase ICP.**
- Suction with caution—only when needed—and limit to 2 passes of 10 seconds each with negative pressure no more than 120 mm Hg. Suction just beyond end of endo/tracheal tube without touching tracheal wall or carina. Administer lidocaine intratracheally (**reduces cough reflex**), hyperoxygenate before suctioning as appropriate **to minimize hypoxia.**
- Maintain patency of urinary drainage system **to reduce risk of hypertension, increased ICP, associated dysreflexia if spinal cord injury is also present and spinal cord shock is past.** (Refer to ND Autonomic Dysreflexia.)
- Weigh as indicated. Calculate fluid balance every shift/daily **to determine fluid needs/maintain hydration and prevent fluid overload.**
- Restrict fluid intake as necessary, administer IV fluids via pump/control device **to prevent inadvertent fluid bolus or vascular overload.**
- Regulate environmental temperature/bed linens, use cooling blanket as indicated **to decrease metabolic and O_2 needs when fever present.**
- Investigate increased restlessness **to determine causative factors and initiate corrective measures early or as indicated.**
- Provide appropriate safety measures/initiate treatment for seizures **to prevent injury/increase of ICP/hypoxia.**
- Administer supplemental oxygen; hyperventilate as indicated when on mechanical ventilation. Monitor arterial blood gases (ABGs), particularly CO_2 and Pao_2 levels. **$Paco_2$ level of 28 to 30 mm Hg decreases cerebral blood flow while maintaining adequate cerebral oxygenation, while a Pao_2 of less than 65 mm Hg may cause cerebral vascular dilation.**
- Administer medications (e.g., antihypertensives, diuretics, analgesics/sedatives, antipyretics, vasopressors, antiseizure drugs, neuromuscular blocking agents, and corticosteroids) as appropriate **to maintain homeostasis.**
- Prepare client for surgery as indicated (e.g., evacuation of hematoma/space-occupying lesion) **to reduce ICP/enhance circulation.**

NURSING PRIORITY NO. 4. To promote wellness (Teaching/Discharge Considerations):

- Discuss with caregivers specific situations (e.g., if client choking or experiencing pain, needing to be repositioned, constipated, blocked urinary flow) and review appropriate interventions **to prevent/limit episodic increases in ICP.**

- Identify signs/symptoms suggesting increased ICP (in client at risk without an ICP monitor), for example, restlessness, deterioration in neurologic responses. Review appropriate interventions.

Documentation Focus

ASSESSMENT/REASSESSMENT

- Neurologic findings noting right/left sides separately (such as pupils, motor response, reflexes, restlessness, nuchal rigidity).
- Response to activities/events (e.g., changes in pressure waveforms/vital signs).
- Presence/characteristics of seizure activity.

PLANNING

- Plan of care and who is involved in planning.
- Teaching plan.

IMPLEMENTATION/EVALUATION

- Response to interventions and actions performed.
- Attainment/progress toward desired outcome(s).
- Modifications to plan of care.

DISCHARGE PLANNING

- Future needs, plan for meeting them, and determining who is responsible for actions.
- Referrals as identified.

SAMPLE NURSING OUTCOMES & INTERVENTIONS CLASSIFICATIONS (NOC/NIC)

NOC—Neurological Status
NIC—Cerebral Edema Management

Knowledge, deficient [Learning Need] (specify)

Taxonomy II: Perception/Cognition—Class 4 Cognition (00126)
[Diagnostic Division: Teaching/Learning]
Submitted 1980

Definition: Absence or deficiency of cognitive information related to specific topic [Lack of specific information necessary for clients/SO(s) to make informed choices regarding condition/treatment/lifestyle changes]

Information that appears in brackets has been added by the authors to clarify and enhance the use of nursing diagnoses.

Related Factors

Lack of exposure
Information misinterpretation
Unfamiliarity with information resources
Lack of recall
Cognitive limitation
Lack of interest in learning
[Client's request for no information]
[Inaccurate/incomplete information presented]

Defining Characteristics

SUBJECTIVE

Verbalization of the problem
[Request for information]
[Statements reflecting misconceptions]

OBJECTIVE

Inaccurate follow-through of instruction
Inadequate performance of test
Inappropriate or exaggerated behaviors (e.g., hysterical, hostile,
    agitated, apathetic)
[Development of preventable complication]

Desired Outcomes/Evaluation Criteria—Client Will:

- Participate in learning process.
- Identify interferences to learning and specific action(s) to deal with them.
- Exhibit increased interest/assume responsibility for own learning and begin to look for information and ask questions.
- Verbalize understanding of condition/disease process and treatment.
- Identify relationship of signs/symptoms to the disease process and correlate symptoms with causative factors.
- Perform necessary procedures correctly and explain reasons for the actions.
- Initiate necessary lifestyle changes and participate in treatment regimen.

Actions/Interventions

NURSING PRIORITY NO. 1. To assess readiness to learn and individual learning needs:

- Ascertain level of knowledge, including anticipatory needs.
- Determine client's ability to learn. (May not be physically, emotionally, or mentally capable at this time.)
- Be alert to signs of avoidance. May need to allow client to

suffer the consequences of lack of knowledge before client is ready to accept information.

- Identify support persons/SO(s) requiring information.

NURSING PRIORITY NO. 2. To determine other factors pertinent to the learning process:

- Note personal factors (e.g., age, sex, social/cultural influences, religion, life experiences, level of education, sense of powerlessness).
- Determine blocks to learning: language barriers (e.g., can't read, speaks/understands only nondominant language); physical factors (e.g., sensory deficits, such as aphasia, dyslexia); physical stability (e.g., acute illness, activity intolerance); difficulty of material to be learned.
- Assess the level of the client's capabilities and the possibilities of the situation. (**May need to help SO[s] and/or caregivers to learn.**)

NURSING PRIORITY NO. 3. To assess the client's/SO's motivation:

- Identify motivating factors for the individual.
- Provide information relevant to the situation.
- Provide positive reinforcement. (**Encourages continuation of efforts.**) Avoid use of negative reinforcers (e.g., criticism and threats).

NURSING PRIORITY NO. 4. To establish priorities in conjunction with client:

- Determine client's most urgent need from both client's and nurse's viewpoint. **Identifies starting point.**
- Discuss client's perception of need. Relate information to client's personal desires/needs and values/beliefs.
- Differentiate "critical" content from "desirable" content. **Identifies information that can be addressed at a later time.**

NURSING PRIORITY NO. 5. To establish the content to be included:

- Identify information that needs to be remembered (cognitive).
- Identify information having to do with emotions, attitudes, and values (affective).
- Identify psychomotor skills that are necessary for learning.

NURSING PRIORITY NO. 6. To develop learner's objectives:

- State objectives clearly in learner's terms **to meet learner's (not instructor's) needs.**
- Identify outcomes (results) to be achieved.
- Recognize level of achievement, time factors, and short-term and long-term goals.
- Include the affective goals (e.g., reduction of stress).

NURSING PRIORITY NO. 7. To identify teaching methods to be used:

- Determine client's method of accessing information (visual, auditory, kinesthetic, gustatory/olfactory) and include in teaching plan **to facilitate learning.**
- Involve the client/SO(s) by using programmed books, questions/dialogue, audiovisual materials.
- Involve with others who have same problems/needs/concerns (e.g., group presentations, support groups). **Provides role model and sharing of information.**
- Provide mutual goal setting and learning contracts. (**Clarifies expectations of teacher and learner.**)
- Use team and group teaching as appropriate.

NURSING PRIORITY NO. 8. To facilitate learning:

- Provide written information/guidelines for client to refer to as necessary. **Reinforces learning process.**
- Pace and time learning sessions and learning activities to individual's needs. Involve and evaluate with client.
- Provide an environment that is conducive to learning.
- Be aware of factors related to teacher in the situation: Vocabulary, dress, style, knowledge of the subject, and ability to impart information effectively.
- Begin with information the client already knows and move to what the client does not know, progressing from simple to complex. **Limits sense of being overwhelmed.**
- Deal with the client's anxiety. Present information out of sequence, if necessary, dealing first with material that is most anxiety-producing **when the anxiety is interfering with the client's learning process.**
- Provide active role for client in learning process. **Promotes sense of control over situation.**
- Provide for feedback (positive reinforcement) and evaluation of learning/acquisition of skills.
- Be aware of informal teaching and role modeling that takes place on an ongoing basis (e.g., answering specific questions/reinforcing previous teaching during routine care).
- Assist client to use information in all applicable areas (e.g., situational, environmental, personal).

NURSING PRIORITY NO. 9. To promote wellness (Teaching/Discharge Considerations):

- Provide phone number of contact person **to answer questions/validate information postdischarge.**
- Identify available community resources/support groups.
- Provide information about additional learning resources (e.g., bibliography, tapes). **May assist with further learning/promote learning at own pace.**

Documentation Focus

ASSESSMENT/REASSESSMENT

- Individual findings/learning style and identified needs, presence of learning blocks (e.g., hostility, inappropriate behavior).

PLANNING

- Plan for learning, methods to be used, and who is involved in the planning.
- Teaching plan.

IMPLEMENTATION/EVALUATION

- Responses of the client/SO(s) to the learning plan and actions performed. How the learning is demonstrated.
- Attainment/progress toward desired outcome(s).
- Modifications to plan of care.

DISCHARGE PLANNING

- Additional learning/referral needs.

SAMPLE NURSING OUTCOMES & INTERVENTIONS CLASSIFICATIONS (NOC/NIC)

NOC—Knowledge: [specify—25 choices]
NIC—Teaching: [specify—14 choices]

Knowledge (specify), readiness for enhanced

Taxonomy II: Perception/Cognition—Class 4 Cognition (00161)
[Diagnostic Division: Teaching/Learning]
Submitted 2002

Definition: The presence or acquisition of cognitive information related to a specific topic is sufficient for meeting health-related goals and can be strengthened

Related Factors

To be developed

Defining Characteristics

SUBJECTIVE

Expresses an interest in learning
Explains knowledge of the topic; describes previous experiences pertaining to the topic

---

Information that appears in brackets has been added by the authors to clarify and enhance the use of nursing diagnoses.

OBJECTIVE

Behaviors congruent with expressed knowledge

Desired Outcomes/Evaluation Criteria—Client will:

- Exhibit responsibility for own learning and seek answers to questions.
- Verify accuracy of informational resources.
- Verbalize understanding of information gained.
- Use information to develop individual plan to meet health-care needs/goals.

Actions/Interventions

NURSING PRIORITY NO. **1.** To develop plan for learning:

- Verify client's level of knowledge about specific topic. **Provides opportunity to assure accuracy and completeness of knowledge base for future learning.**
- Determine motivation/expectations for learning. **Provides insight useful in developing goals and identifying information needs.**
- Assist client to identify learning goals. **Helps to frame or focus content to be learned and provides measure to evaluate learning process.**
- Ascertain preferred methods of learning (e.g., auditory, visual, interactive, or "hands-on"). **Identifies best approaches to facilitate learning process.**
- Note personal factors (e.g., age, sex, social/cultural influences, religion, life experiences, level of education) **that may impact learning style, choice of informational resources.**
- Determine challenges to learning: language barriers (e.g., can't read, speaks/understands only nondominant language); physical factors (e.g., sensory deficits, such as aphasia, dyslexia); physical stability (e.g., acute illness, activity intolerance); difficulty of material to be learned. **Identifies special needs to be addressed if learning is to be successful.**

NURSING PRIORITY NO. **2.** To facilitate learning:

- Identify/provide information in varied formats appropriate to client's learning style (e.g., audiotapes, print materials, videos, classes/seminars). **Use of multiple formats increases learning and retention of material.**
- Provide information about additional/outside learning resources (e.g., bibliography, pertinent Web sites). **Promotes ongoing learning at own pace.**
- Discuss ways to verify accuracy of informational resources. **Encourages independent search for learning opportunities**

while reducing likelihood of acting on erroneous or unproven data that could be detrimental to client's well-being.

- Identify available community resources/support groups. **Provides additional opportunities for role-modeling, skill training, anticipatory problem solving, and so forth.**
- Be aware of informal teaching and role modeling that takes place on an ongoing basis (e.g., community/peer role models, support group feedback, print advertisements, popular music/videos). **Incongruencies may exist creating questions/potentially undermining learning process.**

NURSING PRIORITY NO. 3. To enhance optimum wellness:

- Assist client to identify ways to integrate and use information in all applicable areas (e.g., situational, environmental, personal). **Ability to apply/use information increases desire to learn and retention of information.**
- Encourage client to journal, keep a log or graph as appropriate. **Provides opportunity for self-evaluation of effects of learning, such as better management of chronic condition, reduction of risk factors, acquisition of new skills.**

Documentation Focus

ASSESSMENT/REASSESSMENT

- Individual findings/learning style and identified needs, presence of challenges to learning.

PLANNING

- Plan for learning, methods to be used, and who is involved in the planning.
- Educational plan.

IMPLEMENTATION/EVALUATION

- Responses of the client/SO(s) to the learning plan and actions performed.
- How the learning is demonstrated.
- Attainment/progress toward desired outcome(s).
- Modifications to lifestyle/treatment plan.

DISCHARGE PLANNING

- Additional learning/referral needs.

SAMPLE NURSING OUTCOMES & INTERVENTIONS CLASSIFICATIONS (NOC/NIC)

NOC—Knowledge: [specify—25 choices]
NIC—Teaching: [specify—14 choices]

Loneliness, risk for

Taxonomy II: Self-Perception—Class 1 Self-Concept
(00054)
[Diagnostic Division: Social Interaction]
Submitted 1994

Definition: At risk for experiencing vague dysphoria

Risk Factors

Affectional deprivation
Physical isolation
Cathectic deprivation
Social isolation

> NOTE: A risk diagnosis is not evidenced by signs and symptoms, as
> the problem has not occurred and nursing interventions are
> directed at prevention.

Desired Outcomes/Evaluation Criteria—Client Will:

* Identify individual difficulties and ways to address them.
* Engage in social activities.
* Report involvement in interactions/relationship client views
  as meaningful.

Actions/Interventions

NURSING PRIORITY NO. **1.** To identify causative/precipitating
factors:

* Differentiate between ordinary loneliness and a state of
  constant sense of dysphoria. Note client's age and duration of
  problem, that is, situational (such as leaving home for college)
  or chronic. **Elderly individuals incur multiple losses associ-
  ated with aging, loss of spouse, decline in physical health, and
  changes in roles intensifying feelings of loneliness.**
* Determine degree of distress, tension, anxiety, restlessness
  present. Note history of frequent illnesses, accidents, crises.
* Note presence/proximity of family, SO(s).
* Determine how individual perceives/deals with solitude.
* Review issues of separation from parents as a child, loss of
  SO(s)/spouse.
* Assess sleep/appetite disturbances, ability to concentrate.
* Note expressions of "yearning" for an emotional partnership.

NURSING PRIORITY NO. **2.** To assist client to identify feelings and
situations in which he or she experiences loneliness:

* Establish nurse-client relationship in which client feels free to
  talk about feelings.

Information that appears in brackets has been added by the authors
to clarify and enhance the use of nursing diagnoses.

- Discuss individual concerns about feelings of loneliness and relationship between loneliness and lack of SO(s). Note desire/willingness to change situation. **Motivation can impede—or facilitate—achieving desired outcomes.**
- Support expression of negative perceptions of others and whether client agrees. **Provides opportunity for client to clarify reality of situation, recognize own denial.**
- Accept client's expressions of loneliness as a primary condition and not necessarily as a symptom of some underlying condition.

NURSING PRIORITY NO. 3. To assist client to become involved:

- Discuss reality versus perceptions of situation.
- Discuss importance of emotional bonding (attachment) between infants/young children, parents/caregivers as appropriate.
- Involve in classes, such as assertiveness, language/communication, social skills, **to address individual needs/enhance socialization.**
- Role-play situations to develop interpersonal skills.
- Discuss positive health habits, including personal hygiene, exercise activity of client's choosing.
- Identify individual strengths, areas of interest **that provide opportunities for involvement with others.**
- Encourage attendance at group activities to meet individual needs (e.g., therapy, separation/grief, religion).
- Help client establish plan for progressive involvement, beginning with a simple activity (e.g., call an old friend, speak to a neighbor) and leading to more complicated interactions/activities.
- Provide opportunities for interactions in a supportive environment (e.g., have client accompanied as in a "buddy system") during initial attempts to socialize. **Helps reduce stress, provides positive reinforcement, and facilitates successful outcome.**

NURSING PRIORITY NO. 4. To promote wellness (Teaching/Discharge Considerations):

- Encourage involvement in special-interest groups (computers, bird watchers); charitable services (serving in a soup kitchen, youth groups, animal shelter).
- Suggest volunteering for church committee or choir; attending community events with friends and family; becoming involved in political issues/campaigns; enrolling in classes at local college/continuing education programs.
- Refer to appropriate counselors for help with relationships and so on.
- Refer to NDs Hopelessness; Anxiety; Social Isolation.

Documentation Focus

ASSESSMENT/REASSESSMENT

- Assessment findings, including client's perception of problem, availability of resources/support systems.
- Client's desire/commitment to change.

PLANNING

- Plan of care and who is involved in planning.
- Teaching plan.

IMPLEMENTATION/EVALUATION

- Response to interventions/teaching and actions performed.
- Attainment/progress toward desired outcome(s).
- Modifications to plan of care.

DISCHARGE PLANNING

- Long-term needs, plan for follow-up and who is responsible for actions to be taken.
- Specific referrals made.

SAMPLE NURSING OUTCOMES & INTERVENTIONS CLASSIFICATIONS (NOC/NIC)

NOC—Loneliness
NIC—Socialization Enhancement

Memory, impaired

Taxonomy II: Perception/Cognition—Class 4 Cognition (00131)
[Diagnostic Division: Neurosensory]
Submitted 1994

Definition: Inability to remember or recall bits of information or behavioral skills (Impaired memory may be attributed to physiopathological or situational causes that are either temporary or permanent)

Related Factors

Acute or chronic hypoxia
Anemia
Decreased cardiac output
Fluid and electrolyte imbalance
Neurological disturbances [e.g., brain injury/concussion]
Excessive environmental disturbances; [manic state, fugue, traumatic event]

Information that appears in brackets has been added by the authors to clarify and enhance the use of nursing diagnoses.

[Substance use/abuse; effects of medications]
[Age]

Defining Characteristics

SUBJECTIVE

Reported experiences of forgetting
Inability to recall recent or past events, factual information, [or familiar persons, places, items]

OBJECTIVE

Observed experiences of forgetting
Inability to determine if a behavior was performed
Inability to learn or retain new skills or information
Inability to perform a previously learned skill
Forget to perform a behavior at a scheduled time

Desired Outcomes/Evaluation Criteria—Client Will:

- Verbalize awareness of memory problems.
- Establish methods to help in remembering essential things when possible.
- Accept limitations of condition and use resources effectively.

Actions/Interventions

NURSING PRIORITY NO. 1. To assess causative factor(s)/degree of impairment:

- Determine physical/biochemical factors that may be related to loss of memory.
- Assist with/review results of cognitive testing.
- Evaluate skill proficiency levels, including self-care activities and driving ability.
- Ascertain how client/family view the problem (e.g., practical problems of forgetting and/or role and responsibility impairments related to loss of memory and concentration) **to determine significance/impact of problem.**

NURSING PRIORITY NO. 2. To maximize level of function:

- Implement appropriate memory retraining techniques, such as keeping calendars, writing lists, memory cue games, mnemonic devices, using computers, and so forth.
- Assist in/instruct client and family in associate-learning tasks, such as practice sessions recalling personal information, reminiscing, locating a geographic location (Stimulation Therapy).
- Encourage ventilation of feelings of frustration, helplessness, and so forth. Refocus attention to areas of control and progress **to lessen feelings of powerlessness/hopelessness.**

- Provide for/emphasize importance of pacing learning activities and having appropriate rest **to avoid fatigue.**
- Monitor client's behavior and assist in use of stress-management techniques **to reduce frustration.**
- Structure teaching methods and interventions to client's level of functioning and/or potential for improvement.
- Determine client's response to/effects of medications prescribed to improve attention, concentration, memory processes and to lift spirits/modify emotional responses. **Helpful in deciding whether quality of life is improved when considering side effects/cost of drugs.**

NURSING PRIORITY NO. 3. To promote wellness (Teaching/Discharge Considerations):

- Assist client/SO(s) to establish compensation strategies **to improve functional lifestyle and safety,** such as menu planning with a shopping list, timely completion of tasks on a daily planner, checklists at the front door to ascertain that lights and stove are off before leaving.
- Refer to/encourage follow-up with counselors, rehabilitation programs, job coaches, social/financial support systems **to help deal with persistent/difficult problems.**
- Assist client to deal with functional limitations (such as loss of driving privileges) and identify resources **to meet individual needs, maximizing independence.**

Documentation Focus

ASSESSMENT/REASSESSMENT

- Individual findings, testing results, and perceptions of significance of problem.
- Actual impact on lifestyle and independence.

PLANNING

- Plan of care and who is involved in planning process.
- Teaching plan.

IMPLEMENTATION/EVALUATION

- Responses to interventions/teaching and actions performed.
- Attainment/progress toward desired outcome(s).
- Modifications to plan of care.

DISCHARGE PLANNING

- Long-term needs and who is responsible for actions to be taken.
- Specific referrals made.

SAMPLE NURSING OUTCOMES
& INTERVENTIONS CLASSIFICATIONS (NOC/NIC)

NOC—Memory
NIC—Memory Training

Mobility, impaired bed

Taxonomy II: Activity/Rest—Class 2 Activity/Exercise
(00091)
[Diagnostic Division: Safety]
Submitted 1998

Definition: Limitation of independent movement from
one bed position to another

Related Factors

To be developed
[Neuromuscular impairment]
[Pain/discomfort]

Defining Characteristics

SUBJECTIVE

[Reported difficulty performing activities]

OBJECTIVE

Impaired ability to: turn side to side, move from supine to sitting or
sitting to supine, "scoot" or reposition self in bed, move from supine
to prone or prone to supine, from supine to long-sitting or long-
sitting to supine

Desired Outcomes/Evaluation
Criteria—Client/Caregiver Will:

- Verbalize willingness to/and participate in repositioning
  program.
- Verbalize understanding of situation/risk factors, individual
  therapeutic regimen, and safety measures.
- Demonstrate techniques/behaviors that enable safe repositioning.
- Maintain position of function and skin integrity as
  evidenced by absence of contractures, footdrop, decubitus,
  and so forth.
- Maintain or increase strength and function of affected and/or
  compensatory body part.

Information that appears in brackets has been added by the authors
to clarify and enhance the use of nursing diagnoses.

Actions/Interventions

NURSING PRIORITY NO. 1. To identify causative/contributing factors:

- Determine diagnoses that contribute to immobility (e.g., MS, arthritis, parkinsonism, hemi/para/tetraplegia, fractures/ multiple trauma, mental illness, depression).
- Note individual risk factors and current situation, such as surgery, casts, amputation, traction, pain, age/weakness/debilitation, severe depression, aggravating immobility, head injury, dementia, burns, SCI.
- Determine degree of perceptual/cognitive impairment and/or ability to follow directions.

NURSING PRIORITY NO. 2. To assess functional ability:

- Determine functional level classification 1 to 4 (1 = requires use of equipment or device, 2 = requires help from another person for assistance, 3 = requires help from another person and equipment device, 4 = dependent, does not participate in activity).
- Note emotional/behavioral responses to problems of immobility.
- Note presence of complications related to immobility.

NURSING PRIORITY NO. 3. To promote optimal level of function and prevent complications:

- Include physical and occupational therapists in creating exercise program and identifying assistive devices.
- Turn frequently, reposition in good body alignment, using appropriate support.
- Instruct caregivers in methods of moving client relative to specific situations.
- Observe skin for reddened areas/shearing. Provide regular skin care as appropriate.
- Assist on/off bedpan and into sitting position when possible. **Facilitates elimination.**
- Administer medication prior to activity as needed for pain relief **to permit maximal effort/involvement in activity.**
- Observe for change in strength to do more or less self-care **to adjust care as indicated.**
- Assist with activities of hygiene, toileting, feeding.
- Provide diversional activities as appropriate.
- Ensure call bell is within reach.
- Provide individually appropriate methods to communicate adequately with client.
- Provide extremity protection (padding, exercises, etc.).

NURSING PRIORITY NO. 4. To promote wellness (Teaching/ Discharge Considerations):

- Involve client/SO in determining activity schedule. **Promotes commitment to plan, maximizing outcomes.**
- Encourage continuation of exercises **to maintain/enhance gains in strength/muscle control.**
- Obtain/identify sources for assistive devices. Demonstrate safe use and proper maintenance.

Documentation Focus

ASSESSMENT/REASSESSMENT

- Individual findings, including level of function/ability to participate in specific/desired activities.

PLANNING

- Plan of care and who is involved in the planning.

IMPLEMENTATION/EVALUATION

- Responses to interventions/teaching and actions performed.
- Attainment/progress toward desired outcome(s).
- Modification to plan of care.

DISCHARGE PLANNING

- Discharge/long-range needs, noting who is responsible for each action to be taken.
- Specific referrals made.
- Sources of/maintenance for assistive devices.

SAMPLE NURSING OUTCOMES & INTERVENTIONS CLASSIFICATIONS (NOC/NIC)

NOC—Body Position: Self-Initiated
NIC—Bed Rest Care

Mobility, impaired physical

Taxonomy II: Activity/Rest—Class 2 Activity/Exercise (00085)
[Diagnostic Division: Safety]
Submitted 1973; Nursing Diagnosis Extension and Classification (NDEC) Revision 1998

Definition: Limitation in independent, purposeful physical movement of the body or of one or more extremities

Information that appears in brackets has been added by the authors to clarify and enhance the use of nursing diagnoses.

Related Factors

Sedentary lifestyle, disuse or deconditioning; limited cardiovascular endurance

Decreased muscle strength, control and/or mass; joint stiffness or contracture; loss of integrity of bone structures

Intolerance to activity/decreased strength and endurance

Pain/discomfort

Neuromuscular/musculoskeletal impairment

Sensoriperceptual/cognitive impairment; developmental delay

Depressive mood state or anxiety

Selective or generalized malnutrition; altered cellular metabolism; body mass index above 75th age-appropriate percentile

Lack of knowledge regarding value of physical activity; cultural beliefs regarding age-appropriate activity; lack of physical or social environmental supports

Prescribed movement restrictions; medications

Reluctance to initiate movement

Defining Characteristics

SUBJECTIVE

[Report of pain/discomfort on movement]

OBJECTIVE

Limited range of motion; limited ability to perform gross fine/motor skills; difficulty turning

Slowed movement; uncoordinated or jerky movements, decreased [sic]reaction time

Gait changes (e.g., decreased walking speed; difficulty initiating gait, small steps, shuffles feet; exaggerated lateral postural sway)

Postural instability during performance of routine ADLs

Movement-induced shortness of breath/tremor

Engages in substitutions for movement (e.g., increased attention to other's activity, controlling behavior, focus on preillness/disability activity)

Suggested Functional Level Classification:

0—Completely independent

1—Requires use of equipment or device

2—Requires help from another person for assistance, supervision, or teaching

3—Requires help from another person and equipment device

4—Dependent, does not participate in activity

Desired Outcomes/Evaluation Criteria—Client Will:

• Verbalize willingness to and demonstrate participation in activities.

- Verbalize understanding of situation/risk factors and individual treatment regimen and safety measures.
- Demonstrate techniques/behaviors that enable resumption of activities.
- Maintain position of function and skin integrity as evidenced by absence of contractures, footdrop, decubitus, and so forth.
- Maintain or increase strength and function of affected and/or compensatory body part.

Actions/Interventions

NURSING PRIORITY NO. **1.** To identify causative/contributing factors:

- Determine diagnosis that contributes to immobility (e.g., MS, arthritis, parkinsonism, hemiplegia/paraplegia, depression).
- Note situations such as surgery, fractures, amputation, tubings (chest, catheter, etc.) that may restrict movement.
- Assess degree of pain, listening to client's description.
- Ascertain client's perception of activity/exercise needs.
- Note decreased motor agility related to age.
- Determine degree of perceptual/cognitive impairment and ability to follow directions.
- Assess nutritional status and energy level.

NURSING PRIORITY NO. **2.** To assess functional ability:

- Determine degree of immobility in relation to previously suggested scale.
- Observe movement when client is unaware of observation **to note any incongruencies with reports of abilities.**
- Note emotional/behavioral responses to problems of immobility. **Feelings of frustration/powerlessness may impede attainment of goals.**
- Determine presence of complications related to immobility (e.g., pneumonia, elimination problems, contractures, decubitus, anxiety). Refer to ND Disuse Syndrome, risk for.

NURSING PRIORITY NO. **3.** To promote optimal level of function and prevent complications:

- Assist/have client reposition self on a regular schedule as dictated by individual situation (including frequent shifting of weight when client is wheelchair-bound).
- Instruct in use of siderails, overhead trapeze, roller pads **for position changes/transfers.**
- Support affected body parts/joints using pillows/rolls, foot supports/shoes, air mattress, water bed, and so forth **to maintain position of function and reduce risk of pressure ulcers.**

- Assist with treatment of underlying condition causing pain and/or dysfunction.
- Administer medications prior to activity as needed for pain relief **to permit maximal effort/involvement in activity.**
- Provide regular skin care to include pressure area management.
- Schedule activities with adequate rest periods during the day **to reduce fatigue.** Provide client with ample time to perform mobility-related tasks.
- Encourage participation in self-care, occupational/diversional/recreational activities. **Enhances self-concept and sense of independence.**
- Identify energy-conserving techniques for ADLs. **Limits fatigue, maximizing participation.**
- Discuss discrepancies in movement when client aware/unaware of observation and methods for dealing with identified problems.
- Provide for safety measures as indicated by individual situation, including environmental management/fall prevention.
- Consult with physical/occupational therapist as indicated **to develop individual exercise/mobility program and identify appropriate adjunctive devices.**
- Encourage adequate intake of fluids/nutritious foods. **Promotes well-being and maximizes energy production.**

NURSING PRIORITY NO. **4.** To promote wellness (Teaching/Discharge Considerations):

- Encourage client's/SO's involvement in decision making as much as possible. **Enhances commitment to plan, optimizing outcomes.**
- Assist client to learn safety measures as individually indicated (e.g., use of heating pads, locking wheelchair before transfers, removal or securing of scatter/area rugs).
- Involve client and SO(s) in care, assisting them to learn ways of managing problems of immobility.
- Demonstrate use of adjunctive devices (e.g., walkers, braces, prosthetics). Identify appropriate resources for obtaining and maintaining appliances/equipment. **Promotes independence and enhances safety.**
- Review individual dietary needs. Identify appropriate vitamin/herbal supplements.

Documentation Focus

ASSESSMENT/REASSESSMENT

- Individual findings, including level of function/ability to participate in specific/desired activities.

PLANNING

- Plan of care and who is involved in the planning.
- Teaching plan.

IMPLEMENTATION/EVALUATION

- Responses to interventions/teaching and actions performed.
- Attainment/progress toward desired outcome(s).
- Modifications to plan of care.

DISCHARGE PLANNING

- Discharge/long-range needs, noting who is responsible for each action to be taken.
- Specific referrals made.
- Sources of/maintenance for assistive devices.

SAMPLE NURSING OUTCOMES & INTERVENTIONS CLASSIFICATIONS (NOC/NIC)

NOC—Mobility Level
NIC—Exercise Therapy: Muscle Control

Mobility, impaired wheelchair

Taxonomy II: Activity/Rest—Class 2 Activity/Exercise (00089)
[Diagnostic Division: Safety]
Submitted 1998

Definition: Limitation of independent operation of wheelchair within environment

Related Factors

To be developed

Defining Characteristics

Impaired ability to operate manual or power wheelchair on even or uneven surface, on an incline or decline, on curbs
Note: Specify level of independence (Refer to ND Mobility, impaired physical)

Desired Outcomes/Evaluation Criteria—Client Will:

- Be able to move safely within environment, maximizing independence.
- Identify and use resources appropriately.

Information that appears in brackets has been added by the authors to clarify and enhance the use of nursing diagnoses.

Caregiver Will:

* Provide safe mobility within environment and community.

Actions/Interventions

NURSING PRIORITY NO. **1.** To identify causative/contributing factors:

* Determine diagnosis that contributes to immobility (e.g., ALS, SCI, spastic cerebral palsy, brain injury) and client's functional level/individual abilities.
* Identify factors in environments frequented by the client that contribute to inaccessibility (e.g., uneven floors/surfaces, lack of ramps, steep incline/decline, narrow doorways/ spaces).
* Ascertain access to and appropriateness of public and/or private transportation.

NURSING PRIORITY NO. **2.** To promote optimal level of function and prevent complications:

* Ascertain that wheelchair provides the base mobility to maximize function.
* Provide for client's safety while in a wheelchair (e.g., supports for all body parts, repositioning and transfer assistive devices, and height adjustment).
* Note evenness of surfaces client would need to negotiate and refer to appropriate sources for modifications. Clear pathways of obstructions.
* Recommend/arrange for alterations to home/work or school/recreational settings frequented by client.
* Determine need for and capabilities of assistive persons. Provide training and support as indicated.
* Monitor client's use of joystick, sip and puff, sensitive mechanical switches, and so forth **to provide necessary equipment if condition/capabilities change.**
* Monitor client for adverse effects of immobility (e.g., contractures, muscle atrophy, DVT, pressure ulcers).

NURSING PRIORITY NO. **3.** To promote wellness (Teaching/ Discharge Considerations):

* Identify/refer to medical equipment suppliers **to customize client's wheelchair for size, positioning aids, and electronics suited to client's ability (e.g., sip and puff, head movement, sensitive switches, etc.).**
* Encourage client's/SO's involvement in decision making as much as possible. **Enhances commitment to plan, optimizing outcomes.**
* Involve client/SO(s) in care, assisting them in managing immobility problems. **Promotes independence.**

- Demonstrate/provide information regarding individually appropriate safety measures.
- Refer to support groups relative to specific medical condition/disability; independence/political action groups. **Provides role modeling, assistance with problem solving.**
- Identify community resources **to provide ongoing support.**

Documentation Focus

ASSESSMENT/REASSESSMENT

- Individual findings, including level of function/ability to participate in specific/desired activities.

PLANNING

- Plan of care and who is involved in the planning.
- Teaching plan.

IMPLEMENTATION/EVALUATION

- Responses to interventions/teaching and actions performed.

DISCHARGE PLANNING

- Discharge/long-range needs, noting who is responsible for each action to be taken.
- Specific referrals made.
- Sources of/maintenance for assistive devices.

SAMPLE NURSING OUTCOMES & INTERVENTIONS CLASSIFICATIONS (NOC/NIC)

NOC—Ambulation: Wheelchair
NIC—Positioning: Wheelchair

Nausea

Taxonomy II: Comfort—Class 1 Physical Comfort (00134)
[Diagnostic Division: Food/Fluid]
Submitted 1998; Revised 2002

Definition: A subjective unpleasant, wavelike sensation in the back of the throat, epigastrium, or abdomen that may lead to the urge or need to vomit

Related Factors

TREATMENT RELATED

Gastric irritation: Pharmaceuticals (e.g., aspirin, nonsteroidal anti-inflammatory drugs, steroids, antibiotics), alcohol, iron, and blood

---

Information that appears in brackets has been added by the authors to clarify and enhance the use of nursing diagnoses.

Gastric distention: delayed gastric emptying caused by pharmacological interventions (e.g., narcotics administration, anesthesia agents)

Pharmaceuticals (e.g., analgesics, antiviral for HIV, aspirin, opioids, chemotherapeutic agents)

Toxins (e.g., radiotherapy)

BIOPHYSICAL

Biochemical disorders (e.g., uremia, diabetic ketoacidosis, pregnancy)

Cardiac pain; cancer of stomach or intra-abdominal tumors (e.g., pelvic or colorectal cancers); local tumors (e.g., acoustic neuroma, primary or secondary brain tumors, bone metastases at base of skull)

Toxins (e.g., tumor-produced peptides, abdominal metabolites due to cancer)

Esophageal or pancreatic disease; liver or splenetic capsule stretch

Gastric distention due to delayed gastric emptying, pyloric intestinal obstruction, genitourinary and biliary distension, upper bowel stasis, external compression of the stomach, liver, spleen, or other organ enlargement that slows stomach functioning (squashed stomach syndrome), excess food intake

Gastric irritation due to pharyngeal and/or peritoneal inflammation

Motion sickness, Meniere's disease, or labyrinthitis

Physical factors such as increased intracranial pressure, and meningitis

SITUATIONAL

Psychological factors (e.g., pain, fear, anxiety, noxious odors, taste, unpleasant visual stimulation)

Defining Characteristics

SUBJECTIVE

Reports nausea ("sick to my stomach")

OBJECTIVE

Aversion toward food
Increased salivation, sour taste in mouth
Increased swallowing, gagging sensation

Desired Outcomes/Evaluation Criteria—Client Will:

- Be free of nausea.
- Manage chronic nausea, as evidenced by acceptable level of dietary intake.
- Maintain/regain weight as appropriate.

Actions/Interventions

NURSING PRIORITY NO. 1. To determine causative/contributing factors:

- Assess for presence of conditions of the GI tract (e.g., peptic ulcer disease, cholecystitis, gastritis, ingestion of "problem" foods). **Dietary changes may be sufficient to decrease frequency of nausea.**

- Note systemic conditions that may result in nausea (e.g., pregnancy, cancer treatment, myocardial infarction—MI, hepatitis, systemic infections, drug toxicity, presence of neurogenic causes-stimulation of the vestibular system, CNS trauma/tumor). **Helpful in determining appropriate interventions/need for treatment of underlying condition.**
- Identify situations that client perceives as anxiety inducing, threatening, or distasteful (e.g., "this is nauseating"). **May be able to limit/control exposure to situations or take medication prophylactically.**
- Note psychologic factors, including those that are culturally determined (e.g., eating certain foods considered repulsive in one's own culture).
- Determine if nausea is potentially self-limiting and/or mild (e.g., first trimester of pregnancy, 24-hour GI viral infection) or is severe and prolonged (e.g., cancer treatment, hyperemesis gravidarum). **Indicates degree of effect on fluid/electrolyte balance and nutritional status.**
- Check vital signs, especially for older clients, and note signs of dehydration. **Nausea may occur in the presence of postural hypotension/fluid volume deficit.**

NURSING PRIORITY NO. 2. To promote comfort and enhance intake:

- Administer/monitor response to medications that prevent or relieve nausea. **Provides sedative effect and prevents or relieves nausea. (Older clients are more prone to side effects [e.g., excessive sedation, extrapyramidal movements].)**
- Have client try dry foods such as toast, crackers, dry cereal before arising when nausea occurs in the morning, or throughout the day as appropriate.
- Advise client to drink liquids before or after meals, instead of with meals.
- Provide diet and snacks with substitutions of preferred foods when available (including bland/noncaffeinated carbonated beverages, gelatin, sherbet) **to reduce gastric acidity and improve nutrient intake.** Include bland beverages, gelatin, sherbet. Avoid overly sweet, fried and fatty foods **that may increase nausea/be more difficult to digest.**
- Encourage client to eat small meals spaced throughout the day instead of large meals **so stomach does not feel excessively full.**
- Instruct client to eat and drink slowly, chewing food well **to enhance digestion.**

- Provide clean, pleasant smelling, quiet environment. Avoid offending odors such as cooking smells, smoke, perfumes, mechanical emissions when possible **as they may stimulate or worsen nausea.**
- Provide frequent oral care **to cleanse mouth and minimize "bad tastes."**
- Advise client to suck on ice cubes, tart or hard candies; drink cool, clear liquids, such as light-colored sodas. **Can provide some fluid/nutrient intake.**
- Encourage deep, slow breathing **to promote relaxation and refocus attention away from nausea.**
- Use distraction with music, chatting with family/friends, watching TV **to limit dwelling on unpleasant sensation.**
- Administer antiemetic on regular schedule before/during and after administration of antineoplastic agents **to prevent/ control side effects of medication.**
- Investigate use of acupressure point therapy (e.g., elastic band worn around wrist with small, hard bump that presses against acupressure point). **Some individuals with chronic nausea report this to be helpful and without sedative effect of medication.**
- Time chemotherapy doses **for least interference with food intake.**

NURSING PRIORITY NO. 3. To promote wellness (Teaching/ Discharge Considerations):

- Review individual factors causing nausea and ways to avoid problem. **Provides necessary information for client to manage own care.**
- Instruct in proper use, side effects, and adverse reactions of antiemetic medications. **Enhances client safety and effective management of condition.**
- Advise client to prepare and freeze meals in advance **for days when nausea is severe or cooking is impossible.**
- Discuss potential complications and possible need for medical follow-up or alternative therapies. **Timely recognition and intervention may limit severity of complications (e.g., dehydration).**
- Review signs of dehydration and stress importance of replacing fluids and/or electrolytes (with products such as Gatorade or Pedialyte). **Increases likelihood of preventing potentially serious complication.**

Documentation Focus

ASSESSMENT/REASSESSMENT

- Individual findings, including individual factors causing nausea.

- Baseline weight, vital signs.
- Specific client preferences for nutritional intake.

PLANNING

- Plan of care and who is involved in planning.
- Teaching plan.

IMPLEMENTATION/EVALUATION

- Response to interventions/teaching and actions performed.
- Attainment/progress toward desired outcome(s).
- Modifications to plan of care.

DISCHARGE PLANNING

- Individual long-term needs, noting who is responsible for actions to be taken.
- Specific referrals made.

SAMPLE NURSING OUTCOMES & INTERVENTIONS CLASSIFICATIONS (NOC/NIC)

NOC—Symptom Severity
NIC—Nausea Management

Noncompliance [Adherence, ineffective] [specify]

Taxonomy II: Life Principles—Class 3 Value/Belief/Action Congruence (00079)
[Diagnostic Division: Teaching/Learning]
Submitted 1973; Revised 1998 (by small group work 1996)

Definition: Behavior of person and/or caregiver that fails to coincide with a health-promoting or therapeutic plan agreed on by the person (and/or family and/or community) and healthcare professional; in the presence of an agreed-on health-promoting or therapeutic plan, person's or caregiver's behavior is fully or partially adherent or nonadherent and may lead to clinically ineffective, partially ineffective outcomes

Related Factors

HEALTHCARE PLAN

Duration
SOs; cost; intensity; complexity

Information that appears in brackets has been added by the authors to clarify and enhance the use of nursing diagnoses.

INDIVIDUAL FACTORS

Personal and developmental abilities; knowledge and skill relevant to the regimen behavior; motivational forces

Individual's value system; health beliefs, cultural influences, spiritual values

[Altered thought processes, such as depression, paranoia]

[Difficulty changing behavior, as in addictions]

[Issues of secondary gain]

HEALTH SYSTEM

Individual health coverage; financial flexibility of plan

Credibility of provider; client-provider relationships; provider continuity and regular follow-up; provider reimbursement of teaching and follow-up; communication and teaching skills of the provider

Access and convenience of care; satisfaction with care

NETWORK

Involvement of members in health plan; social value regarding plan

Perceived beliefs of SOs' communication and teaching skills

Defining Characteristics

SUBJECTIVE

Statements by client or SO(s) of failure to adhere (does not perceive illness/risk to be serious, does not believe in efficacy of therapy, unwilling to follow treatment regimen or accept side effects/limitations)

OBJECTIVE

Behavior indicative of failure to adhere (by direct observation)

Objective tests (e.g., physiological measures, detection of physiologic markers)

Failure to progress

Evidence of development of complications/exacerbation of symptoms

Failure to keep appointments

[Inability to set or attain mutual goals]

[Denial]

Desired Outcomes/Evaluation Criteria—Client Will:

- Participate in the development of mutually agreeable goals and treatment plan.
- Verbalize accurate knowledge of condition and understanding of treatment regimen.
- Make choices at level of readiness based on accurate information.
- Access resources appropriately.
- Demonstrate progress toward desired outcomes/goals.

Actions/Interventions

NURSING PRIORITY NO. 1. To determine reason for alteration/disregard of therapeutic regimen/instructions:

- Discuss with client/SO(s) their perception/understanding of the situation (illness/treatment).
- Listen to/Active-listen client's complaints, comments.
- Note language spoken, read, and understood.
- Be aware of developmental level as well as chronological age of client.
- Assess level of anxiety, locus of control, sense of powerlessness, and so forth.
- Note length of illness. (**Clients tend to become passive and dependent in long-term, debilitating illnesses.**)
- Clarify value system: cultural/religious values, health/illness beliefs of the client/SO(s).
- Determine social characteristics, demographic and educational factors, as well as personality of the client.
- Verify psychologic meaning of the behavior (e.g., may be denial). Note issues of secondary gain—**family dynamics, school/workplace issues, involvement in legal system may unconsciously affect client's decision.**
- Assess availability/use of support systems and resources.
- Be aware of nurses'/healthcare providers' attitudes and behaviors toward the client. (Do they have an investment in the client's compliance/recovery? What is the behavior of the client and nurse when client is labeled "noncompliant"?) **Some care providers may be enabling client whereas others' judgmental attitudes may impede treatment progress.**

NURSING PRIORITY NO. 2. To assist client/SO(s) to develop strategies for dealing effectively with the situation:

- Develop therapeutic nurse-client relationship. **Promotes trust, provides atmosphere in which client/SO(s) can freely express views/concerns.**
- Explore client involvement in or lack of mutual goal setting. (**Client will be more likely to follow through on goals he or she participated in developing.**)
- Review treatment strategies. Identify which interventions in the plan of care are most important in meeting therapeutic goals and which are least amenable to compliance. **Sets priorities and encourages problem solving areas of conflict.**
- Contract with the client for participation in care. **Enhances commitment to follow through.**
- Encourage client to maintain self-care, providing for assistance when necessary. Accept client's evaluation of own strengths/limitations while working with client to improve abilities.

- Provide for continuity of care in and out of the hospital/care setting, including long-range plans. **Supports trust, facilitates progress toward goals.**
- Provide information and help client to know where and how to find it on own. **Promotes independence and encourages informed decision making.**
- Give information in manageable amounts, using verbal, written, and audiovisual modes at level of client's ability. **Facilitates learning.**
- Have client paraphrase instructions/information heard. **Helps validate client's understanding and reveals misconceptions.**
- Accept the client's choice/point of view, even if it appears to be self-destructive. Avoid confrontation regarding beliefs **to maintain open communication.**
- Establish graduated goals or modified regimen as necessary (e.g., client with COPD who smokes a pack of cigarettes a day may be willing to reduce that amount). **May improve quality of life, encouraging progression to more advanced goals.**

NURSING PRIORITY NO. 3. To promote wellness (Teaching/Discharge Considerations):

- Stress importance of the client's knowledge and understanding of the need for treatment/medication, as well as consequences of actions/choices.
- Develop a system for self-monitoring **to provide a sense of control and enable the client to follow own progress and assist with making choices.**
- Provide support systems **to reinforce negotiated behaviors.** Encourage client to continue positive behaviors, especially if client is beginning to see benefit.
- Refer to counseling/therapy and/or other appropriate resources.
- Refer to NDs Coping, ineffective; Coping, family: compromised; Knowledge, deficient (specify); Anxiety.

Documentation Focus

ASSESSMENT/REASSESSMENT

- Individual findings/deviation from prescribed treatment plan and client's reasons in own words.
- Consequences of actions to date.

PLANNING

- Plan of care and who is involved in planning.
- Teaching plan.

IMPLEMENTATION/EVALUATION

- Response to interventions/teaching and actions performed.
- Attainment/progress toward desired outcome(s).
- Modifications to plan of care.

DISCHARGE PLANNING

- Long-term needs and who is responsible for actions to be taken.
- Specific referrals made.

SAMPLE NURSING OUTCOMES
& INTERVENTIONS CLASSIFICATIONS (NOC/NIC)

NOC—Compliance Behavior
NIC—Mutual Goal Setting

Nutrition: imbalanced, less than body requirements

Taxonomy II: Nutrition—Class 1 Ingestion (00002)
[Diagnostic Division: Food/Fluid]
Submitted 1975

Definition: Intake of nutrients insufficient to meet metabolic needs

Related Factors

Inability to ingest or digest food or absorb nutrients because of biological, psychological, or economical factors
[Increased metabolic demands, e.g., burns]
[Lack of information, misinformation, misconceptions]

Defining Characteristics

SUBJECTIVE

Reported inadequate food intake less than recommended daily allowances (RDA)
Reported lack of food
Aversion to eating; reported altered taste sensation; satiety immediately after ingesting food
Abdominal pain with or without pathological condition; abdominal cramping
Lack of interest in food; perceived inability to digest food
Lack of information, misinformation, misconceptions [Note: The authors view this as a related factor rather than a defining characteristic.]

Information that appears in brackets has been added by the authors to clarify and enhance the use of nursing diagnoses.

OBJECTIVE

Body weight 20% or more under ideal [for height and frame]
Loss of weight with adequate food intake
Evidence of lack of [available] food
Weakness of muscles required for swallowing or mastication
Sore, inflamed buccal cavity
Poor muscle tone
Capillary fragility
Hyperactive bowel sounds; diarrhea and/or steatorrhea
Pale conjunctiva and mucous membranes
Excessive loss of hair [or increased growth of hair on body (lanugo)];
   [cessation of menses]
[Decreased subcutaneous fat/muscle mass]
[Abnormal laboratory studies (e.g., decreased albumin, total proteins;
   iron deficiency; electrolyte imbalances)]

Desired Outcomes/Evaluation Criteria—Client Will:

- Demonstrate progressive weight gain toward goal.
- Display normalization of laboratory values and be free of signs of malnutrition as reflected in Defining Characteristics.
- Verbalize understanding of causative factors when known and necessary interventions.
- Demonstrate behaviors, lifestyle changes to regain and/or maintain appropriate weight.

Actions/Interventions

NURSING PRIORITY NO. 1. To assess causative/contributing factors:

- Identify clients at risk for malnutrition (e.g., intestinal surgery, hypermetabolic states, restricted intake, prior nutritional deficiencies).
- Determine ability to chew, swallow, taste. Note denture fit; presence of mechanical barriers; lactose intolerance, cystic fibrosis, pancreatic disease (**factors that can affect ingestion and/or digestion of nutrients**).
- Ascertain understanding of individual nutritional needs **to determine what information to provide client/SO.**
- Note availability/use of financial resources and support systems. Determine ability to acquire and store various types of food.
- Discuss eating habits, including food preferences, intolerances/aversions **to appeal to clients likes/desires.**
- Assess drug interactions, disease effects, allergies, use of laxatives, diuretics. (**These factors may be affecting appetite, food intake, or absorption.**)

- Determine psychologic factors, cultural or religious desires/influences **that may affect food choices.**
- Perform psychologic assessment as indicated **to assess body image and congruency with reality.**
- Note occurrence of amenorrhea, tooth decay, swollen salivary glands, and report of constant sore throat (**may be signs of bulimia/affect ability to eat).**
- Review usual activities/exercise program noting repetitive activities (e.g., constant pacing)/inappropriate exercise (e.g., prolonged jogging). **May reveal obsessive nature of weight-control measures.**

NURSING PRIORITY NO. 2. To evaluate degree of deficit:

- Assess weight, age, body build, strength, activity/rest level, and so forth. **Provides comparative baseline.**
- Note total daily intake. Maintain diary of calorie intake, patterns and times of eating **to reveal changes that should be made in client's dietary intake.**
- Calculate basal energy expenditure (BEE) using Harris-Benedict formula and estimate energy and protein requirements.
- Measure/calculate subcutaneous fat and muscle mass via triceps skin fold and midarm muscle circumference or other anthropometric measurements **to establish baseline parameters.**
- Auscultate bowel sounds. Note characteristics of stool (color, amount, frequency, etc.).
- Review indicated laboratory data (e.g., serum albumin/prealbumin, transferrin, amino acid profile, iron, BUN, nitrogen balance studies, glucose, liver function, electrolytes, total lymphocyte count, indirect calorimetry).
- Assist with diagnostic procedures (e.g., Schilling's test, D-xylose test, 72-hour stool fat, GI series).

NURSING PRIORITY NO. 3. To establish a nutritional plan that meets individual needs:

- Assist in developing individualized regimen **to correct/control underlying causative factors (e.g., cancer, malabsorption syndrome, anorexia).**
- Consult dietitian/nutritional team as indicated **to implement interdisciplinary team management.**
- Provide diet modifications as indicated. For example:
  Increase protein, carbohydrates, calories
  Use sauces, butters, creams, or oils in food/beverage, if fat well tolerated
  Small feedings with snacks (easily digested snack at hs)
  Mechanical soft or blenderized tube feedings
  Appetite stimulants (e.g., wine) if indicated

Dietary supplements

Formula tube feedings; parenteral nutrition infusion

• Administer pharmaceutical agents as indicated:

Digestive drugs/enzymes

Vitamin/mineral (iron) supplements

Medications (e.g., antacids, anticholinergics, antiemetics, antidiarrheals)

• Determine whether client prefers/tolerates more calories in a particular meal.

• Use flavoring agents (e.g., lemon and herbs) if salt is restricted **to enhance food satisfaction and stimulate appetite.**

• Encourage use of sugar/honey in beverages if carbohydrates are tolerated well.

• Encourage client to choose foods that are appealing **to stimulate appetite.**

• Avoid foods that cause intolerances/increase gastric motility (e.g., gas-forming foods, hot/cold, spicy, caffeinated beverages, milk products, and the like), according to individual needs.

• Limit fiber/bulk if indicated, **because it may lead to early satiety.**

• Promote pleasant, relaxing environment, including socialization when possible **to enhance intake.**

• Prevent/minimize unpleasant odors/sights. **May have a negative effect on appetite/eating.**

• Provide oral care before/after meals and PM.

• Encourage use of lozenges and so forth **to stimulate salivation when dryness is a factor.**

• Promote adequate/timely fluid intake. (**Limiting fluids 1 hour prior to meal decreases possibility of early satiety.**)

• Weigh weekly and prn **to monitor effectiveness of efforts.**

• Develop individual strategies when problem is mechanical (e.g., wired jaws or paralysis following stroke). Consult occupational therapist **to identify appropriate assistive devices,** or speech therapist **to enhance swallowing ability.** (Refer to ND Swallowing, impaired.)

• Develop structured (behavioral) program of nutrition therapy (e.g., document time/length of eating period, then put food in blender and tube-feed food not eaten), **particularly when problem is anorexia nervosa or bulimia.**

• Recommend/support hospitalization **for controlled environment as indicated in severe malnutrition/life-threatening situations.**

NURSING PRIORITY NO. 4. To promote wellness (Teaching/Discharge Considerations):

• Emphasize importance of well-balanced, nutritious intake.

Provide information regarding individual nutritional needs and ways to meet these needs within financial constraints.

- Develop behavior modification program with client involvement appropriate to specific needs.
- Provide positive regard, love, and acknowledgment of "voice within" guiding client with eating disorder.
- Develop consistent, realistic weight gain goal.
- Weigh weekly and document results **to monitor effectiveness of dietary plan.**
- Consult with dietitian/nutritional support team as necessary **for long-term needs.**
- Develop regular exercise/stress reduction program.
- Review drug regimen, side effects, and potential interactions with other medications/over-the-counter drugs.
- Review medical regimen and provide information/assistance as necessary.
- Assist client to identify/access resources such as food stamps, budget counseling, Meals on Wheels, community food banks, and/or other appropriate assistance programs.
- Refer for dental hygiene/professional care, counseling/psychiatric care, family therapy as indicated.
- Provide/reinforce client teaching regarding preoperative and postoperative dietary needs when surgery is planned.
- Assist client/SO(s) to learn how to blenderize food and/or perform tube feeding.
- Refer to home health resources and so on **for initiation/ supervision of home nutrition therapy when used.**

Documentation Focus

ASSESSMENT/REASSESSMENT

- Baseline and subsequent assessment findings to include signs/symptoms as noted in Defining Characteristics and laboratory diagnostic findings.
- Caloric intake.
- Individual cultural/religious restrictions, personal preferences.
- Availability/use of resources.
- Personal understanding/perception of problem.

PLANNING

- Plan of care and who is involved in planning.
- Teaching plan.

IMPLEMENTATION/EVALUATION

- Client's responses to interventions/teaching and actions performed.

- Results of weekly weigh-in.
- Attainment/progress toward desired outcome(s).
- Modifications to plan of care.

DISCHARGE PLANNING

- Long-term needs/who is responsible for actions to be taken.
- Specific referrals made.

SAMPLE NURSING OUTCOMES
& INTERVENTIONS CLASSIFICATIONS (NOC/NIC)

NOC—Nutritional Status
NIC—Nutrition Management

Nutrition: imbalanced, more than body requirements

Taxonomy II: Nutrition—Class 1 Ingestion (00001)
[Diagnostic Division: Food/Fluid]
Submitted 1975

Definition: Intake of nutrients that exceeds metabolic needs

Related Factors

Excessive intake in relationship to metabolic need

Defining Characteristics

SUBJECTIVE

Reported dysfunctional eating patterns:
Pairing food with other activities
Eating in response to external cues such as time of day, social situation
Concentrating food intake at end of day
Eating in response to internal cues other than hunger, for example, anxiety
Sedentary activity level

OBJECTIVE

Weight 20% over ideal for height and frame [obese]
Triceps skin fold greater than 15 mm in men and 25 mm in women
Weight 10% over ideal for height and frame [overweight]
Observed dysfunctional eating patterns [as noted in subjective]
[Percentage of body fat greater than 22% for trim women and 15% for trim men]

Information that appears in brackets has been added by the authors to clarify and enhance the use of nursing diagnoses.

Desired Outcomes/Evaluation Criteria—Client Will:

- Verbalize a more realistic self-concept/body image (congruent mental and physical picture of self).
- Demonstrate acceptance of self as is rather than an idealized image.
- Demonstrate appropriate changes in lifestyle and behaviors, including eating patterns, food quantity/quality, and exercise program.
- Attain desirable body weight with optimal maintenance of health.

Actions/Interventions

NURSING PRIORITY NO. 1. To identify causative/contributing factors:

- Assess knowledge of nutritional needs and amount of money spent/available for purchasing food.
- Ascertain how client perceives food and the act of eating.
- Review diary of foods/fluids ingested, times and patterns of eating, activities/place, whether alone or with other(s); and feelings before, during, and after eating.
- Calculate total calorie intake.
- Ascertain previous dieting history.
- Discuss client's view of self, including what being fat does for the client. **Active cultural practices may place high importance on food and intake as well as large body size (e.g., Samoan).** Note negative/positive monologues (self-talk) of the individual.
- Obtain body drawing. (Client draws self on wall with chalk, then stands against it and actual body is drawn to determine difference between the two.) **Determines whether client's view of self-body image is congruent with reality.**
- Ascertain occurrence of negative feedback from SO(s). **May reveal control issues, impact motivation for change.**
- Review daily activity and exercise program **to identify areas for modification.**

NURSING PRIORITY NO. 2. To establish weight reduction program:

- Discuss client's motivation for weight loss (e.g., for own satisfaction/self-esteem, or to gain approval from another person). **Helps client determine realistic motivating factors for individual situation (e.g., acceptance of self "as is," improvement of health status).**
- Obtain commitment for weight loss **if contracting is implemented.**

- Record height, weight, body build, gender, and age.
- Calculate calorie requirements based on physical factors and activity.
- Provide information regarding specific nutritional needs. **(Obese individual may be deficient in needed nutrients.)** Assist client in determining type of diet to be used within physician/dietitian guidelines.
- Work with dietitian **to assist in creating/evaluating nutritional program.**
- Set realistic goals for weekly weight loss.
- Discuss eating behaviors (e.g., eating over sink, "nibbling," kinds of activities associated with eating) and identify necessary modifications. Develop appetite-reeducation–plan **to support continuation of behavioral changes.**
- Stress need for adequate fluid intake.
- Encourage involvement in planned activity program of client's choice and within physical abilities.
- Monitor individual drug regimen (e.g., appetite suppressants, hormone therapy, vitamin/mineral supplements).
- Provide positive reinforcement/encouragement for efforts as well as actual weight loss. **Enhances commitment to program.**

NURSING PRIORITY NO. 3. To promote wellness (Teaching/Discharge Considerations):

- Discuss myths client/SO(s) may have about weight and weight loss.
- Assist client to choose nutritious foods that reflect personal likes, meet individual needs, and are within financial budget.
- Identify ways to manage stress/tension during meals. **Promotes relaxation to permit focus on act of eating and awareness of satiety.**
- Review and discuss strategies to deal appropriately with feelings **instead of overeating.**
- Encourage variety and moderation in dietary plan **to decrease boredom.**
- Advise to plan for special occasions (birthday/holidays) by reducing intake before event and/or eating "smart" **to redistribute/reduce calories and allow for participation.**
- Discuss importance of an occasional treat by planning for inclusion in diet **to avoid feelings of deprivation arising from self-denial.**
- Recommend client weigh only once per week, same time/clothes, and graph on chart. Measure/monitor body fat when possible **(more accurate measure).**

- Discuss normalcy of ups and downs of weight loss: plateauing, set point (at which weight is not being lost), hormonal influences, and so forth. **Prevents discouragement when progress stalls.**
- Encourage buying personal items/clothing as a reward for weight loss or other accomplishments. Suggest disposing of "fat clothes" **to encourage positive attitude of permanent change and remove "safety valve" of having wardrobe available "just in case" weight is regained.**
- Involve SO(s) in treatment plan as much as possible **to provide ongoing support and increase likelihood of success.**
- Refer to community support groups/psychotherapy as indicated.
- Provide contact number for dietitian **to address ongoing nutrition/dietary needs.**
- Refer to NDs Body Image, disturbed; Coping, ineffective.

Documentation Focus

ASSESSMENT/REASSESSMENT

- Individual findings, including current weight, dietary pattern; perceptions of self, food, and eating; motivation for loss, support/feedback from SO(s).

PLANNING

- Plan of care/interventions and who is involved in planning.
- Teaching plan.

IMPLEMENTATION/EVALUATION

- Responses to interventions, weekly weight, and actions performed.
- Attainment/progress toward desired outcome(s).
- Modifications to plan of care.

DISCHARGE PLANNING

- Long-term needs and who is responsible for actions to be taken.
- Specific referrals made.

SAMPLE NURSING OUTCOMES & INTERVENTIONS CLASSIFICATIONS (NOC/NIC)

NOC—Weight Control
NIC—Weight Reduction Assistance

Nutrition: imbalanced, risk for more than body requirements

Taxonomy II: Nutrition—Class 1 Ingestion (00003)
[Diagnostic Division: Food/Fluid]
Submitted 1980; Revised 2000

Definition: At risk for an intake of nutrients that exceeds metabolic needs

Risk Factors

Reported/observed obesity in one or both parents[/spouse; hereditary predisposition]

Rapid transition across growth percentiles in infants or children, [adolescents]

Reported use of solid food as major food source before 5 months of age

Reported/observed higher baseline weight at beginning of each pregnancy [frequent, closely spaced pregnancies]

Dysfunctional eating patterns; pairing food with other activities; eating in response to external cues such as time of day, social situation, or internal cues other than hunger (such as anxiety)

Concentrating food intake at end of day

Observed use of food as reward or comfort measure

[Frequent/repeated dieting]

[Socially/culturally isolated; lacking other outlets]

[Alteration in usual activity patterns/sedentary lifestyle]

[Alteration in usual coping patterns]

[Majority of foods consumed are concentrated, high-calorie/fat sources]

[Significant/sudden decline in financial resources, lower socioeconomic status]

NOTE: A risk diagnosis is not evidenced by signs and symptoms, as the problem has not occurred and nursing interventions are directed at prevention.

Desired Outcomes/Evaluation Criteria—Client Will:

- Verbalize understanding of body and energy needs.
- Identify lifestyle/cultural factors that predispose to obesity.
- Demonstrate behaviors, lifestyle changes to reduce risk factors.
- Acknowledge responsibility for own actions and need to "act, not react" to stressful situations.
- Maintain weight at a satisfactory level for height, body build, age, and gender.

Information that appears in brackets has been added by the authors to clarify and enhance the use of nursing diagnoses.

Actions/Interventions

NUTRITION: IMBALANCED, RISK FOR MORE THAN BODY REQUIREMENTS

NURSING PRIORITY NO. **1.** To assess potential factors for undesired weight gain:

- Note presence of factors as listed in Risk Factors. (**A high correlation exists between obesity in parents and children. When one parent is obese, 40% of the children may be over-weight; when both are obese, the proportion may be as high as 80%.**)
- Determine age and activity level/exercise patterns.
- Calculate growth percentiles in infants/children.
- Review laboratory data **for indicators of endocrine/metabolic disorders.**
- Determine weight change patterns, lifestyle, and cultural factors that may predispose to weight gain. **Socio-economic group, amount of money available for purchasing food, proximity of grocery store, and available storage space for food are all factors that may impact food choices and intake.**
- Assess eating patterns in relation to risk factors.
- Determine patterns of hunger and satiety. (**Patterns differ in those who are predisposed to weight gain. Skipping meals decreases the metabolic rate.**)
- Note history of dieting/kinds of diets used. Determine whether yo-yo dieting or bulimia is a factor.
- Identify personality characteristics that may indicate potential for obesity: for example, rigid thinking patterns, external locus of control, negative body image/self-concept, negative monologues (self-talk), dissatisfaction with life.
- Determine psychologic significance of food to the client.
- Listen to concerns and assess motivation to prevent weight gain.

NURSING PRIORITY NO. **2.** To assist client to develop preventive program to avoid weight gain:

- Provide information on balancing calorie intake and energy expenditure.
- Help client develop new eating patterns/habits (e.g., eat slowly, eat when hungry, stop when full, do not skip meals).
- Discuss importance/help client develop a program of exercise and relaxation techniques. **Encourages client to incorporate plan into lifestyle.**
- Assist the client to develop strategies for reducing stressful thinking/actions. **Promotes relaxation, reduces likelihood of stress/comfort eating.**

NURSING PRIORITY NO. **3**. To promote wellness (Teaching/Discharge Considerations):

• Review individual risk factors and provide information **to assist the client with motivation and decision making.**

• Consult with dietitian about specific nutrition/dietary issues.

• Provide information for new mothers about nutrition for developing babies.

• Encourage the client to make a decision to lead an active life and control food habits.

• Assist client in learning to be in touch with own body and to identify feelings that may provoke "comfort eating," such as anger, anxiety, boredom, sadness.

• Develop a system for self-monitoring **to provide a sense of control and enable the client to follow own progress and assist with making choices.**

• Refer to support groups and appropriate community resources for behavior modification as indicated.

Documentation Focus

ASSESSMENT/REASSESSMENT

• Findings related to individual situation, risk factors, current caloric intake/dietary pattern.

PLANNING

• Plan of care and who is involved in the planning.
• Teaching plan.

IMPLEMENTATION/EVALUATION

• Response to interventions/teaching and actions performed.
• Attainment/progress toward desired outcome(s).
• Modifications to plan of care.

DISCHARGE PLANNING

• Long-range needs, noting who is responsible for actions to be taken.
• Specific referrals made.

SAMPLE NURSING OUTCOMES & INTERVENTIONS CLASSIFICATIONS (NOC/NIC)

NOC—Weight Control
NIC—Weight Management

Nutrition, readiness for enhanced

Taxonomy II: Health Awareness—Class 2 Health
Management (00163)
[Diagnostic Division: Food/Fluid]
Submitted 2002

Definition: A pattern of nutrient intake that is sufficient
for meeting metabolic needs and can be strengthened

Related Factors

To be developed

Defining Characteristics

SUBJECTIVE

Expresses willingness to enhance nutrition
Eats regularly
Expresses knowledge of healthy food and fluid choices
Attitude toward eating and drinking is congruent with health goals

OBJECTIVE

Consumes adequate food and fluid
Follows an appropriate standard for intake (e.g., the food pyramid or
    American Diabetic Association Guidelines)
Safe preparation and storage for food and fluids

Desired Outcomes/Evaluation
Criteria—Client Will:

- Demonstrate behaviors to attain/maintain appropriate
  weight.
- Be free of signs of malnutrition.
- Be able to safely prepare and store foods.

Actions/Interventions

NURSING PRIORITY NO. 1. To determine current nutritional
status and eating patterns:

- Assess client's knowledge of current nutritional needs and
  ways client is meeting these needs. **Provides baseline for
  further teaching and/or interventions.**
- Assess eating patterns and food/fluid choices in relation to
  any health-risk factors and health goals. **Helps to identify
  specific strengths and weaknesses that can be addressed.**
- Determine that age-related and developmental needs are
  met. **These factors are constantly present throughout the life
  span, although differing for each age group. For example,
  older adults need same nutrients as younger adults, but in**

Information that appears in brackets has been added by the authors
to clarify and enhance the use of nursing diagnoses.

smaller amounts, and with attention to certain components, such as calcium, fiber, vitamins, protein, and water. Infants/children require small meals and constant attention to needed nutrients for proper growth/development while dealing with child's food preferences and eating habits.

- Evaluate for influence of cultural factors to determine what client considers to be normal dietary practices, as well as to identify food preferences and eating patterns that can be strengthened and/or altered, if indicated.
- Assess how client perceives food, food preparation, and the act of eating to determine client's feeling and emotions regarding food and self-image.
- Ascertain occurrence of/potential for negative feedback from SO(s). May reveal control issues that could impact client's motivation for change.
- Determine patterns of hunger and satiety. Helps identify strengths and weaknesses in eating patterns and potential for change (e.g., person predisposed to weight gain may need a different time for a big meal than evening, or need to learn what foods reinforce feelings of satisfaction).
- Assess client's ability to safely store and prepare foods to determine if health information or resources might be needed.

NURSING PRIORITY NO. 2. To assist client/SO(s) to develop plan to meet individual needs:

- Assist in obtaining/review results of individual testing (e.g., weight/height, body fat percent, lipids, glucose, complete blood count, total protein, etc.) to determine that client is healthy and/or identify dietary changes that may be helpful in attaining health goals.
- Encourage client's beneficial eating patterns/habits (e.g., controlling portion size, eating regular meals, reading product labels, reducing high-fat or fast-food intake, following specific dietary program, drinking water and healthy beverages). Positive feedback promotes continuation of healthy lifestyle habits and new behaviors.
- Discuss use of rewards.
- Provide instruction/reinforce information regarding special needs. Enhances decision-making process and promotes responsibility for meeting own needs.
- Address reading of food labels and instruct in meaning of labeling as indicated to assist client/SO in making healthful choices.
- Review safe preparation and storage of food to avoid food-borne illnesses.
- Consult with and refer to dietitian/physician as indicated.

Client/SO may benefit from advice regarding specific nutrition/dietary issues or may require regular follow-up to determine that needs are being met when following a medically prescribed program.

- Develop a system for self-monitoring **to provide a sense of control and enable the client to follow own progress, and assist in making choices.**

NURSING PRIORITY NO. 3. To promote optimum wellness:

- Review individual risk factors and provide additional information/response to concerns. **Assists the client with motivation and decision making.**
- Provide bibliotherapy and help client/SO(s) identify and evaluate resources they can access on their own. **When referencing the Internet or nontraditional/unproven resources, the individual must exercise some restraint and determine the reliability of the source/information before acting on it.**
- Encourage variety and moderation in dietary plan **to decrease boredom and encourage client in efforts to make healthy choices about eating and food.**
- Assist client to identify/access community resources when indicated. **May benefit from assistance such as food stamps, WIC, budget counseling, Meals on Wheels, community food banks, and/or other assistance programs.**

Documentation Focus

ASSESSMENT/REASSESSMENT

- Assessment findings, including client perception of needs and desire/expectations for improvement.
- Individual cultural/religious restrictions, personal preferences.
- Availability/use of resources.

PLANNING

- Individual goals for enhancement.
- Plan for growth and who is involved in planning.

IMPLEMENTATION/EVALUATION

- Response to activities/learning and actions performed.
- Attainment/progress toward desired outcome(s).
- Modifications to plan.

DISCHARGE PLANNING

- Long-range needs/expectations and plan of action.
- Available resources and specific referrals made.

SAMPLE NURSING OUTCOMES & INTERVENTIONS CLASSIFICATION (NOC/NIC)

NOC—Symptom Control
NIC—Health System Guidance

Oral Mucous Membrane, impaired

Taxonomy II: Safety/Protection—Class 2 Physical Injury
(00045)
[Diagnostic Division: Food/Fluid]
Submitted 1982; Nursing Diagnosis Extension and
Classification (NDEC) Revision 1998

Definition: Disruption of the lips and soft tissue of the
oral cavity

Related Factors

Pathological conditions—oral cavity (radiation to head or neck); cleft
  lip or palate; loss of supportive structures
Trauma
Mechanical (e.g., ill-fitting dentures; braces; tubes [ET, nasogastric],
  surgery in oral cavity)
Chemical (e.g., alcohol, tobacco, acidic foods, regular use of inhalers)
Chemotherapy; immunosuppression/compromised; decreased
  platelets; infection; radiation therapy
Dehydration, malnutrition or vitamin deficiency
NPO for more than 24 hours
Lack of/impaired or decreased salivation; mouth breathing
Ineffective oral hygiene; barriers to oral self-care/professional care
Medication side effects
Stress; depression
Diminished hormone levels (women); aging-related loss of connective,
  adipose, or bone tissue

Defining Characteristics

SUBJECTIVE

Xerostomia (dry mouth)
Oral pain/discomfort
Self-report of bad/diminished or absent taste; difficulty eating or swal-
  lowing

OBJECTIVE

Coated tongue; smooth atrophic, sensitive tongue; geographic tongue
Gingival or mucosal pallor
Stomatitis; hyperemia; bleeding gingival hyperplasia; macroplasia;
  vesicles, nodules, or papules
White patches/plaques, spongy patches or white curdlike exudate,
  oral lesions or ulcers; fissures; cheilitis; desquamation; mucosal
  denudation

Information that appears in brackets has been added by the authors
to clarify and enhance the use of nursing diagnoses.

Edema
Halitosis; [carious teeth]
Gingival recession, pockets deeper than 4 mm
Purulent drainage or exudates; presence of pathogens
Enlarged tonsils beyond what is developmentally appropriate
Red or bluish masses (e.g., hemangiomas)
Difficult speech

Desired Outcomes/Evaluation Criteria—Client Will:

- Verbalize understanding of causative factors.
- Identify specific interventions to promote healthy oral mucosa.
- Demonstrate techniques to restore/maintain integrity of oral mucosa.
- Report/demonstrate a decrease in symptoms/complaints as noted in Defining Characteristics.

Actions/Interventions

NURSING PRIORITY NO. 1. To identify causative/contributing factors to condition:

- Note presence of illness/disease/trauma (e.g., herpes simplex, gingivitis, facial fractures, cancer or cancer therapies, as well as generalized debilitating conditions).
- Determine nutrition/fluid intake and reported changes.
- Note use of tobacco (including smokeless) and alcohol.
- Observe for chipped or sharp-edged teeth. Note fit of dentures or other prosthetic devices when used.
- Assess medication use and possibility of side effects **affecting health or integrity of oral mucous membranes.**
- Determine allergies to food/drugs, other substances.
- Evaluate client's ability to provide self-care and availability of necessary equipment/assistance.
- Review oral hygiene practices: frequency and type (brush/floss/Water Pik); professional dental care.

NURSING PRIORITY NO. 2. To correct identified/developing problems:

- Routinely inspect oral cavity for sores, lesions, and/or bleeding. Recommend client establish regular schedule, such as when performing oral care activities.
- Encourage adequate fluids **to prevent dehydration.**
- Provide for increased humidity, if indicated, by vaporizer or room humidifier.
- Avoid irritating foods/fluids, temperature extremes. Provide soft or pureed diet as required.
- Recommend avoiding alcohol, smoking/chewing tobacco, **which may further irritate mucosa.**

- Encourage use of chewing gum, hard candy, and so forth **to stimulate saliva.**
- Lubricate lips and provide commercially prepared oral lubricant solution.
- Use lemon/glycerin swabs with caution; **may be irritating if mucosa is injured.**
- Provide frequent oral care (including after meals/at bedtime) with alcohol-free mouthwash (especially before meals). May use dilute hydrogen peroxide or 2% sodium perborate (if infection present), sodium chloride, sodium bicarbonate, or alkaline solutions, depending on cause of condition.
- Use soft-bristle brush or sponge/cotton-tip applicators to cleanse teeth and tongue (**limits mucosal/gum irritation**).
- Provide anesthetic lozenges or analgesics such as Stanford solution, viscous lidocaine (Xylocaine), hot pepper (capsaicin) candy, as indicated **to reduce oral discomfort/ pain.**
- Administer antibiotics, as ordered, **when infection is present.**
- Change position of ET tube/airway q8h and prn **to minimize pressure on tissues.**
- Provide adequate nutritional intake when malnutrition is a factor.

NURSING PRIORITY NO. 3. To promote wellness (Teaching/ Discharge Considerations):

- Review current oral hygiene patterns and provide information as required/desired **to correct deficiencies/encourage proper care.**
- Instruct parents in oral hygiene techniques and proper dental care for infants/children (e.g., safe use of pacifier, brushing of teeth and gums, avoidance of sweet drinks and candy, recognition and treatment of thrush). **Encourages early initiation of good oral health practices and timely intervention for treatable problems.**
- Discuss special mouth care required during and after illness/ trauma, or following surgical repair (e.g., cleft lip/palate) **to facilitate healing.**
- Identify need for/demonstrate use of special "appliances" **to perform own oral care.**
- Listen to concerns about appearance and provide accurate information about possible treatments/outcomes. Discuss effect of condition on self-esteem/body image, noting withdrawal from usual social activities/relationships, and/or expressions of powerlessness.
- Review information regarding drug regimen, use of local anesthetics.
- Promote general health/mental health habits. (**Altered immune response can affect the oral mucosa.**)

- Provide nutritional information **to correct deficiencies, reduce irritation/gum disease, prevent dental caries.**
- Stress importance of limiting nighttime regimen of bottle of milk for infant in bed. Suggest pacifier or use of water during night **to prevent bottle syndrome with decaying of teeth.**
- Recommend regular dental checkups/care.
- Identify community resources (e.g., low-cost dental clinics, Meals on Wheels/food stamps, home care aide).

Documentation Focus

ASSESSMENT/REASSESSMENT

- Condition of oral mucous membranes, routine oral care habits and interferences.

PLANNING

- Plan of care and who is involved in planning.
- Teaching plan.

IMPLEMENTATION/EVALUATION

- Responses to interventions/teaching and actions performed.
- Attainment/progress toward desired outcome(s).
- Modifications to plan of care.

DISCHARGE PLANNING

- Long-term needs and who is responsible for actions to be taken.
- Specific referrals made, resources for special appliances.

SAMPLE NURSING OUTCOMES & INTERVENTIONS CLASSIFICATIONS (NOC/NIC)

NOC—Oral Health
NIC—Oral Health Restoration

Pain, acute

Taxonomy II: Comfort—Class 1 Physical Comfort (00132)
[Diagnostic Division: Pain/Comfort]
Submitted 1996

Definition: Unpleasant sensory and emotional experience arising from actual or potential tissue damage or described in terms of such damage (International Association for the Study of Pain); sudden or slow onset of any intensity from mild to severe with an anticipated or predictable end and a duration of less than 6 months

---

Information that appears in brackets has been added by the authors to clarify and enhance the use of nursing diagnoses.

Related Factors

Injuring agents (biological, chemical, physical, psychological)

Defining Characteristics

SUBJECTIVE

Verbal or coded report [may be less from clients younger than age 40, men, and some cultural groups]
Changes in appetite and eating
[Pain unrelieved and/or increased beyond tolerance]

OBJECTIVE

Guarded/protective behavior; antalgic position/gestures
Facial mask; sleep disturbance (eyes lack luster, beaten look, fixed or scattered movement, grimace)
Expressive behavior (restlessness, moaning, crying, vigilance, irritability, sighing)
Distraction behavior (pacing, seeking out other people and/or activities, repetitive activities)
Autonomic alteration in muscle tone (may span from listless [flaccid] to rigid)
Autonomic responses (diaphoresis; blood pressure, respiration, pulse change; pupillary dilation)
Self-focusing
Narrowed focus (altered time perception, impaired thought process, reduced interaction with people and environment)
[Fear/panic]

Desired Outcomes/Evaluation Criteria—Client Will:

• Report pain is relieved/controlled.
• Follow prescribed pharmacological regimen.
• Verbalize methods that provide relief.
• Demonstrate use of relaxation skills and diversional activities as indicated for individual situation.

Actions/Interventions

NURSING PRIORITY NO. 1. To assess etiology/precipitating contributory factors:

• Perform a comprehensive assessment of pain to include location, characteristics, onset/duration, frequency, quality, severity (0 to 10 or faces scale), and precipitating/aggravating factors.
• Determine possible pathophysiologic/psychologic causes of pain (e.g., inflammation, fractures, neuralgia, surgery, influenza, pleurisy, angina, cholecystitis, burns, headache, herniated disc, grief, fear/anxiety).

- Note location of surgical procedures, as this can influence the amount of postoperative pain experienced; for example, vertical/diagonal incisions are more painful than transverse or S-shaped. Presence of known/unknown complication(s) may make the pain more severe than anticipated.
- Assess client's perceptions, along with behavioral and physiologic responses. Note client's attitude toward pain and use of specific pain medications, including any history of substance abuse.
- Note client's locus of control (internal/external). Individuals with external locus of control may take little or no responsibility for pain management.
- Assist in thorough diagnosis, including neurologic and psychologic factors (pain inventory, psychologic interview) as appropriate when pain persists.

NURSING PRIORITY NO. 2. To evaluate client's response to pain:

- Perform pain assessment each time pain occurs. Note and investigate changes from previous reports to rule out worsening of underlying condition/development of complications.
- Accept client's description of pain. (Pain is a subjective experience and cannot be felt by others.) Acknowledge the pain experience and convey acceptance of client's response to pain.
- Note cultural and developmental influences affecting pain response. (Verbal/behavioral cues may have no direct relationship to the degree of pain perceived [e.g., stoic versus exaggerated].)
- Observe nonverbal cues (e.g., how client walks, holds body, sits; facial expression; cool fingertips/toes, which can mean constricted vessels) and other objective. Defining Characteristics as noted, especially in persons who cannot communicate verbally. Observations may/may not be congruent with verbal reports indicating need for further evaluation.
- Assess for referred pain as appropriate to help determine possibility of underlying condition or organ dysfunction requiring treatment.
- Monitor vital signs—usually altered in acute pain.
- Ascertain client's knowledge of and expectations about pain management.
- Review client's previous experiences with pain and methods found either helpful or unhelpful for pain control in the past.

NURSING PRIORITY NO. 3. To assist client to explore methods for alleviation/control of pain:

- Work with client to prevent pain. Use flow sheet to document pain, therapeutic interventions, response, and length of time before pain recurs. Instruct client to report pain as soon as it begins **as timely intervention is more likely to be successful in alleviating pain.**
- Determine client's acceptable level of pain on a 0 to 10 or faces scale.
- Encourage verbalization of feelings about the pain.
- Provide quiet environment, calm activities.
- Provide comfort measures (e.g., back rub, change of position, use of heat/cold) **to provide nonpharmacologic pain management.**
- Instruct in/encourage use of relaxation exercises, such as focused breathing, commercial or individualized tapes (e.g., "white" noise, music, instructional).
- Encourage diversional activities (e.g., TV/radio, socialization with others).
- Review procedures/expectations and tell client when treatment will hurt, use puppets to demonstrate procedure for child **to reduce concern of the unknown and associated muscle tension.**
- Suggest parent be present during procedures **to comfort child.**
- Identify ways of avoiding/minimizing pain (e.g., splinting incision during cough; firm mattress, and/or proper supporting shoes for low back pain, good body mechanics).
- Administer analgesics as indicated to maximal dosage as needed **to maintain "acceptable" level of pain. Notify physician if regimen is inadequate to meet pain control goal.**
- Demonstrate/monitor use of self-administration/client-controlled analgesia (PCA).
- Assist client to alter drug regimen, based on individual needs. **Increasing/decreasing dosage, stepped program (switching from injection to oral route, increased time span as pain lessens) helps in self-management of pain.**
- Note when pain occurs (e.g., only with ambulation, every evening) **to medicate prophylactically as appropriate.**
- Instruct client in use of transcutaneous electrical stimulation (TENS) unit when ordered.
- Assist in treatment of underlying disease processes causing pain. Evaluate effectiveness of periodic therapies (e.g., cortisone injections for joint inflammation).

NURSING PRIORITY NO. 4. To promote wellness (Teaching/Discharge Considerations):

- Encourage adequate rest periods **to prevent fatigue.**
- Review ways to lessen pain, including techniques, such as Therapeutic Touch (TT), biofeedback, self-hypnosis, and relaxation skills.
- Discuss impact of pain on lifestyle/independence and ways to maximize level of functioning.
- Provide for individualized physical therapy/exercise program that can be continued by the client when discharged. **(Promotes active, not passive role.)**
- Discuss with SO(s) ways in which they can assist client and reduce precipitating factors that may cause or increase pain (e.g., participating in household tasks following abdominal surgery).
- Identify specific signs/symptoms and changes in pain requiring medical follow-up.

Documentation Focus

ASSESSMENT/REASSESSMENT

- Individual assessment findings, including client's description of response to pain, specifics of pain inventory, expectations of pain management, and acceptable level of pain.
- Prior medication use; substance abuse.

PLANNING

- Plan of care and who is involved in planning.
- Teaching plan.

IMPLEMENTATION/EVALUATION

- Response to interventions/teaching and actions performed.
- Attainment/progress toward desired outcome(s).
- Modifications to plan of care.

DISCHARGE PLANNING

- Long-term needs, noting who is responsible for actions to be taken.
- Specific referrals made.

SAMPLE NURSING OUTCOMES & INTERVENTIONS CLASSIFICATIONS (NOC/NIC)

NOC—Pain Level
NIC—Pain Management

Pain, chronic

Taxonomy II: Comfort—Class 1 Physical Comfort (00133)
[Diagnostic Division: Pain/Discomfort]
Submitted 1986; Revised 1996

Definition: Unpleasant sensory and emotional experience arising from actual or potential tissue damage or described in terms of such damage (International Association for the Study of Pain); sudden or slow onset of any intensity from mild to severe, constant or recurring without an anticipated or predictable end and a duration of greater than 6 months
[Pain is a signal that something is wrong. Chronic pain can be recurrent and periodically disabling (e.g., migraine headaches) or may be unremitting. While chronic pain syndrome includes various learned behaviors, psychological factors become the primary contribution to impairment. It is a complex entity, combining elements from other NDs, such as Powerlessness; Diversional Activity, deficient; Family Processes, interrupted; Self-Care Deficit; and Disuse Syndrome, risk for.]

Related Factors

Chronic physical/psychosocial disability

Defining Characteristics

SUBJECTIVE

Verbal or coded report
Fear of reinjury
Altered ability to continue previous activities
Changes in sleep patterns; fatigue
[Changes in appetite]
[Preoccupation with pain]
[Desperately seeks alternative solutions/therapies for relief/control of pain]

OBJECTIVE

Observed evidence of: protective/guarding behavior; facial mask; irritability; self-focusing; restlessness; depression
Reduced interaction with people
Anorexia, weight changes
Atrophy of involved muscle group
Sympathetic mediated responses (temperature, cold, changes of body position, hypersensitivity)

Desired Outcomes/Evaluation Criteria—Client Will:

• Verbalize and demonstrate (nonverbal cues) relief and/or control of pain/discomfort.

Information that appears in brackets has been added by the authors
to clarify and enhance the use of nursing diagnoses.

- Verbalize recognition of interpersonal/family dynamics and reactions that affect the pain problem.
- Demonstrate/initiate behavioral modifications of lifestyle and appropriate use of therapeutic interventions.

Family/SO(s) Will:

- Cooperate in pain management program. (Refer to ND Coping, family: readiness for enhanced.)

Actions/Interventions.

NURSING PRIORITY NO. 1. To assess etiology/precipitating factors:

- Identify factors as outlined for ND Pain, acute.
- Assist in thorough diagnosis, including neurologic, psychologic evaluation (Minnesota Multiphasic Personality Inventory—MMPI, pain inventory, psychologic interview).
- Assess for phantom limb pain when amputation has occurred.
- Evaluate emotional/physical components of individual situation. Note codependent components, enabling behaviors of caregivers/family members **that support continuation of the status quo.**
- Determine cultural factors for the individual situation (e.g., how expression of pain is accepted—moaning aloud or enduring in stoic silence; magnification of symptoms to convince others of reality of pain).
- Note sex and age of client. **Current literature suggests there may be differences between women and men as to how they perceive and/or respond to pain. Sensitivity to pain is likely to decline as one gets older.**
- Discuss use of nicotine, sugar, caffeine, white flour as appropriate (**some holistic practitioners believe these items need to be eliminated from the client's diet).**
- Evaluate current and past analgesic/narcotic drug use (including alcohol).
- Determine issues of secondary gain for the client/SO(s) (e.g., financial/insurance, marital/family concern, work issues). **May interfere with progress in pain management/resolution of situation.**
- Make home visit when possible, observing such factors as safety equipment, adequate room, colors, plants, family interactions. Note impact of home environment on the client.

NURSING PRIORITY NO. 2. To determine client response to chronic pain situation:

- Evaluate pain behavior. (**May be exaggerated because client's** perception of pain is not believed or because client believes caregivers are discounting reports of pain.)

- Determine individual client threshold for pain (physical examination, pain profile, and the like).
- Ascertain duration of pain problem, who has been consulted, and what drugs and therapies (including alternative/complementary) have been used.
- Note lifestyle effects of pain (e.g., decreased activity, weight loss or gain, sleep difficulties).
- Assess degree of personal maladjustment of the client, such as isolationism, anger, irritability, loss of work time/job.
- Note availability/use of personal and community resources.
- Acknowledge and assess pain matter-of-factly, avoiding undue expressions of concern.

NURSING PRIORITY NO. **3.** To assist client to deal with pain:

- Include client and SO(s) in establishing pattern of discussing pain for specified length of time **to limit focusing on pain.**
- Use interventions from ND Pain, acute as appropriate (e.g., heat/cold, splinting or exercises, hydrotherapy, electrical stimulation/TENS unit).
- Review client expectations versus reality, **because pain may not be resolved but can be significantly lessened or managed.**
- Discuss the physiologic dynamics of tension/anxiety and how this affects the pain.
- Investigate and use nonpharmacologic methods of pain control (e.g., visualization, guided imagery, Therapeutic Touch [TT], progressive muscle relaxation, biofeedback, massage).
- Assist client to learn breathing techniques (e.g., diaphragmatic breathing) **to assist in muscle and generalized relaxation.**
- Encourage client to use positive affirmations: "I am healing." "I am relaxed." "I love this life." Have client be aware of internal-external dialogue. Say "cancel" when negative thoughts develop.
- Use tranquilizers, narcotics, and analgesics sparingly. **These changes are physically and psychologically addicting, promote sleep disturbances-especially interfering with deep REM (rapid eye movement) sleep, and client may need to be detoxified if many medications are currently used.** Note: Antidepressants have an additional benefit of analgesic effects **because perception of pain decreases as depression is lessened.**
- Encourage right-brain stimulation with activities such as love, laughter, and music **to release endorphins, enhancing sense of well-being.**
- Encourage use of subliminal tapes **to bypass logical part of**

the brain by saying: "I am becoming a more relaxed person." "It is all right for me to relax."

- Assist family in developing a program of positive reinforcement, encouraging client to use own control and diminishing attention given to pain behavior.
- Be alert to changes in pain. **May indicate a new physical problem.**

NURSING PRIORITY NO. 4. To promote wellness (Teaching/Discharge Considerations):

- Assist client and SO(s) to learn how to heal by developing sense of internal control, by being responsible for own treatment, and by obtaining the information and tools to accomplish this.
- Discuss potential for developmental delays in child with chronic pain. Identify current level of function and review appropriate expectations for individual child.
- Review safe use of medications, side effects requiring medical evaluation.
- Assist client to learn to change pain behavior to wellness behavior. "Act as if you are well."
- Encourage and assist family member/SO(s) to learn massage techniques.
- Recommend that client and SO(s) take time for themselves. **Provides opportunity to re-energize and refocus on tasks at hand.**
- Identify and discuss potential hazards of unproved and/or nonmedical therapies/remedies.
- Identify community support groups/resources to meet individual needs (e.g., yard care, home maintenance, alternative transportation). **Proper use of resources may reduce negative pattern of "overdoing" heavy activities, then spending several days in bed recuperating.**
- Refer for counseling and/or marital therapy, Parent Effectiveness classes, and so forth as needed. **Presence of chronic pain affects all relationship/family dynamics.**
- Refer to NDs Coping, ineffective; Coping, family: compromised.

Documentation Focus

ASSESSMENT/REASSESSMENT

- Individual findings, including duration of problem/specific contributing factors, previously/currently used interventions.
- Perception of pain, effects on lifestyle, and expectations of therapeutic regimen.
- Family's/SO's response to client, and support for change.

PLANNING

- Plan of care and who is involved in planning.
- Teaching plan.

IMPLEMENTATION/EVALUATION

- Responses to interventions/teaching and actions performed.
- Attainment/progress toward desired outcome(s).
- Modifications to plan of care.

DISCHARGE PLANNING

- Long-term needs and who is responsible for actions to be taken.
- Specific referrals made.

SAMPLE NURSING OUTCOMES & INTERVENTIONS CLASSIFICATIONS (NOC/NIC)

NOC—Pain Control
NIC—Pain Management

Parental Role Conflict

Taxonomy II: Role Relationships—Class 1 Role
Performance (00064)
[Diagnostic Division: Social Interaction]
Submitted 1988

Definition: Parent experience of role confusion and conflict in response to crisis

Related Factors

Separation from child because of chronic illness [/disability]
Intimidation with invasive or restrictive modalities (e.g., isolation, intubation); specialized care centers, policies
Home care of a child with special needs (e.g., apnea monitoring, postural drainage, hyperalimentation)
Change in marital status
Interruptions of family life because of home-care regimen (treatments, caregivers, lack of respite)

Defining Characteristics

SUBJECTIVE

Parent(s) express(es) concerns/feeling of inadequacy to provide for child's physical and emotional needs during hospitalization or in the home
Parent(s) express(es) concerns about changes in parental role, family functioning, family communication, family health

---

Information that appears in brackets has been added by the authors to clarify and enhance the use of nursing diagnoses.

Expresses concern about perceived loss of control over decisions relating to child

Verbalizes feelings of guilt, anger, fear, anxiety and/or frustrations about effect of child's illness on family process

OBJECTIVE

Demonstrates disruption in caretaking routines

Reluctant to participate in usual caretaking activities even with encouragement and support

Demonstrates feelings of guilt, anger, fear, anxiety, and/or frustrations about the effect of child's illness on family process

Desired Outcomes/Evaluation Criteria—Parent(s) Will:

- Verbalize understanding of situation and expected parent's/child's role.
- Express feelings about child's illness/situation and effect on family life.
- Demonstrate appropriate behaviors in regard to parenting role.
- Assume caretaking activities as appropriate.
- Handle family disruptions effectively.

Actions/Interventions

NURSING PRIORITY NO. 1. To assess causative/contributory factors:

- Assess individual situation and parent's perception of/concern about what is happening and expectations of self as caregiver.
- Note parental status including age and maturity, stability of relationship, other responsibilities. (Increasing numbers of elderly individuals are providing full-time care for young grandchildren whose parents are unavailable or unable to provide care.)
- Ascertain parent's understanding of child's developmental stage and expectations for the future **to identify misconceptions/strengths.**
- Note coping skills currently being used by each individual as well as how problems have been dealt with in the past. **Provides basis for comparison and reference for client's coping abilities.**
- Determine use of substances (e.g., alcohol, other drugs, including prescription medications). **May interfere with individual's ability to cope/problem-solve.**
- Assess availability/use of resources, including extended family, support groups, and financial.
- Perform testing such as Parent-Child Relationship Inventory (PCRI) for further evaluation as indicated.

NURSING PRIORITY NO. 2. To assist parents to deal with current crisis:

- Encourage free verbal expression of feelings (including negative feelings of anger and hostility), setting limits on inappropriate behavior.
- Acknowledge difficulty of situation and normalcy of feeling overwhelmed and helpless. Encourage contact with parents who experienced similar situation with child and had positive outcome.
- Provide information, including technical information when appropriate, **to meet individual needs/correct misconceptions.**
- Promote parental involvement in decision making and care as much as possible/desired. **Enhances sense of control.**
- Encourage interaction/facilitate communication between parent(s) and children.
- Promote use of assertiveness, relaxation skills **to help individuals to deal with situation/crisis.**
- Assist parent to learn proper administration of medications/treatments as indicated.
- Provide for/encourage use of respite care, parent time off **to enhance emotional well-being.**

NURSING PRIORITY NO. 3. To promote wellness (Teaching/Discharge Considerations):

- Provide anticipatory guidance **to encourage making plans for future needs.**
- Encourage setting realistic and mutually agreed-on goals.
- Provide/identify learning opportunities specific to needs (e.g., parenting classes, equipment use/troubleshooting).
- Refer to community resources as appropriate (e.g., visiting nurse, respite care, social services, psychiatric care/family therapy, well-baby clinics, special needs support services).
- Refer to ND Parenting, impaired, for additional interventions.

Documentation Focus

ASSESSMENT/REASSESSMENT

- Findings, including specifics of individual situation/parental concerns, perceptions, expectations.

PLANNING

- Plan of care and who is involved in the planning.
- Teaching plan.

IMPLEMENTATION/EVALUATION

- Parent's responses to interventions/teaching and actions performed.

- Attainment/progress toward desired outcome(s).
- Modifications to plan of care.

DISCHARGE PLANNING

- Long-term needs and who is responsible for each action to be taken.
- Specific referrals made.

SAMPLE NURSING OUTCOMES
& INTERVENTIONS CLASSIFICATIONS (NOC/NIC)

NOC—Parenting
NIC—Parenting Promotion

Parenting, impaired

Taxonomy II: Role Relationships—Class 1 Caregiving Roles (00056)
[Diagnostic Division: Social Interaction]
Submitted 1998; Nursing Diagnosis Extension and Classification (NDEC) Revision 1998

Definition: Inability of the primary caretaker to create, maintain, or regain an environment that promotes the optimum growth and development of the child [Note: It is important to reaffirm that adjustment to parenting in general is a normal maturational process that elicits nursing behaviors to prevent potential problems and to promote health.]

Related Factors

SOCIAL

Presence of stress (e.g., financial, legal, recent crisis, cultural move [e.g., from another country/cultural group within same country]); unemployment or job problems; financial difficulties; relocations; poor home environments
Lack of family cohesiveness; marital conflict, declining satisfaction; change in family unit
Role strain or overload; single parents; father of child not involved
Unplanned or unwanted pregnancy; lack of, or poor, parental role model; low self-esteem
Low socioeconomic class; poverty; lack of resources, access to resources, social support networks, transportation
Inadequate child-care arrangements; lack of value of parenthood; inability to put child's needs before own
Poor problem-solving skills; maladaptive coping strategies
Social isolation
History of being abusive/being abused; legal difficulties

Information that appears in brackets has been added by the authors to clarify and enhance the use of nursing diagnoses.

KNOWLEDGE

Lack of knowledge about child health maintenance, parenting skills, child development; inability to recognize and act on infant cues
Unrealistic expectation for self, infant, partner
Low educational level or attainment; limited cognitive functioning; lack of cognitive readiness for parenthood
Poor communication skills
Preference for physical punishment

PHYSIOLOGICAL

Physical illness

INFANT OR CHILD

Premature birth; multiple births; unplanned or unwanted child; not gender desired
Illness; prolonged separation from parent/separation at birth
Difficult temperament; lack of goodness of fit (temperament) with parental expectations
Handicapping condition or developmental delay; altered perceptual abilities; attention-deficit hyperactivity disorder

PSYCHOLOGICAL

Young age, especially adolescent
Lack of, or late, prenatal care; difficult labor and/or delivery; multiple births; high number or closely spaced pregnancies
Sleep deprivation or disruption; depression
Separation from infant/child
History of substance abuse or dependencies
Disability; history of mental illness

Defining Characteristics

SUBJECTIVE

Parental
Statements of inability to meet child's needs; cannot control child
Negative statements about child
Verbalization of role inadequacy frustration

OBJECTIVE

Infant or Child
Frequent accidents/illness; failure to thrive
Poor academic performance/cognitive development
Poor social competence; behavioral disorders
Incidence of physical and psychological trauma or abuse
Lack of attachment; separation anxiety
Runaway
Parental
Maternal-child interaction deficit; poor parent-child interaction; little cuddling; insecure or lack of attachment to infant
Inadequate child health maintenance; unsafe home environment;

inappropriate child-care arrangements; inappropriate visual, tactile, auditory stimulation

Poor or inappropriate caretaking skills; inconsistent care/behavior management

Inflexibility to meet needs of child, situation

High punitiveness; rejection or hostility to child; child abuse; child neglect; abandonment

Desired Outcomes/Evaluation Criteria—Client Will:

- Verbalize realistic information and expectations of parenting role.
- Verbalize acceptance of the individual situation.
- Identify own strengths, individual needs, and methods/resources to meet them.
- Demonstrate appropriate attachment/parenting behaviors.

Actions/Interventions

NURSING PRIORITY NO. 1. To assess causative/contributing factors:

- Note family constellation; two-parent, single, extended family, or child living with other relative such as grandparent.
- Determine developmental stage of the family (e.g., new child, adolescent, child leaving/returning home).
- Assess family relationships and identify needs of individual members. Report and take necessary actions as legally/professionally indicated if child's safety is a concern.
- Assess parenting skill level, taking into account the individual's intellectual, emotional, and physical strengths and weaknesses. (**Parents with significant impairments may need more education/assistance.**)
- Observe attachment behaviors between parental figure and child. (Refer to ND Attachment, risk for impaired parent/infant/child.)
- Note presence of factors in the child (e.g., birth defects, hyperactivity) **that may affect attachment and caretaking needs.**
- Evaluate physical challenges/limitations. **Might affect the parent's ability to care for a child (e.g., visual/hearing impairment, quadriplegia, severe depression).**
- Determine presence/effectiveness of support systems, role models, extended family, and community resources available to the parent(s).
- Note absence from home setting/lack of child supervision by parent (e.g., working long hours/out of town, multiple responsibilities such as working and attending educational classes).

NURSING PRIORITY NO. 2. To foster development of parenting skills:

- Create an environment in which relationships can be developed and needs of each individual met. (**Learning is more effective when individuals feel safe.**)
- Make time for listening to concerns of the parent(s).
- Emphasize positive aspects of the situation, maintaining a hopeful attitude toward the parent's capabilities and potential for improving the situation.
- Note staff attitudes toward parent/child and specific problem/disability; for example, needs of disabled parent(s) to be seen as an individual and evaluated apart from a stereotype. **Negative attitudes are detrimental to promoting positive outcomes.**
- Encourage expression of feelings, such as helplessness, anger, frustration. Set limits on unacceptable behaviors.
- Acknowledge difficulty of situation and normalcy of feelings. **Enhances feelings of acceptance.**
- Recognize stages of grieving process when the child is disabled or other than anticipated (e.g., girl instead of boy, misshapen head/prominent birthmark). Allow time for parents to express feelings and deal with the "loss."
- Encourage attendance at skill classes (e.g., Parent Effectiveness) **to assist in developing communication and problem-solving techniques.**
- Emphasize parenting functions rather than mothering/fathering skills. **By virtue of gender, each person brings something to the parenting role; however, nurturing tasks can be done by both parents.**

NURSING PRIORITY NO. 3. To promote wellness (Teaching/ Discharge Considerations):

- Involve all available members of the family in learning.
- Provide information appropriate to the situation, including time management, limit setting, and stress-reduction techniques. **Facilitates satisfactory implementation of plan/new behaviors.**
- Develop support systems appropriate to the situation (e.g., extended family, friends, social worker, home care services).
- Assist parent to plan time and conserve energy in positive ways. **Enables individual to cope effectively with difficulties as they arise.**
- Encourage parents to identify positive outlets for meeting their own needs (e.g., going out for dinner, making time for their own interests and each other/dating). **Promotes general well-being, helps reduce burnout.**
- Refer to appropriate support/therapy groups as indicated.

- Identify community resources (e.g., child-care services) to assist with individual needs to provide respite and support.
- Refer to NDs such as Coping, ineffective; Coping, family: compromised; Violence, risk for [specify]; Self-Esteem [specify]; Family Processes, interrupted, and so on.

Documentation Focus

ASSESSMENT/REASSESSMENT

- Individual findings, including parenting skill level, deviations from normal parenting expectations, family makeup, and developmental stages.
- Availability/use of support systems and community resources.

PLANNING

- Plan of care and who is involved in planning.
- Teaching plan.

IMPLEMENTATION/EVALUATION

- Parent(s')/child's responses to interventions/teaching and actions performed.
- Attainment/progress toward desired outcome(s).
- Modification to plan of care.

DISCHARGE PLANNING

- Long-range needs and who is responsible for actions to be taken.
- Specific referrals made.

SAMPLE NURSING OUTCOMES & INTERVENTIONS CLASSIFICATIONS (NOC/NIC)

NOC—Role Performance
NIC—Parenting Promotion

Parenting, readiness for enhanced

Taxonomy II: Role Relationships—Class 1 Caregiving Roles (00164)
[Diagnostic Divisions: Social Interaction]
Submitted 2002

Definition: A pattern of providing an environment for children or other dependent person(s) that is sufficient to nurture growth and development and can be strengthened

Information that appears in brackets has been added by the authors to clarify and enhance the use of nursing diagnoses.

Related Factors

To be developed

Defining Characteristics

SUBJECTIVE

Expresses willingness to enhance parenting
Children or other dependent person(s) express satisfaction with home
    environment

OBJECTIVE

Emotional and tacit support of children or dependent person(s) is
    evident; bonding or attachment evident
Physical and emotional needs of children/dependent person(s) are met
Realistic expectations of children/dependent person(s) exhibited

Desired Outcomes/Evaluation
Criteria—Client Will:

- Verbalize realistic information and expectations of parenting
  role.
- Identify own strengths, individual needs, and methods/
  resources to meet them.
- Demonstrate appropriate attachment/parenting behaviors.

Actions/Interventions

NURSING PRIORITY NO. **1.** To determine need/motivation for
improvement:

- Note family constellation: two-parent, single, extended family,
  or child living with other relative, such as grandparent.
  **Understanding makeup of the family provides information
  about needs to assist them in improving their family connections.**
- Determine developmental stage of the family (e.g., new child,
  adolescent, child leaving/returning home, retirement). **These
  maturational crises bring changes in the family, which can
  provide opportunity for enhancing parenting skills and
  improving family interactions.**
- Assess family relationships and identify needs of individual
  members, noting any special concerns that exist, such as, birth
  defects, illness, hyperactivity. **The family is a system and when
  members make decision to improve parenting skills, the
  changes affect all parts of the system. Identifying needs,
  special situations, and relationships can help to develop plan
  to bring about effective change.**
- Assess parenting skill level, taking into account the individual's intellectual, emotional, and physical strengths and weaknesses. **Identifies areas of need for education, skill training,**

and information on which to base plan for enhancing parenting skills.

- Observe attachment behaviors between parent(s) and child(ren), recognizing cultural background which may influence expected behaviors. Behaviors such as eye-to-eye contact, use of en-face position, talking to infant in high-pitched voice are indicative of attachment behaviors in American culture but may not be appropriate in another culture. Failure to bond is thought to affect subsequent parent-child interactions.
- Determine presence/effectiveness of support systems, role models, extended family, and community resources available to the parent(s). Parents desiring to enhance abilities and improve family life can benefit by role models that help them develop own style of parenting.
- Note cultural/religious influences on parenting, expectations of self/child, sense of success or failure. Expectations may vary with different cultures (e.g., Arab-Americans hold children to be sacred but child-rearing is based on negative rather than positive reinforcements and parents are more strict with girls than boys). These beliefs may interfere with desire to improve parenting skills when there is conflict between the two.

NURSING PRIORITY NO. 2. To foster improvement of parenting skills:

- Create an environment in which relationships can be developed and needs of each individual family member can be met. A safe environment in which individuals can freely express their thoughts and feelings optimizes learning and positive interactions among family members enhancing relationships.
- Make time for listening to concerns of the parent(s). Promotes sense of importance and of being heard and identifies accurate information regarding needs of the family for enhancing relationships.
- Encourage expression of feelings, such as helplessness, anger while setting limits on unacceptable behaviors. Identification of feelings promotes understanding of self and enhances connections with others in the family. Unacceptable behaviors result in feelings of anger and diminished self-esteem and can lead to problems in the family relationships.
- Emphasize parenting functions rather than mothering/fathering skills. By virtue of gender, each person brings something to the parenting role; however, nurturing tasks can be done by both parents, enhancing family relationships.

- Encourage attendance at skill classes, such as Parent Effectiveness Training. Assists in developing communication skills of Active-listening, I-messages, and problem-solving techniques to improve family relationships and promote a win-win environment.

NURSING PRIORITY NO. 3. To promote optimal wellness:

- Involve all members of the family in learning. The family system benefits from all members participating in learning new skills to enhance family relationships.
- Encourage parents to identify positive outlets for meeting their own needs. Activities, such as going out for dinner, making time for their own interests and each other/dating promotes general well-being, enhance family relationships and improve family functioning.
- Provide information as indicated, including time management, stress-reduction techniques. Learning about positive parenting skills, understanding growth and developmental expectations, and ways to reduce stress and anxiety promotes individual's ability to deal with problems that may arise in the course of family relationships.
- Discuss current 'family rules,' identifying areas of needed change. Rules may be imposed by adults, rather than through a democratic process involving all family members, leading to conflict and angry confrontations. Setting positive family rules with all family members participating can promote an effective, functional family.
- Discuss need for long-term planning and ways in which family can maintain desired positive relationships. Each stage of life brings its own challenges and understanding and preparing for each one enables family members to move through them in positive ways, promoting family unity and resolving inevitable conflicts with win-win solutions.

Documentation Focus

ASSESSMENT/REASSESSMENT

- Individual findings, including parenting skill level, parenting expectations, family makeup, and developmental stages.
- Availability/use of support systems and community resources.

PLANNING

- Plan for enhancement, who is involved in planning.

IMPLEMENTATION/EVALUATION

- Family members responses to interventions/teaching and actions performed.

- Attainment/progress toward desired outcome(s).
- Modifications to plan.

DISCHARGE PLANNING

- Long-range needs and who is responsible for actions to be taken.
- Modification to plan.

SAMPLE NURSING OUTCOMES
& INTERVENTIONS CLASSIFICATIONS (NOC/NIC)

NOC—Parenting
NIC—Parenting Promotion

Parenting, risk for impaired

Taxonomy II: Role Relationships—Class 1 Caregiving Roles (00057)
[Diagnostic Division: Social Interaction]
Submitted 1978; Nursing Diagnosis Extension and Classification (NDEC) Revision 1998

Definition: Risk for inability of the primary caretaker to create, maintain, or regain an environment that promotes the optimum growth and development of the child. [**Note:** It is important to reaffirm that adjustment to parenting in general is a normal maturational process that elicits nursing behaviors to prevent potential problems and to promote health.]

Risk Factors

Lack of role identity; lack of available role model, ineffective role model

SOCIAL

Stress [e.g., financial, legal, recent crisis, cultural move (e.g., from another country/cultural group within same country)]; unemployment or job problems; financial difficulties; relocations; poor home environments
Lack of family cohesiveness; marital conflict, declining satisfaction; change in family unit
Role strain/overload; single parents; father of child not involved
Unplanned or unwanted pregnancy; lack of, or poor, parental role model; low self-esteem
Low socioeconomic class; poverty; lack of: [resources], access to resources, social support networks, transportation
Inadequate child-care arrangements; lack of value of parenthood; inability to put child's needs before own
Poor problem-solving skills; maladaptive coping strategies

Information that appears in brackets has been added by the authors to clarify and enhance the use of nursing diagnoses.

Social isolation

History of being abusive/being abused; legal difficulties

KNOWLEDGE

Lack of knowledge about child health maintenance, parenting skills, child development; inability to recognize and act on infant cues

Unrealistic expectation of child

Low educational level or attainment; low cognitive functioning; lack of cognitive readiness for parenthood

Poor communication skills

Preference for physical punishment

PHYSIOLOGICAL

Physical illness

INFANT OR CHILD

Premature birth; multiple births; unplanned or unwanted child; not gender desired

Illness; prolonged separation from parent/separation at birth

Difficult temperament; lack of goodness of fit (temperament) with parental expectations

Handicapping condition or developmental delay; altered perceptual abilities; attention-deficit hyperactivity disorder

PSYCHOLOGICAL

Young age, especially adolescent

Lack of, or late, prenatal care; difficult labor and/or delivery; multiple births; high number or closely spaced pregnancies

Sleep deprivation or disruption; depression

Separation from infant/child

History of substance abuse or dependencies

Disability; history of mental illness

NOTE: A risk diagnosis is not evidenced by signs and symptoms, as the problem has not occurred and nursing interventions are directed at prevention.

Desired Outcomes/Evaluation Criteria—Client Will:

- Verbalize awareness of individual risk factors.
- Identify own strengths, individual needs, and methods/resources to meet them.
- Demonstrate behavior/lifestyle changes to reduce potential for development of problem or reduce/eliminate effects of risk factors.
- Participate in activities, classes to promote growth.

Refer to Parenting, impaired or Attachment, risk for impaired parent/infant/child, for interventions and documentation focus.

NOC—Parenting
NIC—Parenting Promotion

Peripheral Neurovascular Dysfunction, risk for

Taxonomy II: Safety/Protection—Class 2 Physical Injury
(00086)
[Diagnostic Division: Neurosensory]
Submitted 1992

Definition: At risk for disruption in circulation, sensation, or motion of an extremity

Risk Factors

Fractures
Mechanical compression (e.g., tourniquet, cast, brace, dressing, or restraint)
Orthopedic surgery; trauma
Immobilization
Burns
Vascular obstruction

NOTE: A risk diagnosis is not evidenced by signs and symptoms, as the problem has not occurred and nursing interventions are directed at prevention.

Desired Outcomes/Evaluation Criteria—Client Will:

- Maintain function as evidenced by sensation/movement within normal range for the individual.
- Identify individual risk factors.
- Demonstrate/participate in behaviors and activities to prevent complications.
- Relate signs/symptoms that require medical reevaluation.

Actions/Interventions

NURSING PRIORITY NO. **1.** To determine significance/degree of potential for compromise:

- Note individual risk factors, such as history of previous problems in extremity(ies), immobility/paralysis, duration/progression of condition.
- Assess presence, location, and degree of swelling/edema

Information that appears in brackets has been added by the authors to clarify and enhance the use of nursing diagnoses.

formation. Measure affected extremity and compare with unaffected extremity.

- Note position/location of casts, braces, traction apparatus.
- Review recent/current drug regimen, noting use of anticoagulants and vasoactive agents.

NURSING PRIORITY NO. 2. To prevent deterioration/maximize circulation of affected limb(s):

- Remove jewelry from affected limb.
- Limit/avoid use of restraints. Pad limb and evaluate status frequently, if restraints are required.
- Monitor entire length of injured extremity for swelling/edema formation. Note appearance, spread of hematoma.
- Monitor presence/quality of peripheral pulse distal to injury or impairment via palpation/Doppler. **Occasionally a pulse may be palpated even though circulation is blocked by a soft clot through which pulsations may be felt; or perfusion through larger arteries may continue after increased compartment pressure has collapsed the arteriole/venule circulation in the muscle.**
- Assess capillary return, skin color, and warmth in the limb(s) at risk and compare with unaffected extremities. **Peripheral pulses, capillary refill, skin color, and sensation may be normal even in the presence of compartmental syndrome, because superficial circulation is usually not compromised.**
- Perform neurovascular assessments, noting changes in motor/sensory function. Ask client to localize pain/discomfort, and to report numbness and tingling; presence of pain with exercise or rest (atherosclerotic changes). Refer to ND Tissue Perfusion, ineffective (specify type: renal, cerebral, cardiopulmonary, gastrointestinal, peripheral), as appropriate.
- Test sensation of peroneal nerve by pinch/pinprick in the dorsal web between first and second toe, and assess ability to dorsiflex toes if indicated (e.g., presence of leg fracture).
- Inspect tissues around cast edges for rough places, pressure points. Investigate reports of "burning sensation" under cast.
- Observe position/location of supporting ring of splints/sling. Readjust as indicated.
- Maintain elevation of injured extremity(ies) unless contraindicated by confirmed presence of compartment syndrome. **In presence of increased compartment pressure, elevation of extremity actually impedes arterial flow, decreasing perfusion.**
- Apply ice bags around injury/fracture site as indicated.
- Investigate sudden signs of limb ischemia (e.g., decreased skin temperature, pallor, increased pain), reports of pain that is extreme for type of injury, increased pain on passive move-

ment of extremity, development of paresthesia, muscle tension/tenderness with erythema, change in pulse quality distal to injury. Place limb in neutral position, avoiding elevation. Report symptoms to physician at once **to provide for timely intervention.**

- Split/bivalve cast, reposition traction/restraints as appropriate **to release pressure.**
- Assist with measurements of/monitor intracompartmental pressures as indicated. **Provides for early intervention/evaluates effectiveness of therapy.**
- Prepare for surgical intervention (e.g., fibulectomy/fasciotomy) as indicated **to relieve pressure/restore circulation.**
- Use techniques, such as repositioning/padding, to relieve pressure.
- Encourage client to routinely exercise digits/joints distal to injury. Encourage ambulation as soon as possible.
- Evaluate for tenderness, swelling, pain on dorsiflexion of foot (positive Homans' sign).
- Keep linens off affected extremity with bed cradle.
- Apply antiembolic hose/sequential pressure device as indicated.
- Monitor Hb/Hct, coagulation studies (e.g., prothrombin time).
- Administer IV fluids, blood products as needed **to maintain circulating volume/tissue perfusion.**
- Administer anticoagulants as indicated for thrombotic vascular obstructions.

NURSING PRIORITY NO. **3.** To promote wellness (Teaching/Discharge Considerations):

- Review proper body alignment, elevation of limbs as appropriate.
- Discuss necessity of avoiding constrictive clothing, sharp angulation of legs/crossing legs.
- Demonstrate proper use of antiembolic hose.
- Review safe use of heat/cold therapy as indicated.
- Instruct client/SO(s) to check shoes, socks for proper fit and/or wrinkles, and so on.
- Demonstrate/recommend continuation of exercises **to maintain function and circulation of limbs.**

Documentation Focus

ASSESSMENT/REASSESSMENT

- Specific risk factors, nature of injury to limb.
- Assessment findings, including comparison of affected/unaffected limb, characteristics of pain in involved area.

PLANNING

- Plan of care and who is involved in the planning.
- Teaching plan.

IMPLEMENTATION/EVALUATION

- Response to interventions/teaching and actions performed.
- Attainment/progress toward desired outcome(s).
- Modification of plan of care.

DISCHARGE PLANNING

- Long-term needs/referrals and who is responsible for actions to be taken.
- Specific referrals made.

SAMPLE NURSING OUTCOMES
& INTERVENTIONS CLASSIFICATIONS (NOC/NIC)

NOC—Tissue Perfusion: Peripheral
NIC—Peripheral Sensation Management

Personal Identity, disturbed

Taxonomy II: Self-Perception—Class 1 Self-Concept
(00121)
[Diagnostic Division: Ego Integrity]
Submitted1978

Definition: Inability to distinguish between self and nonself

Related Factors

To be developed
[Organic brain syndrome]
[Poor ego differentiation, as in schizophrenia]
[Panic/dissociative states]
[Biochemical body change]

Defining Characteristics

To be developed

SUBJECTIVE

[Confusion about sense of self, purpose or direction in life, sexual identification/preference]

Information that appears in brackets has been added by the authors to clarify and enhance the use of nursing diagnoses.

OBJECTIVE

[Difficulty in making decisions]
[Poorly differentiated ego boundaries]
[See ND Anxiety for additional characteristics]

Desired Outcomes/Evaluation Criteria—Client Will:

- Acknowledge threat to personal identity.
- Integrate threat in a healthy, positive manner (e.g., state anxiety is reduced, make plans for the future).
- Verbalize acceptance of changes that have occurred.
- State ability to identify and accept self (long-term outcome).

Actions/Interventions

NURSING PRIORITY NO. 1. To assess causative/contributing factors:

- Ascertain client's perception of the extent of the threat to self and how client is handling the situation.
- Determine speed of occurrence of threat. **An event that has happened quickly may be more threatening.**
- Define disturbed body image. (**Body image is the basis of personal identity.**)
- Be aware of physical signs of panic state. (Refer to ND Anxiety.)
- Note age of client. **An adolescent may struggle with the developmental task of personal/sexual identity, whereas an older person may have more difficulty accepting/dealing with a threat to identity, such as progressive loss of memory.**
- Assess availability and use of support systems. Note response of family/SO(s).
- Note withdrawn/automatic behavior, regression to earlier developmental stage, general behavioral disorganization, or display of self-mutilation behaviors in adolescent or adult; delayed development, preference for solitary play, display of self-stimulation in child.
- Determine presence of hallucinations/delusions, distortions of reality.

NURSING PRIORITY NO. 2. To assist client to manage/deal with threat:

- Make time to listen to client, encouraging appropriate expression of feelings, including anger and hostility.
- Provide calm environment.
- Use crisis-intervention principles **to restore equilibrium when possible.**

- Assist client to develop strategies to cope with threat to identity. **Helps reduce anxiety and promotes self-awareness and self-esteem.**
- Engage client in activities to help in identifying self as an individual (e.g., use of mirror for visual feedback, tactile stimulation).
- Provide for simple decisions, concrete tasks, calming activities.
- Allow client to deal with situation in small steps because **may be unable to cope with larger picture when in stress overload.**
- Assist client in developing/participating in an individualized exercise program (walking is an excellent beginning program).
- Provide concrete assistance as needed (e.g., help with ADLs, providing food).
- Take advantage of opportunities to promote growth. Realize that client will have difficulty learning while in a dissociative state.
- Maintain reality orientation without confronting client's irrational beliefs. **Client may become defensive, blocking opportunity to look at other possibilities.**
- Use humor judiciously when appropriate.
- Discuss options for dealing with issues of sexual gender (e.g., therapy/gender-change surgery when client is a transsexual).
- Refer to NDs Body Image, disturbed; Self-Esteem [specify]; Spiritual Distress.

NURSING PRIORITY NO. 3. To promote wellness (Teaching/ Discharge Considerations):

- Provide accurate information about threat to and potential consequences for individual.
- Assist client and SO(s) to acknowledge and integrate threat into future planning (e.g., wearing ID bracelet when prone to mental confusion; change of lifestyle to accommodate change of gender for transsexual client).
- Refer to appropriate support groups (e.g., day-care program, counseling/psychotherapy, gender identity).

Documentation Focus

ASSESSMENT/REASSESSMENT

- Findings, noting degree of impairment.
- Nature of and client's perception of the threat.

PLANNING

- Plan of care and who is involved in the planning.
- Teaching plan.

- Client's response to interventions/teaching and actions performed.
- Attainment/progress toward desired outcome(s).
- Modifications to plan of care.

DISCHARGE PLANNING

- Long-term needs and who is responsible for actions to be taken.
- Specific referrals made.

SAMPLE NURSING OUTCOMES
& INTERVENTIONS CLASSIFICATIONS (NOC/NIC)

NOC—Identity
NIC—Self-Esteem Enhancement

Poisoning, risk for

Taxonomy II: Safety/Protection—Class 4 Environmental
Hazards (00037)
[Diagnostic Division: Safety]
Submitted 1980

Definition: At accentuated risk of accidental exposure
to or ingestion of drugs or dangerous products in doses
sufficient to cause poisoning [or the adverse effects of
prescribed medication/drug use]

Risk Factors

INTERNAL (INDIVIDUAL)

Reduced vision
Lack of safety or drug education
Lack of proper precaution; [unsafe habits, disregard for safety measures, lack of supervision]
Insufficient finances
Verbalization of occupational setting without adequate safeguards
Cognitive or emotional difficulties; [behavioral]
[Age (e.g., young child, elderly person)]
[Chronic disease state, disability]
[Cultural or religious beliefs/practices]

EXTERNAL (ENVIRONMENTAL)

Large supplies of drugs in house
Medicines stored in unlocked cabinets accessible to children or
confused persons

Information that appears in brackets has been added by the authors
to clarify and enhance the use of nursing diagnoses.

Availability of illicit drugs potentially contaminated by poisonous additives

Flaking, peeling paint or plaster in presence of young children

Dangerous products placed or stored within the reach of children or confused persons

Unprotected contact with heavy metals or chemicals

Paint, lacquer, and so forth in poorly ventilated areas or without effective protection

Chemical contamination of food and water

Presence of poisonous vegetation

Presence of atmospheric pollutants, [proximity to industrial chemicals/pattern of prevailing winds]

[Therapeutic margin of safety of specific drugs (e.g., therapeutic versus toxic level, half-life, method of uptake and degradation in body, adequacy of organ function)]

[Use of multiple herbal supplements or megadosing]

NOTE: A risk diagnosis is not evidenced by signs and symptoms, as the problem has not occurred and nursing interventions are directed at prevention.

Desired Outcomes/Evaluation Criteria—Client Will:

- Verbalize understanding of dangers of poisoning.
- Identify hazards that could lead to accidental poisoning.
- Correct environmental hazards as identified.
- Demonstrate necessary actions/lifestyle changes to promote safe environment.

Actions/Interventions

NURSING PRIORITY NO. 1. To assess causative/contributing factors:

- Determine presence of internal/external risk factors in client's environment, including presence of allergens/pollutants that may affect client's condition.
- Assess client's knowledge of safety hazards of drugs/herbal supplements/environment and ability to respond to potential threat.
- Determine use of legal/illegal drugs, for example, alcohol, marijuana, heroin, prescription/OTC drugs. Review results of laboratory tests/toxicology screening as indicated.

NURSING PRIORITY NO. 2. To assist in correcting factors that can lead to accidental poisoning:

- Discuss safety cap and/or lockup of medicines, cleaning products, paint/solvents, and so forth.
- Administer children's medications as drugs, not candy. Recap medication containers immediately after obtaining current dosage. **Open containers increase risk of accidental ingestion.**

- Stress importance of supervising infant/child or individuals with cognitive limitations.
- Code medicines for the visually impaired.
- Have responsible SO(s)/home health nurse supervise medication regimen/prepare medications for the cognitively or visually impaired, or obtain prefilled med box from pharmacy.
- Encourage discarding outdated/unused drug safely (disposing in hazardous waste collection areas, not down drain/toilet).
- Refer identified health/safety violations to the appropriate resource (e.g., health department, Occupational Safety and Health Administration—OSHA).
- Repair/replace/correct unsafe household items/situations (e.g., storage of solvents in soda bottles, flaking/peeling paint or plaster).

NURSING PRIORITY NO. **3.** To promote wellness (Teaching/ Discharge Considerations):

- Institute community programs to assist individuals to identify and correct risk factors in own environment.
- Review drug side effects/potential interactions with client/ SO(s). Discuss use of OTC drugs/herbal supplements and possibilities of misuse, drug interactions, and overdosing as with vitamin megadosing, and so on.
- Educate client to outdoor hazards, both local and vacation, for example, vegetation (poison ivy), ticks, and bees. Encourage susceptible person to carry kit with a prefilled syringe of epinephrine and an epinephrine nebulizer for immediate use when necessary.
- Encourage periodic inspection of well water/tap water to identify possible contaminants.
- Review sources of possible water contamination (e.g., sewage disposal, agricultural/industrial runoff).
- Review pertinent job-related health department/OSHA regulations.
- Refer to resources that provide information about air quality (e.g., pollen index, "bad air days").
- Provide list of emergency numbers placed by telephone for use if poisoning occurs.
- Encourage parent to place safety stickers on drugs/chemicals to warn children of harmful contents.
- Instruct in first aid measures or ascertain that client/SO has access to written literature when potential exists for accidents/trauma.
- Stress avoidance of use of ipecac syrup in home. May be used inappropriately. Cause adverse effects.
- Refer substance abuser to detoxification programs, inpatient/ outpatient rehabilitation, counseling, support groups, and psychotherapy.

- Encourage emergency measures, awareness and education (e.g., CPR/first aid class, community safety programs, ways to access emergency medical personnel).

Documentation Focus

ASSESSMENT/REASSESSMENT

- Identified risk factors noting internal/external concerns.

PLANNING

- Plan of care and who is involved in the planning.
- Teaching plan.

IMPLEMENTATION/EVALUATION

- Response to interventions/teaching and actions performed.
- Attainment/progress toward desired outcome(s).
- Modification to plan of care.

DISCHARGE PLANNING

- Long-term needs and who is responsible for actions to be taken.
- Specific referrals made.

SAMPLE NURSING OUTCOMES & INTERVENTIONS CLASSIFICATIONS (NOC/NIC)

NOC—Risk Control: Drug Use
NIC—Environmental Management: Safety

Post-Trauma Syndrome [specify stage]

Taxonomy II: Coping/Stress Tolerance—Class 1 Post-Trauma Responses (00141)
[Diagnostic Division: Ego Integrity]
Submitted 1986; Nursing Diagnosis Extension and Classification (NDEC) Revision 1998

Definition: Sustained maladaptive response to a traumatic, overwhelming event

Related Factors

Events outside the range of usual human experience
Serious threat or injury to self or loved ones; serious accidents; industrial and motor-vehicle accidents
Physical and psychosocial abuse; rape
Witnessing mutilation, violent death, or other horrors; tragic occurrence involving multiple deaths

---

Information that appears in brackets has been added by the authors to clarify and enhance the use of nursing diagnoses.

Natural and/or human-made disasters; sudden destruction of one's
home or community; epidemics

Wars; military combat; being held prisoner of war or criminal victim-
ization (torture)

Defining Characteristics

SUBJECTIVE

Intrusive thoughts/dreams; nightmares; flashbacks

Palpitations; headaches; [loss of interest in usual activities, loss of feeling of intimacy/sexuality]

Hopelessness; shame

[Excessive verbalization of the traumatic event, verbalization of
survival guilt or guilt about behavior required for survival]

Gastric irritability; [changes in appetite; sleep disturbance/insomnia;
chronic fatigue/easy fatigability]

OBJECTIVE

Anxiety; fear

Hypervigilant; exaggerated startle response; neurosensory irritability;
irritability

Grief; guilt

Difficulty in concentrating; depression

Anger and/or rage; aggression

Avoidance; repression; alienation; denial; detachment; psychogenic
amnesia; numbing

Altered mood states; [poor impulse control/irritability and explosive-
ness]; panic attacks; horror

Substance abuse; compulsive behavior

Enuresis (in children)

[Difficulty with interpersonal relationships; dependence on others;
work/school failure]

[Stages:

ACUTE SUBTYPE: Begins within 6 months and does not last
longer than 6 months.

CHRONIC SUBTYPE: Lasts more than 6 months.

DELAYED SUBTYPE: Period of latency of 6 months or more
before onset of symptoms.]

Desired Outcomes/Evaluation
Criteria—Client Will:

- Express own feelings/reactions, avoiding projection.
- Verbalize a positive self-image.
- Report reduced anxiety/fear when memories occur.
- Demonstrate ability to deal with emotional reactions in an
individually appropriate manner.
- Demonstrate appropriate changes in behavior/lifestyle (e.g.,
share experiences with others, seek/get support from SO(s) as
needed, change in job/residence).

- Report absence of physical manifestations (such as pain, chronic fatigue).
- Refer to ND Rape-Trauma Syndrome for additional outcomes when trauma is the result of rape.

Actions/Interventions

NURSING PRIORITY NO. 1. To assess causative factor(s) and individual reaction:

ACUTE

- Observe for and elicit information about physical or psychological injury and note associated stress-related symptoms such as "numbness," headache, tightness in chest, nausea, pounding heart, and so forth.
- Identify psychologic responses: anger, shock, acute anxiety, confusion, denial. Note laughter, crying; calm or agitated, excited (hysterical) behavior; expressions of disbelief and/or self-blame, lability of emotional changes.
- Assess client's knowledge of and anxiety related to the situation. Note ongoing threat to self (e.g., contact with perpetrator and/or associates).
- Identify social aspects of trauma/incident (e.g., disfigurement, chronic conditions/permanent disabilities).
- Ascertain ethnic, background/cultural and religious perceptions and beliefs about the occurrence (e.g., retribution from God).
- Determine degree of disorganization.
- Identify whether incident has reactivated preexisting or coexisting situations (physical/psychological). **Affects how the client views the trauma.**
- Determine disruptions in relationships (e.g., family, friends, coworkers, SOs). **Support persons may not know how to deal with client/situation (e.g., be oversolicitous or withdraw).**
- Note withdrawn behavior, use of denial, and use of chemical substances or impulsive behaviors (e.g., chain-smoking, overeating).
- Be aware of signs of increasing anxiety (e.g., silence, stuttering, inability to sit still). **Increasing anxiety may indicate risk for violence.**
- Note verbal/nonverbal expressions of guilt or self-blame when client has survived trauma in which others died.
- Assess signs/stage of grieving for self and others.
- Identify development of phobic reactions to ordinary articles (e.g., knives); situations (e.g., walking in groups of people, strangers ringing doorbell).

CHRONIC (IN ADDITION TO PREVIOUS ASSESSMENT)

- Evaluate continued somatic complaints (e.g., gastric irritation, anorexia, insomnia, muscle tension, headache). Investigate reports of new/changes in symptoms.
- Note manifestations of chronic pain or pain symptoms in excess of degree of physical injury.
- Be aware of signs of severe/prolonged depression; note presence of flashbacks, intrusive memories, and/or nightmares.
- Assess degree of dysfunctional coping (e.g., use of chemical substances/substance abuse) and consequences.

NURSING PRIORITY NO. 2. To assist client to deal with situation that exists:

ACUTE

- Provide a calm, safe environment. **Promotes sense of trust and safety.**
- Assist with documentation for police report, as indicated, and stay with the client.
- Listen to/investigate physical complaints. **Emotional reactions may limit client's ability to recognize physical injury.**
- Identify supportive persons for this individual.
- Remain with client, listen as client recounts incident/concerns—possibly repeatedly. (If client does not want to talk, accept silence.) **Provides psychologic support.**
- Provide environment in which client can talk freely about feelings, fear (including concerns about relationship with/response of SO), and experiences/sensations (e.g., loss of control, "near-death experience").
- Help child to express feelings about event using techniques appropriate to developmental level (e.g., play for young child, stories/puppets for preschooler, peer group for adolescent). **Children are more likely to express in play what they may not be able to verbalize directly.**
- Assist with practical realities (e.g., temporary housing, money, notifications of family members, or other needs).
- Be aware of and assist client to use ego strengths in a positive way by acknowledging ability to handle what is happening. **Enhances self-concept, reduces sense of helplessness.**
- Allow the client to work through own kind of adjustment. If the client is withdrawn or unwilling to talk, do not force the issue.
- Listen for expressions of fear of crowds and/or people.

CHRONIC

- Continue listening to expressions of concern. **May need to continue to talk about the incident.**

- Permit free expression of feelings (may continue from the crisis phase). Do not rush client through expressions of feelings too quickly and do not reassure inappropriately. **Client may believe pain and/or anguish is misunderstood and may be depressed. Statements such as "You don't understand" or "You weren't there" are a defense, a way of pushing others away.**
- Encourage client to talk out experience, expressing feelings of fear, anger, loss/grief. (Refer to ND Grieving, dysfunctional).
- Ascertain/monitor sleep pattern of children as well as adults. Sleep disturbances/nightmares may develop delaying resolution, impairing coping abilities.
- Encourage client to become aware of and accepting of own feelings and reactions when identified.
- Acknowledge reality of loss of self, which existed before the incident. Assist client to move toward an acceptance of the potential for growth that exists within client.
- Continue to allow client to progress at own pace.
- Give "permission" to express/deal with anger at the assailant/situation in acceptable ways.
- Keep discussion on practical and emotional level rather than intellectualizing the experience, **which allows client to avoid dealing with feelings.**
- Assist in dealing with practical concerns and effects of the incident, such as court appearances, altered relationships with SO(s), employment problems.
- Provide for sensitive, trained counselors/therapists and engage in therapies, such as psychotherapy in conjunction with medications, Implosive Therapy (flooding), hypnosis, relaxation, Rolfing, memory work, cognitive restructuring, Eye Movement Desensitization and Reprocessing (EMDR), physical and occupational therapies.
- Discuss use of medication (e.g., antidepressants). **Lithium may be used to reduce explosiveness; low-dose psychotropics may be used when loss of contact with reality is a problem.**

NURSING PRIORITY NO. **3.** To promote wellness (Teaching/Discharge Considerations):

- Assist client to identify and monitor feelings while therapy is occurring.
- Provide information about what reactions client may expect during each phase. Let client know these are common reactions. Be sure to phrase in neutral terms of "You may or you may not...." **Helps reduce fear of the unknown.**
- Assist client to identify factors that may have created a vulnerable situation and that he or she may have power to change **to protect self in the future.**

- Avoid making value judgments.
- Discuss lifestyle changes client is contemplating and how they may contribute to recovery. **Helps client evaluate appropriateness of plans.**
- Assist with learning stress-management techniques.
- Discuss recognition of and ways to manage "anniversary reactions," letting client know normalcy of recurrence of thoughts and feelings at this time.
- Suggest support group for SO(s) **to assist with understanding of and ways to deal with client.**
- Encourage psychiatric consultation, especially if client is unable to maintain control, is violent, is inconsolable, or does not seem to be making an adjustment. **Participation in a group may be helpful.**
- Refer to family/marital counseling if indicated.
- Refer to NDs Powerlessness; Coping, ineffective; Grieving, anticipatory/dysfunctional.

Documentation Focus

ASSESSMENT/REASSESSMENT

- Individual findings, noting current dysfunction and behavioral/emotional responses to the incident.
- Specifics of traumatic event.
- Reactions of family/SO(s).

PLANNING

- Plan of care and who is involved in the planning.
- Teaching plan.

IMPLEMENTATION/EVALUATION

- Responses to interventions/teaching and actions performed.
- Emotional changes.
- Attainment/progress toward desired outcome(s).
- Modifications to plan of care.

DISCHARGE PLANNING

- Long-term needs and who is responsible for actions to be taken.
- Specific referrals made.

SAMPLE NURSING OUTCOMES & INTERVENTIONS CLASSIFICATIONS (NOC/NIC)

NOC—Fear Control
NIC—Support System Enhancement

Post-Trauma Syndrome, risk for

Taxonomy II: Coping/Stress Tolerance—Class 1 Post-Trauma Responses (00145)
[Diagnostic Division: Ego Integrity]
Submitted 1998; Nursing Diagnosis Extension and Classification (NDEC) Submission 1998

Definition: At risk for sustained maladaptive response to a traumatic, overwhelming event

Risk Factors

Occupation (e.g., police, fire, rescue, corrections, emergency room staff, mental health worker, [and their family members])
Perception of event; exaggerated sense of responsibility; diminished ego strength
Survivor's role in the event
Inadequate social support; nonsupportive environment; displacement from home
Duration of the event

> NOTE: A risk diagnosis is not evidenced by signs and symptoms, as the problem has not occurred and nursing interventions are directed at prevention.

Desired Outcomes/Evaluation Criteria—Client Will:

- Be free of severe anxiety.
- Demonstrate ability to deal with emotional reactions in an individually appropriate manner.
- Report absence of physical manifestations (pain, nightmares/flashbacks, fatigue) associated with event.

Actions/Interventions°

NURSING PRIORITY NO. **1.** To assess contributing factors and individual reaction:

- Note occupation (e.g., police, fire, emergency room, etc.), as listed in Risk Factors.
- Assess client's knowledge of and anxiety related to potential or recurring situations.
- Identify how client's past experiences may affect current situation.
- Listen for comments of taking on responsibility (e.g., "I should have been more careful/gone back to get her").
- Evaluate for life factors/stressors currently or recently occurring, such as displacement from home due to catastrophic event (e.g., illness/injury, fire/flood/violent storm/earthquake).

Information that appears in brackets has been added by the authors to clarify and enhance the use of nursing diagnoses.

- Identify client's coping mechanisms.
- Determine availability/usefulness of client's support systems, family, social, community, and so forth. (Note: Family members can also be at risk.)

NURSING PRIORITY NO. 2. To assist client to deal with situation that exists:

- Educate high-risk persons/families about signs/symptoms of post-trauma response, especially if it is likely to occur in their occupation/life.
- Identify and discuss client's strengths (e.g., very supportive family, usually copes well with stress, etc.) as well as vulnerabilities (e.g., client tends toward alcohol/other drugs for coping, client has witnessed a murder, etc.)
- Discuss how individual coping mechanisms have worked in past traumatic events.
- Evaluate client's perceptions of events and personal significance (e.g., policeman/parent investigating death of a child).
- Provide emotional and physical presence **to strengthen client's coping abilities.**
- Encourage expression of feelings. Note whether feelings expressed appear congruent with events the client experienced. **Incongruency may indicate deeper conflict and can impede resolution.**
- Observe for signs and symptoms of stress responses, such as nightmares, reliving an incident, poor appetite, irritability, numbness and crying, family/relationship disruption. **These responses are normal in the early postincident time frame. If prolonged and persistent, the client may be experiencing post-traumatic stress disorder.**

NURSING PRIORITY NO. 3. To promote wellness (Teaching/Discharge Considerations):

- Provide a calm, safe environment **in which client can deal with disruption of life.**
- Encourage client to identify and monitor feelings on an ongoing basis. **Promotes awareness of changes in ability to deal with stressors.**
- Encourage learning stress-management techniques **to help with resolution of situation.**
- Recommend participation in debriefing sessions that may be provided following major events. **Dealing with the stressor promptly may facilitate recovery from event/prevent exacerbation.**
- Identify employment, community resource groups. **Provides opportunity for ongoing support to deal with recurrent stressors.**
- Refer for individual/family counseling as indicated.

Documentation Focus

ASSESSMENT/REASSESSMENT

- Identified risk factors noting internal/external concerns.
- Client's perception of event and personal significance.

PLANNING

- Plan of care and who is involved in the planning.
- Teaching plan.

IMPLEMENTATION/EVALUATION

- Response to interventions/teaching and actions performed.
- Attainment/progress toward desired outcome(s).

DISCHARGE PLANNING

- Long-term needs and who is responsible for actions to be taken.
- Specific referrals made.

SAMPLE NURSING OUTCOMES & INTERVENTIONS CLASSIFICATIONS (NOC/NIC)

NOC—Grief Resolution
NIC—Crisis Intervention

Powerlessness [specify level]

Taxonomy II: Self-Perception—Class 1 Self-Concept
(00125)
[Diagnostic Division: Ego Integrity]
Submitted 1982

Definition: Perception that one's own action will not significantly affect an outcome; a perceived lack of control over a current situation or immediate happening

Related Factors

Healthcare environment [e.g., loss of privacy, personal possessions, control over therapies]
Interpersonal interaction [e.g., misuse of power, force; abusive relationships]
Illness-related regimen [e.g., chronic/debilitating conditions]
Lifestyle of helplessness [e.g., repeated failures, dependency]

Information that appears in brackets has been added by the authors to clarify and enhance the use of nursing diagnoses.

Defining Characteristics

SUBJECTIVE

Severe
Verbal expressions of having no control or influence over situation, outcome, or self-care
Depression over physical deterioration that occurs despite client compliance with regimens
Moderate
Expressions of dissatisfaction and frustration over inability to perform previous tasks and/or activities
Expression of doubt regarding role performance
Reluctance to express true feelings; fear of alienation from caregivers
Low
Expressions of uncertainty about fluctuating energy levels

OBJECTIVE

Severe
Apathy [withdrawal, resignation, crying]
[Anger]
Moderate
Does not monitor progress
Nonparticipation in care or decision making when opportunities are provided
Dependence on others that may result in irritability, resentment, anger, and guilt
Inability to seek information regarding care
Does not defend self-care practices when challenged
Passivity
Low
Passivity

Desired Outcomes/Evaluation Criteria—Client Will:

- Express sense of control over the present situation and future outcome.
- Make choices related to and be involved in care.
- Identify areas over which individual has control.
- Acknowledge reality that some areas are beyond individual's control.

Actions/Interventions

NURSING PRIORITY NO. **1.** To assess causative/contributing factors:

- Identify situational circumstances (e.g., strange environment, immobility, diagnosis of terminal/chronic illness, lack of support system(s), lack of knowledge about situation).
- Determine client's perception/knowledge of condition and treatment plan.

- Ascertain client response to treatment regimen. Does client see reason(s) and understand it is in the client's interest or is client compliant and helpless?
- Identify client locus of control: internal (expressions of responsibility for self and ability to control outcomes "I didn't quit smoking") or external (expressions of lack of control over self and environment—"Nothing ever works out"; "What bad luck to get lung cancer").
- Assess degree of mastery client has exhibited in life.
- Determine if there has been a change in relationships with SO(s).
- Note availability/use of resources.
- Investigate caregiver practices. Do they support client control/responsibility?

NURSING PRIORITY NO. **2.** To assess degree of powerlessness experienced by the client/SO(s):

- Listen to statements client makes: "They don't care"; "It won't make any difference"; "Are you kidding?"
- Note expressions that indicate "giving up," such as "It won't do any good."
- Note behavioral responses (verbal and nonverbal) including expressions of fear, interest or apathy, agitation, withdrawal.
- Note lack of communication, flat affect, and lack of eye contact.
- Identify the use of manipulative behavior and reactions of client and caregivers. (**Manipulation is used for management of powerlessness because of distrust of others, fear of intimacy, search for approval, and validation of sexuality.**)

NURSING PRIORITY NO. **3.** To assist client to clarify needs relative to ability to meet them:

- Show concern for client as a person.
- Make time to listen to client's perceptions and concerns and encourage questions.
- Accept expressions of feelings, including anger and hopelessness.
- Avoid arguing or using logic with hopeless client. **Client will not believe it can make a difference.**
- Express hope for the client. (**There is always hope of something.**)
- Identify strengths/assets and past coping strategies that were successful. **Helps client to recognize own ability to deal with difficult situation.**
- Assist client to identify what he or she can do for self. Identify things the client can/cannot control.

- Encourage client to maintain a sense of perspective about the situation.

NURSING PRIORITY NO. **4.** To promote independence:

- Use client's locus of control to develop individual plan of care (e.g., for client with internal control, encourage client to take control of own care and for those with external control, begin with small tasks and add as tolerated).
- Develop contract with client specifying goals agreed on. **Enhances commitment to plan, optimizing outcomes.**
- Treat expressed decisions and desires with respect. (Avoid critical parenting behaviors.)
- Provide client opportunities to control as many events as energy and restrictions of care permit.
- Discuss needs openly with client and set up agreed-on routines for meeting identified needs. **Minimizes use of manipulation.**
- Minimize rules and limit continuous observation to the degree that safety permits **to provide sense of control for the client.**
- Support client efforts to develop realistic steps to put plan into action, reach goals, and maintain expectations.
- Provide positive reinforcement for desired behaviors.
- Direct client's thoughts beyond present state to future when appropriate.
- Schedule frequent brief visits to check on client, deal with client needs, and let client know someone is available.
- Involve SO(s) in client care as appropriate.

NURSING PRIORITY NO. **5.** To promote wellness (Teaching/ Discharge Considerations):

- Instruct in/encourage use of anxiety and stress-reduction techniques.
- Provide accurate verbal and written information about what is happening and discuss with client/SO(s). Repeat as often as necessary.
- Assist client to set realistic goals for the future.
- Assist client to learn/use assertive communication skills.
- Facilitate return to a productive role in whatever capacity possible for the individual. Refer to occupational therapist/ vocational counselor as indicated.
- Encourage client to think productively and positively and take responsibility for choosing own thoughts.
- Problem-solve with client/SO(s).
- Suggest periodic review of own needs/goals.
- Refer to support groups, counseling/therapy, and so forth as indicated.

Documentation Focus

ASSESSMENT/REASSESSMENT

• Individual findings, noting degree of powerlessness, locus of control, individual's perception of the situation.

PLANNING

• Plan of care and who is involved in the planning.
• Teaching plan.

IMPLEMENTATION/EVALUATION

• Responses to interventions/teaching and actions performed.
• Specific goals/expectations.
• Attainment/progress toward desired outcome(s).
• Modifications to plan of care.

DISCHARGE PLANNING

• Long-term needs and who is responsible for actions to be taken.
• Specific referrals made.

SAMPLE NURSING OUTCOMES & INTERVENTIONS CLASSIFICATIONS (NOC/NIC)

NOC—Health Beliefs: Perceived Control
NIC—Self-Responsibility Facilitation

Powerlessness, risk for

Taxonomy II: Self-Perception—Class 1 Self-Concept (00125)
[Diagnostic Division: Ego Integrity]
Submitted 2000

Definition: At risk for perceived lack of control over a situation and/or one's ability to significantly affect an outcome

Risk Factors

Physiological
    Chronic or acute illness (hospitalization, intubation, ventilator, suctioning); dying
    Acute injury or progressive debilitating disease process (e.g., spinal cord injury, multiple sclerosis)
    Aging (e.g., decreased physical strength, decreased mobility)
Psychosocial
    Lack of knowledge of illness or healthcare system

Information that appears in brackets has been added by the authors to clarify and enhance the use of nursing diagnoses.

Lifestyle of dependency with inadequate coping patterns
Absence of integrality (e.g., essence of power)
Decreased self-esteem; low or unstable body image

> NOTE: A risk diagnosis is not evidenced by signs and symptoms, as the problem has not occurred and nursing interventions are directed at prevention.

Desired Outcomes/Evaluation Criteria—Client Will:

- Express sense of control over the present situation and hopefulness about future outcomes.
- Make choices related to and be involved in care.
- Identify areas over which individual has control.
- Acknowledge reality that some areas are beyond individual's control.

Actions/Interventions

NURSING PRIORITY NO. **1.** To assess causative/contributing factors:

- Identify situational circumstances (e.g., acute illness, sudden hospitalization, diagnosis of terminal or debilitating/chronic illness, very young or aging with decreased physical strength and mobility, lack of knowledge about illness, healthcare system).
- Determine client's perception/knowledge of condition and proposed treatment plan.
- Identify client's locus of control: Internal (expressions of responsibility for self and environment) or external (expressions of lack of control over self and environment).
- Assess client's self-esteem and degree of mastery client has exhibited in life situations.
- Note availability and use of resources.
- Listen to statements client makes which might indicate feelings of powerlessness (e.g., "They don't care"; "It won't make a difference"; "It won't do any good").
- Observe behavioral responses (verbal and nonverbal) for expressions of fear, disinterest or apathy, or withdrawal.
- Be alert for signs of manipulative behavior and note reactions of client and caregivers. (**Manipulation may be used for management of powerlessness because of fear and distrust.**)

NURSING PRIORITY NO. **2.** To assist client to clarify needs and ability to meet them:

- Show concern for client as a person. Encourage questions.
- Make time to listen to client's perceptions of the situation as well as concerns.

- Accept expressions of feelings, including anger and reluctance to try to work things out.
- Express hope for client and encourage review of past experiences with successful strategies.
- Assist client to identify what he or she can do to help self and what situations can/cannot be controlled.

NURSING PRIORITY NO. **3.** To promote wellness (Teaching/Discharge Considerations):

- Encourage client to be active in own healthcare management and to take responsibility for choosing own actions and reactions.
- Plan and problem-solve with client and SO(s).
- Support client efforts to develop realistic steps to put plan into action, reach goals, and maintain expectations.
- Provide accurate verbal and written instructions about what is happening and what realistically might happen.
- Suggest periodic review of own needs/goals.
- Refer to support groups or counseling/therapy as appropriate.

Documentation Focus

ASSESSMENT/REASSESSMENT

- Individual findings, noting potential for powerlessness, locus of control, individual's perception of the situation.

PLANNING

- Plan of care and who is involved in the planning.
- Teaching plan.

IMPLEMENTATION/EVALUATION

- Responses to interventions/teaching and actions performed.
- Specific goals/expectations.
- Modifications to plan of care.

DISCHARGE PLANNING

- Long-term needs and who is responsible for actions to be taken.
- Specific referrals made.

SAMPLE NURSING OUTCOMES & INTERVENTIONS CLASSIFICATIONS (NOC/NIC)

NOC—Health Beliefs: Perceived Control
NIC—Self-Responsibility Facilitation

Protection, ineffective

Taxonomy II: Safety/Protection—Class 2 Physical Injury
(00043)
[Diagnostic Division: Safety]
Submitted 1990

Definition: Decrease in the ability to guard self from
internal or external threats such as illness or injury

Related Factors

Extremes of age
Inadequate nutrition
Alcohol abuse
Abnormal blood profiles (e.g., leukopenia, thrombocytopenia, anemia,
coagulation)
Drug therapies (e.g., antineoplastic, corticosteroid, immune, anticoag-
ulant, thrombolytic)
Treatments (e.g., surgery, radiation)
Diseases, such as cancer and immune disorders

Defining Characteristics

SUBJECTIVE

Neurosensory alterations
Chilling
Itching
Insomnia; fatigue; weakness
Anorexia

OBJECTIVE

Deficient immunity
Impaired healing; altered clotting
Maladaptive stress response
Perspiring [inappropriately]
Dyspnea; cough
Restlessness; immobility
Disorientation
Pressure sores

Authors' note: The purpose of this diagnosis seems to
combine multiple NDs under a single heading for ease of planning care when a number of variables may be present.
Outcomes/evaluation criteria and interventions are specifically
tied to individual related factors that are present, such as:

Extremes of age: Concerns may include body temperature/
thermoregulation or thought process/sensory-perceptual
alterations, as well as risk for trauma, suffocation, or
poisoning; and fluid volume imbalances.

Inadequate nutrition: Brings up issues of nutrition, less than
body requirements; infection, altered thought processes,
trauma, ineffective coping, and altered family processes.

Information that appears in brackets has been added by the authors
to clarify and enhance the use of nursing diagnoses.　　**411**

Alcohol abuse: May be situational or chronic with problems ranging from ineffective breathing patterns, decreased cardiac output, and fluid volume deficit to nutritional problems, infection, trauma, altered thought processes, and coping/family process difficulties.

Abnormal blood profile: Suggests possibility of fluid volume deficit, decreased tissue perfusion, impaired gas exchange, activity intolerance, or risk for infection.

Drug therapies, treatments, and disease concerns: Would include risk for infection, fluid volume imbalances, altered skin/tissue integrity, pain, nutritional problems, fatigue, and emotional responses.

It is suggested that the user refer to specific NDs based on identified related factors and individual concerns for this client to find appropriate outcomes and interventions.

SAMPLE NURSING OUTCOMES & INTERVENTIONS CLASSIFICATIONS (NOC/NIC)

NOC—Cognitive Orientation
NIC—Postanesthesia Care

Rape-Trauma Syndrome [specify]

Taxonomy II: Coping/Stress Tolerance—Class 1 Post-Trauma Responses (see A, B, C, following)
[Diagnostic Division: Ego Integrity]
Submitted 1980

Definition: Sustained maladaptive response to a forced, violent sexual penetration against the victim's will and consent. Note: This syndrome includes the following three subcomponents: [A] Rape-Trauma; [B] Compound Reaction; and [C] Silent Reaction

NOTE: Although attacks are most often directed toward women, men also may be victims.

Related Factors

Rape [actual/attempted forced sexual penetration]

Defining Characteristics

[A] RAPE-TRAUMA—TAXONOMY II (00142)
NURSING DIAGNOSIS EXTENSION AND CLASSIFICATION (NDEC) REVISION 1998

SUBJECTIVE

Embarrassment; humiliation; shame; guilt; self-blame
Loss of self-esteem; helplessness; powerlessness

Information that appears in brackets has been added by the authors to clarify and enhance the use of nursing diagnoses.

Shock; fear; anxiety; anger; revenge
Nightmare and sleep disturbances
Change in relationships; sexual dysfunction

OBJECTIVE

Physical trauma (e.g., bruising, tissue irritation); muscle tension
and/or spasms
Confusion; disorganization; inability to make decisions
Agitation; hyperalertness; aggression
Mood swings; vulnerability; dependence; depression
Substance abuse; suicide attempts
Denial; phobias; paranoia; dissociative disorders

[B] COMPOUND REACTION—TAXONOMY II (00143)

The trauma syndrome that develops from this attack or attempted
attack includes an acute phase of disorganization of the victim's
lifestyle and a long-term process of reorganization of lifestyle.

Related Factors

To be developed

Defining Characteristics

ACUTE PHASE. Emotional reactions (e.g., anger, embarrassment, fear of
physical violence and death, humiliation, self-blame, revenge)
Multiple physical symptoms (e.g., gastrointestinal irritability, genitourinary discomfort, muscle tension, sleep pattern disturbance)
Reactivated symptoms of such previous conditions (i.e., physical/
psychiatric illness); reliance on alcohol and/or drugs
LONG-TERM PHASE. Changes in lifestyle (e.g., changes in residence, dealing with repetitive nightmares and phobias, seeking family/social
network support)

[C] SILENT REACTION—TAXONOMY II (00141)

Related Factors

To be developed

Defining Characteristics

Abrupt changes in relationships with men
Increase in nightmares
Increasing anxiety during interview (i.e., blocking of associations, long
periods of silence; minor stuttering, physical distress)
Pronounced changes in sexual behavior
No verbalization of the occurrence of rape
Sudden onset of phobic reactions

Desired Outcomes/Evaluation Criteria—Client Will:

- Deal appropriately with emotional reactions as evidenced by
behavior and expression of feelings.

- Report absence of physical complications, pain, and discomfort.
- Verbalize a positive self-image.
- Verbalize recognition that incident was not of own doing.
- Identify behaviors/situations within own control that may reduce risk of recurrence.
- Deal with practical aspects (e.g., court appearances).
- Demonstrate appropriate changes in lifestyle (e.g., change in job/residence) as necessary and seek/obtain support from SO(s) as needed.
- Interact with individuals/groups in desired and acceptable manner.

Actions/Interventions

NURSING PRIORITY NO. 1. To assess trauma and individual reaction, noting length of time since occurrence of event:

- Observe for and elicit information about physical injury and assess stress-related symptoms, such as numbness, headache, tightness in chest, nausea, pounding heart, and so forth.
- Identify psychologic responses: anger, shock, acute anxiety, confusion, denial. Note laughter, crying, calm or agitated, excited (hysterical) behavior, expressions of disbelief, and/or self-blame.
- Note signs of increasing anxiety (e.g., silence, stuttering, inability to sit still).
- Determine degree of disorganization.
- Identify whether incident has reactivated preexisting or coexisting situations (physical/psychological). **Can affect how the client views the trauma.**
- Determine disruptions in relationships with men and with others (e.g., family, friends, coworkers, SO[s]).
- Identify development of phobic reactions to ordinary articles (e.g., knives) and situations (e.g., walking in groups of people, strangers ringing doorbell).
- Note degree of intrusive repetitive thoughts, sleep disturbances.
- Assess degree of dysfunctional coping (e.g., use of alcohol, other drugs, suicidal/homicidal ideation, marked change in sexual behavior).

NURSING PRIORITY NO. 2. To assist client to deal with situation that exists:

- Explore own feelings (nurse/caregiver) regarding rape/incest issue prior to interacting with the client. **Need to recognize own biases to prevent imposing them on the client.**

ACUTE PHASE

- Stay with the client/do not leave child unattended. Provides reassurance/sense of safety.
- Involve rape response team when available. Provide same-sex examiner when appropriate.
- Evaluate infant/child/adolescent as dictated by age, sex, and developmental level.
- Assist with documentation of incident for police/child-protective services reports, maintain sequencing and collection of evidence (chain of evidence), label each specimen, and store/package properly.
- Provide environment in which client can talk freely about feelings and fears, including concerns about relationship with/response of SO(s), pregnancy, sexually transmitted diseases.
- Provide psychologic support by listening and remaining with client. If client does not want to talk, accept silence. **May indicate Silent Reaction.**
- Listen to/investigate physical complaints. Assist with medical treatments as indicated. **Emotional reactions may limit client's ability to recognize physical injury.**
- Assist with practical realities (e.g., safe temporary housing, money, or other needs).
- Be aware of client's ego strengths and assist client to use them in a positive way by acknowledging client's ability to handle what is happening.
- Identify supportive persons for this individual.

POSTACUTE PHASE

- Allow the client to work through own kind of adjustment. **May be withdrawn or unwilling to talk;** do not force the issue.
- Listen for expressions of fear of crowds, men, and so forth. **May reveal developing phobias.**
- Discuss specific concerns/fears. Identify appropriate actions (e.g., diagnostic testing for pregnancy, sexually transmitted diseases) and provide information as indicated.
- Include written instructions that are concise and clear regarding medical treatments, crisis support services, and so on. **Reinforces teaching, provides opportunity to deal with information at own pace.**

LONG-TERM PHASE

- Continue listening to expressions of concern. **May need to continue to talk about the assault.** Note persistence of somatic complaints (e.g., nausea, anorexia, insomnia, muscle tension, headache).

- Permit free expression of feelings (may continue from the crisis phase). Do not rush client through expressions of feelings too quickly and do not reassure inappropriately. **Client may believe pain and/or anguish is misunderstood and depression may limit responses.**
- Acknowledge reality of loss of self that existed before the incident. Assist client to move toward an acceptance of the potential for growth that exists within individual.
- Continue to allow client to progress at own pace.
- Give "permission" to express/deal with anger at the perpetrator/situation in acceptable ways. Set limits on destructive behaviors. **Facilitates resolution of feelings without diminishing self-concept.**
- Keep discussion on practical and emotional level rather than intellectualizing the experience, **which allows client to avoid dealing with feelings.**
- Assist in dealing with ongoing concerns about and effects of the incident, such as court appearance, pregnancy, sexually transmitted disease, relationship with SO(s), and so forth.
- Provide for sensitive, trained counselors, considering individual needs. (**Male/female counselors may be best determined on an individual basis as counselor's gender may be an issue for some clients, affecting ability to disclose.**)

NURSING PRIORITY NO. 3. To promote wellness (Teaching/Discharge Considerations):

- Provide information about what reactions client may expect during each phase. Let client know these are common reactions. Be sure to phrase in neutral terms of "You may or may not…" (Be aware that, although male rape perpetrators are usually heterosexual, the male victim may be concerned about his own sexuality and may exhibit a homophobic response.)
- Assist client to identify factors that may have created a vulnerable situation and that she or he may have power to change **to protect self in the future.**
- Avoid making value judgments.
- Discuss lifestyle changes client is contemplating and how they will contribute to recovery. **Helps client evaluate appropriateness of plans.**
- Encourage psychiatric consultation if client is violent, inconsolable, or does not seem to be making an adjustment. **Participation in a group may be helpful.**
- Refer to family/marital counseling as indicated.
- Refer to NDs Powerlessness; Coping, ineffective; Grieving, anticipatory/dysfunctional; Anxiety; Fear.

Documentation Focus

ASSESSMENT/REASSESSMENT

- Individual findings, including nature of incident, individual reactions/fears, degree of trauma (physical/emotional), effects on lifestyle.
- Reactions of family/SO(s).
- Samples gathered for evidence and disposition/storage (chain of evidence).

PLANNING

- Plan of action and who is involved in planning.
- Teaching plan.

IMPLEMENTATION/EVALUATION

- Responses to interventions/teaching and actions performed.
- Attainment/progress toward desired outcome(s).
- Modifications to plan of care.

DISCHARGE PLANNING

- Long-term needs and who is responsible for actions to be taken.
- Specific referrals made.

SAMPLE NURSING OUTCOMES & INTERVENTIONS CLASSIFICATION (NOC/NIC)—RAPE-TRAUMA SYNDROME

NOC—Abuse Recovery: Emotional
NIC—Rape Trauma Treatment

COMPOUND REACTION

NOC—Coping
NIC—Crises Intervention

SILENT REACTION

NOC—Abuse Recovery: Sexual
NIC—Counseling

Relocation Stress Syndrome

Taxonomy II: Coping/Stress Tolerance—Class 1 Post-Trauma Responses (00114)
[Diagnostic Division: Ego Integrity]
Submitted 1992; Revised 2000

Definition: Physiological and/or psychosocial disturbance following transfer from one environment to another

---

Information that appears in brackets has been added by the authors to clarify and enhance the use of nursing diagnoses.

Related Factors

Past, concurrent, and recent losses
Feeling of powerlessness
Lack of adequate support system; lack of predeparture counseling;
    unpredictability of experience
Isolation from family/friends; language barrier
Impaired psychosocial health; passive coping
Decreased health status

Defining Characteristics

SUBJECTIVE

Anxiety (e.g., separation); anger
Insecurity; worry; fear
Loneliness; depression
Unwillingness to move, or concern over relocation
Sleep disturbance

OBJECTIVE

Temporary or permanent move; voluntary/involuntary move
Increased [frequency of] verbalization of needs
Pessimism; frustration
Increased physical symptoms/illness (e.g., gastrointestinal distur-
    bances; weight change)
Withdrawal; aloneness; alienation; [hostile behavior/outbursts]
Loss of identity, self-worth, or self-esteem; dependency
[Increased confusion/cognitive impairment]

Desired Outcomes/Evaluation Criteria—Client Will:

- Verbalize understanding of reason(s) for change.
- Demonstrate appropriate range of feelings and lessened fear.
- Participate in routine and special/social events as able.
- Verbalize acceptance of situation.
- Experience no catastrophic event.

Actions/Interventions

NURSING PRIORITY NO. 1. To assess degree of stress as perceived/experienced by client and determine issues of safety:

- Ascertain client's perceptions about change(s) and expectations for the future, noting client's age. (**Children can be traumatized by transfer to new school/loss of peers; elderly persons may be affected by loss of long-term home/neighborhood setting and support persons.**)

- Monitor behavior, noting presence of suspiciousness/ paranoia, irritability, defensiveness. Compare with SO's/ staff's description of customary responses. **May temporarily exacerbate mental deterioration (cognitive inaccessibility) and further impair communication (social inaccessibility).**
- Note signs of increased stress, reports of "new" physical discomfort/pain, or presence of fatigue.
- Determine involvement of family/SO(s). Note availability/use of support systems and resources.
- Determine presence of cultural and/or religious concerns/ conflicts.

NURSING PRIORITY NO. 2. To assist client to deal with situation/changes:

- Encourage visit to new surroundings prior to transfer when possible. **Provides opportunity to "get acquainted" with new situation, reducing fear of unknown.**
- Orient to surroundings/schedules. Introduce to staff members, roommate/residents. Provide clear, honest information about actions/events.
- Encourage free expression of feelings. Acknowledge reality of situation and maintain hopeful attitude regarding move/ change.
- Identify strengths/successful coping behaviors the individual has used previously. **Incorporating these into problem solving builds on past successes.**
- Encourage individual/family to personalize area with pictures, own belongings, and the like as appropriate. **Enhances sense of belonging/personal space.**
- Determine client's usual schedule of activities and incorporate into facility routine as possible. **Reinforces sense of importance of individual.**
- Introduce diversional activities, such as art therapy, music, and so on. **Involvement increases opportunity to interact with others, decreasing isolation.**
- Place in private room, if appropriate, and include SO(s)/ family into care activities, meal time, and so on.
- Encourage hugging and use of touch unless client is paranoid or agitated at the moment. **Human connection reaffirms acceptance of individual.**
- Deal with aggressive behavior by imposing calm, firm limits. Control environment and protect others from client's disruptive behavior. **Promotes safety for client/others.**
- Remain calm, place in a quiet environment, providing time-out, **to prevent escalation into panic state and violent behavior.**

NURSING PRIORITY NO. 3. To promote wellness (Teaching/ Discharge Considerations):

- Involve client in formulating goals and plan of care when possible. **Supports independence and commitment to achieving outcomes.**
- Discuss benefits of adequate nutrition, rest, and exercise **to maintain physical well-being.**
- Involve in anxiety- and stress-reduction activities as able to enhance psychologic well-being.
- Encourage participation in activities/hobbies/personal interactions as appropriate. **Promotes creative endeavors, stimulating the mind.**
- Support self-responsibility and coping strategies to foster sense of control and self-worth.

Documentation Focus

ASSESSMENT/REASSESSMENT

- Assessment findings, individual's perception of the situation/changes, specific behaviors.
- Safety issues.

PLANNING

- Note plan of care, who is involved in planning, and who is responsible for proposed actions.
- Teaching plan.

IMPLEMENTATION/EVALUATION

- Response to interventions (especially time-out/seclusion)/ teaching and actions performed.
- Sentinel events.
- Attainment/progress toward desired outcome(s).
- Modifications to plan of care.

DISCHARGE PLANNING

- Long-term needs and who is responsible for actions to be taken.
- Specific referrals made.

SAMPLE NURSING OUTCOMES & INTERVENTIONS CLASSIFICATIONS (NOC/NIC)

NOC—Psychosocial Adjustment: Life Change
NIC—Coping Enhancement

Taxonomy II: Coping/Stress Tolerance—Class 1 Post-Trauma Responses (00149)
[Diagnostic Division: Ego Integrity]
Submitted 2000

Definition: At risk for physiological and/or psychosocial disturbance following transfer from one environment to another

Risk Factors

Moderate to high degree of environmental change (e.g., physical, ethnic, cultural)

Temporary and/or permanent moves; voluntary/involuntary move

Lack of adequate support system/group; lack of predeparture counseling

Passive coping; feelings of powerlessness

Moderate mental competence (e.g., alert enough to experience changes)

Unpredictability of experiences

Decreased psychosocial or physical health status

Past, current, recent losses

NOTE: A risk diagnosis is not evidenced by signs and symptoms, as the problem has not occurred and nursing interventions are directed at prevention.

Desired Outcomes/Evaluation Criteria—Client Will:

- Verbalize understanding of reason(s) for change.
- Express feelings and concerns openly and appropriately.
- Experience no catastrophic event.

Actions/Interventions

NURSING PRIORITY NO. 1. To assess causative/contributing factors:

- Evaluate client for current and potential losses related to relocation, noting age, developmental level, role in family, and physical/emotional health status.
- Ascertain client's perception about change(s) and expectations for the future, noting client's age. (**Transfer to new school/loss of peers can traumatize children; elderly individuals may be affected by loss of long-term home/neighborhood setting and support persons.**)
- Note whether relocation will be temporary (e.g., extended care for rehabilitation therapies) or long-term/permanent (e.g., move from home of many years, placement in nursing home).

Information that appears in brackets has been added by the authors to clarify and enhance the use of nursing diagnoses.

- Evaluate client/caregiver's resources and coping abilities. Determine family/SO degree of involvement and willingness to be involved.
- Determine issues of safety that may be involved.

NURSING PRIORITY NO. 2. To prevent/minimize adverse response to change: Refer to Relocation Stress Syndrome for additional Action/Interventions and Documentation Focus.

Role Performance, ineffective

Taxonomy II: Role Relationships—Class 3 Role Performance (00055)
[Diagnostic Division: Social Interaction]
Submitted 1978; Revised 1996, 1998

Definition: Patterns of behavior and self-expression that do not match the environmental context, norms, and expectations. Note: There is a typology of roles: sociopersonal (friendship, family, marital, parenting, community), home management, intimacy (sexuality, relationship building), leisure/exercise/recreation, self-management, socialization (developmental transitions), community contributor, and religious

Related Factors

SOCIAL

Inadequate role socialization (e.g., role model, expectations, responsibilities)
Young age, developmental level
Lack of resources; low socioeconomic status; poverty
Stress and conflict; job schedule demands
Family conflict; domestic violence
Inadequate support system; lack of rewards
Inadequate or inappropriate linkage with the healthcare system

KNOWLEDGE

Lack of knowledge about role/role skills; lack of or inadequate role model
Inadequate role preparation (e.g., role transition, skill, rehearsal, validation); lack of opportunity for role rehearsal
Education attainment level; developmental transitions
Role transition
Unrealistic role expectations

PHYSIOLOGICAL

Health alterations (e.g., physical health, body image, self-esteem, mental health, psychosocial health, cognition, learning style, neurological health); fatigue; pain; low self-esteem; depression

Information that appears in brackets has been added by the authors to clarify and enhance the use of nursing diagnoses.

Substance abuse
Inadequate/inappropriate linkage with healthcare system

Defining Characteristics

SUBJECTIVE

Altered role perceptions/change in self-perception of role/usual
    patterns of responsibility/capacity to resume role/other's perception
    of role
Inadequate opportunities for role enactment
Role dissatisfaction; overload; denial
Discrimination [by others]; powerlessness

OBJECTIVE

Inadequate knowledge; role competency and skills; adaptation to
    change or transition; inappropriate developmental expectations
Inadequate confidence; motivation; self-management; coping
Inadequate opportunities/external support for role enactment
Role strain; conflict; confusion; ambivalence; [failure to assume role]
Uncertainty; anxiety or depression; pessimistic
Domestic violence; harassment; system conflict

Desired Outcomes/Evaluation Criteria—Client Will:

- Verbalize realistic perception and acceptance of self in changed role.
- Verbalize understanding of role expectations/obligations.
- Talk with family/SO(s) about situation and changes that have occurred and limitations imposed.
- Develop realistic plans for adapting to new role/role changes.

Actions/Interventions

NURSING PRIORITY NO. 1. To assess causative/contributing factors:

- Identify type of role dysfunction, for example, developmental (adolescent to adult); situational (husband to father, gender identity); health-illness transitions.
- Determine client role in family constellation.
- Identify how client sees self as a man/woman in usual lifestyle/role functioning.
- Ascertain client's view of sexual functioning (e.g., loss of childbearing ability following hysterectomy).
- Identify cultural factors relating to individual's sexual roles.
- Determine client's perceptions/concerns about current situation. **May believe current role is more appropriate for the**

opposite sex (e.g., passive role of the patient may be somewhat less threatening for women).

• Interview SO(s) regarding their perceptions and expectations.

NURSING PRIORITY NO. 2. To assist client to deal with existing situation:

• Discuss perceptions and significance of the situation as seen by client.
• Maintain positive attitude toward the client.
• Provide opportunities for client to exercise control over as much as possible. **Enhances self-concept and promotes commitment to goals.**
• Offer realistic assessment of situation and communicate hope.
• Discuss and assist the client/SO(s) to develop strategies for dealing with changes in role related to past transitions, cultural expectations, and value/belief challenges. **Helps those involved deal with differences between individuals (e.g., adolescent task of separation in which parents clash with child's choices).**
• Acknowledge reality of situation related to role change and help client to express feelings of anger, sadness, and grief. Encourage celebration of positive aspects of change and expressions of feelings.
• Provide open environment for client to discuss concerns about sexuality. **Embarrassment can block discussion of sensitive subject.** (Refer to NDs Sexual Dysfunction; Sexuality Pattern, ineffective.)
• Identify role model for the client. Educate about role expectations using written and audiovisual materials.
• Use the techniques of role rehearsal to help the client develop new skills **to cope with changes.**

NURSING PRIORITY NO. 3. To promote wellness (Teaching/ Discharge Considerations):

• Make information available for client to learn about role expectations/demands that may occur. **Provides opportunity to be proactive in dealing with changes.**
• Accept client in changed role. Encourage and give positive feedback for changes and goals achieved. **Provides reinforcement and facilitates continuation of efforts.**
• Refer to support groups, employment counselors, Parent Effectiveness classes, counseling/psychotherapy as indicated by individual need(s). **Provides ongoing support to sustain progress.**
• Refer to NDs Self-Esteem [specify] and the Parenting diagnoses.

Documentation Focus

ASSESSMENT/REASSESSMENT

- Individual findings, including specifics of predisposing crises/situation, perception of role change.
- Expectations of SO(s).

PLANNING

- Plan of care and who is involved in planning.
- Teaching plan.

IMPLEMENTATION/EVAULATION

- Responses to interventions/teaching and actions performed.
- Attainment/progress toward desired outcome(s).
- Modifications plan of care.

DISCHARGE PLANNING

- Long-term needs and who is responsible for actions to be taken.
- Specific referrals made.

SAMPLE NURSING OUTCOMES & INTERVENTIONS CLASSIFICATIONS (NOC/NIC)

NOC—Role Performance
NIC—Role Enhancement

Self-Care deficit: bathing/hygiene, dressing/grooming, feeding, toileting

Taxonomy II: Activity/Rest—Class 2 Activity/Exercise (Bathing/Hygiene 00108, Dressing/Grooming 00109, Feeding 00102, Toileting 00110)
[Diagnostic Division: Hygiene]
Submitted 1980; Nursing Diagnosis Extension and Classification (NDEC) Revision 1998

Definition: Impaired ability to perform feeding, bathing/hygiene, dressing and grooming, or toileting activities for oneself [on a temporary, permanent, or progressing basis] [**Note:** Self-care also may be expanded to include the practices used by the client to promote health, the individual responsibility for self, a way of thinking. Refer to NDs Home Maintenance, impaired; Health Maintenance, ineffective.]

Related Factors

Weakness or tiredness; decreased or lack of motivation
Neuromuscular/musculoskeletal impairment

Information that appears in brackets has been added by the authors to clarify and enhance the use of nursing diagnoses. **425**

Environmental barriers
Severe anxiety
Pain, discomfort
Perceptual or cognitive impairment
Inability to perceive body part or spatial relationship
    [bathing/hygiene]
Impaired transfer ability (self-toileting)
Impaired mobility status (self-toileting)
[Mechanical restrictions such as cast, splint, traction, ventilator]

Defining Characteristics

SELF-FEEDING DEFICIT*

Inability to:
Prepare food for ingestion; open containers
Handle utensils; get food onto utensil safely; bring food from
    a receptacle to the mouth
Ingest food safely; manipulate food in mouth; chew/swallow
    food
Pick up cup or glass
Use assistive device
Ingest sufficient food; complete a meal
Ingest food in a socially acceptable manner

SELF-BATHING/HYGIENE DEFICIT*

Inability to:
Get bath supplies
Wash body or body parts
Obtain or get to water source; regulate temperature or flow of
    bath water
Get in and out of bathroom [tub]
Dry body

SELF-DRESSING/GROOMING DEFICIT*

Inability to choose clothing, pick up clothing, use assistive
    devices
Impaired ability to obtain or replace articles of clothing; put on
    or take off necessary items of clothing on upper/lower body;
    fasten clothing/use zippers; put on socks/shoes
Inability to maintain appearance at a satisfactory level

SELF-TOILETING DEFICIT*

Inability to:
Get to toilet or commode
Manipulate clothing
Sit on or rise from toilet or commode

---

*[Refer to ND Mobility, impaired physical, for suggested functional
level classification.]

Carry out proper toilet hygiene
Flush toilet or [empty] commode

Desired Outcomes/Evaluation Criteria—Client Will:

- Identify individual areas of weakness/needs.
- Verbalize knowledge of healthcare practices.
- Demonstrate techniques/lifestyle changes to meet self-care needs.
- Perform self-care activities within level of own ability.
- Identify personal/community resources that can provide assistance.

Actions/Interventions

NURSING PRIORITY NO. **1.** To identify causative/contributing factors:

- Determine existing conditions/extremes of age/developmental level affecting ability of individual to care for own needs: CVA, MS, Alzheimer's, and so forth.
- Note concomitant medical problems that may be factors for care (e.g., high BP, heart disease, malnutrition, pain, and/or medications client is taking).
- Note other etiologic factors present, including language barriers, speech impairment, visual acuity/hearing problem, emotional stability/ability.
- Assess barriers to participation in regimen (e.g., lack of information, insufficient time for discussion; psychologic and/or intimate family problems that may be difficult to share; fear of appearing stupid or ignorant; social/economic; work/home environment problems).

NURSING PRIORITY NO. **2.** To assess degree of disability:

- Identify degree of individual impairment/functional level according to scale (noted in ND Mobility, impaired physical).
- Assess memory/intellectual functioning. Note developmental level to which client has regressed/progressed.
- Determine individual strengths and skills of the client.
- Note whether deficit is temporary or permanent, should decrease or increase with time.

NURSING PRIORITY NO. **3.** To assist in correcting/dealing with situation:

- Establish "contractual" partnership with client/SO(s).
- Promote client/SO participation in problem identification and decision making. **Enhances commitment to plan, optimizing outcomes.**
- Develop plan of care appropriate to individual situation, scheduling activities to conform to client's normal schedule.

- Plan time for listening to the client/SO(s) **to discover barriers to participation in regimen.**
- Provide for communication among those who are involved in caring for/assisting the client. **Enhances coordination and continuity of care.**
- Establish remotivation/resocialization programs when indicated.
- Assist with rehabilitation program **to enhance capabilities.**
- Provide privacy during personal care activities.
- Allow sufficient time for client to accomplish tasks to fullest extent of ability. Avoid unnecessary conversation/interruptions.
- Assist with necessary adaptations to accomplish ADLs. Begin with familiar, easily accomplished tasks **to encourage client and build on successes.**
- Arrange for assistive devices as necessary (e.g., raised toilet seat/grab bars, buttonhook, modified eating utensils).
- Identify energy-saving behaviors (e.g., sitting instead of standing when possible).
- Implement bowel or bladder training/retraining programs as indicated.
- Encourage food and fluid choices reflecting individual likes and abilities that meet nutritional needs. Provide assistive devices/alternate feeding methods as appropriate.
- Assist with medication regimen as necessary, noting potential for/presence of side effects.
- Make home visit **to assess environmental/discharge needs.**

NURSING PRIORITY NO. 4. To promote wellness (Teaching/Discharge Considerations):

- Assist the client to become aware of rights and responsibilities in health/healthcare and to assess own health strengths— physical, emotional, and intellectual.
- Support client in making health-related decisions and assist in developing self-care practices and goals that promote health.
- Provide for ongoing evaluation of self-care program, identifying progress and needed changes.
- Review/modify program periodically to accommodate changes in client's abilities. **Assists client to adhere to plan of care to fullest extent.**
- Encourage keeping a journal of progress.
- Review safety concerns. Modify activities/environment **to reduce risk of injury.**
- Refer to home care provider, social services, physical/occupational therapy, rehabilitation and counseling resources as indicated.
- Identify additional community resources (e.g., senior services, Meals on Wheels).

- Review instructions from other members of the healthcare team and provide written copy. **Provides clarification, reinforcement, and periodic review by client/caregivers.**
- Give family information about respite/other care options. **Allows them free time away from the care situation to renew themselves.**
- Assist/support family with alternative placements as necessary. **Enhances likelihood of finding individually appropriate situation to meet client's needs.**
- Be available for discussion of feelings about situation (e.g., grieving, anger).
- Refer to NDs Injury/Trauma, risk for; Coping, ineffective; Coping, family: compromised; Self-Esteem, situational low; Constipation; Bowel Incontinence; Urinary Elimination, impaired; Mobility, impaired physical; Activity intolerance; Powerlessness.

Documentation Focus

ASSESSMENT/REASSESSMENT

- Individual findings, functional level, and specifics of limitation(s).
- Needed resources/adaptive devices.

PLANNING

- Plan of care and who is involved in planning.
- Teaching plan.

IMPLEMENTATION/EVALUATION

- Response to interventions/teaching and actions performed.
- Attainment/progress toward desired outcome(s).
- Modifications of plan of care.

DISCHARGE PLANNING

- Long-term needs and who is responsible for actions to be taken.
- Type of and source for assistive devices.
- Specific referrals made.

SAMPLE NURSING OUTCOMES & INTERVENTIONS CLASSIFICATIONS (NOC/NIC)

BATHING/HYGIENE DEFICIT

NOC—Self-Care Bathing
NIC—Self-Care Assistance: Bathing/Hygiene

DRESSING/GROOMING DEFICIT

NOC—Self-Care Dressing
NIC—Self-Care Assistance: Dressing/Grooming

NOC—Self-Care Eating
NIC—Self-Care Assistance: Feeding

TOILETING DEFICIT

NOC—Self-Care Toileting
NIC—Self-Care Assistance: Toileting

Self-Concept, readiness for enhanced

Taxonomy II: Self-Perception—Class 1 Self-Concept
(00167)
[Diagnostic Divisions: Ego Integrity]
Submitted 2002

Definition: A pattern of perceptions or ideas about the self that is sufficient for well-being and can be strengthened

Related Factors

To be developed

Defining Characteristics

SUBJECTIVE

Expresses willingness to enhance self-concept
Expresses satisfaction with thoughts about self, sense of worthiness, role performance, body image, and personal identity; confidence in abilities
Accepts strengths and limitations

OBJECTIVE

Actions are congruent with expressed feelings and thoughts

Desired Outcomes/Evaluation Criteria—Client Will:

- Verbalize understanding of own sense of self-concept.
- Participate in programs and activities to enhance self-esteem.
- Demonstrate behaviors/lifestyle changes to promote positive self-esteem.
- Participate in family/group/community activities to enhance self-concept.

Actions/Interventions

NURSING PRIORITY NO. **1.** To assess current situation and desire for improvement:

- Determine current status of individual's belief about self. Self-concept consists of the physical self (body image), personal self (identity) and self-esteem, and information about client's

---

Information that appears in brackets has been added by the authors **430** to clarify and enhance the use of nursing diagnoses.

current thinking about self provides a beginning for making changes to improve self.

- Determine availability/quality of family/SO(s) support. **Presence of supportive people who reflect positive attitudes regarding the individual promotes a positive sense of self.**
- Identify family dynamics, present and past. Self-esteem begins in early childhood and is influenced by the perceptions of how the individual is viewed by significant others. **Provides information about family functioning that will help to develop plan of care for enhancing client's self-concept.**
- Note willingness to seek assistance, motivation for change. **Individuals who have a sense of their own self-image and are willing to look at themselves realistically will be able to progress in the desire to improve.**
- Determine client's concept of self in relation to cultural/religious ideals/beliefs.
- Observe nonverbal behaviors and note congruence with verbal expressions. Discuss cultural meanings of nonverbal communication. **Incongruencies between verbal and nonverbal communication require clarification. Interpretation of nonverbal expressions is culturally determined and needs to be identified to avoid misinterpretation.**

NURSING PRIORITY NO. **2.** To facilitate personal growth:

- Develop therapeutic relationship. Be attentive, validate client's communication, provide encouragement for efforts, maintain open communication, use skills of Active-listening and I-messages. **Promotes trusting situation in which client is free to be open and honest with self and others.**
- Accept client's perceptions/view of current status. **Avoids threatening existing self-esteem and provides opportunity for client to develop realistic plan for improving self-concept.**
- Be aware that people are not programmed to be rational. **They must seek information, choosing to learn, to think rather than merely accepting/reacting in order to have respect for self, facts, honesty, and to develop positive self-esteem.**
- Discuss client perception of self, confronting misconceptions and identifying negative self-talk. Address distortions in thinking, such as self-referencing (beliefs that others are focusing on individual's weaknesses/limitations); filtering (focusing on negative and ignoring positive); catastrophizing (expecting the worst outcomes). **Addressing these issues openly allows client to identify things that may negatively affect self-esteem and provides opportunity for change.**
- Have client list current/past successes and strengths. **Emphasizes fact that client is and has been successful in many actions taken.**
- Use positive I-messages rather than praise. **Praise is a form of**

external control, coming from outside sources, whereas I-messages allow the client to develop internal sense of self-esteem.

- Discuss what behavior does for client (positive intention). Ask what options are available to the client/SO(s)? **Encourages thinking about what inner motivations are and what actions can be taken to enhance self-esteem.**
- Give reinforcement for progress noted. **Positive words of encouragement support development of effective coping behaviors.**
- Allow client to progress at own rate. **Adaptation to a change in self-concept depends on its significance to the individual and disruption to lifestyle.**
- Involve in activities/exercise program of choice, promote socialization. **Enhances sense of well-being/can help to energize client.**

NURSING PRIORITY NO. 3. To promote optimum sense of self-worth and happiness:

- Assist client to identify goals that are personally achievable. Provide positive feedback for verbal and behavioral indications of improved self-view. **Increases likelihood of success and commitment to change.**
- Refer to vocational/employment counselor, educational resources as appropriate. **Assists with improving development of social/vocational skills.**
- Encourage participation in classes/activities/hobbies that client enjoys or would like to experience. **Provides opportunity for learning new information/skills that can enhance feelings of success, improving self-esteem.**
- Reinforce that current decision to improve self-concept is ongoing. **Continued work and support are necessary to sustain behavior changes/personal growth.**
- Suggest assertiveness training classes. **Promotes learning to assist with developing new skills to promote self-esteem.**
- Emphasize importance of grooming and personal hygiene and assist in developing skills to improve appearance and dress for success. **Looking your best improves sense of self-esteem and presenting a positive appearance enhances how others see you.**

Documentation Focus

ASSESSMENT/REASSESSMENT

- Individual findings, including evaluations of self and others, current and past successes.
- Interactions with others/lifestyle.
- Motivation for/willingness to change

PLANNING

- Plan of care and who is involved in planning.
- Educational plan.

IMPLEMENTATION/EVALUATION

- Responses to interventions/teaching and actions performed.
- Attainment/progress toward desired outcome(s).
- Modifications to plan of care.

DISCHARGE PLANNING

- Long-term needs and who is responsible for actions to be taken.
- Specific referrals made.

SAMPLE NURSING OUTCOMES & INTERVENTIONS CLASSIFICATIONS (NOC/NIC)

NOC—Self-Esteem
NIC—Coping Enhancement

Self-Esteem, chronic low

Taxonomy II: Self-Perception—Class 2 Self-Esteem (00119)
[Diagnostic Division: Ego Integrity]
Submitted 1988; Revised 1996

Definition: Long-standing negative self-evaluation/feelings about self or self-capabilities

Related Factors

To be developed
[Fixation in earlier level of development]
[Continual negative evaluation of self/capabilities from childhood]
[Personal vulnerability]
[Life choices perpetuating failure; ineffective social/occupational functioning]
[Feelings of abandonment by SO; willingness to tolerate possibly life-threatening domestic violence]
[Chronic physical/psychiatric conditions; antisocial behaviors]

Defining Characteristics

SUBJECTIVE

(Long-standing or chronic:)
Self-negating verbalization
Expressions of shame/guilt
Evaluates self as unable to deal with events
Rationalizes away/rejects positive feedback and exaggerates negative feedback about self

---

Information that appears in brackets has been added by the authors to clarify and enhance the use of nursing diagnoses. **433**

OBJECTIVE

Hesitant to try new things/situations (long-standing or chronic)
Frequent lack of success in work or other life events
Overly conforming, dependent on others' opinions
Lack of eye contact
Nonassertive/passive; indecisive
Excessively seeks reassurance

Desired Outcomes/Evaluation Criteria—Client Will:

- Verbalize understanding of negative evaluation of self and reasons for this problem.
- Participate in treatment program to promote change in self-evaluation.
- Demonstrate behaviors/lifestyle changes to promote positive self-esteem.
- Verbalize increased sense of self-esteem in relation to current situation.
- Participate in family/group/community activities to enhance change.

Actions/Interventions

NURSING PRIORITY NO. 1. To assess causative/contributing factors:

- Determine factors of low self-esteem related to current situation (e.g., family crises, physical disfigurement, social isolation), noting age and developmental level of individual.
- Assess content of negative self-talk. Note client's perceptions of how others view him or her.
- Determine availability/quality of family/SO(s) support.
- Identify family dynamics, present and past.
- Note nonverbal behavior (e.g., nervous movements, lack of eye contact). **Incongruencies between verbal/nonverbal communication require clarification.**
- Determine degree of participation and cooperation with therapeutic regimen (e.g., maintaining scheduled medications such as antidepressants/antipsychotics).
- Note willingness to seek assistance, motivation for change.
- Be alert to client's concept of self in relation to cultural/religious ideal(s).

NURSING PRIORITY NO. 2. To promote client sense of self-esteem in dealing with situation:

- Develop therapeutic relationship. Be attentive, validate client's communication, provide encouragement for efforts, maintain open communication, use skills of Active-listening and

I-messages. **Promotes trusting situation in which client is free to be open and honest with self and therapist.**

- Address presenting medical/safety issues.
- Accept client's perceptions/view of situation. Avoid threatening existing self-esteem.
- Be aware that people are not programmed to be rational. **They must seek information—choosing to learn; to think rather than merely accepting/reacting—in order to have respect for self, facts, honesty, and to develop positive self-esteem.**
- Discuss client perceptions of self related to what is happening; confront misconceptions and negative self-talk. Address distortions in thinking, such as self-referencing (belief that others are focusing on individual's weaknesses/limitations), filtering (focusing on negative and ignoring positive), catastrophizing (expecting the worst outcomes). **Addressing these issues openly provides opportunity for change.**
- Emphasize need to avoid comparing self with others. Encourage client to focus on aspects of self that can be valued.
- Have client list current/past successes and strengths.
- Use positive I-messages rather than praise. **Assists client to develop internal sense of self-esteem.**
- Discuss what behavior does for client (positive intention). What options are available to the client/SO(s)?
- Assist client to deal with sense of powerlessness. Refer to ND Powerlessness.
- Set limits on aggressive or problem behaviors such as acting out, suicide preoccupation, or rumination. Put self in client's place (empathy not sympathy).
- Give reinforcement for progress noted. **Positive words of encouragement support development of coping behaviors.**
- Allow client to progress at own rate. **Adaptation to a change in self-concept depends on its significance to individual, disruption to lifestyle, and length of illness/debilitation.**
- Assist client to recognize and cope with events, alterations, and sense of loss of control by incorporating changes accurately into self-concept.
- Involve in activities/exercise program, promote socialization. **Enhances sense of well-being/can help energize client.**

NURSING PRIORITY NO. 3. To promote wellness (Teaching/Discharge Considerations):

- Discuss inaccuracies in self-perception with client/SO(s).
- Prepare client for events/changes that are expected, when possible.
- Provide structure in daily routine/care activities.

- Emphasize importance of grooming and personal hygiene. Assist in developing skills as indicated (e.g., makeup classes, dress for success). **People feel better about themselves when they present a positive outer appearance.**
- Assist client to identify goals that are personally achievable. Provide positive feedback for verbal and behavioral indications of improved self-view. **Increases likelihood of success and commitment to change.**
- Refer to vocational/employment counselor, educational resources as appropriate. **Assists with development of social/ vocational skills.**
- Encourage participation in classes/activities/hobbies that client enjoys or would like to experience.
- Reinforce that this therapy is a brief encounter in overall life of the client/SO(s), with continued work and ongoing support being necessary **to sustain behavior changes/personal growth.**
- Refer to classes **to assist with new learning skills to promote self-esteem** (e.g., **assertiveness training, positive self-image, communication skills**).
- Refer to counseling/therapy, mental health, and special needs support groups as indicated.

Documentation Focus

ASSESSMENT/REASSESSMENT

- Individual findings, including early memories of negative evaluations (self and others), subsequent/precipitating failure events.
- Effects on interactions with others/lifestyle.
- Specific medical/safety issues.
- Motivation for/willingness to change.

PLANNING

- Plan of care and who is involved in planning.
- Teaching plan.

IMPLEMENTATION/EVALUATION

- Responses to interventions/teaching and actions performed.
- Attainment/progress toward desired outcome(s).
- Modifications to plan of care.

DISCHARGE PLANNING

- Long-term needs and who is responsible for actions to be taken.
- Specific referrals made.

SAMPLE NURSING OUTCOMES & INTERVENTIONS CLASSIFICATIONS (NOC/NIC)

NOC—Self-Esteem
NIC—Self-Esteem Enhancement

Self-Esteem, situational low

Taxonomy II: Self-Perception—Class 2 Self-Esteem (00120)
[Diagnostic Division: Ego Integrity]
Submitted 1988; Revised 1996, 2000

Definition: Development of a negative perception of self-worth in response to a current situation (specify)

Related Factors

Developmental changes (specify); [maturational transitions, adolescence, aging]
Functional impairments; disturbed body image
Loss (specify)[e.g., loss of health status, body part, independent functioning; memory deficit/cognitive impairment]
Social role changes (specify)
Failures/rejections; lack of recognition/rewards; [feelings of abandonment by SO]
Behavior inconsistent with values

Defining Characteristics

SUBJECTIVE

Reports current situational challenge to self-worth
Expressions of helplessness and uselessness
Evaluation of self as unable to deal with situations or events

OBJECTIVE

Self-negating verbalizations
Indecisive, nonassertive behavior

Desired Outcomes/Evaluation Criteria—Client Will:

- Verbalize understanding of individual factors that precipitated current situation.
- Identify feelings and underlying dynamics for negative perception of self.
- Express positive self-appraisal.
- Demonstrate behaviors to restore positive self-esteem.
- Participate in treatment regimen/activities to correct factors that precipitated crisis.

Information that appears in brackets has been added by the authors to clarify and enhance the use of nursing diagnoses.

Actions/Interventions

NURSING PRIORITY NO. 1. To assess causative/contributing factors:

- Determine individual situation (e.g., family crisis, physical disfigurement) related to low self-esteem in the present circumstances.
- Identify basic sense of self-esteem of client, image client has of self: existential, physical, psychological.
- Assess degree of threat/perception of client in regard to crisis.
- Be aware of sense of control client has (or perceives to have) over self and situation.
- Determine client's awareness of own responsibility for dealing with situation, personal growth, and so forth.
- Assess family/SO(s) dynamics and support of client.
- Be alert to client's concept of self in relation to cultural/religious ideals.
- Note client's locus of control (internal/external).
- Determine past coping skills in relation to current episode.
- Assess negative attitudes and/or self-talk.
- Note nonverbal body language. **Incongruencies between verbal/nonverbal communication requires clarification.**
- Assess for self-destructive/suicidal behavior. (Refer to ND Suicide, risk for as appropriate.)
- Identify previous adaptations to illness/disruptive events in life. **(May be predictive of current outcome.)**

NURSING PRIORITY NO. 2. To assist client to deal with loss/change and recapture sense of positive self-esteem:

- Assist with treatment of underlying condition when possible. **For example, cognitive restructuring and improved concentration in mild brain injury often result in restoration of positive self-esteem.**
- Encourage expression of feelings, anxieties. **Facilitates grieving the loss.**
- Active-listen client's concerns/negative verbalizations without comment or judgment.
- Identify individual strengths/assets and aspects of self that remain intact, can be valued. Reinforce positive traits, abilities, self-view.
- Help client identify own responsibility and control or lack of control in situation.
- Assist client to problem-solve situation, developing plan of action and setting goals to achieve desired outcome. **Enhances commitment to plan, optimizing outcomes.**
- Convey confidence in client's ability to cope with current situation.
- Mobilize support systems.

- Provide opportunity for client to practice alternative coping strategies, including progressive socialization opportunities.
- Encourage use of visualization, guided imagery, and relaxation to promote positive sense of self.
- Provide feedback of client's self-negating remarks/behavior, using I-messages **to allow the client to experience a different view.**
- Encourage involvement in decisions about care when possible.

NURSING PRIORITY NO. **3.** To promote wellness (Teaching/Discharge Considerations):

- Encourage client to set long-range goals for achieving necessary lifestyle changes. **Supports view that this is an ongoing process.**
- Support independence in ADLs/mastery of therapeutic regimen. **Individuals who are confident are more secure and positive in self-appraisal.**
- Promote attendance in therapy/support group as indicated.
- Involve extended family/SO(s) in treatment plan. **Increases likelihood they will provide appropriate support to client.**
- Provide information to assist client in making desired changes.
- Suggest participation in group/community activities (e.g., assertiveness classes, volunteer work, support groups).

Documentation Focus

ASSESSMENT/REASSESSMENT

- Individual findings, noting precipitating crisis, client's perceptions, effects on desired lifestyle/interaction with others.

PLANNING

- Plan of care and who is involved in planning.
- Teaching plan.

IMPLEMENTATION/EVALUATION

- Responses to interventions/teaching, actions performed, and changes that may be indicated.
- Attainment/progress toward desired outcome(s).
- Modifications to plan of care.

DISCHARGE PLANNING

- Long-term needs/goals and who is responsible for actions to be taken.
- Specific referrals made.

SAMPLE NURSING OUTCOMES
& INTERVENTIONS CLASSIFICATIONS (NOC/NIC)

NOC—Self-Esteem
NIC—Self-Esteem Enhancement

Self-Esteem, risk for situational low

Taxonomy II: Self-Perception—Class 2 Self-Esteem
(00153)
[Diagnostic Division: Ego Integrity]
Submitted 2000

Definition: At risk for developing negative perception
of self-worth in response to a current situation (specify)

Risk Factors

Developmental changes (specify)
Disturbed body image; functional impairment (specify); loss (specify)
Social role changes (specify)
History of learned helplessness; neglect, or abandonment
Unrealistic self-expectations
Behavior inconsistent with values
Lack of recognition/rewards; failures/rejections
Decreased power/control over environment
Physical illness (specify)

> NOTE: A risk diagnosis is not evidenced by signs and symptoms, as
> the problem has not occurred and nursing interventions are
> directed at prevention.

Desired Outcomes/Evaluation
Criteria—Client Will:

- Acknowledge factors that lead to possibility of feelings of low
  self-esteem.
- Verbalize view of self as a worthwhile, important person who
  functions well both interpersonally and occupationally.
- Demonstrate self-confidence by setting realistic goals and
  actively participating in life situation.

Actions/Interventions

NURSING PRIORITY NO. **1.** To assess causative/contributing
factors:

- Determine individual factors that may contribute to diminished self-esteem.
- Identify basic sense of self-worth of client, image client has of
  self: existential, physical, psychological.

Information that appears in brackets has been added by the authors
to clarify and enhance the use of nursing diagnoses.

- Note client's perception of threat to self in current situation.
- Be aware of sense of control client has (or perceives to have) over self and situation.
- Determine client awareness of own responsibility for dealing with situation, personal growth, and so forth.
- Assess family/SO(s) dynamics and support of client.
- Note client concept of self in relation to cultural/religious ideals.
- Assess negative attitudes and/or self-talk. **Contributes to view of situation as hopeless, difficult.**
- Listen for self-destructive/suicidal verbalizations, noting behaviors that indicate these thoughts.
- Note nonverbal body language. **Incongruencies between verbal/nonverbal communication require clarification.**
- Identify previous adaptations to illness/disruptive events in life. **May be predictive of current outcome.**

Refer to NDs, Self-Esteem, situational low, and Self-Esteem, chronic low, as appropriate for additional nursing priorities/interventions.

Documentation Focus

ASSESSMENT/REASSESSMENT

- Individual findings, including individual expressions of lack of self-esteem, effects on interactions with others/lifestyle.
- Underlying dynamics and duration (situational or situational exacerbating chronic).

PLANNING

- Plan of care and who is involved in planning.
- Teaching plan.

IMPLEMENTATION/EVALUATION

- Responses to interventions/teaching, actions performed, and changes that may be indicated.
- Attainment/progress toward desired outcome(s).
- Modifications to plan of care.

DISCHARGE PLANNING

- Long-term needs/goals and who is responsible for actions to be taken.
- Specific referrals made.

SAMPLE NURSING OUTCOMES & INTERVENTIONS CLASSIFICATIONS (NOC/NIC)

NOC—Self-Esteem
NIC—Self-Esteem Enhancement

Self-Mutilation

Self-Mutilation

Taxonomy II: Safety/Protection—Class 3 Violence (00151)
[Diagnostic Division: Safety]
Submitted 2000

Definition: Deliberate self-injurious behavior causing
tissue damage with the intent of causing nonfatal injury
to attain relief of tension

Related Factors

History of self-injurious behavior; family history of self-destructive
behaviors

Feelings of depression, rejection, self-hatred, separation anxiety, guilt,
depersonalization

Low or unstable self-esteem/body image; labile behavior (mood
swings); feels threatened with actual or potential loss of significant
relationship (e.g., loss of parent/parental relationship)

Perfectionism; emotionally disturbed; battered child; substance abuse;
eating disorders; sexual identity crisis; childhood illness or surgery;
childhood sexual abuse

Adolescence; peers who self-mutilate; isolation from peers

Family divorce; family alcoholism; violence between parental figures

History of inability to plan solutions or see long-term consequences;
inadequate coping

Mounting tension that is intolerable; needs quick reduction of stress;
impulsivity; irresistible urge to cut/damage self

Use of manipulation to obtain nurturing relationship with others;
chaotic/disturbed interpersonal relationships; poor parentadolescent
communication; lack of family confidant

Experiences dissociation or depersonalization; psychotic state
(command hallucinations); character disorders; borderline personality disorders; developmentally delayed or autistic individuals

Foster, group, or institutional care; incarceration

Defining Characteristics

SUBJECTIVE

Self-inflicted burns (e.g., eraser, cigarette)
Ingestion/inhalation of harmful substances/objects

OBJECTIVE

Cuts/scratches on body
Picking at wounds
Biting; abrading; severing
Insertion of object(s) into body orifice(s)
Hitting
Constricting a body part

Information that appears in brackets has been added by the authors
to clarify and enhance the use of nursing diagnoses.

Desired Outcomes/Evaluation Criteria—Client Will:

- Verbalize understanding of reasons for occurrence of behavior.
- Identify precipitating factors/awareness of arousal state that occurs prior to incident.
- Express increased self-concept/self-esteem.
- Seeks help when feeling anxious and having thoughts of harming self.

Actions/Interventions

NURSING PRIORITY NO. 1. To assess causative/contributing factors:

- Determine underlying dynamics of individual situation as listed in Related Factors. Note previous episodes of self-mutilation behavior. **Although some body piercing (e.g., ears) is generally accepted as decorative, piercing of multiple sites often is an attempt to establish individuality, addressing issues of separation and belonging.**
- Identify previous history of self-mutilative behavior and relationship to stressful events.
- Determine presence of inflexible, maladaptive personality traits that reflect personality/character disorder (e.g., impulsive, unpredictable, inappropriate behaviors, intense anger or lack of control of anger).
- Evaluate history of mental illness (e.g., borderline personality, identity disorder).
- Note use/abuse of addicting substances.
- Review laboratory findings (e.g., blood alcohol, polydrug screen, glucose, and electrolyte levels). **Drug use may affect behavior.**

NURSING PRIORITY NO. 2. To structure environment to maintain client safety:

- Assist client to identify feelings leading up to desire for self-mutilation. **Early recognition of recurring feelings provides opportunity to seek other ways of coping.**
- Provide external controls/limit setting. **May decrease the opportunity to self-mutilate.**
- Include client in development of plan of care. **Commitment to plan promotes likelihood of adherence.**
- Encourage appropriate expression of feelings. **Identifies feelings and promotes understanding of what leads to development of tension.**
- Note feelings of healthcare providers/family, such as frustration, anger, defensiveness, need to rescue. **Client may be**

manipulative, evoking defensiveness and conflict. These feelings need to be identified, recognized, and dealt with openly with staff and client.

- Provide care for client's wounds, when self-mutilation occurs, in a matter-of-fact manner. Do not offer sympathy or additional attention that could provide reinforcement for maladaptive behavior and may encourage its repetition. A matter-of-fact approach can convey empathy/concern.

NURSING PRIORITY NO. 3. To promote movement toward positive changes:

- Involve client in developing plan of care. Enhances commitment to goals, optimizing outcomes.
- Develop a contract between client and counselor to enable the client to stay physically safe, such as "I will not cut or harm myself for the next 8 hours." Renew contract on a regular basis and have both parties sign and date each contract.
- Provide avenues of communication for times when client needs to talk to avoid cutting or damaging self.
- Assist client to learn assertive behavior. Include the use of effective communication skills, focusing on developing self-esteem by replacing negative self-talk with positive comments.
- Use interventions that help the client to reclaim power in own life (e.g., experiential and cognitive).

NURSING PRIORITY NO. 4. To promote wellness (Teaching/Discharge Considerations):

- Discuss commitment to safety and ways in which client will deal with precursors to undesired behavior.
- Promote the use of healthy behaviors, identifying the consequences and outcomes of current actions.
- Identify support systems.
- Discuss living arrangements when client is discharged. May need assistance with transition to changes required to avoid recurrence of self-mutilating behaviors.
- Involve family/SO(s) in planning for discharge and involve in group therapies as appropriate. Promotes coordination and continuation of plan, commitment to goals.
- Provide information and discuss the use of medication as appropriate. Antidepressant medications may be useful, but they need to be weighed against the potential for overdosing.
- Refer to NDs Anxiety; Social Interaction, impaired; Self-Esteem, (specify).

Documentation Focus

ASSESSMENT/REASSESSMENT

- Individual findings, including risk factors present, underlying dynamics, prior episodes.

PLANNING

- Plan of care and who is involved in planning.
- Teaching plan.

IMPLEMENTATION/EVALUATION

- Response to interventions/teaching and actions performed.
- Attainment/progress toward desired outcome(s).
- Modifications to plan of care.

DISCHARGE PLANNING

- Long-range needs and who is responsible for actions to be taken.
- Community resources, referrals made.

SAMPLE NURSING OUTCOMES & INTERVENTIONS CLASSIFICATIONS (NOC/NIC)

NOC—Self-Mutilation Restraint
NIC—Behavior Management: Self-Harm

Self-Mutilation, risk for

Taxonomy II: Safety/Protection—Class 3 Violence (00139)
[Diagnostic Division: Safety]
Submitted 1992; Revised 2000

Definition: At risk for deliberate self-injurious behavior causing tissue damage with the intent of causing nonfatal injury to attain relief of tension

Risk Factors

Feelings of depression, rejection, self-hatred, separation anxiety, guilt, and depersonalization
Low or unstable self-esteem/body image
Adolescence; isolation from peers; peers who self-mutilate
Perfectionism; childhood illness or surgery; eating disorders; substance abuse; sexual identity crisis
Emotionally disturbed and/or battered children; childhood sexual abuse; developmentally delayed or autistic individual
Inadequate coping; loss of control over problem-solving situations; history of inability to plan solutions or see long-term consequences

---

Information that appears in brackets has been added by the authors to clarify and enhance the use of nursing diagnoses.

Experiences mounting tension that is intolerable; inability to express tension verbally; needs quick reduction of stress

Experiences irresistible urge to cut/damage self; history of self-injurious behavior

Chaotic/disturbed interpersonal relationships; use of manipulation to obtain nurturing relationship with others

Family alcoholism; divorce; history of self-destructive behaviors; violence between parental figures

Loss of parent/parental relationships; feels threatened with actual or potential loss of significant relationship

Character disorders; borderline personality disorders; experiences dissociation or depersonalization; psychotic state (command hallucinations)

Foster, group, or institutional care; incarceration

> NOTE: A risk diagnosis is not evidenced by signs and symptoms, as the problem has not occurred and nursing interventions are directed at prevention.

Desired Outcomes/Evaluation Criteria—Client Will:

- Verbalize understanding of reasons for occurrence of behavior.
- Identify precipitating factors/awareness of arousal state that occurs prior to incident.
- Express increased self-concept/self-esteem.
- Demonstrate self-control as evidenced by lessened (or absence of) episodes of self-mutilation.
- Engage in use of alternative methods for managing feelings/individuality.

Actions/Interventions

NURSING PRIORITY NO. 1. To assess causative/contributing factors:

- Determine underlying dynamics of individual situation as listed in Risk Factors. Note previous episodes of self-mutilating behavior (e.g., cutting, scratching, bruising, unconventional body piercings). **Although some body piercing (e.g., ears) is generally accepted as decorative, piercing of multiple sites often is an attempt to establish individuality, addressing issues of separation and belonging.**
- Identify conditions that may interfere with ability to control own behavior (e.g., psychotic state, mental retardation, autism).
- Note beliefs, cultural/religious practices that may be involved in choice of behavior.
- Determine use/abuse of addictive substances.
- Assess presence of inflexible, maladaptive personality traits **that reflect personality/character disorder** (e.g., impulsive,

unpredictable, inappropriate behaviors, intense anger or lack of control of anger).

- Note degree of impairment in social and occupational functioning. **May dictate treatment setting (e.g., specific outpatient program, short-stay inpatient).**
- Review laboratory findings (e.g., blood alcohol, polydrug screen, glucose, electrolyte levels).

NURSING PRIORITY NO. 2. To structure environment to maintain client safety:

- Assist client to identify feelings and behaviors that precede desire for self-mutilation. **Early recognition of recurring feelings provides client opportunity to seek other ways of coping.**
- Provide external controls/limit setting **to decrease the need to self-mutilate.**
- Include client in development of plan of care **to reestablish ego boundaries, strengthen commitment to goals and participation in therapy.**
- Encourage client to recognize and appropriately express feelings verbally.
- Keep client in continuous staff view and do special observation checks **to promote safety.**
- Develop schedule of alternative healthy, success-oriented activities, as in groups such as Overeaters Anonymous (OA) or similar 12-step program based on individual needs, self-esteem activities including positive affirmations, visiting with friends, and exercise.
- Structure inpatient milieu to maintain positive, clear, open communication among staff and clients, with an understanding that "secrets are not tolerated" and will be confronted.
- Note feelings of healthcare providers/family, such as frustration, anger, defensiveness, distraction, despair and powerlessness, need to rescue. **Client may be manipulating/splitting providers/family members, which evokes defensiveness and resultant conflict. These feelings need to be identified, recognized, and dealt with openly with staff and client.**

NURSING PRIORITY NO. 3. To promote movement toward positive actions:

- Encourage client involvement in developing plan of care. **Enhances commitment to goals, optimizing outcomes.**
- Assist client to learn assertive behavior rather than nonassertive/aggressive behavior. Include use of effective communication skills, focusing on developing self-esteem by replacing negative self-talk with positive comments.
- Develop a contract between client and counselor **to enable the**

client to stay physically safe, such as "I will not cut or harm myself for the next 8 hours." Contract is renewed on a regular basis and signed and dated by both parties. Contingency arrangements need to be made so client can talk to counselor as needed.

- Discuss with client/family normalcy of adolescent task of separation and ways of achieving.
- Promote the use of healthy behaviors, identifying the consequences and outcomes of current actions: "Does this get you what you want?" "How does this behavior help you achieve your goals?"
- Use interventions that help the client to reclaim power in own life (e.g., experiential and cognitive).
- Involve client/family in group therapies as appropriate.

NURSING PRIORITY NO. 4. To promote wellness (Teaching/Discharge Considerations):

- Discuss commitment to safety and ways in which client will deal with precursors to undesired behavior.
- Mobilize support systems.
- Identify living circumstances client will be going to once discharged. May need assistance with transition to changes required to avoid recurrence of self-mutilating behaviors.
- Arrange for continued involvement in group therapy(ies).
- Involve family/SO(s) in planning for discharge. Promotes coordination and continuation of plan, commitment to goals.
- Discuss and provide information about the use of medication as appropriate. Antidepressant medications may be useful, but use needs to be weighed against potential for overdosing.
- Refer to NDs Anxiety; Social Interaction, impaired; Self-Esteem (specify).

Documentation Focus

ASSESSMENT/REASSESSMENT

- Individual findings, including risk factors present, underlying dynamics, prior episodes.

PLANNING

- Plan of care and who is involved in planning.
- Teaching plan.

IMPLEMENTATION/EVALUATION

- Response to interventions/teaching and actions performed.
- Attainment/progress toward desired outcome(s).
- Modifications to plan of care.

- Long-range needs and who is responsible for actions to be taken.
- Community resources, referrals made.

SAMPLE NURSING OUTCOMES & INTERVENTIONS CLASSIFICATIONS (NOC/NIC)

NOC—Self-Mutilation Restraint
NIC—Behavior Management: Self-Harm

Sensory Perception, disturbed (specify: visual, auditory, kinesthetic, gustatory, tactile, olfactory)

Taxonomy II: Perception/Cognition—Class 3 Sensation/Perception (00122)
[Diagnostic Division: Neurosensory]
Submitted 1978; Revised 1980, 1998 (by small group work 1996)

Definition: Change in the amount or patterning of incoming stimuli accompanied by a diminished, exaggerated, distorted, or impaired response to such stimuli

Related Factors

Excessive/insufficient environmental stimuli
[Therapeutically restricted environments (e.g., isolation, intensive care, bedrest, traction, confining illnesses, incubator)]
[Socially restricted environment (e.g., institutionalization, homebound, aging, chronic/terminal illness, infant deprivation); stigmatized (e.g., mentally ill/retarded/handicapped); bereaved]
[Excessive noise level, such as work environment, client's immediate environment (ICU with support machinery and the like)]
Altered sensory reception, transmission, and/or integration:
[Neurological disease, trauma, or deficit]
[Altered status of sense organs]
[Inability to communicate, understand, speak, or respond]
[Sleep deprivation]
[Pain, (phantom limb)]
Biochemical imbalances; electrolyte imbalance; biochemical imbalances for sensory distortion (e.g., illusions, hallucinations)[elevated BUN, elevated ammonia, hypoxia]; [drugs, e.g., stimulants or depressants, mind-altering drugs]
Psychological stress [narrowed perceptual fields caused by anxiety]
Altered sensory perception

Information that appears in brackets has been added by the authors to clarify and enhance the use of nursing diagnoses.

Defining Characteristics

SUBJECTIVE

Reported change in sensory acuity [e.g., photosensitivity, hypoesthe-sias/hyperesthesias, diminished/altered sense of taste, inability to tell position of body parts (proprioception)]
Visual/auditory distortions
[Distortion of pain, e.g., exaggerated, lack of]

OBJECTIVE

Measured change in sensory acuity
Change in usual response to stimuli, [rapid mood swings, exaggerated emotional responses, anxiety/panic state, motor incoordination, altered sense of balance/falls (e.g., Ménierè's syndrome)]
Change in problem-solving abilities; poor concentration
Disoriented in time, in place, or with people
Altered communication patterns
Change in behavior pattern
Restlessness, irritability
Hallucinations; [illusions]; [bizarre thinking]

Desired Outcomes/Evaluation Criteria—Client Will:

- Regain/maintain usual level of cognition.
- Recognize and correct/compensate for sensory impairments.
- Verbalize awareness of sensory needs and presence of overload and/or deprivation.
- Identify/modify external factors that contribute to alterations in sensory/perceptual abilities.
- Use resources effectively and appropriately.
- Be free of injury.

Actions/Interventions

NURSING PRIORITY NO. 1. To assess causative/contributing factors and degree of impairment:

- Identify underlying reason for alterations in sensory perception, as noted in Related Factors.
- Be aware of clients at risk for loss/alterations in sensory/perceptual senses (e.g., increased intraocular pressure after eye surgery), drug toxicity side effects (e.g., halos around lights, ringing in ears), middle-ear disturbances (altered sense of balance).
- Review laboratory values (e.g., electrolytes, chemical profile, ABGs, serum drug levels).
- Assess ability to speak and respond to simple commands.
- Evaluate sensory awareness: Stimulus of hot/cold, dull/sharp; awareness of motion, and location of body parts, visual acui-

ty and hearing. Investigate reports of feeling cold—**may indicate decrease in peripheral circulation/cellular catabolism.**

- Determine response to painful stimuli, **to note whether response is appropriate to stimulus, immediate, or delayed.**
- Observe for behavioral responses (e.g., illusions/hallucinations, delusions, withdrawal, hostility, crying, inappropriate affect, confusion/disorientation).
- Ascertain client's perception of problem/changes.
- Interview SO(s) regarding his or her observations of changes that have occurred/responses of client to changes.

NURSING PRIORITY NO. 2. To promote normalization of response to stimuli:

- Note degree of alteration/involvement (single/multiple senses).
- Listen to and respect client's expressions of deprivation. Take these into consideration in planning care.
- Provide means of communication as indicated.
- Provide a stable environment with continuity of care by same personnel as much as possible. Have personnel wear name tags/reintroduce self as appropriate.
- Avoid isolation of client, physically or emotionally, **to prevent sensory deprivation/limit confusion.**
- Provide feedback to assist client to separate reality from fantasy/altered perception.
- Reorient to time, place, staff, and events as necessary (especially when vision is impaired).
- Explain procedures/activities, expected sensations, and outcomes.
- Minimize discussion of negatives (e.g., client and personnel problems) within client's hearing. **Client may misinterpret and believe references are to himself/herself.**
- Eliminate extraneous noise/stimuli, including nonessential equipment, alarms/audible monitor signals when possible.
- Provide undisturbed rest/sleep periods.
- Arrange bed, personal articles, and food trays to take advantage of functional vision. **Enhances independence and safety.**
- Describe food when client cannot see and assist as necessary.
- Speak to visually impaired or unresponsive client during care **to provide auditory stimulation and prevent startle reflex.**
- Provide tactile stimulation as care is given. **Communicates presence/connection with other human being, because touching is an important part of caring and a deep psychologic need.**
- Provide sensory stimulation, including familiar smells/

sounds, tactile stimulation with a variety of objects, changing of light intensity and other cues (e.g., clocks, calendars).

- Encourage SO(s) to bring in familiar objects, talk to, and touch the client frequently.
- Provide diversional activities as able (e.g., TV/radio, conversation, large-print or talking books). (Refer to ND Diversional Activity, deficient.)
- Involve other health-team members in providing stimulating modalities, such as music therapy, sensory training, remotivation therapy.
- Identify and encourage use of resources/prosthetic devices (e.g., hearing aids, computerized visual aid/glasses with a level plumbline for balance). **Useful for augmenting senses.**
- Limit/carefully monitor use of sedation, especially in older population.

NURSING PRIORITY NO. 3. To prevent injury/complications:

- Place call bell within reach and be sure client knows where it is/how to use it.
- Provide safety measures (e.g., siderails, bed in low position, ambulate with assistance). Protect from thermal injury (e.g., monitor use of heating pads/lights, ice packs). Note perceptual deficit on chart **so caregivers are aware.**
- Position doors and furniture so they are out of travel path for client with impaired vision, or strategically place items/grab bars **to aid in maintaining balance.**
- Ambulate with assistance/devices **to enhance balance.**
- Describe where affected areas of body are when moving the client.
- Limit activities that may increase intraocular pressure when indicated: Avoid sudden movement of the head, rubbing eyes, bending/stooping, use of bedpan (**may be more strain than getting up to the bathroom**).
- Monitor drug regimen postsurgically (e.g., antiemetics, miotics, sympathomimetics, beta blockers) **to prevent increase in or to reduce intraocular pressure.**
- Refer to NDs Injury, risk for; Trauma, risk for.

NURSING PRIORITY NO. 4. To promote wellness (Teaching/Discharge Considerations):

- Assist client/SO(s) to learn effective ways of coping with and managing sensory disturbances, anticipating safety needs according to client's sensory deficits and developmental level.
- Identify alternative ways of dealing with perceptual deficits (e.g., compensation techniques).
- Provide explanations of and plan care with client, involving SO(s) as much as possible. **Enhances commitment to and continuation of plan, optimizing outcomes.**

- Review home safety measures pertinent to deficits.
- Discuss drug regimen, noting possible toxic side effects of both prescription and OTC drugs. **Prompt recognition of side effects allows for timely intervention/change in drug regimen.**
- Demonstrate use/care of sensory prosthetic devices. **Identify resources/community programs for acquiring and maintaining devices.**
- Promote meaningful socialization. (Refer to ND Social Isolation.)
- Encourage out-of-bed/out-of-room activities.
- Refer to appropriate helping resources, such as Society for the Blind, Self-Help for the Hard of Hearing (SHHH), or local support groups, screening programs, and so forth.
- Refer to additional NDs Anxiety; Thought Processes, disturbed; Unilateral Neglect; Confusion, acute/chronic, as appropriate.

Documentation Focus

ASSESSMENT/REASSESSMENT

- Individual findings, noting specific deficit/associated symptoms, perceptions of client/SO(s).
- Assistive device needs.

PLANNING

- Plan of care, including who is involved in planning.
- Teaching plan.

IMPLEMENTATION/EVALUATION

- Responses to interventions/teaching and actions performed.
- Attainment/progress toward desired outcome(s).
- Modifications to plan of care.

DISCHARGE PLANNING

- Long-term needs and who is responsible for actions to be taken.
- Available resources; specific referrals made.

SAMPLE NURSING OUTCOMES & INTERVENTIONS CLASSIFICATIONS (NOC/NIC)

AUDITORY

NOC—Hearing Compensation Behavior
NIC—Communication Enhancement: Hearing Deficit

VISUAL

NOC—Vision Compensation Behavior
NIC—Communication Enhancement: Visual Deficit

GUSTATORY/OLFACTORY

NOC—Distorted Thought Control
NIC—Nutrition Management

KINESTHETIC

NOC—Balance
NIC—Body Mechanics Promotion

TACTILE

NOC—Sensory Function: Cutaneous
NIC—Peripheral Sensation Management

Sexual Dysfunction

Taxonomy II: Sexuality—Class 2 Sexual Function (00059)
[Diagnostic Division: Sexuality]
Submitted 1980

Definition: Change in sexual function that is viewed as
unsatisfying, unrewarding, inadequate

Related Factors

Biopsychosocial alteration of sexuality:
    Ineffectual or absent role models; lack of SO
    Vulnerability
    Misinformation or lack of knowledge
    Physical abuse; psychosocial abuse (e.g., harmful relationships)
    Values conflict
    Lack of privacy
    Altered body structure or function (pregnancy, recent childbirth,
        drugs, surgery, anomalies, disease process, trauma, [paraplegia/
        quadriplegia], radiation, [effects of aging])

Defining Characteristics

SUBJECTIVE

Verbalization of problem [e.g., loss of sexual desire, disruption of
    sexual response patterns such as premature ejaculation, dyspareu-
    nia, vaginismus]
Actual or perceived limitation imposed by disease and/or therapy
Inability to achieve desired satisfaction
Alterations in achieving perceived sex role
Conflicts involving values
Alterations in achieving sexual satisfaction
Seeking confirmation of desirability

Information that appears in brackets has been added by the authors
to clarify and enhance the use of nursing diagnoses.

Alteration in relationship with SO
Change of interest in self and others

Desired Outcomes/Evaluation Criteria—Client Will:

- Verbalize understanding of sexual anatomy/function and alterations that may affect function.
- Verbalize understanding of individual reasons for sexual problems.
- Identify stressors in lifestyle that may contribute to the dysfunction.
- Identify satisfying/acceptable sexual practices and some alternative ways of dealing with sexual expression.
- Discuss concerns about body image, sex role, desirability as a sexual partner with partner/SO.

Actions/Interventions

NURSING PRIORITY NO. **1.** To assess causative/contributing factors:

- Obtain sexual history, including usual pattern of functioning and level of desire. Note vocabulary used by the individual **to maximize communication/understanding.**
- Have client describe problem in own words.
- Determine importance of sex to individual/partner and client's motivation for change.
- Be alert to comments of client **as sexual concerns are often disguised as humor, sarcasm, and/or offhand remarks.**
- Assess knowledge of client/SO regarding sexual anatomy/ function and effects of current situation/condition.
- Determine preexisting problems that may be factors in current situation (e.g., marital/job stress, role conflicts).
- Identify current stress factors in individual situation. **These factors may be producing enough anxiety to cause depression or other psychologic reaction(s) that would cause physiologic symptoms.**
- Discuss cultural/religious value factors or conflicts present.
- Determine pathophysiology, illness/surgery/trauma involved, and impact on (perception of) individual/SO.
- Review medication regimen/drug use (prescription, OTC, illegal, alcohol) and cigarette use. **Antihypertensives may cause erectile dysfunction; MAO inhibitors and tricyclics can cause erection/ejaculation problems and anorgasmia in women; narcotics/alcohol produce impotence and inhibit orgasm; smoking creates vasoconstriction and may be a factor in erectile dysfunction.**

- Observe behavior/stage of grieving when related to body changes or loss of a body part (e.g., pregnancy, obesity, amputation, mastectomy).
- Assist with diagnostic studies to determine cause of erectile dysfunction. (**More than half of the cases have a physical cause such as diabetes, vascular problems, etc.**) Monitor penile tumescence during REM sleep **to assist in determining physical ability.**
- Explore with client the meaning of client's behavior. (**Masturbation, for instance, may have many meanings/ purposes, such as for relief of anxiety, sexual deprivation, pleasure, a nonverbal expression of need to talk, way of alienating.**)
- Avoid making value judgments **as they do not help the client to cope with the situation. Note:** Nurse needs to be aware of and be in control of own feelings and response to client expressions and/or concerns.

NURSING PRIORITY NO. **2.** To assist client/SO(s) to deal with individual situation:

- Establish therapeutic nurse-client relationship **to promote treatment and facilitate sharing of sensitive information/ feelings.**
- Assist with treatment of underlying medical conditions, including changes in medication regimen, weight management, cessation of smoking, and so forth.
- Provide factual information about individual condition involved. **Promotes informed decision making.**
- Determine what client wants to know **to tailor information to client needs. Note:** Information affecting client safety/consequences of actions may need to be reviewed/reinforced.
- Encourage and accept expressions of concern, anger, grief, fear.
- Assist client to be aware/deal with stages of grieving for loss/change.
- Encourage client to share thoughts/concerns with partner and to clarify values/impact of condition on relationship.
- Provide for/identify ways to obtain privacy **to allow for sexual expression for individual and/or between partners without embarrassment and/or objections of others.**
- Assist client/SO(s) to problem-solve alternative ways of sexual expression.
- Provide information about availability of corrective measures such as medication (e.g., papaverine or sildenafil—Viagra— for erectile dysfunction) or reconstructive surgery (e.g., penile/breast implants) when indicated.

- Refer to appropriate resources as need indicates (e.g., health-care coworker with greater comfort level and/or knowledge-able clinical nurse specialist or professional sex therapist, family counseling).

NURSING PRIORITY NO. 3. To promote wellness (Teaching/Discharge Considerations):

- Provide sex education, explanation of normal sexual functioning when necessary.
- Provide written material appropriate to individual needs (include list of books related to client's needs) **for reinforcement at client's leisure/readiness to deal with sensitive materials.**
- Encourage ongoing dialogue and take advantage of teachable moments that occur.
- Demonstrate and assist client to learn relaxation and/or visualization techniques.
- Assist client to learn regular self-examination as indicated (e.g., breast/testicular examinations).
- Identify community resources for further assistance (e.g., Reach for Recovery, CanSurmount, Ostomy Association).
- Refer for further professional assistance concerning relationship difficulties, low sexual desire/other sexual concerns (such as premature ejaculation, vaginismus, painful intercourse).
- Identify resources for assistive devices/sexual "aids."

Documentation Focus

ASSESSMENT/REASSESSMENT

- Individual findings including nature of dysfunction, predisposing factors, perceived effect on sexuality/relationships.
- Response of SO(s).
- Motivation for change.

PLANNING

- Plan of care and who is involved in planning.
- Teaching plan.

IMPLEMENTATION/EVALUATION

- Response to interventions/teaching and actions performed.
- Attainment/progress toward desired outcome(s).
- Modifications to plan of care.

DISCHARGE PLANNING

- Long-term needs/referrals and who is responsible for actions to be taken.
- Community resources, specific referrals made.

SAMPLE NURSING OUTCOMES
& INTERVENTIONS CLASSIFICATIONS (NOC/NIC)

NOC—Sexual Functioning
NIC—Sexual Counseling

Sexuality Pattern, ineffective

Taxonomy II: Sexuality—Class 2 Sexual Function (00065)
[Diagnostic Division: Sexuality]
Submitted 1986

Definition: Expressions of concern regarding own
sexuality

Related Factors

Knowledge/skill deficit about alternative responses to health-related
    transitions, altered body function or structure, illness or medical
    treatment
Lack of privacy
Impaired relationship with a SO; lack of SO
Ineffective or absent role models
Conflicts with sexual orientation or variant preferences
Fear of pregnancy or of acquiring a sexually transmitted disease

Defining Characteristics

SUBJECTIVE

Reported difficulties, limitations, or changes in sexual behaviors or
    activities
[Expressions of feeling alienated, lonely, loss, powerless, angry]

Desired Outcomes/Evaluation
Criteria—Client Will:

- Verbalize understanding of sexual anatomy and function.
- Verbalize knowledge and understanding of sexual limitations,
  difficulties, or changes that have occurred.
- Verbalize acceptance of self in current (altered) condition.
- Demonstrate improved communication and relationship
  skills.
- Identify individually appropriate method of contraception.

Actions/Interventions

NURSING PRIORITY NO. 1. To assess causative/contributing
factors:

- Obtain sexual history, as indicated, including perception of

---

Information that appears in brackets has been added by the authors
to clarify and enhance the use of nursing diagnoses.

normal function, use of vocabulary (assessing basic knowledge). Note comments/concerns about sexual identity.

- Determine importance of sex and a description of the problem in the client's own words. Be alert to comments of client/SO (e.g., discount of overt or covert sexual expressions such as "He's just a dirty old man"). **Sexual concerns are often disguised as sarcasm, humor, or in offhand remarks.**
- Note cultural/religious value factors and conflicts that may exist.
- Assess stress factors in client's environment that might cause anxiety or psychologic reactions (power issues involving SO, adult children, aging, employment, loss of prowess).
- Explore knowledge of effects of altered body function/limitations precipitated by illness and/or medical treatment of alternative sexual responses and expressions (e.g., undescended testicle in young male, gender change/reassignment procedure, mutilating cancer surgery).
- Review substance use history (prescription medication, OTC drugs, alcohol, and illicit drugs).
- Explore issues and fears associated with sex (pregnancy, sexually transmitted diseases, trust/control issues, inflexible beliefs, preference confusion, altered performance).
- Determine client's interpretation of the altered sexual activity or behavior (e.g., a way of controlling, relief of anxiety, pleasure, lack of partner). **These behaviors (when related to body changes, including pregnancy or weight loss/gain, or loss of body part) may reflect a stage of grieving.**
- Assess life-cycle issues, such as adolescence, young adulthood, menopause, aging.
- Avoid value judgments—**they do not help the client to cope with the situation. Note:** Nurse needs to be aware of and in control of own feelings and responses to the client's expressions and/or concerns.

NURSING PRIORITY NO. 2. To assist client/SO to deal with individual situation:

- Provide atmosphere in which discussion of sexual problems is encouraged/permitted. Sense of trust/comfort enhances ability to discuss sensitive matters.
- Provide information about individual situation, determining client needs and desires.
- Encourage discussion of individual situation with opportunity for expression of feelings without judgment.
- Provide specific suggestions about interventions directed toward the identified problems.
- Identify alternative forms of sexual expression that might be acceptable to both partners.

- Discuss ways to manage individual devices/appliances (e.g., ostomy bag, breast prostheses, urinary collection device) when change in body image/medical condition is involved.
- Provide anticipatory guidance about losses that are to be expected (e.g., loss of known self when transsexual surgery is planned).
- Introduce client to individuals who have successfully managed a similar problem. **Provides positive role model, support for problem solving.**

NURSING PRIORITY NO. 3. To promote wellness (Teaching/Discharge Considerations):

- Provide factual information about problem(s) as identified by the client.
- Engage in ongoing dialogue with the client and SO(s) as situation permits.
- Discuss methods/effectiveness/side effects of contraceptives if indicated.
- Refer to community resources (e.g., Planned Parenthood, gender-identity clinic, social services, others) as indicated.
- Refer for intensive individual/group psychotherapy, which may be combined with couple/family and/or sex therapy, as appropriate.
- Refer to NDs Sexual Dysfunction; Body Image, disturbed; Self-Esteem [specify].

Documentation Focus

ASSESSMENT/REASSESSMENT

- Individual findings, including nature of concern, perceived difficulties/limitations or changes, specific needs/desires.
- Response of SO(s).

PLANNING

- Plan of care and who is involved in the planning.
- Teaching plan.

IMPLEMENTATION/EVALUATION

- Response to interventions/teaching and actions performed.
- Attainment/progress toward desired outcome(s).
- Modifications to plan of care.

DISCHARGE PLANNING

- Long-term needs/teaching and referrals and who is responsible for actions to be taken.
- Community resources, specific referrals made.

SAMPLE NURSING OUTCOMES & INTERVENTIONS CLASSIFICATIONS (NOC/NIC)

NOC—Sexual Identity: Acceptance
NIC—Teaching: Sexuality

Skin Integrity, impaired

Taxonomy II: Safety/Protection—Class 2 Physical Injury
(00046)
[Diagnostic Division: Safety]
Submitted 1975; Revised 1998 (by small group work
1996)

Definition: Altered epidermis and/or dermis [The
integumentary system is the largest multifunctional
organ of the body.]

Related Factors

EXTERNAL

Hyperthermia or hypothermia
Chemical substance; radiation; medications
Physical immobilization
Humidity; moisture; [excretions/secretions]
Altered fluid status
Mechanical factors (e.g., shearing forces, pressure, restraint), [trauma:
    injury/surgery]
Extremes in age

INTERNAL

Altered nutritional state (e.g., obesity, emaciation); metabolic state;
    fluid status
Skeletal prominence; alterations in turgor (change in elasticity); [pres-
    ence of edema]
Altered circulation; sensation; pigmentation
Developmental factors
Immunological deficit
[Psychogenic]

Defining Characteristics

SUBJECTIVE

[Reports of itching, pain, numbness of affected/surrounding area]

OBJECTIVE

Disruption of skin surface (epidermis)
Destruction of skin layers (dermis)
Invasion of body structures

Information that appears in brackets has been added by the authors
to clarify and enhance the use of nursing diagnoses.

Desired Outcomes/Evaluation Criteria—Client Will:

- Display timely healing of skin lesions/wounds/pressure sores without complication.
- Maintain optimal nutrition/physical well-being.
- Participate in prevention measures and treatment program.
- Verbalize feelings of increased self-esteem and ability to manage situation.

Actions/Interventions

NURSING PRIORITY NO. 1. To assess causative/contributing factors:

- Identify underlying condition/pathology involved (e.g., skin and other cancers, burns, scleroderma, lupus, psoriasis, acne, diabetes, occupational hazards, steroid therapy, familial history, trauma, surgical incision/amputation, radiation therapy, communicable diseases).
- Note general debilitation, reduced mobility, changes in skin/muscle mass associated with aging/chronic disease, presence of incontinence/problems with self-care.
- Assess blood supply and sensation (nerve damage) of affected area.
- Determine nutritional status and areas at risk for injury because of malnutrition (e.g., pressure points on emaciated and/or elderly client).
- Evaluate risks for injury (e.g., the use of restraints, long-term immobility).
- Note laboratory results pertinent to causative factors (e.g., studies such as Hb/Hct, blood glucose, albumin/protein).

NURSING PRIORITY NO. 2. To assess extent of involvement/injury:

- Obtain a history of condition, including age at onset, date of first episode, how long it lasted, original site, characteristics of lesions, and any changes that have occurred.
- Note changes in skin color, texture, and turgor. Assess areas of least pigmentation for color changes (e.g., sclera, conjunctiva, nailbeds, buccal mucosa, tongue, palms, and soles of feet).
- Palpate skin lesions for size, shape, consistency, texture, temperature, and hydration.
- Determine depth of injury/damage to integumentary system (epidermis, dermis, and/or underlying tissues).
- Measure length, width, depth of ulcers. Note extent of tunneling/undermining, if present.
- Inspect surrounding skin for erythema, induration, maceration.

- Photograph lesion(s) as appropriate **to document status/ provide visual baseline for future comparisons.**
- Note odors emitted from the skin/area of injury.
- Classify ulcer using tool such as Wagner Ulcer Classification System. **Provides consistent terminology for documentation.**

NURSING PRIORITY NO. 3. To determine impact of condition:

- Ascertain attitudes of individual/SO(s) about condition (e.g., cultural values, stigma). Note misconceptions. **Identifies areas to be addressed in teaching plan and potential referral needs.**
- Obtain psychologic assessment of client's emotional status, noting potential or sexual problems arising from presence of condition.
- Note presence of compromised vision, hearing, or speech. **Skin is a particularly important avenue of communication for these people and, when compromised, may affect responses.**

NURSING PRIORITY NO. 4. To assist client with correcting/minimizing condition and promote optimal healing:

- Inspect skin on a daily basis, describing lesions and changes observed.
- Periodically remeasure/photograph wound and observe for complications (e.g., infection, dehiscence) **to monitor progress of wound healing.**
- Keep the area clean/dry, carefully dress wounds, support incision (e.g., use of Steri-Strips, splinting when coughing), prevent infection, and stimulate circulation to surrounding areas **to assist body's natural process of repair.**
- Assist with débridement/enzymatic therapy as indicated (e.g., burns, severe pressures sores).
- Use appropriate barrier dressings, wound coverings, drainage appliances, and skin-protective agents for open/draining wounds and stomas **to protect the wound and/or surrounding tissues.** Expose lesions/ulcer to air and light as indicated.
- Limit/avoid use of plastic material (e.g., rubber sheet, plastic-backed linen savers). Remove wet/wrinkled linens promptly. **Moisture potentiates skin breakdown.**
- Develop repositioning schedule for client, involving client in reasons for and decisions about times and positions in conjunction with other activities **to enhance understanding and cooperation.**
- Use appropriate padding devices (e.g., air/water mattress, sheepskin) when indicated **to reduce pressure on/enhance circulation to compromised tissues.**
- Encourage early ambulation/mobilization. **Promotes circulation and reduces risks associated with immobility.**

- Calculate ankle-brachial index for clients with potential for/ actual impairment of circulation to lower extremities. **Result less than 0.9 indicates need for close monitoring/more aggressive intervention (e.g., tighter blood glucose and weight control in diabetic client).**
- Obtain specimen from draining wounds when appropriate for culture/sensitivities/Gram's stain **to determine appropriate therapy.**
- Provide optimum nutrition and increased protein intake **to provide a positive nitrogen balance to aid in healing and to maintain general good health.**
- Monitor periodic laboratory studies relative to general well-being and status of specific problem.
- Consult with wound specialist as indicated **to assist with developing plan of care for problematic or potentially serious wounds.**

NURSING PRIORITY NO. **5.** To promote wellness (Teaching/Discharge Considerations):

- Review importance of skin and measures to maintain proper skin functioning.
- Discuss importance of early detection of skin changes and/or complications.
- Assist the client/SO(s) in understanding and following medical regimen and developing program of preventive care and daily maintenance. **Enhances commitment to plan, optimizing outcomes.**
- Review measures to avoid spread/reinfection of communicable disease/conditions.
- Emphasize importance of proper fit of clothing/shoes, use of specially lined shock-absorbing socks or pressure-reducing insoles for shoes **in presence of reduced sensation/circulation.**
- Identify safety factors for use of equipment/appliances (e.g., heating pad, ostomy appliances, padding straps of braces).
- Encourage client to verbalize feelings and discuss how/if condition affects self-concept/self-esteem. (Refer to NDs Body Image, disturbed, Self-Esteem, situational low.)
- Assist client to work through stages of grief and feelings associated with individual condition.
- Lend psychologic support and acceptance of client, using touch, facial expressions, and tone of voice.
- Assist client to learn stress reduction and alternate therapy techniques **to control feelings of helplessness and deal with situation.**
- Refer to dietitian or certified diabetes educator as appropriate **to enhance healing, reduce risk of recurrence of diabetic ulcers.**

Documentation Focus

ASSESSMENT/REASSESSMENT

- Characteristics of lesion(s)/condition, ulcer classification.
- Causative/contributing factors.
- Impact of condition.

PLANNING

- Plan of care and who is involved in planning.
- Teaching plan.

IMPLEMENTATION/EVALUATION

- Responses to interventions/teaching and actions performed.
- Attainment/progress toward desired outcome(s).
- Modifications to plan of care.

DISCHARGE PLANNING

- Long-term needs/referrals and who is responsible for actions to be taken.
- Specific referrals made.

SAMPLE NURSING OUTCOMES & INTERVENTIONS CLASSIFICATIONS (NOC/NIC)

NOC—Tissue Integrity: Skin & Mucous Membranes
NIC—Skin Care: Topical Treatments

Skin Integrity, risk for impaired

Taxonomy II: Safety/Protection—Class 2 Physical Injury (00047)
[Diagnostic Division: Safety]
Submitted 1975; Revised 1998 (by small group work 1996)

Definition: At risk for skin being adversely altered

Note: Risk should be determined by the use of a risk assessment tool (e.g., Braden Scale)

Risk Factors

EXTERNAL

Chemical substance; radiation
Hypothermia or hyperthermia
Physical immobilization
Excretions and/or secretions; humidity; moisture
Mechanical factors (e.g., shearing forces, pressure, restraint)
Extremes of age

Information that appears in brackets has been added by the authors to clarify and enhance the use of nursing diagnoses.

INTERNAL

Medication

Alterations in nutritional state (e.g., obesity, emaciation), metabolic state, [fluid status]

Skeletal prominence; alterations in skin turgor (change in elasticity); [presence of edema]

Altered circulation, sensation, pigmentation

Developmental factors

Psychogenic

Immunologic

> NOTE: A risk diagnosis is not evidenced by signs and symptoms, as the problem has not occurred and nursing interventions are directed at prevention.

Desired Outcomes/Evaluation Criteria—Client Will:

- Identify individual risk factors.
- Verbalize understanding of treatment/therapy regimen.
- Demonstrate behaviors/techniques to prevent skin breakdown.

Actions/Interventions

NURSING PRIORITY NO. **1.** To assess causative/contributing factors:

- Note general debilitation, reduced mobility, changes in skin and muscle mass associated with aging, poor nutritional status or chronic diseases, incontinence and/or problems of self-care and/or medication/therapy, and so forth.
- Note laboratory results pertinent to causative factors (e.g., Hg/Hct, blood glucose, albumin/total protein).
- Calculate ankle-brachial index as appropriate (diabetic clients or others with impaired circulation to lower extremities). **Result less than 0.9 indicates need for more aggressive preventive interventions (e.g., closer blood glucose and weight control).**

NURSING PRIORITY NO. **2.** To maintain skin integrity at optimal level:

- Handle infant (especially premature infants) gently. **Epidermis of infants and very young children is thin and lacks subcutaneous depth that will develop with age.**
- Maintain strict skin hygiene, using mild nondetergent soap, drying gently and thoroughly and lubricating with lotion or emollient as indicated.
- Massage bony prominences gently and avoid friction when moving client.
- Change position in bed/chair on a regular schedule.

Encourage participation with active and assistive range-of-motion exercises.

- Provide adequate clothing/covers; protect from drafts **to prevent vasoconstriction.**
- Keep bedclothes dry, use nonirritating materials, and keep bed free of wrinkles, crumbs, and so forth.
- Provide protection by use of pads, pillows, foam mattress, water bed, and so forth **to increase circulation and alter/eliminate excessive tissue pressure.**
- Inspect skin surfaces/pressure points routinely.
- Observe for reddened/blanched areas and institute treatment immediately. **Reduces likelihood of progression to skin breakdown.**
- Provide for safety measures during ambulation and other therapies that might cause dermal injury (e.g., properly fitting hose/footwear, use of heating pads/lamps, restraints).

NURSING PRIORITY NO. **3.** To promote wellness (Teaching/Discharge Considerations):

- Provide information to client/SO(s) about the importance of regular observation and effective skin care in preventing problems.
- Emphasize importance of adequate nutritional/fluid intake **to maintain general good health and skin turgor.**
- Encourage continuation of regular exercise program (active/assistive) **to enhance circulation.**
- Recommend elevation of lower extremities when sitting **to enhance venous return and reduce edema formation.**
- Encourage restriction/abstinence from tobacco, **which can cause vasoconstriction.**
- Suggest use of ice, colloidal bath, lotions **to decrease irritable itching.**
- Recommend keeping nails short or wearing gloves **to reduce risk of dermal injury when severe itching is present.**
- Discuss importance of avoiding exposure to sunlight in specific conditions (e.g., systemic lupus, tetracycline/psychotropic drug use, radiation therapy) as well as potential for development of skin cancer.
- Counsel diabetic and neurologically impaired client about importance of skin care, especially of lower extremities.
- Perform periodic assessment using a tool such as Braden Scale **to determine changes in risk status and need for alterations in the plan of care.**

Documentation Focus

ASSESSMENT/REASSESSMENT

- Individual findings, including individual risk factors.

PLANNING

- Plan of care and who is involved in planning.
- Teaching plan.

IMPLEMENTATION/EVALUATION

- Responses to interventions/teaching and actions performed.
- Attainment/progress toward desired outcome(s).
- Modifications to plan of care.

DISCHARGE PLANNING

- Long-term needs and who is responsible for actions to be taken.

SAMPLE NURSING OUTCOMES & INTERVENTIONS CLASSIFICATIONS (NOC/NIC)

NOC—Risk Control
NIC—Pressure Management

Sleep Deprivation

Taxonomy II: Activity/Rest—Class 1 Sleep/Rest (00096)
[Diagnostic Division: Activity/Rest]
Nursing Diagnosis Extension and Classification (NDEC)
Submission 1998

Definition: Prolonged periods of time without sleep (sustained natural, periodic suspension of relative consciousness)

Related Factors

Sustained environmental stimulation; unfamiliar or uncomfortable sleep environment

Inadequate daytime activity; sustained circadian asynchrony; aging-related sleep stage shifts; non–sleep-inducing parenting practices

Sustained inadequate sleep hygiene; prolonged use of pharmacological or dietary antisoporifics

Prolonged physical/psychological discomfort; periodic limb movement (e.g., restless leg syndrome, nocturnal myoclonus); sleep-related: enuresis; painful erections

Nightmares; sleepwalking; sleep terror

Sleep apnea

Sundowner's syndrome; dementia

Idiopathic CNS hypersomnolence; narcolepsy; familial sleep paralysis

---

Information that appears in brackets has been added by the authors to clarify and enhance the use of nursing diagnoses.

Defining Characteristics

SUBJECTIVE

Daytime drowsiness; decreased ability to function
Malaise; tiredness; lethargy
Anxious
Perceptual disorders (e.g., disturbed body sensation, delusions, feeling afloat); heightened sensitivity to pain

OBJECTIVE

Restlessness; irritability
Inability to concentrate; slowed reaction
Listlessness; apathy
Mild, fleeting nystagmus; hand tremors
Acute confusion; transient paranoia; agitated or combative; hallucinations

Desired Outcomes/Evaluation Criteria—Client Will:

- Identify individually appropriate interventions to promote sleep.
- Verbalize understanding of sleep disorders.
- Adjust lifestyle to accommodate chronobiological rhythms.
- Report improvement in sleep/rest pattern.

Family Will:

- Deal appropriately with parasomnias.

Actions/Interventions

NURSING PRIORITY NO. 1. To assess causative/contributing factors:

- Determine presence of physical or psychological stressors, including night-shift working hours, pain, advanced age, current/recent illness, death of a spouse.
- Note medical diagnoses that affect sleep (e.g., dementia, encephalitis, brain injury, narcolepsy, depression, asthma, sleep-induced respiratory disorders/obstructive sleep apnea, nocturnal myoclonus).
- Evaluate for use of medications and/or other drugs affecting sleep (e.g., diet pills, antidepressives, antihypertensives, alcohol, stimulants, sedatives, diuretics, narcotics).
- Note environmental factors affecting sleep (e.g., unfamiliar or uncomfortable sleep environment, excessive noise and light, uncomfortable temperature, roommate irritations/actions— e.g., snoring, watching TV late at night).
- Determine presence of parasomnias: nightmares/terrors or somnambulism (e.g., sitting, sleepwalking, or other complex behavior during sleep).

• Note reports of terror, brief periods of paralysis, sense of body being disconnected from the brain. **Occurrence of sleep paralysis, though not widely recognized in the United States, has been well documented elsewhere and may result in feelings of fear/reluctance to go to sleep.**

NURSING PRIORITY NO. 2. To assess degree of impairment:

• Determine client's usual sleep pattern and expectations. **Provides comparative baseline.**
• Ascertain duration of current problem and effect on life/functional ability.
• Listen to subjective reports of sleep quality.
• Observe physical signs of fatigue (e.g., restlessness, reports of feeling not rested or being exhausted, irritability, changes in behavior/performance, disorientation, frequent yawning).
• Determine interventions client has tried to date. **Helps identify appropriate options.**
• Distinguish client's beneficial bedtime habits from detrimental ones (e.g., drinking late-evening milk versus drinking late-evening coffee).
• Instruct client and/or bed partner to keep a sleep-wake log **to document symptoms and identify factors that are interfering with sleep.**
• Do a chronological chart **to determine peak performance rhythms.**

NURSING PRIORITY NO. 3. To assist client to establish optimal sleep pattern:

• Encourage client to develop plan to restrict caffeine, alcohol, and other stimulating substances from late afternoon/evening intake, and avoid eating large evening/late-night meals. **These factors are known to disrupt sleep patterns.**
• Recommend bedtime snack (protein, simple carbohydrate, and low fat) for young children 15 to 30 minutes before retiring. **Sense of fullness and satiety promotes sleep and reduces likelihood of gastric upset.**
• Promote adequate physical exercise activity during day. **Enhances expenditure of energy/release of tension so that client feels ready for sleep/rest.**
• Review medications being taken and their effect on sleep, suggesting modifications in regimen, **if medications are found to be interfering.**
• Suggest abstaining from daytime naps **because they impair ability to sleep at night.**
• Investigate anxious feelings **to help determine basis and appropriate anxiety-reduction techniques.**
• Recommend quiet activities, such as reading/listening to

soothing music in the evening, **to reduce stimulation so client can relax.**
- Instruct in relaxation techniques, music therapy, meditation, and so forth to decrease tension, prepare for rest/sleep.
- Limit evening fluid intake if nocturia is present **to reduce need for nighttime elimination.**
- Discuss/implement effective age-appropriate bedtime rituals (e.g., going to bed at same time each night, drinking warm milk, rocking, story reading, cuddling, favorite blanket/toy) **to enhance client's ability to fall asleep, reinforce that bed is a place to sleep, and promote sense of security for child.**
- Provide calm, quiet environment and manage controllable sleep-disrupting factors (e.g., noise, light, room temperature).
- Administer sedatives/other sleep medications when indicated, noting client's response. Time pain medications for peak effect/duration **to reduce need for redosing during prime sleep hours.**
- Instruct client to get out of bed, leave bedroom, engage in relaxing activities if unable to fall asleep, and not return to bed until feeling sleepy.
- Review with the client the physician's recommendations for medications or surgery (alteration of facial structures/ tracheotomy) and/or apneic oxygenation therapy—continuous positive airway pressure (CPAP) such as Respironics— **when sleep apnea is severe as documented by sleep disorder studies.**

NURSING PRIORITY NO. 4. To promote wellness (Teaching/ Discharge Considerations):
- Review possibility of next-day drowsiness/"rebound" insomnia and temporary memory loss **that may be associated with prescription sleep medications.**
- Discuss use/appropriateness of OTC sleep medications/herbal supplements. Note possible side effects and drug interactions.
- Refer to support group/counselor to help deal with psychologic stressors (e.g., grief, sorrow). Refer to NDs Grieving, dysfunctional; Sorrow, chronic.
- Encourage family counseling **to help deal with concerns arising from parasomnias.**
- Refer to sleep specialist/laboratory **when problem is unresponsive to interventions.**

Documentation Focus

ASSESSMENT/REASSESSMENT
- Assessment findings, including specifics of sleep pattern (current and past) and effects on lifestyle/level of functioning.

- Medications/interventions, previous therapies.
- Family history of similar problem.

PLANNING

- Plan of care and who is involved in planning.
- Teaching plan.

IMPLEMENTATION/EVALUATION

- Client's response to interventions/teaching and actions performed.
- Attainment/progress toward desired outcome(s).
- Modifications to plan of care.

DISCHARGE PLANNING

- Long-term needs and who is responsible for actions to be taken.
- Specific referrals made.

SAMPLE NURSING OUTCOMES & INTERVENTIONS CLASSIFICATIONS (NOC/NIC)

NOC—Sleep
NIC—Sleep Enhancement

Sleep Pattern, disturbed

Taxonomy II: Activity/Rest—Class 1 Sleep/Rest (00095)
[Diagnostic Division: Activity/Rest]
Nursing Diagnosis Extension and Classification (NDEC)
Revision 1998

Definition: Time-limited disruption of sleep (natural, periodic suspension of consciousness) amount and quality

Related Factors

PSYCHOLOGICAL

Daytime activity pattern; fatigue; dietary; body temperature
Social schedule inconsistent with chronotype; shift work;
    daylight/darkness exposure
Frequently changing sleep-wake schedule/travel across time zones;
    circadian asynchrony
Childhood onset; aging-related sleep shifts; periodic gender-related
    hormonal shifts
Inadequate sleep hygiene; maladaptive conditioned wakefulness

---

Information that appears in brackets has been added by the authors
to clarify and enhance the use of nursing diagnoses.

Ruminative presleep thoughts; anticipation; thinking about home
Preoccupation with trying to sleep; fear of insomnia
Biochemical agents; medications; sustained use of antisleep agents
Temperament; loneliness; grief; anxiety; fear; boredom; depression
Separation from SO(s); loss of sleep partner, life change
Delayed or advanced sleep phase syndrome

ENVIRONMENTAL

Excessive stimulation; noise; lighting; ambient temperature, humidity; noxious odors; sleep partner
Unfamiliar sleep furnishings
Interruptions for therapeutics, monitoring, laboratory tests; other-generated awakening
Physical restraint
Lack of sleep privacy/control

PARENTAL

Mother's sleep-wake pattern/emotional support
Parent-infant interaction

PHYSIOLOGICAL

Position
Gastroesophageal reflux; nausea
Shortness of breath; stasis of secretions; fever
Urinary urgency, incontinence

Defining Characteristics

SUBJECTIVE

Verbal complaints [reports] of difficulty falling asleep/not feeling well rested; dissatisfaction with sleep
Sleep onset greater than 30 minutes
Three or more nighttime awakenings; prolonged awakenings
Awakening earlier or later than desired; early morning insomnia
Decreased ability to function; [falling asleep during activities]

OBJECTIVE

Less than age-normed total sleep time
Increased proportion of stage 1 sleep
Decreased proportion of stages 3 and 4 sleep (e.g., hyporesponsiveness, excess sleepiness, decreased motivation)
Decreased proportion of REM sleep (e.g., REM rebound, hyperactivity, emotional lability, agitation and impulsivity, atypical polysomnographic features)
Sleep maintenance insomnia
Self-induced impairment of normal pattern
[Changes in behavior and performance (increasing irritability, disorientation, listlessness, restlessness, lethargy)]
[Physical signs (mild fleeting nystagmus, ptosis of eyelid, slight hand tremor, expressionless face, dark circles under eyes, changes in posture, frequent yawning)]

Desired Outcomes/Evaluation Criteria—Client Will:

- Verbalize understanding of sleep disturbance.
- Identify individually appropriate interventions to promote sleep.
- Adjust lifestyle to accommodate chronobiological rhythms.
- Report improvement in sleep/rest pattern.
- Report increased sense of well-being and feeling rested.

Actions/Interventions

NURSING PRIORITY NO. **1.** To identify causative/contributing factors:

- Identify presence of factors as listed in Related Factors, including factors that can contribute to insomnia (such as chronic pain); metabolic diseases (such as hyperthyroidism and diabetes); prescribed/OTC drug use; aging (**a high percentage of elderly are affected by sleep problems**).
- Assess sleep pattern disturbances that are associated with specific underlying illnesses (e.g., nocturia occurring with benign prostatic hypertrophy).
- Observe parent-infant interactions/provision of emotional support. Note mother's sleep-wake pattern. **Lack of knowledge of infant cues/problem relationships may create tension interfering with sleep. Structured sleep routines based on adult schedules may not meet child's needs.**
- Ascertain presence/frequency of enuresis.
- Review psychologic assessment, noting individual and personality characteristics.
- Determine recent traumatic events in client's life (e.g., a death in family, loss of job).
- Evaluate use of caffeine and alcoholic beverages (**overindulgence interferes with REM sleep**).
- Assist with diagnostic testing (e.g., EEG, sleep studies).

NURSING PRIORITY NO. **2.** To evaluate sleep pattern and dysfunction(s):

- Observe and/or obtain feedback from client/SO(s) regarding usual bedtime, rituals/routines, number of hours of sleep, time of arising, and environmental needs **to determine usual sleep pattern and provide comparative baseline.**
- Determine client's/SO's expectations of adequate sleep. **Provides opportunity to address misconceptions/unrealistic expectations.**
- Investigate whether client snores and in what position(s) this occurs.
- Listen to subjective reports of sleep quality.
- Identify circumstances that interrupt sleep and frequency.

- Note alteration of habitual sleep time such as change of work pattern/rotating shifts, change in normal bedtime (hospitalization).
- Observe physical signs of fatigue (e.g., restlessness, hand tremors, thick speech).
- Do a chronological chart **to determine peak performance rhythm.**
- Graph "circadian" rhythms of individual's biological internal chemistry per protocol as indicated. (**Note: Studies have shown sleep cycles are affected by body temperature at onset of sleep.**)

NURSING PRIORITY NO. 3. To assist client to establish optimal sleep/rest patterns:

- Arrange care to provide for uninterrupted periods for rest, especially allowing for longer periods of sleep at night when possible. Do as much care as possible without waking client.
- Explain necessity of disturbances for monitoring vital signs and/or other care when client is hospitalized.
- Provide quiet environment and comfort measures (e.g., back rub, washing hands/face, cleaning and straightening sheets) in preparation for sleep.
- Discuss/implement effective age-appropriate bedtime rituals (e.g., going to bed at same time each night, drinking warm milk, rocking, story reading, cuddling, favorite blanket/toy) **to enhance client's ability to fall asleep, reinforce that bed is a place to sleep, and promote sense of security for child.**
- Recommend limiting intake of chocolate and caffeine/alcoholic beverages, especially prior to bedtime.
- Limit fluid intake in evening if nocturia is a problem **to reduce need for nighttime elimination.**
- Explore other sleep aids (e.g., warm bath/milk, protein intake before bedtime).
- Administer pain medications (if required) 1 hour before sleep **to relieve discomfort and take maximum advantage of sedative effect.**
- Monitor effects of drug regimen—amphetamines or stimulants (e.g., Methylphenidate—Ritalin used in narcolepsy).
- Use barbiturates and/or other sleeping medications sparingly. **Research indicates long-term use of these medications can actually induce sleep disturbances.**
- Develop behavioral program for insomnia:
  Establish routine bedtime and arising.
  Think relaxing thoughts when in bed.
  Do not nap in the daytime.
  Do not read in bed; get out of bed if not asleep in 15 minutes.
  Limit sleep to 7 hours a night.
  Get up the same time each day—even on weekends/days off.

- Assure client that occasional sleeplessness should not threaten health.

NURSING PRIORITY NO. 4. To promote wellness (Teaching/Discharge Considerations):

- Assist client to develop individual program of relaxation. Demonstrate techniques (e.g., biofeedback, self-hypnosis, visualization, progressive muscle relaxation).
- Encourage participation in regular exercise program during day **to aid in stress control/release of energy. Exercise at bedtime may stimulate rather than relax client and actually interfere with sleep.**
- Recommend inclusion of bedtime snack (e.g., milk or mild juice, crackers, protein source such as cheese/peanut butter) in dietary program **to reduce sleep interference from hunger/hypoglycemia.**
- Suggest that bed/bedroom be used only for sleep, not for working, watching TV.
- Provide for child's (or impaired individual's) sleep time safety (e.g., infant placed on back, bedrails/bed in low position, nonplastic sheets).
- Investigate use of aids to block out light/noise, such as sleep mask, darkening shades/curtains, earplugs, monotonous sounds such as low-level background noise (white noise).
- Participate in program to "reset" the body's sleep clock (chronotherapy) **when client has delayed sleep-onset insomnia.**
- Assist individual to develop schedules that take advantage of peak performance times as identified in chronobiological chart.
- Recommend midmorning nap if one is required. **Napping, especially in the afternoon, can disrupt normal sleep patterns.**
- Assist client to deal with grieving process when loss has occurred. (Refer to ND Grieving, dysfunctional.)
- Refer to sleep specialist/laboratory for treatment when indicated.

Documentation Focus

ASSESSMENT/REASSESSMENT

- Assessment findings, including specifics of sleep pattern (current and past) and effects on lifestyle/level of functioning.
- Medications/interventions, previous therapies

PLANNING

- Plan of care and who is involved in planning.
- Teaching plan.

IMPLEMENTATION/EVALUATION

- Client's response to interventions/teaching and actions performed.
- Attainment/progress toward desired outcome(s).
- Modifications to plan of care.

DISCHARGE PLANNING

- Long-term needs and who is responsible for actions to be taken.
- Specific referrals made.

SAMPLE NURSING OUTCOMES & INTERVENTIONS CLASSIFICATIONS (NOC/NIC)

NOC—Sleep
NIC—Sleep Enhancement

Sleep, readiness for enhanced

Taxonomy II: Activity/Rest—Class 1 Sleep/Rest (00165)
[Diagnostic Division: Activity/Rest]
Submitted 2002

Definition: A pattern of natural, periodic suspension of consciousness that provides adequate rest, sustains a desired lifestyle, and can be strengthened

Related Factors

To be developed

Defining Characteristics

SUBJECTIVE

Expresses willingness to enhance sleep
Expresses a feeling of being rested after sleep
Follows sleep routines that promote sleep habits

OBJECTIVE

Amount of sleep and REM sleep is congruent with developmental needs
Occasional or infrequent use of medications to induce sleep

Desired Outcomes/Evaluation Criteria—Client Will:

- Identify individually appropriate interventions to promote sleep.

Information that appears in brackets has been added by the authors to clarify and enhance the use of nursing diagnoses.

- Verbalize feeling rested after sleep.
- Adjust lifestyle to accommodate routines that promote sleep.

Actions/Interventions

NURSING PRIORITY NO. **1.** To determine motivation for continued growth:

- Listen to client's reports of sleep quantity and quality. Determine client's/SO's expectations of adequate sleep. **Reveals client's experience and expectations. Provides opportunity to address misconceptions/unrealistic expectations and plan for interventions.**
- Observe and/or obtain feedback from client/SO(s) regarding usual bedtime, desired rituals and routines, number of hours of sleep, time of arising, and environmental needs **to determine usual sleep pattern and provide comparative baseline for improvements.**
- Note client report of potential for alteration of habitual sleep time (e.g., change of work pattern/rotating shifts) or change in normal bedtime (e.g., hospitalization). **Helps identify circumstances that are known to interrupt sleep patterns and which could disrupt the person's biological rhythms.**

NURSING PRIORITY NO. **2.** To assist client to enhance sleep/rest:

- Discuss adult client's usual bedtime rituals, expectations for obtaining good sleep time. **Provides information on client's management of the situation and identifies areas that might be modified.**
- Discuss/implement effective age-appropriate bedtime rituals for infant/child (e.g., rocking, story reading, cuddling, favorite blanket/toy). **Rituals can enhance ability to fall asleep, reinforces that bed is a place to sleep and promote sense of security for child.**
- Assist client in use of necessary equipment, instructing as necessary. **Client may use oxygen or CPAP system to improve sleep/rest if hypoxia or sleep apnea diagnosed.**
- Investigate use of sleep mask, darkening shades/curtains, earplugs, low-level background (white) noise. **Aids in blocking out light and disturbing noise.**
- Arrange care **to provide for uninterrupted periods for rest.** Explain necessity of disturbances for monitoring vital signs and/or other care when client is hospitalized. Do as much care as possible without waking client, during night. **Allows for longer periods of uninterrupted sleep, especially during night.**
- Provide quiet environment and comfort measures (e.g., back rub, washing hands/face, cleaning and straightening sheets). **Promotes relaxation and readiness for sleep.**

- Explore/implement use of warm bath, comfortable room temperature, use of soothing music, favorite calming TV show. **Nonpharmaceutical aids may enhance falling asleep.**
- Recommend limiting intake of chocolate and caffeine/alcoholic beverages, especially prior to bedtime. **Substances known to impair falling or staying asleep. Use of alcohol at bedtime may help individual fall asleep, but ensuing sleep is then fragmented.**
- Limit fluid intake in evening if nocturia or bedwetting is a problem **to reduce need for nighttime elimination.**

NURSING PRIORITY NO. **3.** To promote optimum wellness:

- Assure client that occasional sleeplessness should not threaten health. **Knowledge that occasional insomnia is universal and usually not harmful, may promote relaxation and relief from worry.**
- Encourage client to develop individual program of relaxation (e.g., biofeedback, self-hypnosis, visualization, progressive muscle relaxation). **Methods that reduce sympathetic response and decrease stress can help in inducing sleep, particularly in persons suffering from chronic and long-term sleep disturbances.**
- Encourage participation in regular exercise program during day **to aid in stress control/release of energy. Note: Exercise at bedtime may stimulate rather than relax client and actually interfere with sleep.**
- Recommend inclusion of bedtime snack (e.g., milk or mild juice, crackers, protein source, such as cheese/peanut butter) in dietary program **to reduce sleep interference from hunger/hypoglycemia.**
- Advise using barbiturates and/or other sleeping medications sparingly. **These medications, while useful for promoting sleep in the short-term, can interfere with REM sleep.**

Documentation Focus

ASSESSMENT/REASSESSMENT

- Assessment findings, including specifics of sleep pattern (current and past) and effects on lifestyle/level of functioning.
- Medications/interventions, previous therapies.

PLANNING

- Plan of care and who is involved in planning.
- Teaching plan.

IMPLEMENTATION/EVALUATION

- Client's response to interventions/teaching and actions performed.

- Attainment/progress toward desired outcome(s).
- Modifications to plan of care.

DISCHARGE PLANNING

- Long-term needs and who is responsible for actions to be taken.
- Specific referrals made.

SAMPLE NURSING OUTCOMES & INTERVENTIONS CLASSIFICATION (NOC/NIC)

NOC—Sleep
NIC—Sleep Enhancement

Social Interaction, impaired

Taxonomy II: Role Relationship—Class 3 Role Performance (00052)
[Diagnostic Division: Social Interaction]
Submitted 1986

Definition: Insufficient or excessive quantity or ineffective quality of social exchange

Related Factors

Knowledge/skill deficit about ways to enhance mutuality
Communication barriers [including head injury, stroke, other neurological conditions affecting ability to communicate]
Self-concept disturbance
Absence of available SO(s) or peers
Limited physical mobility [e.g., neuromuscular disease]
Therapeutic isolation
Sociocultural dissonance
Environmental barriers
Altered thought processes

Defining Characteristics

SUBJECTIVE

Verbalized discomfort in social situations
Verbalized inability to receive or communicate a satisfying sense of belonging, caring, interest, or shared history
Family report of change of style or pattern of interaction

OBJECTIVE

Observed discomfort in social situations
Observed inability to receive or communicate a satisfying sense of belonging, caring, interest, or shared history

---

Information that appears in brackets has been added by the authors to clarify and enhance the use of nursing diagnoses.

Observed use of unsuccessful social interaction behaviors
Dysfunctional interaction with peers, family, and/or others

Desired Outcomes/Evaluation Criteria—Client Will:

- Verbalize awareness of factors causing or promoting impaired social interactions.
- Identify feelings that lead to poor social interactions.
- Express desire/be involved in achieving positive changes in social behaviors and interpersonal relationships.
- Give self positive reinforcement for changes that are achieved.
- Develop effective social support system; use available resources appropriately.

Actions/Interventions

NURSING PRIORITY NO. 1. To assess causative/contributing factors:

- Review social history with client/SO(s) and go back far enough in time to note when changes in social behavior or patterns of relating occurred/began, for example, loss or long-term illness of loved one; failed relationships; loss of occupation, financial, or political (power) position; change in status in family hierarchy (job loss, aging, illness); poor coping/adjustment to developmental stage of life, as with marriage, birth/adoption of child, or children leaving home.
- Ascertain ethnic/cultural or religious implications for the client **because these impact choice of behaviors.**
- Review medical history noting stressors of physical/long-term illness (e.g., stroke, cancer, MS, head injury, Alzheimer's disease), mental illness (e.g., schizophrenia), medications/drugs, debilitating accidents.
- Determine family patterns of relating and social behaviors. Explore possible family scripting of behavioral expectations in the children and how the client was affected. (**May result in conforming or rebellious behaviors.**)
- Observe client while relating to family/SO(s) and note observations of prevalent patterns.
- Encourage client to verbalize feeling of discomfort about social situations. Note any causative factors, recurring precipitating patterns, and barriers to using support systems.
- Note effects of changes on socioeconomic level, ethnic/religious practices.

NURSING PRIORITY NO. 2. To assess degree of impairment:

- Encourage client to verbalize problems and perceptions of reasons for problems. Active-listen to note indications of hopelessness, powerlessness, fear, anxiety, grief, anger, feeling unloved or unlovable; problems with sexual identity; hate (directed or not).

- Observe and describe social/interpersonal behaviors in objective terms, noting speech patterns, body language (a) in the therapeutic setting and (b) in normal areas of daily functioning (if possible): family, job, social/entertainment settings.
- Determine client's use of coping skills and defense mechanisms. **(Affects ability to be involved in social situations.)**
- Evaluate possibility of client being the victim of or using destructive behaviors against self or others. (Refer to ND Violence, [actual/]risk for other-directed/self-directed.)
- Interview family, SO(s), friends, spiritual leaders, coworkers, as appropriate, **to obtain observations of client's behavioral changes.**

NURSING PRIORITY NO. 3. To assist client/SO(s) to recognize/ make positive changes in impaired social and interpersonal interactions:

- Establish therapeutic relationship using positive regard for the person, Active-listening, and providing safe environment for self-disclosure.
- Have client list behaviors that cause discomfort. **Once recognized, client can choose to change.**
- Have family/SO(s) list client's behaviors that are causing discomfort for them.
- Review/list negative behaviors observed previously by caregivers, coworkers, and so forth.
- Compare lists and validate reality of perceptions. Help client prioritize those behaviors needing change.
- Explore with client and role-play means of making changes in social interactions/behaviors (as determined earlier).
- Role-play random social situations in therapeutically controlled environment with "safe" therapy group. Have group note behaviors, both positive and negative, and discuss these and any changes needed.
- Role-play changes and discuss impact. Include family/SO(s) as indicated. **Enhances comfort with new behaviors.**
- Provide positive reinforcement for improvement in social behaviors and interactions. **Encourages continuation of desired behaviors/efforts for change.**
- Participate in multidisciplinary client-centered conferences to evaluate progress. Involve everyone associated with client's care, family members, SO(s), and therapy group.
- Work with the client to alleviate underlying negative self-concepts **because they often impede positive social interactions.**
- Involve neurologically impaired client in individual and/or group interactions as situation allows.

- Refer for family therapy as indicated **because social behaviors and interpersonal relationships involve more than the individual.**

NURSING PRIORITY NO. **4.** To promote wellness (Teaching/Discharge Considerations):

- Encourage client to keep a daily journal in which social interactions of each day can be reviewed and the comfort/discomfort experienced noted with possible causes/precipitating factors. **Helps client to identify responsibility for own behavior(s).**
- Assist the client to develop positive social skills through practice of skills in real social situations accompanied by a support person. Provide positive feedback during interactions with client.
- Seek community programs for client involvement that promote positive behaviors the client is striving to achieve.
- Encourage classes, reading materials, community support groups, and lectures for self-help in alleviating negative self-concepts that lead to impaired social interactions.
- Encourage ongoing family or individual therapy as long as it is promoting growth and positive change. (Be alert to possibility of therapy being used as a crutch.)
- Provide for occasional follow-up **for reinforcement of positive behaviors after professional relationship has ended.**
- Refer to/involve psychiatric clinical nurse specialist for additional assistance when indicated.

Documentation Focus

ASSESSMENT/REASSESSMENT

- Individual findings, including factors affecting interactions, nature of social exchanges, specifics of individual behaviors.
- Perceptions/response of others.

PLANNING

- Plan of care and who is involved in the planning.
- Teaching plan.

IMPLEMENTATION/EVALUATION

- Responses to interventions/teaching and actions performed.
- Attainment/progress toward desired outcome(s).
- Modifications to plan of care.

DISCHARGE PLANNING

- Long-term needs and who is responsible for actions to be taken.
- Community resources, specific referrals made.

NOC—Social Interaction Skills
NIC—Socialization Enhancement

Social Isolation

Taxonomy II: Comfort—Class 3 Social Comfort (00053)
[Diagnostic Division: Social Interaction]
Submitted 1982

Definition: Aloneness experienced by the individual
and perceived as imposed by others and as a negative
or threatened state

Related Factors

Factors contributing to the absence of satisfying personal relationships
   (e.g., delay in accomplishing developmental tasks); immature
   interests
Alterations in physical appearance/mental status
Altered state of wellness
Unaccepted social behavior/values
Inadequate personal resources
Inability to engage in satisfying personal relationships
[Traumatic incidents or events causing physical and/or emotional
   pain]

Defining Characteristics

SUBJECTIVE

Expresses feelings of aloneness imposed by others
Expresses feelings of rejection
Expresses values acceptable to the subculture but unacceptable to the
   dominant cultural group
Inability to meet expectations of others
Experiences feelings of difference from others
Inadequacy in or absence of significant purpose in life
Expresses interests inappropriate to developmental age/stage
Insecurity in public

OBJECTIVE

Absence of supportive SO(s)—family, friends, group
Sad, dull affect
Inappropriate or immature interests/activities for developmental
   age/stage
Hostility projected in voice, behavior
Evidence of physical/mental handicap or altered state of wellness
Uncommunicative; withdrawn; no eye contact

Information that appears in brackets has been added by the authors
to clarify and enhance the use of nursing diagnoses.

Preoccupation with own thoughts; repetitive meaningless actions
Seeking to be alone or existing in a subculture
Showing behavior unaccepted by dominant cultural group

Desired Outcomes/Evaluation Criteria—Client Will:

- Identify causes and actions to correct isolation.
- Verbalize willingness to be involved with others.
- Participate in activities/programs at level of ability/desire.
- Express increased sense of self-worth.

Actions/Interventions

NURSING PRIORITY NO. 1. To assess causative/contributing factors:

- Determine presence of factors as listed in Related Factors and other concerns (e.g., elderly; female; adolescent; ethnic/racial minority; economically/educationally disadvantaged).
- Identify blocks to social contacts (e.g., physical immobility, sensory deficits, housebound, incontinence).
- Assess factors in client's life that may contribute to sense of helplessness (e.g., loss of spouse/parent).
- Listen to comments of client regarding sense of isolation. Differentiate isolation from solitude and loneliness **which may be acceptable or by choice.**
- Assess client's feelings about self, sense of ability to control situation, sense of hope, and coping skills.
- Identify support systems available to the client including presence of/relationship with extended family.
- Determine drug use (legal/illicit).
- Identify behavior response of isolation (e.g., excessive sleeping/daydreaming, substance use), **which also may potentiate isolation.**
- Review history and elicit information about traumatic events that may have occurred. (Refer to ND Post-Trauma Syndrome.)

NURSING PRIORITY NO. 2. To alleviate conditions that contribute to client's sense of isolation:

- Establish therapeutic nurse-client relationship. **Promotes trust, allowing client to feel free to discuss sensitive matters.**
- Note onset of physical/mental illness and where recovery is anticipated or condition is chronic/progressive.
- Spend time visiting with client, and identify other resources available (e.g., volunteer, social worker, chaplain).
- Develop plan of action with client: Look at available resources; support risk-taking behaviors, financial planning, appropriate medical care/self-care, and so forth.

- Introduce client to those with similar/shared interests and other supportive people. **Provides role models, encourages problem solving.**
- Provide positive reinforcement when client makes move(s) toward other(s). **Encourages continuation of efforts.**
- Provide for placement in sheltered community when necessary.
- Assist client to problem-solve solutions to short-term/imposed isolation (e.g., communicable disease measures, including compromised host).
- Encourage open visitation when possible and/or telephone contacts **to maintain involvement with others.**
- Provide environmental stimuli (e.g., open curtains, pictures, TV, and radio).
- Promote participation in recreational/special interest activities in setting that client views as safe.
- Identify foreign-language resources, such as interpreter, newspaper, radio programming, as appropriate.

NURSING PRIORITY NO. 3. To promote wellness (Teaching/Discharge Considerations):

- Assist client to learn skills (e.g., problem solving, communication, social skills, self-esteem, ADLs).
- Encourage and assist client to enroll in classes as needed (e.g., assertiveness, vocational, sex education).
- Help client differentiate between isolation and loneliness/aloneness and not slip into an undesired state.
- Involve client in programs directed to correction and prevention of identified causes of problem (e.g., senior citizen services, daily telephone contact, house sharing, pets, day-care centers, church resources).
- Refer to therapists as appropriate **to facilitate grief work, relationship building, and so on.**
- Involve children and adolescents in programs/activities **to promote socialization skills and peer contact.**

Documentation Focus

ASSESSMENT/REASSESSMENT

- Individual findings, including precipitating factors, effect on lifestyle/relationships, and functioning.
- Client's perception of situation.

PLANNING

- Plan of care and who is involved in planning.
- Teaching plan.

IMPLEMENTATION/EVALUATION

- Responses to interventions/teaching and actions performed.
- Attainment/progress toward desired outcome(s).
- Modifications to plan of care.

DISCHARGE PLANNING

- Long-term needs/referrals and who is responsible for actions to be taken.
- Available resources, specific referrals made.

SAMPLE NURSING OUTCOMES & INTERVENTIONS CLASSIFICATIONS (NOC/NIC)

NOC—Social Involvement
NIC—Social Enhancement

Sorrow, chronic

Taxonomy II: Coping/Stress Tolerance—Class 2 Coping Responses (00137)
[Diagnostic Division: Ego Integrity]
Submitted1998

Definition: Cyclical, recurring, and potentially progressive pattern of pervasive sadness experienced (by a parent or caregiver, individual with chronic illness or disability) in response to continual loss, throughout the trajectory of an illness or disability

Related Factors

Death of a loved one
Experiences chronic physical or mental illness or disability (e.g., mental retardation, MS, prematurity, spina bifida or other birth defects, chronic mental illness, infertility, cancer, Parkinson's disease); one or more trigger events (e.g., crises in management of the illness, crises related to developmental stages, missed opportunities or milestones that bring comparisons with developmental, social, or personal norms)
Unending caregiving as a constant reminder of loss

Defining Characteristics

SUBJECTIVE

Expresses one or more of the following feelings: anger, being misunderstood, confusion, depression, disappointment, emptiness, fear, frustration, guilt/self-blame, helplessness, hopelessness, loneliness, low self-esteem, recurring loss, overwhelmed
Client expresses periodic, recurrent feelings of sadness

Information that appears in brackets has been added by the authors to clarify and enhance the use of nursing diagnoses.

OBJECTIVE

Feelings that vary in intensity, are periodic, may progress and intensify over time, and may interfere with the client's ability to reach his or her highest level of personal and social well-being

Desired Outcomes/Evaluation Criteria—Client Will:

- Acknowledge presence/impact of sorrow.
- Demonstrate progress in dealing with grief.
- Participate in work and/or self-care ADLs as able.
- Verbalize a sense of progress toward resolution of sorrow and hope for the future.

Actions/Interventions

NURSING PRIORITY NO. 1. To assess causative/contributing factors:

- Determine current/recent events or conditions contributing to client's state of mind, as listed in Related Factors (e.g., death of loved one, chronic physical or mental illness or disability, etc.).
- Look for cues of sadness (e.g., sighing, faraway look, unkempt appearance, inattention to conversation, refusing food, etc.).
- Determine level of functioning, ability to care for self.
- Be aware of avoidance behaviors (e.g., anger, withdrawal, denial).
- Identify cultural factors/religious conflicts.
- Ascertain response of family/SO(s) to client's situation. Assess needs of family/SO.
- Refer to Grieving, dysfunctional; Caregiver Role Strain; Coping, ineffective, as appropriate.

NURSING PRIORITY NO. 2. To assist client to move through sorrow:

- Encourage verbalization about situation (helpful in beginning resolution and acceptance). Active-listen feelings and be available for support/assistance.
- Encourage expression of anger/fear/anxiety. Refer to appropriate NDs.
- Acknowledge reality of feelings of guilt/blame, including hostility toward spiritual power. (Refer to ND Spiritual Distress.) **Helps client to take steps toward resolution.**
- Provide comfort and availability as well as caring for physical needs.
- Discuss ways individual has dealt with previous losses. Reinforce use of previously effective coping skills.
- Instruct/encourage use of visualization and relaxation skills.

- Assist SO to cope with client response. (Family/SO may not be dysfunctional but may be intolerant.)
- Include family/SO in setting realistic goals for meeting individual needs.

NURSING PRIORITY NO. **3**. To promote wellness (Teaching/ Discharge Considerations):

- Discuss healthy ways of dealing with difficult situations.
- Have client identify familial, religious, and cultural factors that have meaning for him or her. **May help bring loss or distressing situation into perspective and promote grief/ sorrow resolution.**
- Encourage involvement in usual activities, exercise, and socialization within limits of physical and psychological state.
- Introduce concept of mindfulness (living in the moment). **Promotes feelings of capability and belief that this moment can be dealt with.**
- Refer to other resources (e.g., pastoral care, counseling, psychotherapy, respite-care providers, support groups). **Provides additional help when needed to resolve situation, continue grief work.**

Documentation Focus

ASSESSMENT/REASSESSMENT

- Physical/emotional response to conflict.
- Reactions of family/SO.

PLANNING

- Plan of care and who is involved in planning.
- Teaching plan.

IMPLEMENTATION/EVALUATION

- Response to interventions/teaching and actions performed.
- Attainment/progress toward desired outcome(s).
- Modifications to plan of care.

DISCHARGE PLANNING

- Long-term needs and who is responsible for actions to be taken.
- Available resources, specific referrals made.

SAMPLE NURSING OUTCOMES & INTERVENTIONS CLASSIFICATIONS (NOC/NIC)

NOC—Depression Level
NIC—Hope Instillation

Spiritual Distress

Taxonomy II: Life Principles—Class 3 Value/Belief/Action
Congruence (00066)
[Diagnostic Division: Ego Integrity]
Submitted 1978; Revised 2002

Definition: Impaired ability to experience and integrate
meaning and purpose in life through a person's connectedness with self, others, art, music, literature, nature, or
a power greater than oneself.

Related Factors

Loneliness/social alienation; self-alienation; sociocultural deprivation
Anxiety; pain
Life change
Chronic illness of self or others; death and dying of self or others
[Challenged belief/value system (e.g., moral/ethical implications of
therapy)]

Defining Characteristics

SUBJECTIVE

Connections to Self
Expresses lack of: Hope; meaning and purpose in life; peace/
serenity; love; acceptance; forgiveness of self; courage
[Expresses] anger; guilt
Connections to Others
Refuses interactions with friends, family/spiritual leaders
Verbalizes being separated from their support system
Expresses alienation
Connections with Art, Music, Literature, Nature
Inability to express previous state of creativity (singing/
listening to music/writing)
No interest in nature
No interest in reading spiritual literature
Connections with Power Greater Than Self
Inability to pray/participate in religious activities; sudden
changes in spiritual practices
Expresses being abandoned by or having anger toward God;
without hope, suffering
Request to see a religious leader

OBJECTIVE

Connections to Self
Poor coping
Connections with Power Greater Than Self
Inability to be introspective/inward turning; to experience
the transcendent

Information that appears in brackets has been added by the authors
490 to clarify and enhance the use of nursing diagnoses.

Desired Outcomes/Evaluation Criteria—Client Will:

- Verbalize increased sense of connectedness and hope for future.
- Demonstrate ability to help self/participate in care.
- Participate in activities with others, actively seek relationships.
- Discuss beliefs/values about spiritual issues.
- Verbalize acceptance of self as not deserving illness/situation, "no one is to blame."

Actions/Interventions

NURSING PRIORITY NO. 1. To assess causative/contributing factors:

- Determine client's religious/spiritual orientation, current involvement, presence of conflicts. **Individual spiritual practices/restrictions may affect client care or create conflict between spiritual beliefs and treatment.**
- Listen to client/SO's reports/expressions of anger/concern, alienation from God, belief that illness/situation is a punishment for wrongdoing, and so forth. **Identifies need for spiritual advisor to address client's belief system.**
- Determine sense of futility, feelings of hopelessness and helplessness, lack of motivation to help self. **Indicators that client may see no, or only limited, options/alternatives or personal choices available and lacks energy to deal with situation.**
- Note expressions of inability to find meaning in life, reason for living. Evaluate suicidal ideation. **Crisis of the spirit/loss of will-to-live places client at increased risk for inattention to personal well-being/harm to self.**
- Note recent changes in behavior (e.g., withdrawal from others/creative or religious activities, dependence on alcohol/medications). **Helpful in determining severity/duration of situation and possible need for additional referrals, such as substance withdrawal.**
- Assess sense of self-concept, worth, ability to enter into loving relationships. **Lack of connectedness with self/others impairs client's ability to trust others or feel worthy of trust from others.**
- Observe behavior indicative of poor relationships with others (e.g., manipulative, nontrusting, demanding). **Manipulation is used for management of client's sense of powerlessness because of distrust of others.**
- Determine support systems available to client/SO(s) and how they are used. **Provides insight to client's willingness to pursue outside resources.**

- Be aware of influence of caregiver's belief system. (**It is still possible to be helpful to client while remaining neutral/not espousing own beliefs.**)

NURSING PRIORITY NO. **2.** To assist client/SO(s) to deal with feelings/situation:

- Develop therapeutic nurse-client relationship. Ask how you can be most helpful. Convey acceptance of client's spiritual beliefs/concerns. **Promotes trust and comfort, encouraging client to be open about sensitive matters.**
- Identify inappropriate coping behaviors and associated consequences. **Recognizing consequences of actions may enhance desire to change.**
- Ascertain past coping behaviors **to determine approaches used previously that may be more effective in dealing with current situation.**
- Problem-solve solutions/identify areas for compromise **that may be useful in resolving possible conflicts.**
- Establish environment that promotes free expression of feelings and concerns.
- Provide calm, peaceful setting when possible. **Promotes relaxation and enhances opportunity for reflection on situation/discussions with others, meditation.**
- Set limits on acting-out behavior that is inappropriate/destructive. **Promotes safety for client/others and helps prevent loss of self-esteem.**
- Make time for nonjudgmental discussion of philosophic issues/questions about spiritual impact of illness/situation and/or treatment regimen. **Open communication can assist client in reality checks of perceptions and identifying personal options.**
- Involve client in refining healthcare goals and therapeutic regimen as appropriate. **Enhances commitment to plan, optimizing outcomes.**
- Discuss difference between grief and guilt and help client to identify and deal with each. Point out consequences of actions based on guilt. **Aids client in assuming responsibility for own actions and avoiding acting out of false guilt.**
- Use therapeutic communication skills of reflection and Active-listening. **Helps client find own solutions to concerns.**
- Identify role models (e.g., nurse, individual experiencing similar situation). **Provides opportunities for sharing of experiences/hope and identifying options to deal with situation.**
- Suggest use of journaling. **Can assist in clarifying values/ideas, recognizing and resolving feelings/situation.**
- Assist client to learn use of meditation/prayer and forgiveness **to heal past hurts.**

- Provide information that anger with God is a normal part of the grieving process. **Realizing these feelings are not unusual can reduce sense of guilt, encourage open expression, and facilitate resolution of conflict.**
- Provide time and privacy to engage in spiritual growth/religious activities (e.g., prayer, meditation, scripture reading, listening to music). **Allows client to focus on self and seek connectedness.**
- Encourage/facilitate outings to neighborhood park/nature walks. **Sunshine, fresh air and activity can stimulate release of endorphins promoting sense of well-being.**
- Provide play therapy for child that encompasses spiritual data. **Interactive pleasurable activity promotes open discussion and enhances retention of information. Also provides opportunity for child to practice what has been learned.**
- Abide by parents' wishes in discussing and implementing child's spiritual support. **Limits confusion for child and prevents conflict of values/beliefs.**
- Refer to appropriate resources (e.g., pastoral/parish nurse or religious counselor, crisis counselor, hospice; psychotherapy; Alcoholics/Narcotics Anonymous). **Useful in dealing with immediate situation and identifying long-term resources for support to help foster sense of connectedness.**
- Refer to NDs Coping, ineffective; Powerlessness; Self-Esteem [specify]; Social Isolation; Suicide, risk for.

NURSING PRIORITY NO. 3. To promote wellness (Teaching/ Discharge Considerations):

- Assist client to develop goals for dealing with life/illness situation. **Enhances commitment to goal, optimizing outcomes.**
- Encourage life-review by client. Help client find a reason for living. **Promotes sense of hope and willingness to continue efforts to improve situation.**
- Assist in developing coping skills **to deal with stressors of illness/necessary changes in lifestyle.**
- Assist client to identify SO(s) and people who could provide support as needed. **Ongoing support is required to enhance sense of connectedness and continue progress toward goals.**
- Assist client to identify spiritual resources that could be helpful (e.g., contact spiritual advisor who has qualifications/ experience in dealing with specific problems, such as death/dying, relationship problems, substance abuse, suicide). **Provides answers to spiritual questions, assists in the journey of self-discovery, and can help client learn to accept and forgive self.**

Documentation Focus

ASSESSMENT/REASSESSMENT

- Individual findings, including nature of spiritual conflict, effects of participation in treatment regimen.
- Physical/emotional responses to conflict.

PLANNING

- Plan of care and who is involved in planning.
- Teaching plan.

IMPLEMENTATION/EVALUATION

- Responses to interventions/teaching and actions performed.
- Attainment/progress toward desired outcome(s).
- Modifications to plan of care.

DISCHARGE PLANNING

- Long-term needs and who is responsible for actions to be taken.
- Available resources, specific referrals made.

SAMPLE NURSING OUTCOMES & INTERVENTIONS CLASSIFICATION (NOC/NIC)

NOC—Spiritual Well-Being
NIC—Spiritual Support

Spiritual Distress, risk for

Taxonomy II: Life Principles—Class 3 Value/Belief/Action Congruence (00067)
[Diagnostic Division: Ego Integrity]
Nursing Diagnosis Extension and Classification (NDEC) Submission 1998

Definition: At risk for an altered sense of harmonious connectedness with all of life and the universe in which dimensions that transcend and empower the self may be disrupted

Risk Factors

Physical or psychological stress; energy-consuming anxiety; physical/mental illness
Situation/maturational losses; loss of loved one
Blocks to self-love; low self-esteem; poor relationships; inability to forgive
Substance abuse
Natural disasters

Information that appears in brackets has been added by the authors to clarify and enhance the use of nursing diagnoses.

NOTE: A risk diagnosis is not evidenced by signs and symptoms, as the problem has not occurred and nursing interventions are directed at prevention.

Desired Outcomes/Evaluation Criteria—Client Will:

- Identify meaning and purpose in one's life that reinforces hope, peace, and contentment.
- Verbalize acceptance of self as being worthy, not deserving of illness/situation, and so forth.
- Identify and use resources appropriately.

Actions/Interventions

NURSING PRIORITY NO. 1. To assess causative/contributing factors:

- Ascertain current situation (e.g., natural disaster, death of a spouse, personal injustice).
- Listen to client's/SO's reports/expressions of anger/concern, belief that illness/situation is a punishment for wrongdoing, and so forth.
- Note reason for living and whether it is directly related to situation (e.g., home and business washed away in a flood, parent whose only child is terminally ill).
- Determine client's religious/spiritual orientation, current involvement, presence of conflicts, especially in current circumstances.
- Assess sense of self-concept, worth, ability to enter into loving relationships.
- Observe behavior indicative of poor relationships with others (e.g., manipulative, nontrusting, demanding).
- Determine support systems available to and used by client/SO(s).
- Ascertain substance use/abuse. (**Affects ability to deal with problems in a positive manner.**)

NURSING PRIORITY NO. 2. To assist client/SO(s) to deal with feeling/situation:

- Establish environment that promotes free expression of feelings and concerns.
- Have client identify and prioritize current/immediate needs. **Helps client focus on what needs to be done and identify manageable steps to take.**
- Make time for nonjudgmental discussion of philosophical issues/questions about spiritual impact of illness/situation and/or treatment regimen.
- Discuss difference between grief and guilt and help client to identify and deal with each, assuming responsibility for own

actions, expressing awareness of the consequences of acting out of false guilt.

- Use therapeutic communication skills of reflection and Active-listening. **Helps client find own solutions to concerns.**
- Review coping skills used and their effectiveness in current situation. **Identifies strengths to incorporate into plan and techniques needing revision.**
- Provide role model (e.g., nurse, individual experiencing similar situation/disease). **Sharing of experiences/hope assists client to deal with reality.**
- Suggest use of journaling. **Can assist in clarifying values/ ideas, recognizing and resolving feelings/situation.**
- Refer to appropriate resources for help (e.g., crisis counselor, governmental agencies; pastoral/parish nurse or spiritual advisor who has qualifications/experience dealing with specific problems, such as death/dying, relationship problems, substance abuse, suicide; hospice, psychotherapy, Alcoholics/Narcotics Anonymous).

NURSING PRIORITY NO. 3. To promote wellness (Teaching/ Discharge Considerations):

- Role-play new coping techniques **to enhance integration of new skills/necessary changes in lifestyle.**
- Assist client to identify SO(s) and individuals/support groups who could provide ongoing support **because this is a daily need requiring lifelong commitment.**
- Abide by parents' wishes in discussing and implementing child's spiritual support.
- Discuss benefit of family counseling as appropriate. **Issues of this nature (e.g., situational losses, natural disasters, difficult relationships) affect family dynamics.**

Documentation Focus

ASSESSMENT/REASSESSMENT

- Individual findings, including risk factors, nature of current distress.
- Physical/emotional responses to distress.
- Access to/use of resources.

PLANNING

- Plan of care and who is involved in planning.
- Teaching plan.

IMPLEMENTATION/EVALUATION

- Responses to interventions/teaching and actions performed.
- Attainment/progress toward desired outcome(s).
- Modifications to plan of care.

- Long-term needs and who is responsible for actions to be taken.
- Available resources, specific referrals made.

SAMPLE NURSING OUTCOMES & INTERVENTIONS CLASSIFICATIONS (NOC/NIC)

NOC—Spiritual Well-Being
NIC—Spiritual Support

Spiritual Well-Being, readiness for enhanced

Taxonomy II: Life Principles—Class 2 Beliefs (00068)
[Diagnostic Division: Ego Integrity]
Submitted 1994; Revised 2002

Definition: Ability to experience and integrate meaning and purpose in life through a person's connectedness with self, others, art, music, literature, nature, or a power greater than oneself

Related Factors

To be developed

Defining Characteristics

SUBJECTIVE

Connections to Self
    Desire for enhanced: Hope; meaning and purpose in life; peace/serenity; acceptance; surrender; love; forgiveness of self; satisfying philosophy of life; joy; courage
    Meditation
Connections with Others
    Requests interactions with friends, family/spiritual leaders
    Provides service to others
    Requests forgiveness of others
Connections with Powers Greater Than Self
    Participates in religious activities; prays
    Expresses reverence, [awe]; reports mystical experiences

OBJECTIVE

Connections to Self
    Heightened coping
Connections with Others
    Provides service to others

Information that appears in brackets has been added by the authors to clarify and enhance the use of nursing diagnoses.

Connections with Art, Music, Literature, Nature
Displays creative energy (e.g., writing, poetry); sings/listens to music; reads spiritual literature; spends time outdoors

Desired Outcomes/Evaluation Criteria—Client Will:

* Acknowledge the stabilizing and strengthening forces in one's life needed for balance and well-being of the whole person.
* Identify meaning and purpose in one's life that reinforces hope, peace, and contentment.
* Verbalize a sense of peace/contentment and comfort of spirit.
* Demonstrate behavior congruent with verbalizations that lend support and strength for daily living.

Actions/Interventions

NURSING PRIORITY NO. 1. To determine spiritual state/motivation for growth:

* Ascertain client's perception of current state/degree of connectedness and expectations. **Provides insight as to where client is currently and what hopes for the future may be.**
* Review spiritual/religious history, activities/rituals and frequency of participation. **Provides basis to build on for growth/change.**
* Determine relational values of support systems to one's spiritual centeredness. **The client's family of origin may have differing beliefs from those espoused by the individual that may be a source of conflict for the client. Comfort can be gained when family and friends share client's beliefs and support search for spiritual knowledge.**
* Explore meaning/interpretation and relationship of spirituality, life/death, and illness to life's journey. **Identifying the meaning of these issues is helpful for the client to use the information in forming a belief system that will enable him or her to move forward and live life to the fullest.**
* Clarify the meaning of one's spiritual beliefs/religious practice and rituals to daily living. **Discussing these issues allows client to explore spiritual needs and decide what fits own view of the world to enhance life.**
* Explore ways that spirituality/religious practices have affected one's life and given meaning and value to daily living. Note consequences as well as benefits. **Understanding that there is a difference between spirituality and religion and how each can be useful will help the client begin to use the information in the most useful ways.**
* Discuss life's/God's plan for the individual. **Helpful in determining individual goals/choosing specific options.**

NURSING PRIORITY NO. 2. To assist client to integrate values and beliefs to achieve a sense of wholeness and optimum balance in daily living:

- Explore ways beliefs give meaning and value to daily living. **As client develops understanding of these issues, they will provide support for dealing with current/future concerns.**
- Clarify reality/appropriateness of client's self-perceptions and expectations. **Necessary to provide firm foundation for growth.**
- Determine influence of cultural beliefs/values. **Most individuals are strongly influenced by the spiritual/religious orientation of their family of origin, which can be a very strong determinate for client's choice of activities/receptiveness to various options.**
- Discuss the importance and value of connections to one's daily life. **The contact that one has with others maintains a feeling of belonging and connection and promotes feelings of wholeness and well-being.**
- Identify ways to achieve connectedness or harmony with self, others, nature, higher power (e.g., meditation, prayer, talking/sharing oneself with others; being out in nature/gardening/walking; attending religious activities). **This is a highly individual and personal decision, and no action is too trivial to be considered.**

NURSING PRIORITY NO. 3. To enhance optimum wellness:

- Encourage client to take time to be introspective in the search for peace and harmony. **Finding peace within oneself will carry over to relationships with others and one's outlook on life.**
- Discuss use of relaxation/meditative activities (e.g., yoga, tai chi, prayer). **Helpful in promoting general well-being and sense of connectedness with self/nature/spiritual power.**
- Suggest attendance/involvement in dream-sharing group **to develop/enhance learning of the characteristics of spiritual awareness and facilitate the individual's growth.**
- Identify ways for spiritual/religious expression. **There are multiple options for enhancing spirituality through connectedness with self/others (e.g., volunteering time to community projects, mentoring, singing in the choir, painting, or spiritual writings).**
- Encourage participation in desired religious activities, contact with minister/spiritual advisor. **Validating one's beliefs in an external way can provide support and strengthen the inner self.**
- Discuss and role-play, as necessary, ways to deal with alternative view/conflict that may occur with family/SO(s)/society/cultural group. **Provides opportunity to try out**

different behaviors in a safe environment and be prepared for potential eventualities.

- Provide bibliotherapy, list of relevant resources (e.g., study groups, parish nurse, poetry society), and possible Web sites for later reference/self-paced learning and ongoing support.

Documentation Focus

ASSESSMENT/REASSESSMENT

- Assessment findings, including client perception of needs and desire/expectations for growth/enhancement.

PLANNING

- Plan for growth and who is involved in planning.

IMPLEMENTATION/EVALUATION

- Response to activities/learning and actions performed.
- Attainment/progress toward desired outcome(s).
- Modifications to plan.

DISCHARGE PLANNING

- Long-range needs/expectations and plan of action.
- Specific referrals made.

SAMPLE NURSING OUTCOMES & INTERVENTIONS CLASSIFICATION (NOC/NIC)

NOC—Spiritual Well-Being
NIC—Spiritual Growth Facilitation

Suffocation, risk for

Taxonomy II: Safety/Protection—Class 2 Physical Injury (00036)
[Diagnostic Division: Safety]
Submitted 1980

Definition: Accentuated risk of accidental suffocation (inadequate air available for inhalation)

Risk Factors

INTERNAL (INDIVIDUAL)

Reduced olfactory sensation
Reduced motor abilities
Lack of safety education, precautions
Cognitive or emotional difficulties [e.g., altered consciousness/ mentation]
Disease or injury process

Information that appears in brackets has been added by the authors to clarify and enhance the use of nursing diagnoses.

EXTERNAL (ENVIRONMENTAL)

Pillow/propped bottle placed in an infant's crib
Pacifier hung around infant's head
Children playing with plastic bag or inserting small objects into their
  mouths or noses
Children left unattended in bathtubs or pools
Discarded or unused refrigerators or freezers without removed doors
Vehicle warming in closed garage [/faulty exhaust system]; use of fuel-
  burning heaters not vented to outside
Household gas leaks; smoking in bed
Low-strung clothesline
Person who eats large mouthfuls [or pieces] of food

NOTE: A risk diagnosis is not evidenced by signs and symptoms, as
the problem has not occurred and nursing interventions are
directed at prevention.

Desired Outcomes/Evaluation
Criteria—Client Will:

- Verbalize knowledge of hazards in the environment.
- Identify interventions appropriate to situation.
- Correct hazardous situations to prevent/reduce risk of suffo-
  cation.
- Demonstrate CPR skills and how to access emergency assis-
  tance.

Actions/Interventions

NURSING PRIORITY NO. 1. To assess causative/contributing
factors:

- Note presence of internal/external factors in individual situation (e.g., seizure activity, inadequate supervision of small
  children, comatose client).
- Determine client's/SO's knowledge of safety factors/hazards
  present in the environment.
- Identify level of concern/awareness and motivation of
  client/SO(s) to correct safety hazards and improve individual
  situation.
- Assess neurologic status and note factors that have potential
  to compromise airway or affect ability to swallow (e.g., stroke,
  cerebral palsy, MS, ALS).
- Determine use of antiepileptics and how well epilepsy is
  controlled.
- Note reports of sleep disturbance and fatigue; **may be indicative of sleep apnea (airway obstruction).**

NURSING PRIORITY NO. 2. To reverse/correct contributing
factors:

- Identify/encourage safety measures (such as seizure

precautions; not smoking in bed, propping baby bottle, or running automobile in closed garage) **to prevent/minimize injury.**

- Recommend storing plastic bags out of reach of infants/young children. Avoid use of plastic mattress or crib covers, comforter or fluffy pillows in cribs **to reduce risk of accidental suffocation.**
- Use proper positioning, suctioning, use of adjuncts as indicated for comatose client **to protect/maintain airway.** (Tracheotomy may be necessary.)
- Provide diet modifications as indicated by degree of swallowing disability, cognition **to reduce risk of aspiration.**
- Monitor medication regimen (e.g., anticonvulsants, analgesics, sedatives), noting potential for interaction and oversedation.
- Discuss with client/SO(s) identified environmental safety hazards and problem-solve methods for resolution.
- Emphasize importance of periodic evaluation and repair of gas appliances/furnace, automobile exhaust system **to prevent exposure to carbon monoxide.**

NURSING PRIORITY NO. 3. To promote wellness (Teaching/Discharge Considerations):

- Review safety factors identified in individual situation and methods for remediation.
- Develop plan with client/caregiver for long-range management of situation to avoid injuries. **Enhances commitment to plan, optimizing outcomes.**
- Review importance of chewing carefully, taking small amounts of food, using caution when talking or drinking while eating. Discuss possibility of choking **because of throat muscle relaxation and impaired judgment when drinking alcohol and eating.**
- Emphasize the importance of getting help when beginning to choke; instead of leaving table, remain calm and make gesture across throat, making sure someone recognizes the emergency.
- Promote public education in techniques for clearing blocked airways, Heimlich maneuver, CPR.
- Assist individuals to learn to read package labels and identify safety hazards such as toys with small parts.
- Promote pool safety and use of approved flotation equipment.
- Discuss safety measures regarding use of heaters, household gas appliances, old/discarded appliances.
- Refer to NDs Airway Clearance, ineffective; Aspiration, risk for; Breathing Pattern, ineffective; Sleep Pattern, disturbed; Parenting, impaired.

Documentation Focus

ASSESSMENT/REASSESSMENT

- Individual risk factors, including individual's cognitive status and level of knowledge.
- Level of concern/motivation for change.
- Equipment/airway adjunct needs.

PLANNING

- Plan of care and who is involved in planning.
- Teaching plan.

IMPLEMENTATION/EVALUATION

- Responses to interventions/teaching and actions performed.
- Attainment/progress toward desired outcome(s).
- Modifications to plan of care.

DISCHARGE PLANNING

- Long-term needs/referrals, appropriate preventive measures, and who is responsible for actions to be taken.
- Specific referrals made.

SAMPLE NURSING OUTCOMES & INTERVENTIONS CLASSIFICATIONS (NOC/NIC)

NOC—Risk Control
NIC—Airway Management

Suicide, risk for

Taxonomy II: Safety/Protection—Class 3 Violence (00150)
[Diagnostic Division: Safety]
Submitted 2000

Definition: At risk for self-inflicted, life-threatening injury

Risk Factors/[Indicators]

BEHAVIORAL

History of prior suicide attempt
Buying a gun; stockpiling medicines
Making or changing a will; giving away possessions
Sudden euphoric recovery from major depression
Impulsiveness; marked changes in behavior, attitude, school performance

Information that appears in brackets has been added by the authors to clarify and enhance the use of nursing diagnoses.

VERBAL

Threats of killing oneself; states desire to die/end it all

SITUATIONAL

Living alone; retired; relocation, institutionalization; economic instability
Presence of gun in home
Adolescents living in nontraditional settings (e.g., juvenile detention
center, prison, half-way house, group home)

PSYCHOLOGICAL

Family history of suicide; abuse in childhood
Alcohol and substance use/abuse
Psychiatric illness/disorder (e.g., depression, schizophrenia, bipolar
disorder)
Guilt
Gay or lesbian youth

DEMOGRAPHIC

Age: elderly, young adult males, adolescents
Race: Caucasian, Native-American
Gender: male
Divorced, widowed

PHYSICAL

Physical/terminal illness; chronic pain

SOCIAL

Loss of important relationship; disrupted family life; poor support
systems; social isolation
Grief, bereavement; loneliness
Hopelessness; helplessness
Legal or disciplinary problem
Cluster suicides

NOTE: A risk diagnosis is not evidenced by signs and symptoms, as
the problem has not occurred and nursing interventions are
directed at prevention.

Desired Outcomes/Evaluation
Criteria—Client Will:

- Acknowledge difficulties perceived in current situation.
- Identify current factors that can be dealt with.
- Be involved in planning course of action to correct existing
  problems.

Actions/Interventions

NURSING PRIORITY NO. 1. To assess causative/contributing
factors:

- Identify degree of risk/potential for suicide and seriousness of threat. Use a scale of 1 to 10 and prioritize according to severity of threat, availability of means. (**Risk of suicide is greater in teens and the elderly, but there is a rising awareness of risk in early childhood.**)
- Note behaviors indicative of intent (e.g., gestures, presence of means, such as guns, threats, giving away possessions, previous attempts, and presence of hallucinations or delusions).
- Ask directly if person is thinking of acting on thoughts/feelings **to determine intent.**
- Reevaluate potential for suicide periodically at key times (e.g., mood changes, increasing withdrawal), as well as when client is feeling better and discharge planning becomes active. **The highest risk is when the client has both suicidal ideation and sufficient energy with which to act.**
- Determine presence of SO(s)/friends who are available for support.
- Note withdrawal from usual activities, lack of social interactions.
- Identify conditions, such as acute/chronic brain syndrome; panic state; hormonal imbalance (e.g., PMS, postpartum psychosis, drug-induced) **that may interfere with ability to control own behavior.**
- Review laboratory findings (e.g., blood alcohol, blood glucose, ABGs, electrolytes, renal function tests), **to identify factors that may affect reasoning ability.**
- Assess physical complaints (e.g., sleeping difficulties, lack of appetite).
- Note family history of suicidal behavior. (**Individual risk is increased.**)
- Assess coping behaviors presently used. Note: Client may believe there is no alternative except suicide.
- Determine drug use, involvement with judicial system.

NURSING PRIORITY NO. 2. To assist clients to accept responsibility for own behavior and prevent suicide:

- Develop therapeutic nurse-client relationship, providing consistent caregiver. **Promotes sense of trust, allowing individual to discuss feelings openly.**
- Maintain straightforward communication **to avoid reinforcing manipulative behavior.**
- Explain concern for safety and willingness to help client stay safe.
- Encourage expression of feelings and make time to listen to concerns. **Acknowledges reality of feelings and that they are OK. Helps individual sort out thinking and begin to develop understanding of situation.**

- Give permission to express angry feelings in acceptable ways and let client know someone will be available to assist in maintaining control. **Promotes acceptance and sense of safety.**
- Acknowledge reality of suicide as an option. Discuss consequences of actions if they follow through on intent. Ask how it will help individual to resolve problems. **Helps to focus on consequences of actions and possibility of other options.**
- Maintain observation of client and check environment for hazards that could be used to commit suicide **to increase client safety/reduce risk of impulsive behavior.**
- Help client identify more appropriate solutions/behaviors (e.g., motor activities/exercise) **to lessen sense of anxiety and associated physical manifestations.**
- Provide directions for actions client can take, avoiding negative statements, such as "do nots." **Promotes a positive attitude.**

NURSING PRIORITY NO. **3.** To assist client to plan course of action to correct/deal with existing situation:

- Gear interventions to individual involved (e.g., age, relationship, and current situation).
- Negotiate contract with client regarding willingness not to do anything lethal for a stated period of time. Specify what caregiver will be responsible for and what client responsibilities are.
- Specify alternative actions necessary if client is unwilling to negotiate contract.
- Discuss losses client has experienced and meaning of those losses. **Unresolved issues may be contributing to thoughts of hopelessness.**

NURSING PRIORITY NO. **4.** To promote wellness (Teaching/Discharge Considerations):

- Promote development of internal control by helping client look at new ways to deal with problems.
- Assist with learning problem solving, assertiveness training, and social skills.
- Engage in physical activity programs. **Promotes feelings of self-worth and improves sense of well-being.**
- Determine nutritional needs and help client to plan for meeting them.
- Involve family/SO in planning **to improve understanding and support.**
- Refer to formal resources as indicated (e.g., individual/group/marital psychotherapy, substance abuse treatment program, and social services).

Documentation Focus

ASSESSMENT/REASSESSMENT

- Individual findings, including nature of concern (e.g., suicidal/behavioral risk factors and level of impulse control, plan of action/means to carry out plan).
- Client's perception of situation, motivation for change.

PLANNING

- Plan of care and who is involved in the planning.
- Details of contract regarding suicidal ideation/plans.
- Teaching plan.

IMPLEMENTATION/EVALUATION

- Actions taken to promote safety.
- Response to interventions/teaching and actions performed.
- Attainment/progress toward desired outcome(s).
- Modifications to plan of care.

DISCHARGE PLANNING

- Long-range needs and who is responsible for actions to be taken.
- Available resources, specific referrals made.

SAMPLE NURSING OUTCOMES & INTERVENTIONS CLASSIFICATIONS (NOC/NIC)

NOC—Suicide Self-Restraint
NIC—Suicide Prevention

Surgical Recovery, delayed

Taxonomy II: Activity/Rest—Class 2 Activity/Exercise
(00100)
[Diagnostic Division: Safety]
Submitted 1998

Definition: Extension of the number of postoperative days required to initiate and perform activities that maintain life, health, and well-being

Related Factors

To be developed

Defining Characteristics

SUBJECTIVE

Perception more time needed to recover
Report of pain/discomfort; fatigue

Information that appears in brackets has been added by the authors to clarify and enhance the use of nursing diagnoses. **507**

Loss of appetite with or without nausea
Postpones resumption of work/employment activities

OBJECTIVE

Evidence of interrupted healing of surgical area (e.g., red, indurated, draining, immobile)
Difficulty in moving about; requires help to complete self-care

Desired Outcomes/Evaluation Criteria—Client Will:

- Display complete healing of surgical area.
- Be able to perform desired self-care activities.
- Report increased energy, able to participate in usual (work/employment) activities.

Actions/Interventions

NURSING PRIORITY NO. 1. To assess causative/contributing factors:

- Determine extent of injury/damage to tissues and general state of health.
- Identify underlying condition/pathology involved (e.g., skin/other cancers, burns, diabetes, steroid therapy, multiple trauma, infections, radiation therapy), **which may affect healing/recovery.**
- Note odors emitted from wound, presence of fever, or other signs **suggesting localized/systemic infections.**
- Assess circulation and sensation in affected area **(possible loss of blood flow/nerve damage).**
- Determine nutritional status and current intake.
- Ascertain attitudes of individual about condition (e.g., cultural values, stigma regarding condition, lack of motivation to return to usual role/activities).

NURSING PRIORITY NO. 2. To determine impact of delayed recovery:

- Note length of hospitalization to date and compare with expected length of stay for procedure and situation.
- Determine energy level and current participation in ADLs. Compare with usual level of function.
- Ascertain whether client usually requires assistance in home setting and who provides it/current availability and capability.
- Obtain psychologic assessment of client's emotional status, noting potential problems arising from current situation.

NURSING PRIORITY NO. 3. To promote optimal recovery:

- Inspect incisions/wounds routinely, describing changes (e.g., deepening or healing wound measurements, presence/type of drainage, development of necrosis).

- Observe for complications (e.g., infection, dehiscence).
- Assist with wound care as indicated (e.g., débridement, barrier dressings, wound coverings, skin-protective agents for open/draining wounds).
- Include wound care specialist/stomal therapist as appropriate **to problem-solve healing difficulties.**
- Limit/avoid use of plastics or latex materials. (**Client may be sensitive.**)
- Provide optimal nutrition and adequate protein intake **to provide a positive nitrogen balance aiding in healing and to achieve general good health.**
- Encourage ambulation, regular exercise **to promote circulation, improve strength, and reduce risks associated with immobility.**
- Recommend alternating activity with adequate rest periods **to prevent fatigue.**
- Administer medications as indicated (e.g., client may be experiencing stubborn infection requiring IV antibiotics or management of chronic pain).
- Encourage client to adhere to medical regimen and follow-up care **to monitor healing process and provide for timely intervention as needed.**

NURSING PRIORITY NO. 4. To promote wellness (Teaching/ Discharge Considerations):

- Discuss reality of recovery process and client's/SO's expectations. **Individuals are often unrealistic regarding energy and time required for healing and own abilities/responsibilities to facilitate process.**
- Involve client/SO(s) in setting incremental goals. **Enhances commitment to plan and reduces likelihood of frustration blocking progress.**
- Refer to physical/occupational therapists as indicated **to identify assistive devices to facilitate independence in ADLs.**
- Identify suppliers for dressings/wound care items and assistive devices as needed.
- Consult dietitian for individual dietary plan **to meet increased nutritional needs that reflect personal situation/resources.**
- Determine home situation (e.g., lives alone, bedroom/bathroom on second floor, availability of assistance). **Identifies necessary adjustments, such as moving bedroom to first floor, arranging for commode during recovery, obtaining a Lifeline emergency call system.**
- Discuss alternative placement (e.g., convalescent/rehabilitation center as appropriate).
- Identify community resources (e.g., visiting nurse, home healthcare agency, Meals on Wheels, respite care). **Facilitates adjustment to home setting.**

- Refer for counseling/support. **May need additional help to overcome feelings of discouragement, deal with changes in life.**

Documentation Focus

ASSESSMENT/REASSESSMENT

- Assessment findings, including individual concerns, family involvement, and support factors/availability of resources.

PLANNING

- Plan of care and who is involved in planning.
- Teaching plan.

IMPLEMENTATION/EVALUATION

- Responses of client/SO(s) to plan/interventions/teaching and actions performed.
- Attainment/progress toward desired outcome(s).
- Modifications to plan of care.

DISCHARGE PLANNING

- Long-range needs and who is responsible for actions to be taken.
- Specific referrals made.

SAMPLE NURSING OUTCOMES & INTERVENTIONS CLASSIFICATIONS (NOC/NIC)

NOC—Self-Care: Activities of Daily Living (ADL)
NIC—Self-Care Assistance

Swallowing, impaired

Taxonomy II: Nutrition—Class 1 Ingestion (00103)
[Diagnostic Division: Food/Fluid]
Submitted 1986; Nursing Diagnosis Extension and
Classification (NDEC) Revision 1998

Definition: Abnormal functioning of the swallowing mechanism associated with deficits in oral, pharyngeal, or esophageal structure or function

Related Factors

CONGENITAL DEFICITS

Upper airway anomalies; mechanical obstruction (e.g., edema, tracheostomy tube, tumor); history of tube feeding

Information that appears in brackets has been added by the authors to clarify and enhance the use of nursing diagnoses.

Neuromuscular impairment (e.g., decreased or absent gag reflex, decreased strength or excursion of muscles involved in mastication, perceptual impairment, facial paralysis); conditions with significant hypotonia; cranial nerve involvement

Respiratory disorders; congenital heart disease

Behavioral feeding problems; self-injurious behavior

Failure to thrive or protein energy malnutrition

NEUROLOGICAL PROBLEMS

External/internal traumas; acquired anatomic defects

Nasal or nasopharyngeal cavity defects

Oral cavity or oropharynx abnormalities

Upper airway/laryngeal anomalies; tracheal, laryngeal, esophageal defects

Gastroesophageal reflux disease; achalasia

Premature infants; traumatic head injury; developmental delay; cerebral palsy

Defining Characteristics

SUBJECTIVE

Esophageal Phase Impairment
Complaints [reports] of "something stuck"; odynophagia
Food refusal or volume limiting
Heartburn or epigastric pain
Nighttime coughing or awakening

OBJECTIVE

Oral Phase Impairment
Weak suck resulting in inefficient nippling
Slow bolus formation; lack of tongue action to form bolus; premature entry of bolus
Incomplete lip closure; food pushed out of/falls from mouth
Lack of chewing
Coughing, choking, gagging before a swallow
Piecemeal deglutition; abnormality in oral phase of swallow study
Inability to clear oral cavity; pooling in lateral sulci; nasal reflux; sialorrhea or drooling
Long meals with little consumption
Pharyngeal Phase Impairment
Food refusal
Altered head positions; delayed/multiple swallows; inadequate laryngeal elevation; abnormality in pharyngeal phase by swallow study
Choking, coughing, or gagging; nasal reflux; gurgly voice quality
Unexplained fevers; recurrent pulmonary infections
Esophageal Phase Impairment
Observed evidence of difficulty in swallowing (e.g., stasis of food in oral cavity, coughing/choking); abnormality in esophageal phase by swallow study
Hyperextension of head, arching during or after meals
Repetitive swallowing or ruminating; bruxism
Unexplained irritability surrounding mealtime

Acidic smelling breath; regurgitation of gastric contents or wet burps; vomitus on pillow; vomiting; hematemesis

Desired Outcomes/Evaluation Criteria—Client Will:

- Verbalize understanding of causative/contributing factors.
- Identify individually appropriate interventions/actions to promote intake and prevent aspiration.
- Demonstrate feeding methods appropriate to the individual situation.
- Pass food and fluid from mouth to stomach safely.
- Maintain adequate hydration as evidenced by good skin turgor, moist mucous membranes, and individually appropriate urine output.
- Achieve and/or maintain desired body weight.

Caregiver/SO(s) Will:

- Demonstrate emergency measures in the event of choking.

Actions/Interventions

NURSING PRIORITY NO. 1. To assess causative/contributing factors and degree of impairment:

- Assess sensory-perceptual status (sensory awareness, orientation, concentration, motor coordination).
- Inspect oropharyngeal cavity for edema, inflammation, altered integrity of oral mucosa, adequacy of oral hygiene.
- Ascertain presence and strength of cough and gag reflex.
- Evaluate ability to swallow using crushed ice or small sips of water.
- Auscultate breath sounds **to evaluate the presence of aspiration.**
- Assess strength and excursion of muscles involved in mastication and swallowing.
- Verify proper fit of dentures.
- Record current weight/recent changes.
- Prepare for/assist with diagnostic testing of swallowing activity.

NURSING PRIORITY NO. 2. To prevent aspiration and maintain airway patency:

- Identify individual factors that can precipitate aspiration/compromise airway.
- Raise head to a 90-degree angle with head in anatomic alignment and slightly flexed forward during feeding. Keep HOB elevated for 30 to 45 minutes after feeding, if possible.
- Position client on the unaffected side, placing food in this side

of mouth and having client use the tongue to assist with managing the food when one side of the mouth is affected by the condition (e.g., hemiplegia).

- Suction oral cavity prn. Teach client self-suction when appropriate. **Promotes independence/sense of control.**

NURSING PRIORITY NO. 3. To enhance swallowing ability to meet fluid and caloric body requirements:

- Refer to gastroenterologist as indicated. (**Esophageal dilatation may be necessary when impaired sphincter function or esophageal strictures impede swallowing.**)
- Refer to speech therapist **to identify specific techniques to enhance client efforts/safety measures as indicated.**
- Provide cognitive cues (e.g., remind client to chew/swallow as indicated) **to enhance concentration and performance of swallowing sequence.**
- Encourage a rest period before meals **to minimize fatigue.**
- Provide analgesics prior to feeding as indicated **to enhance comfort, being cautious to avoid decreasing awareness/ sensory perception.**
- Focus attention on feeding/swallowing activity and decreasing environmental stimuli, **which may be distracting during feeding.**
- Determine food preferences of client **to incorporate as possible enhancing intake.** Present foods in an appealing, attractive manner.
- Ensure temperature (hot or cold versus tepid) of foods/fluid, **which will stimulate sensory receptors.**
- Provide a consistency of food/fluid that is most easily swallowed (can be formed into a bolus before swallowing), such as gelatin desserts prepared with less water than usual, pudding, and custard; thickened liquids (addition of thickening agent, or yogurt, cream soups prepared with less water); thinned purees (hot cereal with water added); or thick drinks, such as nectars; fruit juices that have been frozen into "slush" consistency (**thin fluids are most difficult to control**); medium-soft boiled or scrambled eggs; canned fruit; soft-cooked vegetables. Avoid milk products and chocolate, **which may thicken oral secretions.**
- Feed one consistency and/or texture of food at a time.
- Place food midway in oral cavity; provide medium-sized bites (about 15 mL) **to adequately trigger the swallowing reflex.**
- Instruct to chew food on unaffected side as appropriate.
- Massage the laryngopharyngeal musculature (sides of trachea and neck) gently **to stimulate swallowing.**
- Observe oral cavity after each bite and have client check around cheeks with tongue for remaining food. Remove food if unable to swallow.

NURSING DIAGNOSES IN ALPHABETICAL ORDER **513**

- Incorporate client's eating style and pace when feeding to avoid fatigue and frustration with process.
- Allow ample time for eating (feeding).
- Remain with client during meal to reduce anxiety and offer assistance.
- Use a glass with a nose cutout to avoid posterior head tilting while drinking. Never pour liquid into the mouth. Avoid "washing food down" with liquid.
- Monitor intake, output, and body weight to evaluate adequacy of fluid and caloric intake.
- Provide positive feedback for client's efforts.
- Provide oral hygiene following each feeding.
- Consider tube feedings/parenteral solutions as indicated for the client unable to achieve adequate nutritional intake.
- Consult with dysphagia specialist/rehabilitation team as indicated.

NURSING PRIORITY NO. 4. To promote wellness (Teaching/Discharge Considerations):

- Consult with dietitian to establish optimum dietary plan.
- Place medication in gelatin, jelly, or puddings. Consult with pharmacist to determine if pills may be crushed or if liquids/capsules are available.
- Assist client and/or SO in learning specific feeding techniques and swallowing exercises.
- Instruct client and/or SO in emergency measures in event of choking.
- Encourage continuation of facial exercise program to maintain/improve muscle strength.
- Establish routine schedule for monitoring weight.
- Refer to ND Nutrition: imbalanced, risk for less than body requirements.

Documentation Focus

ASSESSMENT/REASSESSMENT

- Individual findings, including degree/characteristics of impairment, current weight/recent changes.
- Effects on lifestyle/socialization and nutritional status.

PLANNING

- Plan of care and who is involved in planning.
- Teaching plan.

IMPLEMENTATION/EVALUATION

- Response to interventions/teaching and actions performed.
- Attainment/progress toward desired outcome(s).
- Modifications to plan of care.

- Long-term needs and who is responsible for actions to be taken.
- Available resources and specific referrals made.

SAMPLE NURSING OUTCOMES & INTERVENTIONS CLASSIFICATIONS (NOC/NIC)

NOC—Swallowing Status
NIC—Swallowing Therapy

Therapeutic Regimen Management: community, ineffective

Taxonomy II: Health Promotion—Class 2 Health Management (0081)
[Diagnostic Division: Teaching/Learning]
Submitted 1994

Definition: Pattern of regulating and integrating into community processes programs for treatment of illness and the sequelae of illness that are unsatisfactory for meeting health-related goals

Related Factors

To be developed
[Lack of safety for community members]
[Economic insecurity]
[Healthcare not available]
[Unhealthy environment]
[Education not available for all community members]
[Does not possess means to meet human needs for recognition, fellowship, security, and membership]

Defining Characteristics

SUBJECTIVE

[Community members/agencies verbalize inability to meet therapeutic needs of all members]
[Community members/agencies verbalize overburdening of resources for meeting therapeutic needs of all members]

OBJECTIVE

Deficits in people and programs to be accountable for illness care of aggregates
Deficits in advocates for aggregates
Deficit in community activities for [primary medical care/prevention]/secondary and tertiary prevention

---

Information that appears in brackets has been added by the authors to clarify and enhance the use of nursing diagnoses.

Illness symptoms above the norm expected for the number and type of population; unexpected acceleration of illness(es)

Number of healthcare resources insufficient[/unavailable] for the incidence or prevalence of illness(es)

[Deficits in community for collaboration and development of coalitions to address programs for treatment of illness and the sequelae of illness]

Desired Outcomes/Evaluation Criteria—Community Will:

- Identify both negative and positive factors affecting community treatment programs for meeting health-related goals.
- Participate in problem solving of factors interfering with regulating and integrating community programs.
- Report illness symptoms moving toward norm expected for the incidence or prevalence of illness(es).

Actions/Interventions

NURSING PRIORITY NO. **1.** To identify causative/precipitating factors:

- Evaluate community healthcare resources for illness/sequelae of illness.
- Note reports from members of the community regarding ineffective/inadequate community functioning.
- Investigate unexpected acceleration of illness in the community.
- Identify strengths/limitations of community resources and community commitment to change.
- Ascertain effect of related factors on community activities.
- Determine knowledge/understanding of treatment regimen.

NURSING PRIORITY NO. **2.** To assist community to develop strategies to improve community functioning/management:

- Foster cooperative spirit of community without negating individuality of members/groups.
- Involve community in determining healthcare goals and prioritize them **to facilitate planning process.**
- Plan together with community health and social agencies **to problem-solve solutions to identified and anticipated problems/needs.**
- Identify specific populations at risk or underserved **to actively involve them in process.**
- Create teaching plan/form speakers' bureau **to disseminate information to community members regarding value of treatment/preventive programs.**

NURSING PRIORITY NO. **3.** To promote wellness (Teaching/Discharge Considerations):

- Assist community to develop a plan for continuing assessment of community needs/functioning and effectiveness of plan. **Promotes proactive approach.**
- Encourage community to form partnerships within the community and between the community and the larger society **to aid in long-term planning for anticipated/projected needs/concerns.**

Documentation Focus

ASSESSMENT/REASSESSMENT

- Assessment findings, including members' perceptions of community problems.

PLANNING

- Plan of care and who is involved in planning.
- Teaching plan.

IMPLEMENTATION/EVALUATION

- Community's response to plan/interventions and actions performed.
- Attainment/progress toward desired outcome(s).
- Modifications to plan of care.

DISCHARGE PLANNING

- Long-range goals and who is responsible for actions to be taken.
- Specific referrals made.

SAMPLE NURSING OUTCOMES & INTERVENTIONS CLASSIFICATIONS (NOC/NIC)

NOC—Community Competence
NIC—Community Health Development

Therapeutic Regimen Management: effective

Taxonomy II: Health Promotion—Class 2 Health Management (00082)
[Diagnostic Division: Teaching/Learning]
Submitted 1994

Definition: Pattern of regulating and integrating into daily living a program for treatment of illness and its sequelae that is satisfactory for meeting specific health goals

---

Information that appears in brackets has been added by the authors to clarify and enhance the use of nursing diagnoses.

Related Factors

To be developed
[Complexity of healthcare management; therapeutic regimen]
[Added demands made on individual or family]
[Adequate social supports]

Defining Characteristics

SUBJECTIVE

Verbalized desire to manage the treatment of illness and prevention of
sequelae
Verbalized intent to reduce risk factors for progression of illness and
sequelae

OBJECTIVE

Appropriate choices of daily activities for meeting the goals of a treatment or prevention program
Illness symptoms are within a normal range of expectation

Desired Outcomes/Evaluation Criteria—Individual Will:

- Verbalize understanding of therapeutic regimen for
  illness/condition.
- Demonstrate effective problem solving in integration of therapeutic regimen into lifestyle.
- Identify/use available resources.
- Remain free of preventable complications/progression of
  illness and sequelae.

Actions/Interventions

NURSING PRIORITY NO. **1**. To assess situation and individual
needs:

- Ascertain client's knowledge/understanding of condition and
  treatment needs. Note specific health goals.
- Identify individual's perceptions of adaptation to treat-
  ment/anticipated changes.
- Note treatments added to present regimen and client's/SO's
  associated learning needs.
- Discuss present resources used by client to note whether
  changes need to be arranged (e.g., increased hours of home
  care assistance; access to case manager to support
  complex/long-term program).

NURSING PRIORITY NO. **2**. To assist client/SO(s) in developing
strategies to meet increased demands of therapeutic regimen:

- Identify steps necessary to reach desired health goal(s).
- Accept client's evaluation of own strengths/limitations while

working together to improve abilities. **Promotes sense of self-esteem and confidence to continue efforts.**

- Provide information/bibliotherapy and help client/SO(s) identify and evaluate resources they can access on their own. **When referencing the Internet or nontraditional/unproven resources, the individual must exercise some restraint and determine the reliability of the source/information provided before acting on it.**
- Acknowledge individual efforts/capabilities **to reinforce movement toward attainment of desired outcomes.**

NURSING PRIORITY NO. 3. To promote wellness (Teaching/Discharge Considerations):

- Promote client/caregiver choices and involvement in planning and implementing added tasks/responsibilities.
- Provide for follow-up contact/home visit as appropriate.
- Assist in implementing strategies for monitoring progress/responses to therapeutic regimen. **Promotes proactive problem solving.**
- Mobilize support systems, including family/SO(s), social, financial, and so on.
- Refer to community resources as needed/desired.

Documentation Focus

ASSESSMENT/REASSESSMENT

- Findings, including dynamics of individual situation.
- Individual strengths/additional needs.

PLANNING

- Plan of care and who is involved in planning.
- Teaching plan.

IMPLEMENTATION/EVALUATION

- Response to interventions/teaching and actions performed.
- Attainment/progress toward desired outcome(s).
- Modifications to plan of care.

DISCHARGE PLANNING

- Short-range and long-range needs and who is responsible for actions.
- Available resources, specific referrals made.

SAMPLE NURSING OUTCOMES & INTERVENTIONS CLASSIFICATIONS (NOC/NIC)

NOC—Symptom Control
NIC—Health System Guidance

Therapeutic Regimen Management: family, ineffective

Taxonomy II: Health Promotion—Class 2 Health
Management (00080)
[Diagnostic Division: Teaching/Learning]
Submitted 1994

Definition: Pattern of regulating and integrating into
family processes a program for treatment of illness and
the sequelae of illness that is unsatisfactory for meeting
specific health goals

Related Factors

Complexity of healthcare system
Complexity of therapeutic regimen
Decisional conflicts
Economic difficulties
Excessive demands made on individual or family
Family conflicts

Defining Characteristics

SUBJECTIVE

Verbalized difficulty with regulation/integration of one or more effects
or prevention of complication; [inability to manage treatment
regimen]
Verbalized desire to manage the treatment of illness and prevention of
the sequelae
Verbalizes that family did not take action to reduce risk factors for
progression of illness and sequelae

OBJECTIVE

Inappropriate family activities for meeting the goals of a treatment or
prevention program
Acceleration (expected or unexpected) of illness symptoms of a family
member
Lack of attention to illness and its sequelae

Desired Outcomes/Evaluation
Criteria—Family Will:

- Identify individual factors affecting regulation/integration of
  treatment program.
- Participate in problem solving of factors.
- Verbalize acceptance of need/desire to change actions to
  achieve agreed-on outcomes or goals of treatment or prevention program.
- Demonstrate behaviors/changes in lifestyle necessary to
  maintain therapeutic regimen.

Information that appears in brackets has been added by the authors
to clarify and enhance the use of nursing diagnoses.

Actions/Interventions

NURSING PRIORITY NO. **1.** To identify causative/precipitating factors:

- Ascertain family's perception of efforts to date.
- Evaluate family activities as related to appropriate family functioning/activities—looking at frequency/effectiveness of family communication, promotion of autonomy, adaptation to meet changing needs, health of home environment/lifestyle, problem-solving abilities, ties to community.
- Note family health goals and agreement of individual members. (**Presence of conflict interferes with problem solving.**)
- Determine understanding of and value of the treatment regimen to the family.
- Identify availability and use of resources.

NURSING PRIORITY NO. **2.** To assist family to develop strategies to improve management of therapeutic regimen:

- Provide information to aid family **in understanding the value of the treatment program.**
- Assist family members to recognize inappropriate family activities. Help the members identify both togetherness and individual needs and behavior **so that effective interactions can be enhanced and perpetuated.**
- Make a plan jointly with family members to deal with complexity of healthcare regimen/system and other related factors. **Enhances commitment to plan, optimizing outcomes.**
- Identify community resources as needed using the three strategies of education, problem solving, and resource linking **to address specific deficits.**

NURSING PRIORITY NO. **3.** To promote wellness as related to future health of family members:

- Help family identify criteria to promote ongoing self-evaluation of situation/effectiveness and family progress. **Provides opportunity to be proactive in meeting needs.**
- Make referrals to and/or jointly plan with other health/social and community resources. **Problems often are multifaceted, requiring involvement of numerous providers/agencies.**
- Provide contact person/case manager for one-to-one assistance as needed **to coordinate care, provide support, assist with problem solving, and so forth.**
- Refer to NDs Caregiver Role Strain; Therapeutic Regimen Management: ineffective, as indicated.

Documentation Focus

ASSESSMENT/REASSESSMENT

- Individual findings, including nature of problem/degree of impairment, family values/health goals, and level of participation and commitment of family members.
- Availability and use of resources.

PLANNING

- Plan of care and who is involved in planning.
- Teaching plan.

IMPLEMENTATION/EVALUATION

- Response to interventions/teaching and actions performed.
- Attainment/progress toward desired outcome(s).
- Modifications of plan of care.

DISCHARGE PLANNING

- Long-term needs, plan for meeting, and who is responsible for actions.
- Specific referrals made.

SAMPLE NURSING OUTCOMES & INTERVENTIONS CLASSIFICATIONS (NOC/NIC)

NOC—Family Participation in Professional Care
NIC—Family Involvement Promotion

Therapeutic Regimen Management: ineffective

Taxonomy II: Health Promotion—Class 2 Health Management (00078)
[Diagnostic Division: Teaching/Learning]
Submitted 1992

Definition: Pattern of regulating and integrating into daily living a program for treatment of illness and the sequelae of illness that is unsatisfactory for meeting specific health goals

Related Factors

Complexity of healthcare system/therapeutic regimen
Decisional conflicts
Economic difficulties
Excessive demands made on individual or family

Information that appears in brackets has been added by the authors to clarify and enhance the use of nursing diagnoses.

Family conflict
Family patterns of healthcare
Inadequate number and types of cues to action
Knowledge deficits
Mistrust of regimen and/or healthcare personnel
Perceived seriousness/susceptibility/barriers/benefits
Powerlessness
Social support deficits

Defining Characteristics

SUBJECTIVE

Verbalized desire to manage the treatment of illness and prevention of sequelae

Verbalized difficulty with regulation/integration of one or more prescribed regimens for treatment of illness and its effects or prevention of complications

Verbalized that did not take action to include treatment regimens in daily routines/reduce risk factors for progression of illness and sequelae

OBJECTIVE

Choice of daily living ineffective for meeting the goals of a treatment or prevention program

Acceleration (expected or unexpected) of illness symptoms

Desired Outcomes/Evaluation Criteria—Client Will:

- Verbalize acceptance of need/desire to change actions to achieve agreed-on outcomes.
- Verbalize understanding of factors/blocks involved in individual situation.
- Participate in problem solving of factors interfering with integration of therapeutic regimen.
- Demonstrate behaviors/changes in lifestyle necessary to maintain therapeutic regimen.
- Identify/use available resources.

Actions/Interventions

NURSING PRIORITY NO. 1. To identify causative/contributing factors:

- Ascertain client's knowledge/understanding of condition and treatment needs.
- Determine client's/family's health goals and patterns of healthcare.
- Identify individual perceptions and expectations of treatment regimen.
- Note availability/use of resources for assistance, caregiving/respite care.

NURSING PRIORITY NO. 2. To assist client/SO(s) to develop strategies to improve management of therapeutic regimen:

- Use therapeutic communication skills **to assist client to problem-solve solution(s).**
- Explore client involvement in or lack of mutual goal setting.
- Identify steps necessary to reach desired goal(s).
- Contract with the client for participation in care.
- Accept client's evaluation of own strengths/limitations while working together to improve abilities. State belief in client's ability to cope and/or adapt to situation.
- Provide positive reinforcement for efforts **to encourage continuation of desired behaviors.**
- Provide information as well as help client to know where and how to find it on own. Reinforce previous instructions and rationale, using a variety of learning modalities, including role playing, demonstration, written materials, and so forth.

NURSING PRIORITY NO. 3. To promote wellness (Teaching/ Discharge Considerations):

- Emphasize importance of client knowledge and understanding of the need for treatment/medication as well as consequences of actions/choices.
- Promote client/caregiver/SO(s) participation in planning and evaluating process. **Enhances commitment to plan, optimizing outcomes.**
- Assist client to develop strategies for monitoring therapeutic regimen. **Promotes early recognition of changes, allowing proactive response.**
- Mobilize support systems, including family/SO(s), social, financial, and so on.
- Refer to counseling/therapy (group and individual) as indicated.
- Identify home- and community-based nursing services **for assessment, follow-up care, and education in client's home.**

Documentation Focus

ASSESSMENT/REASSESSMENT

- Findings, including underlying dynamics of individual situation, client's perception of problem/needs.
- Family involvement/needs.
- Individual strengths/limitations.
- Availability/use of resources.

PLANNING

- Plan of care and who is involved in planning.
- Teaching plan.

IMPLEMENTATION/EVALUATION

- Response to interventions/teaching and actions performed.
- Attainment/progress toward desired outcome(s).
- Modifications to plan of care.

DISCHARGE PLANNING

- Long-range needs and who is responsible for actions to be taken.
- Available resources, specific referrals made.

SAMPLE NURSING OUTCOMES & INTERVENTIONS CLASSIFICATIONS (NOC/NIC)

NOC—Treatment Behavior: Illness or Injury
NIC—Self-Modification Assistance

Therapeutic Regimen Management: readiness for enhanced

Taxonomy II: Health Promotion—Class 2 Health Management (00162)
[Diagnostic Division: Teaching/Learning]
Submitted 2002

Definition: A pattern of regulating and integrating into daily living a program(s) for treatment of illness and its sequelae that is sufficient for meeting health-related goals and can be strengthened

Related Factors

To be developed

Defining Characteristics

SUBJECTIVE

Expresses desire to manage the treatment of illness and prevention of sequelae
Expresses little to no difficulty with regulation/integration of one or more prescribed regimens for treatment of illness or prevention of complications
Describes reduction of risk factors for progression of illness and sequelae

OBJECTIVE

Choices of daily living are appropriate for meeting the goals of treatment or prevention
No unexpected acceleration of illness symptoms

Information that appears in brackets has been added by the authors to clarify and enhance the use of nursing diagnoses.

Desired Outcomes/Evaluation Criteria—Client Will:

- Assume responsibility for managing treatment regimen.
- Demonstrate proactive management by anticipating and planning for eventualities of condition/potential complications.
- Identify/use additional resources as appropriate.
- Remain free of preventable complications/progression of illness and sequelae.

Actions/Interventions

NURSING PRIORITY NO. 1. To determine motivation for continued growth:

- Verify client's level of knowledge/understanding of therapeutic regimen. Note specific health goals. **Provides opportunity to assure accuracy and completeness of knowledgebase for future learning.**
- Identify individual's expectations of long-term treatment needs/anticipated changes.
- Discuss present resources used by client, **to note whether changes can be arranged (e.g., increased hours of home care assistance; access to case manager to support complex/long-term program).**

NURSING PRIORITY NO. 2. To assist client/SO(s) to develop plan to meet individual needs:

- Identify steps necessary to reach desired health goal(s). **Understanding the process enhances commitment and the likelihood of achieving the goals.**
- Accept client's evaluation of own strengths/limitations while working together to improve abilities. **Promotes sense of self-esteem and confidence to continue efforts.**
- Provide information/bibliotherapy and help client/SO(s) identify and evaluate resources they can access on their own. **When referencing the Internet or nontraditional/unproven resources, the individual must exercise some restraint and determine the reliability of the source/information provided before acting on it.**
- Acknowledge individual efforts/capabilities to reinforce movement toward attainment of desired outcomes. **Provides positive reinforcement encouraging continued progress toward desired goals.**

NURSING PRIORITY NO. 3. To promote optimum wellness:

- Promote client/caregiver choices and involvement in planning for and implementing added tasks/responsibilities.
- Assist in implementing strategies for monitoring progress/

responses to therapeutic regimen. **Promotes proactive problem solving.**

- Identify additional community resources/support groups. **Provides additional opportunities for role-modeling, skill training, anticipatory problem solving, and so forth.**

Documentation Focus

ASSESSMENT/REASSESSMENT

- Findings, including dynamics of individual situation.
- Individual strengths/additional needs.

PLANNING

- Plan of care and who is involved in planning.
- Teaching plan.

IMPLEMENTATION/EVALUATION

- Response to interventions/teaching and actions performed.
- Attainment/progress toward desired outcome(s).
- Modifications to plan of care.

DISCHARGE PLANNING

- Short-range and long-range needs and who is responsible for actions.
- Available resources, specific referrals made.

SAMPLE NURSING OUTCOMES & INTERVENTIONS CLASSIFICATION (NOC/NIC)

NOC—Symptom Control
NIC—Health System Guidance

Thermoregulation, ineffective

Taxonomy II: Safety/Protection—Class 6
Thermoregulation (00008)
[Diagnostic Division: Safety]
Submitted 1986

Definition: Temperature fluctuation between hypothermia and hyperthermia

Related Factors

Trauma or illness [e.g., cerebral edema, CVA, intracranial surgery, or head injury]
Immaturity, aging [e.g., loss/absence of brown adipose tissue]
Fluctuating environmental temperature

Information that appears in brackets has been added by the authors to clarify and enhance the use of nursing diagnoses. **527**

[Changes in hypothalamic tissue causing alterations in emission of thermosensitive cells and regulation of heat loss/production]

[Changes in metabolic rate/activity; changes in level/action of thyroxine and catecholamines]

[Chemical reactions in contracting muscles]

Defining Characteristics

OBJECTIVE

Fluctuations in body temperature above or below the normal range
Tachycardia

Reduction in body temperature below normal range; cool skin; pallor (moderate); shivering (mild); piloerection; cyanotic nailbeds; slow capillary refill; hypertension

Warm to touch; flushed skin; increased respiratory rate; seizures/convulsions

Desired Outcomes/Evaluation Criteria—Client/Caregiver Will:

- Verbalize understanding of individual factors and appropriate interventions.
- Demonstrate techniques/behaviors to correct underlying condition/situation.
- Maintain body temperature within normal limits.

Actions/Interventions

NURSING PRIORITY NO. 1. To identify causative/contributing factors:

- Assist with measures to identify causative factor(s)/underlying condition (e.g., obtaining history concerning present symptoms, correlation with past history/family history, diagnostic studies).

NURSING PRIORITY NO. 2. To assist with measures to correct/treat underlying cause:

- Refer to NDs Hypothermia and Hyperthermia **to restore/maintain body temperature within normal range.**
- Administer fluids, electrolytes, and medications as indicated **to restore or maintain body/organ function.**
- Prepare client for/assist with procedures (e.g., surgical intervention, neoplastic agent, antibiotics) **to treat underlying cause of hypothermia or hyperthermia.**

NURSING PRIORITY NO. 3. To promote wellness (Teaching/Discharge Considerations):

- Review causative/related factors, if appropriate, with client/SO(s).
- Provide information concerning disease processes, current

therapies, and postdischarge precautions as appropriate to situation.
- Refer to teaching in NDs Hypothermia; Hyperthermia.

Documentation Focus

ASSESSMENT/REASSESSMENT

- Individual findings, including nature of problem, degree of impairment/fluctuations in temperature.

PLANNING

- Plan of care and who is involved in planning.
- Teaching plan.

IMPLEMENTATION/EVALUATION

- Responses to interventions/teaching actions performed.
- Attainment/progress toward desired outcome(s).
- Modifications to plan of care.

DISCHARGE PLANNING

- Long-term needs and who is responsible for actions to be taken.
- Specific referrals made.

SAMPLE NURSING OUTCOMES & INTERVENTIONS CLASSIFICATIONS (NOC/NIC)

NOC—Thermoregulation
NIC—Temperature Regulation

Thought Processes, disturbed

Taxonomy II: Perception/Cognition—Class 4 Cognition (00130)
[Diagnostic Division: Neurosensory]
Submitted 1973; Revised 1996

Definition: Disruption in cognitive operations and activities

Related Factors

To be developed
[Physiological changes, aging, hypoxia, head injury, malnutrition, infections]
[Biochemical changes, medications, substance abuse]
[Sleep deprivation]
[Psychological conflicts, emotional changes, mental disorders]

Information that appears in brackets has been added by the authors to clarify and enhance the use of nursing diagnoses. **529**

Defining Characteristics

SUBJECTIVE

[Ideas of reference, hallucinations, delusions]

OBJECTIVE

Inaccurate interpretation of environment
Inappropriate/nonreality-based thinking
Memory deficit/problems, [disorientation to time, place, person,
    circumstances and events, loss of short-term/remote memory]
Hypervigilance or hypovigilance
Cognitive dissonance, [decreased ability to grasp ideas, make decisions,
    problem-solve, use abstract reasoning or conceptualize, calculate;
    disordered thought sequencing]
Distractibility, [altered attention span]
Egocentricity
[Confabulation]
[Inappropriate social behavior]

Desired Outcomes/Evaluation Criteria—Client Will:

- Recognize changes in thinking/behavior.
- Verbalize understanding of causative factors when known/
  able.
- Identify interventions to deal effectively with situation.
- Demonstrate behaviors/lifestyle changes to prevent/minimize
  changes in mentation.
- Maintain usual reality orientation.

Actions/Interventions

NURSING PRIORITY NO. 1. To assess causative/contributing
factors:

- Identify factors present, for example, acute/chronic brain
  syndrome (recent CVA/Alzheimer's); increased intracranial
  pressure; infections; malnutrition; sensory deprivation;
  delirium.
- Determine drug use (prescription/OTC/illicit). **May have side
  and/or cumulative effects that alter thought processes and
  sensory-perception.**
- Note schedule of drug administration (**may be significant
  when evaluating cumulative effects**).
- Assess dietary intake/nutritional status.
- Monitor laboratory values for abnormalities, such as metabolic alkalosis, hypokalemia, anemia, elevated ammonia
  levels, and signs of infection.

NURSING PRIORITY NO. 2. To assess degree of impairment:

- Evaluate mental status according to age and developmental

capacity, noting extent of impairment in thinking ability, memory (remote/recent), orientation to person/place/time, insight and judgment.

- Assess attention span/distractibility and ability to make decisions or problem-solve. (**Determines ability to participate in planning/executing care.**)
- Note discrepancies in child's age and mastery of developmental milestones.
- Test ability to receive, send, and appropriately interpret communications.
- Note behavior such as untidy personal habits; slowing and/or slurring of speech.
- Note occurrence of paranoia and delusions, hallucinations.
- Interview SO(s) to determine usual thinking ability, changes in behavior, length of time problem has existed, and other pertinent information **to provide baseline for comparison.**
- Assess client's anxiety level in relation to situation.
- Assist with in-depth testing of specific functions as appropriate.

NURSING PRIORITY NO. **3.** To prevent further deterioration, maximize level of function:

- Assist with treatment for underlying problems such as anorexia (nervosa/other), increased intracranial pressure, sleep disorders, biochemical imbalances. (**Cognition often improves with correction of medical problems.**)
- Establish alternate means for self-expression if unable to communicate verbally.
- Monitor and document vital signs periodically as appropriate.
- Perform neurologic assessments as indicated and compare with baseline. Note changes in level of consciousness and cognition, such as increased lethargy, confusion, drowsiness, irritability; changes in ability to communicate. **Early recognition of changes promotes proactive modifications to plan of care.**
- Reorient to time/place/person as needed. (**Inability to maintain orientation is a sign of deterioration.**)
- Have client write name periodically; keep this record for comparison and report differences.
- Note behavior that may be indicative of potential for violence and take appropriate actions.
- Provide safety measures (e.g., siderails, padding as necessary; close supervision, seizure precautions) as indicated.
- Schedule structured activity and rest periods. **Provides stimulation without undue fatigue.**
- Monitor medication regimen. Ascertain that physician is informed of all medications client is taking, noting possible interactions/cumulative effects.

- Encourage family/SO(s) to participate in reorientation and provide ongoing input (e.g., current news and family happening).
- Refer to appropriate rehabilitation providers (e.g., cognitive retraining program, speech therapist, psychosocial resources, biofeedback, counselor).

NURSING PRIORITY NO. 4. To create therapeutic milieu and assist client/SO(s) to develop coping strategies (especially when condition is irreversible):

- Provide opportunities for SO(s) to ask questions and obtain information.
- Maintain a pleasant, quiet environment and approach in a slow, calm manner. **Client may respond with anxious or aggressive behaviors if startled or overstimulated.**
- Give simple directions, using short words and simple sentences.
- Listen with regard **to convey interest and worth to individual.**
- Maintain reality-oriented relationship and environment (clocks, calendars, personal items, seasonal decorations).
- Present reality concisely and briefly and do not challenge illogical thinking—**defensive reactions may result.**
- Reduce provocative stimuli, negative criticism, arguments, and confrontations **to avoid triggering fight/flight responses.**
- Refrain from forcing activities and communications. **Client may feel threatened and may withdraw or rebel.**
- Respect individuality and personal space.
- Use touch judiciously, respecting personal needs, but keeping in mind physical and psychological importance of touch.
- Provide for nutritionally well-balanced diet incorporating client's preferences as able. Encourage client to eat. Provide pleasant environment and allow sufficient time to eat. **Enhances intake and general well-being.**
- Allow more time for client to respond to questions/comments and make simple decisions.
- Assist client/SO(s) with grieving process for loss of self/abilities as in Alzheimer's disease.
- Encourage participation in resocialization activities/groups when available.

NURSING PRIORITY NO. 5. To promote wellness (Teaching/Discharge Considerations):

- Assist in identifying ongoing treatment needs/rehabilitation program for the individual **to maintain gains and continue progress if able.**
- Stress importance of cooperation with therapeutic regimen.
- Promote socialization within individual limitations.
- Identify problems related to aging that are remediable and

assist client/SO(s) to seek appropriate assistance/access resources. **Encourages problem solving to improve condition rather than accept the status quo.**

- Help client/SO(s) develop plan of care when problem is progressive/long term.
- Refer to community resources (e.g., day-care programs, support groups, drug/alcohol rehabilitation).
- Refer to NDs Confusion, acute; Self-Care Deficit; Grieving, anticipatory/dysfunctional; Sensory Perception, disturbed; Tissue Perfusion, ineffective.

Documentation Focus

ASSESSMENT/REASSESSMENT

- Individual findings, including nature of problem, current and previous level of function, effect on independence and lifestyle.

PLANNING

- Plan of care and who is involved in planning.
- Teaching plan.

IMPLEMENTATION/EVALUATION

- Response to interventions/teaching and actions performed.
- Attainment/progress toward desired outcome(s).
- Modifications to plan of care.

DISCHARGE PLANNING

- Long-term needs/referrals and who is responsible for actions to be taken.
- Available resources, specific referrals made.

SAMPLE NURSING OUTCOMES & INTERVENTIONS CLASSIFICATIONS (NOC/NIC)

NOC—Distorted Thought Control
NIC—Dementia Management

Tissue Integrity, impaired

Taxonomy II: Safety/Protection—Class 2 Physical Injury (00044)
[Diagnostic Division: Safety]
Submitted 1986; Revised 1998 (by small group work 1996)

Definition: Damage to mucous membrane, corneal, integumentary, or subcutaneous tissues

---

Information that appears in brackets has been added by the authors to clarify and enhance the use of nursing diagnoses.

Related Factors

Altered circulation
Nutritional deficit/excess; [metabolic, endocrine dysfunction]
Fluid deficit/excess
Knowledge deficit
Impaired physical mobility
Irritants, chemical (including body excretions, secretions, medications); radiation (including therapeutic radiation)
Thermal (temperature extremes)
Mechanical (e.g., pressure, shear, friction), [surgery]
Knowledge deficit
[Infection]

Defining Characteristics

OBJECTIVE

Damaged or destroyed tissue (e.g., cornea, mucous membrane, integumentary, or subcutaneous)

Desired Outcomes/Evaluation Criteria—Client Will:

- Verbalize understanding of condition and causative factors.
- Identify interventions appropriate for specific condition.
- Demonstrate behaviors/lifestyle changes to promote healing and prevent complications/recurrence.
- Display progressive improvement in wound/lesion healing.

Actions/Interventions

NURSING PRIORITY NO. 1. To identify causative/contributing factors:

- Review history for possible causes: occupational, sports, and ADL hazards; familial history, illness, use of prosthetic devices (false limbs/eye, contacts, dentures, tracheal airways, indwelling catheters, esophageal dilators, etc.).
- Note poor health practices (e.g., lack of cleanliness, frequent use of enemas, poor nutrition, unsafe sexual practices, poor dental hygiene); emotional/psychological problems; cultural/religious practices.
- Assess environmental location of home/work in past and present as well as recent travel. (**Some areas of a country or city seem to be more susceptible to certain disease entities/environmental pollutants.**)
- Note race/ethnic background for genetic/sociocultural factors.
- Note evidence of other organ/tissue involvement (e.g., draining fistula through the integumentary and subcutaneous tissue may involve a bone infection).

- Assess adequacy of blood supply and innervation of the affected tissue.

NURSING PRIORITY NO. 2. To assess degree of impairment:

- Obtain history of condition: characteristics of previous episode(s), if any; when occurred, how many episodes, sites of past episodes; how episode starts/ends; other symptoms that have accompanied episodes; characteristics of lesions and changes/differences between lesions/episodes; duration this episode.
- Record size (depth, width), color, smell, location, temperature, texture, consistency of wounds/lesions if possible. **Provides comparative baseline. (Note:** Full extent of lesions of mucous membranes or subcutaneous tissue may not be discernible.)
- Observe for other distinguishing characteristics of inflamed tissue (e.g., exudate; granulation; cyanosis/pallor; tight, shiny skin).
- Assist with diagnostic procedures (e.g., cultures, oscopy, scans, biopsies); may be necessary **to determine extent of impairment.**
- Determine psychologic effects of condition on the client and family.

NURSING PRIORITY NO. 3. To assist client to correct/minimize impairment and to promote healing:

- Modify/eliminate factors contributing to condition, if possible. Assist with treatment of underlying condition(s) as appropriate.
- Inspect lesions/wounds daily for changes (e.g., signs of infection/complications or healing). **Promotes timely intervention/revision of plan of care.**
- Promote good nutrition with adequate protein and calorie intake, and vitamin/mineral supplements as indicated **to facilitate healing.**
- Encourage adequate periods of rest and sleep, including uninterrupted periods of sufficient duration; meeting comfort needs; limiting/avoiding use of caffeine/alcohol and medications affecting REM sleep.
- Promote early mobility. Provide position changes, active/passive and assistive exercises **to promote circulation and prevent excessive tissue pressure.**
- Provide devices such as eye pads/protective goggles, humidifiers, padding, air/water mattresses, splints, dressings, oral rinses, and so on **to aid in comfort/healing.**
- Practice aseptic technique for cleansing/dressing/medicating lesions. **Reduces risk of cross-contamination.**

- Obtain specimens of culture exudate/lesions for repeat cultures, sensitivity and Gram's stain when appropriate.
- Monitor laboratory studies (e.g., CBC, electrolytes, glucose, cultures) **for changes indicative of healing/infection/complications.**
- Provide safe environment when vision is affected.

NURSING PRIORITY NO. 4. To promote wellness (Teaching/Discharge Considerations):

- Encourage verbalizations of feelings and expectations regarding present condition.
- Help client and family to identify effective coping mechanisms and to begin to implement them.
- Discuss importance of early detection and reporting of changes in condition or any unusual physical discomforts/changes. **Promotes early detection of developing complications.**
- Emphasize need for adequate nutritional/fluid intake.
- Instruct in aseptic/clean techniques for dressing changes and proper disposal of soiled dressings **to prevent spread of infectious agent.**
- Review medical regimen (e.g., proper use of topical sprays, creams, ointments, soaks, or irrigations).
- Identify required changes in lifestyle, occupation, or environment **necessitated by limitations imposed by condition or to avoid causative factors.**
- Refer to community/governmental resources as indicated (e.g., Public Health Department, OSHA, National Association for the Prevention of Blindness).
- Refer to NDs dependent on individual situation (e.g., Skin Integrity, impaired; Oral Mucous Membrane, impaired; Injury, risk for perioperative positioning; Mobility, impaired physical/bed; Sensory Perception, disturbed: visual; Tissue Perfusion, ineffective; Trauma, risk for; Infection, risk for).

Documentation Focus

ASSESSMENT/REASSESSMENT

- Individual findings, including history of condition, characteristics of wound/lesion, evidence of other organ/tissue involvement.
- Impact on functioning/lifestyle.

PLANNING

- Plan of care and who is involved in planning.
- Teaching plan.

IMPLEMENTATION/EVALUATION

- Responses to interventions/teaching, actions performed.
- Attainment/progress toward desired outcome(s).
- Modifications to plan of care.

DISCHARGE PLANNING

- Long-term needs/referrals and who is responsible for actions to be taken.
- Specific referrals made.

SAMPLE NURSING OUTCOMES & INTERVENTIONS CLASSIFICATIONS (NOC/NIC)

NOC—Tissue Integrity: Skin & Mucous Membranes
NIC—Wound Care

Tissue Perfusion, ineffective (specify type: renal, cerebral, cardiopulmonary, gastrointestinal, peripheral)

Taxonomy II: Activity/Rest—Class 4
Cardiovascular/Pulmonary Responses (00024)
[Diagnostic Division: Circulation]
Submitted 1980; Revised 1998 (by small group work 1996)

Definition: Decrease in oxygen resulting in the failure to nourish the tissues at the capillary level [Tissue perfusion problems can exist without decreased cardiac output; however, there may be a relationship between cardiac output and tissue perfusion.]

Related Factors

Interruption of flow—arterial, venous
Exchange problems
Hypervolemia, hypovolemia
Mechanical reduction of venous and/or arterial blood flow
Decreased Hb concentration in blood
Altered affinity of hemoglobin for O_2; enzyme poisoning
Impaired transport of the O_2 across alveolar and/or capillary membrane
Mismatch of ventilation with blood flow
Hypoventilation

Information that appears in brackets has been added by the authors to clarify and enhance the use of nursing diagnoses.

Defining Characteristics

RENAL

Objective
Altered blood pressure outside of acceptable parameters
Oliguria or anuria; hematuria
Arterial pulsations, bruits
Elevation in BUN/Cr ratio

CEREBRAL

Objective
Altered mental status; speech abnormalities
Behavioral changes; [restlessness]; changes in motor response; extremity weakness or paralysis
Changes in pupillary reactions
Difficulty in swallowing

CARDIOPULMONARY

Subjective
Chest pain
Dyspnea
Sense of "impending doom"
Objective
Dysrhythmias
Capillary refill longer than 3 sec
Altered respiratory rate outside of acceptable parameters
Use of accessory muscles; chest retraction; nasal flaring
Bronchospasms
Abnormal ABGs
[Hemoptysis]

GASTROINTESTINAL

Subjective
Nausea
Abdominal pain or tenderness

OBJECTIVE

Hypoactive or absent bowel sounds
Abdominal distention
[Melena]

PERIPHERAL

Subjective
Claudication

OBJECTIVE

Altered skin characteristics (hair, nails, moisture)
Skin temperature changes
Skin discolorations; color diminished; color pale on elevation, color does not return on lowering the leg
Altered sensations

BP changes in extremities; weak or absent pulses; diminished arterial pulsations; bruits
Edema
Delayed healing
Positive Homans' sign

Desired Outcomes/Evaluation Criteria—Client Will:

- Verbalize understanding of condition, therapy regimen, side effects of medications, and when to contact healthcare provider.
- Demonstrate behaviors/lifestyle changes to improve circulation (e.g., cessation of smoking, relaxation techniques, exercise/dietary program).
- Demonstrate increased perfusion as individually appropriate (e.g., skin warm/dry, peripheral pulses present/strong, vital signs within client's normal range, alert/oriented, balanced intake/output, absence of edema, free of pain/discomfort).

Actions/Interventions

NURSING PRIORITY NO. 1. To assess causative/contributing factors:

- Determine factors related to individual situation, for example, previous history of/at risk for formation of thrombus or emboli, fractures, diagnosis of Raynaud's or Buerger's disease. In addition, note situations that can affect all body systems (e.g., SLE, the glucocorticoids in Addison's disease, congestive heart failure, pheochromocytoma/other endocrine imbalances, and sepsis).
- Identify changes related to systemic and/or peripheral alterations in circulation (e.g., altered mentation, vital signs, postural BPs, pain, changes in skin/tissue/organ function, signs of metabolic imbalances).
- Evaluate for signs of infection especially when immune system is compromised.
- Observe for signs of pulmonary emboli: sudden onset of chest pain, cyanosis, respiratory distress, hemoptysis, diaphoresis, hypoxia, anxiety, restlessness.

NURSING PRIORITY NO. 2. To note degree of impairment/organ involvement:

- Determine duration of problem/frequency of recurrence, precipitating/aggravating factors.
- Note customary baseline data (e.g., usual BP, weight, mentation, ABGs, and other appropriate laboratory study values). **Provides comparison with current findings.**
- Ascertain impact on functioning/lifestyle.

RENAL

- Ascertain usual voiding pattern; compare with current situation.
- Note characteristics of urine; measure specific gravity.
- Review laboratory studies (e.g., BUN/Cr levels, proteinuria, specific gravity, serum electrolytes).
- Note mentation (**may be altered by increased BUN/Cr**).
- Auscultate BP, ascertain client's usual range (**decreased glomerular filtration rate—GFR—may increase renin and raise BP**).
- Note presence, location, intensity, duration of pain.
- Observe for dependent/generalized edema.

CEREBRAL

- Determine presence of visual, sensory/motor changes, headache, dizziness, altered mental status, personality changes.
- Note history of brief/intermittent periods of confusion/blackout. (**Suggests transient ischemic attacks—TIAs.**)
- Interview SO(s) regarding their perception of situation.

CARDIOPULMONARY

- Investigate reports of chest pain/angina; note precipitating factors, changes in characteristics of pain episodes.
- Note presence/degree of dyspnea, cyanosis, hemoptysis.
- Determine cardiac rhythm, presence of dysrhythmias.
- Review baseline ABGs, electrolytes, BUN/Cr, cardiac enzymes.

GASTROINTESTINAL

- Note reports of nausea/vomiting, location/type/intensity of pain.
- Auscultate bowel sounds; measure abdominal girth; ascertain client's customary waist size/belt length; note changes in stool/presence of blood.
- Observe for symptoms of peritonitis, ischemic colitis, abdominal angina.

PERIPHERAL

- Ascertain history/characteristics of pain, for example, with/without activity, temperature/color changes, paresthesia, time (day/night), precipitated by heat, and so forth.
- Measure circumference of extremities as indicated. (**Useful in identifying edema in involved extremity.**)
- Assess lower extremities, noting skin texture, presence of edema, ulcerations.
- Measure capillary refill; palpate for presence/absence and quality of pulses.

- Auscultate for systolic/continuous bruits below obstruction in extremities.
- Check for calf tenderness (Homans' sign), swelling, and redness, **which may indicate thrombus formation.**
- Review laboratory studies (e.g., clotting times, Hb/Hct).
- Observe for signs of shock/sepsis. Note presence of bleeding or signs of DIC.

NURSING PRIORITY NO. 3. To maximize tissue perfusion:

RENAL

- Monitor vital signs.
- Measure urine output on a regular schedule. (Intake may be calculated against output.) Weigh daily.
- Administer medication (e.g., anticoagulants in presence of thrombosis, steroids in membranous nephropathy).
- Provide for diet restrictions, as indicated, while providing adequate calories to meet the body's needs. (**Restriction of protein helps limit BUN.**)
- Provide psychologic support for client/SO(s), especially when progression of disease and resultant treatment (dialysis) may be long term.

CEREBRAL

- Elevate HOB (e.g., 10 degrees) and maintain head/neck in midline or neutral position **to promote circulation/venous drainage.**
- Administer medications (e.g., steroids/diuretics may be used to decrease edema, anticoagulants).
- Assist with/monitor hypothermia therapy, **which may be used to decrease metabolic and O_2 needs.**
- Prepare client for surgery as indicated (e.g., carotid endarterectomy, evacuation of hematoma/space-occupying lesion).
- Refer to ND Intracranial Adaptive Capacity, decreased.

CARDIOPULMONARY

- Monitor vital signs, hemodynamics, heart sounds, and cardiac rhythm.
- Encourage quiet, restful atmosphere. **Conserves energy/lowers tissue O_2 demands.**
- Caution client to avoid activities that increase cardiac workload (e.g., straining at stool). Review ways of avoiding constipation.
- Administer medications (e.g., antidysrhythmics, fibrinolytic agents).
- Note signs of ischemia secondary to drug effects.
- Refer to ND Cardiac Output, decreased.

GASTROINTESTINAL

- Maintain gastric/intestinal decompression and measure output periodically.
- Provide small/easily digested food and fluids when tolerated.
- Encourage rest after meals **to maximize blood flow to stomach enhancing digestion.**
- Prepare client for surgery as indicated. (May be a surgical emergency, e.g., resection, bypass graft, mesenteric endarterectomy.)
- Refer to ND Nutrition: imbalanced, less than body requirements.

PERIPHERAL

- Perform assistive/active range-of-motion exercises (Buerger and Buerger-Allen).
- Encourage early ambulation when possible. **Enhances venous return.**
- Discourage sitting/standing for long periods, wearing constrictive clothing, crossing legs.
- Elevate the legs when sitting, but avoid sharp angulation of the hips or knees.
- Avoid use of knee gatch on bed; elevate entire foot as indicated.
- Provide air mattress, sheepskin padding, bed/foot cradle **to protect the extremities.**
- Elevate HOB at night **to increase gravitational blood flow.**
- Apply antithromboembolic hose/Ace bandages to lower extremities before arising from bed **to prevent venous stasis.**
- Use paper tape instead of adhesive.
- Avoid massaging the leg **when at risk for embolus.**
- Exercise caution in use of hot water bottles or heating pads; **tissues may have decreased sensitivity due to ischemia. (Heat also increases the metabolic demands of already compromised tissues.)**
- Monitor circulation above/below casts. Apply ice and elevate limb as appropriate **to reduce edema.**
- Encourage client to limit/quit smoking.
- Assist with/prepare for medical procedures (e.g., sympathectomy, vein graft) **to improve peripheral circulation.**
- Monitor closely for signs of shock when sympathectomy is done **(result of unmediated vasodilation).**
- Administer medications with caution (e.g., vasodilators, papaverine, antilipemics, anticoagulants). **Drug response, half-life, toxic levels may be altered by decreased tissue perfusion.**
- Monitor for signs of bleeding during use of fibrinolytic agents.

NURSING PRIORITY NO. **4.** To promote wellness (Teaching/ Discharge Considerations):

- Discuss the risk factors and potential outcomes of atherosclerosis. (**Information necessary for client to make informed choices and commit to lifestyle changes as appropriate.**)
- Encourage discussion of feelings regarding prognosis/long-term effects of condition.
- Identify necessary changes in lifestyle and assist client to incorporate disease management into ADLs.
- Encourage client to quit smoking, join Smoke-out, other stop-smoking programs. (**Smoking causes vasoconstriction and may further compromise perfusion.**)
- Demonstrate/encourage use of relaxation techniques, exercises/**techniques to decrease tension level.** Establish regular exercise program.
- Review specific dietary changes/restrictions with client (e.g., reduction of cholesterol and triglycerides, high or low in protein, avoidance of rye in Buerger's disease).
- Discuss care of dependent limbs, body hygiene, foot care when circulation is impaired.
- Recommend avoidance of vasoconstricting drugs.
- Discourage massaging of calf in presence of varicose veins/thrombophlebitis **to prevent embolization.**
- Emphasize importance of avoiding use of aspirin, some OTC drugs, vitamins containing potassium, mineral oil, or alcohol when taking anticoagulants.
- Review medical regimen and appropriate safety measures (e.g., use of electric razor when taking anticoagulants).
- Discuss preventing exposure to cold, dressing warmly, and use of natural fibers to retain heat more efficiently.
- Provide preoperative teaching appropriate for the situation.
- Refer to specific support groups, counseling as appropriate.

Documentation Focus

ASSESSMENT/REASSESSMENT

- Individual findings, noting nature/extent and duration of problem, effect on independence/lifestyle.
- Characteristics of pain, precipitators, and what relieves pain.
- Vital signs, cardiac rhythm/dysrhythmias.
- Pulses/BP, including above/below suspected lesion as appropriate.
- I/O and weight as indicated.

PLANNING

- Plan of care and who is involved in planning.
- Teaching plan.

Tissue Perfusion, ineffective (specify type: renal, cerebral, cardiopulmonary, gastrointestinal, peripheral)

IMPLEMENTATION/EVALUATION

• Response to interventions/teaching and actions performed.
• Attainment/progress toward desired outcome(s).
• Modifications to plan of care.

DISCHARGE PLANNING

• Long-term needs and who is responsible for actions to be taken.
• Available resources, specific referrals made.

SAMPLE NURSING OUTCOMES & INTERVENTIONS CLASSIFICATIONS (NOC/NIC)

CARDIOPULMONARY

NOC—Tissue Perfusion: Cardiac
NIC—Cardiac Care

CEREBRAL

NOC—Tissue Perfusion: Cerebral
NIC—Cerebral Perfusion Promotion

RENAL

NOC—Urinary
NIC—Fluid/Electrolyte Management

GASTROINTESTINAL

NOC—Tissue Perfusion: Abdominal Organ
NIC—Nutrition Management

PERIPHERAL

NOC—Tissue Perfusion: Peripheral
NIC—Circulatory Care: Arterial Insufficiency

Transfer Ability, impaired

Taxonomy II: Activity/Rest—Class 2 Activity/Exercise (00090)
[Diagnostic Division: Activity/Rest]
Submitted 1998

Definition: Limitation of independent movement between two nearby surfaces

Related Factors

To be developed
[Conditions that result in poor muscle tone]
[Cognitive impairment]
[Fractures, trauma, spinal cord injury]

Information that appears in brackets has been added by the authors **544** to clarify and enhance the use of nursing diagnoses.

Defining Characteristics

SUBJECTIVE OR OBJECTIVE

Impaired ability to transfer: from bed to chair and chair to bed, chair to car or car to chair, chair to floor or floor to chair, standing to floor or floor to standing; on or off a toilet or commode; in and out of tub or shower, between uneven levels

Specify level of independence—[refer to ND Mobility, impaired physical, for suggested functional level classification]

Desired Outcomes/Evaluation Criteria—Client/Caregiver Will:

- Verbalize understanding of situation and appropriate safety measures.
- Master techniques of transfer successfully.
- Make desired transfer safely.

Actions/Interventions

NURSING PRIORITY NO. 1. To assess causative/contributing factors:

- Determine diagnosis that contributes to transfer problems (e.g., MS, fractures, back injuries, quadriplegia/paraplegia, agedness, dementias, brain injury, etc.).
- Note current situations such as surgery, amputation, contractures, traction apparatus, mechanical ventilation, multiple tubings that restrict movement.

NURSING PRIORITY NO. 2. To assess functional ability:

- Evaluate degree of impairment using 0 to 4 functional level classification.
- Note emotional/behavioral responses of client/SO to problems of immobility.
- Determine presence/degree of perceptual/cognitive impairment and ability to follow directions.

NURSING PRIORITY NO. 3. To promote optimal level of movement:

- Assist with treatment of underlying condition causing dysfunction.
- Consult with PT/OT/rehabilitation team in developing mobility aids and adjunctive devices.
- Instruct in use of siderails, overhead trapeze, safety grab bars, cane walker, devices on the bed/chair that protect client (e.g., call light, bed-positioning switch in easy reach), wheelchair, crutches, assisting as necessary.
- Provide instruction/reinforce information for client and caregivers regarding positioning to improve/maintain balance when transferring.

- Monitor body alignment and balance and encourage wide base of support when standing to transfer.
- Use full-length mirror as needed **to facilitate client's view of own postural alignment.**
- Demonstrate/reinforce safety measures as indicated, such as transfer board, gait belt, supportive footwear, good lighting, clearing floor of clutter, and so forth **to avoid possibility of fall and subsequent injury.**

NURSING PRIORITY NO. 4. To promote wellness (Teaching/Discharge Considerations):

- Assist client/caregivers to learn safety measures as individually indicated (e.g., locking wheelchair before transfer, having scatter rugs removed from floor, using properly placed Hoyer lift, etc.).
- Refer to appropriate community resources for evaluation and modification of environment (e.g., shower/tub, uneven floor surfaces/steps, use of ramps/standing tables/lifts, etc.).

Documentation Focus

ASSESSMENT/REASSESSMENT

- Individual findings, including level of function/ability to participate in desired transfers.

PLANNING

- Plan of care and who is involved in the planning.
- Teaching plan.

IMPLEMENTATION/EVALUATION

- Responses to interventions/teaching and actions performed.
- Attainment/progress toward desired outcome(s).
- Modifications to plan of care.

DISCHARGE PLANNING

- Discharge/long-range needs, noting who is responsible for each action to be taken.
- Specific referrals made.
- Sources of/maintenance for assistive devices.

SAMPLE NURSING OUTCOMES & INTERVENTIONS CLASSIFICATIONS (NOC/NIC)

NOC—Transfer Performance
NIC—Transport

Trauma, risk for

Taxonomy II: Safety/Protection—Class 2 Physical Injury
(00038)
[Diagnostic Division: Safety]
Submitted 1980

Definition: Accentuated risk of accidental tissue injury
(e.g., wound, burn, fracture)

Risk Factors

INTERNAL (INDIVIDUAL)

Weakness; balancing difficulties; reduced large- or small-muscle coor-
   dination, hand/eye coordination
Poor vision
Reduced temperature and/or tactile sensation
Lack of safety education/precautions
Insufficient finances to purchase safety equipment or to effect repairs
Cognitive or emotional difficulties
History of previous trauma

EXTERNAL (ENVIRONMENTAL) [INCLUDES
BUT IS NOT LIMITED TO]:

Slippery floors (e.g., wet or highly waxed; unanchored rug; litter or
   liquid spills on floors or stairways; snow or ice collected on stairs,
   walkways)
Bathtub without handgrip or antislip equipment
Use of unsteady ladder or chairs
Obstructed passageways; entering unlighted rooms
Unsturdy or absent stair rails; children playing without gates at top of
   stairs
Unanchored electric wires
High beds; inappropriate call-for-aid mechanisms for bed-resting
   client
Unsafe window protection in homes with young children
Pot handles facing toward front of stove; bathing in very hot water
   (e.g., unsupervised bathing of young children)
Potential igniting gas leaks; delayed lighting of gas burner or oven
Unscreened fires or heaters; wearing plastic apron or flowing clothing
   around open flames; highly flammable children's toys or clothing
Smoking in bed or near O_2; grease waste collected on stoves
Children playing with matches, candles, cigarettes
Playing with fireworks or gunpowder; guns or ammunition stored
   unlocked
Experimenting with chemical or gasoline; inadequately stored
   combustibles or corrosives (e.g., matches, oily rags, lye; contact with
   acids or alkalis)
Overloaded fuse boxes; faulty electrical plugs, frayed wires, or defective
   appliances; overloaded electrical outlets
Exposure to dangerous machinery; contact with rapidly moving
   machinery, industrial belts, or pulleys

Information that appears in brackets has been added by the authors
to clarify and enhance the use of nursing diagnoses.

Sliding on coarse bed linen or struggling within bed[/chair] restraints

Contact with intense cold; overexposure to sun, sunlamps, radio-therapy

Use of thin or worn-out pot holders [or mitts]

Use of cracked dishware or glasses

Knives stored uncovered; children playing with sharp-edged toys

Large icicles hanging from roof

High-crime neighborhood and vulnerable clients

Driving a mechanically unsafe vehicle; driving at excessive speeds; driving without necessary visual aids

Driving after partaking of alcoholic beverages or [other] drugs

Children riding in the front seat of car, nonuse or misuse of seat restraints/[unrestrained infant/child riding in car]

Misuse [or nonuse] of necessary headgear for motorized cyclists or young children carried on adult bicycles

Unsafe road or road-crossing conditions; playing or working near vehicle pathways (e.g., driveways, lanes, railroad tracks)

> NOTE: A risk diagnosis is not evidenced by signs and symptoms, as the problem has not occurred and nursing interventions are directed at prevention.

Desired Outcomes/Evaluation Criteria—Client/Caregiver Will:

- Identify and correct potential risk factors in the environment.
- Demonstrate appropriate lifestyle changes to reduce risk of injury.
- Identify resources to assist in promoting a safe environment.
- Recognize need for/seek assistance to prevent accidents/injuries.

Actions/Interventions

NURSING PRIORITY NO. 1. To assess causative/contributing factors:

- Determine factors related to individual situation and extent of risk/injuries sustained.
- Note age of individual, mentation, agility, impairment of mobility.
- Evaluate environment (home/work/transportation) for safety hazards.
- Assess interest and knowledge of the client/caregivers regarding safety needs.
- Note history of accidents during given period, noting circumstances of the accident (e.g., time of day that falls occur, activities going on, who was present).
- Assess influence of stress on potential for injury.
- Review potential risk factors (e.g., noise level/use of headphones, various inhalants and length of exposure time).

- Review laboratory studies and observe for signs/symptoms of endocrine/electrolyte imbalances **that may result in/exacerbate conditions, such as confusion, tetany, pathological fractures, and so on.**
- Determine presence/potential for hypothermia or hyperthermia, for example, induced (coma therapy/surgery) or accidental.

NURSING PRIORITY NO. 2. To promote safety measures required by individual situation:

- Orient client to environment.
- Make arrangement for call system for bedridden client in home and in hospital setting. Demonstrate use and place call bell/light within client's reach.
- Keep bed in low position or place mattress on floor as appropriate.
- Use and pad siderails as indicated.
- Provide seizure precautions.
- Lock wheels on bed/movable furniture. Clear travel paths. Provide adequate area lighting.
- Assist with activities and transfers as needed.
- Provide well-fitting, nonskid footwear.
- Demonstrate/monitor use of assistive devices, such as cane, walker, crutches, wheelchair, safety bars.
- Provide supervision while client is smoking.
- Provide for appropriate disposal of potentially injurious items (e.g., needles, scalpel blades).
- Apply/monitor use of restraints when required (e.g., vest, limb, belt, mitten).
- Refer to specific NDs as appropriate (e.g., Hypothermia; Mobility, impaired physical; Skin Integrity, impaired; Sensory Perception, disturbed; Thought Processes, disturbed; Body Temperature, risk for imbalanced; Home Maintenance, impaired).

NURSING PRIORITY NO. 3. To treat underlying medical/psychiatric condition:

- Provide positioning as required by situation (e.g., postcorneal lens surgery, immobilization of fractures).
- Assist with treatments for endocrine/electrolyte imbalance conditions. **(May improve cognition/muscle tone and general well-being.)**
- Provide quiet environment and reduced stimulation as indicated. **Helps limit confusion or overstimulation for clients at risk for such conditions as seizures, tetany, autonomic hyperreflexia.**
- Rewarm client gradually when hypothermia is present. (Refer to ND Hypothermia.)

- Refer to counseling/psychotherapy, as need indicates, especially when individual is "accident-prone"/self-destructive behavior is noted. (Refer to NDs Violence, [actual/] risk for other-directed/self-directed.)

NURSING PRIORITY NO. 4. To promote wellness (Teaching/ Discharge Considerations):

- Stress importance of changing position slowly and obtaining assistance when weak and when problems of balance, coordination, or postural hypotension are present **to reduce risk of syncope/falls.**
- Encourage use of warm-up/stretching exercises before engaging in athletic activity **to prevent muscle injuries.**
- Recommend use of seat belts, fitted helmets for cyclists, approved infant seat; avoidance of hitchhiking.
- Refer to accident prevention programs (e.g., driver training, parenting classes, firearms safety, etc.).
- Develop fire safety program (e.g., family fire drills; use of smoke detectors; yearly chimney cleaning; purchase of fire-retardant clothing, especially children's nightwear; fireworks safety).
- Problem-solve with client/parent to provide adequate child supervision after school, during working hours, and on school holidays.
- Discuss necessary environmental changes (e.g., decals on glass doors to show when they are closed, lowering temperature on hot water heater, adequate lighting of stairways) **to prevent/reduce risk of accidents.**
- Identify community resources (e.g., financial **to assist with necessary corrections/improvements/purchases**).
- Recommend involvement in community self-help programs, such as Neighborhood Watch, Helping Hand.

Documentation Focus

ASSESSMENT/REASSESSMENT

- Individual risk factors, past/recent history of injuries, awareness of safety needs.

PLANNING

- Plan of care and who is involved in the planning.
- Teaching plan.

IMPLEMENTATION/EVALUATION

- Responses to interventions/teaching, actions performed.
- Attainment/progress toward desired outcome(s).
- Modifications to plan of care.

- Long-term needs and who is responsible for actions to be taken.
- Available resources, specific referrals made.

SAMPLE NURSING OUTCOMES & INTERVENTIONS CLASSIFICATIONS (NOC/NIC)

NOC—Safety Status: Physical Injury
NIC—Environmental Management: Safety

Unilateral Neglect

Taxonomy II: Perception/Cognition—Class 1 Attention (00123)
[Diagnostic Division: Neurosensory]
Submitted 1986

Definition: Lack of awareness and attention to one side of the body

Related Factors

Effects of disturbed perceptual abilities (e.g., [homonymous] hemi-anopsia, one-sided blindness; [or visual inattention])
Neurological illness or trauma
[Impaired cerebral blood flow]

Defining Characteristics

SUBJECTIVE

[Reports feeling that part does not belong to own self]

OBJECTIVE

Consistent inattention to stimuli on an affected side
Inadequate self-care [inability to satisfactorily perform ADLs]
[Lack of] positioning and/or safety precautions in regard to the affected side
Does not look toward affected side; [does not touch affected side]
Leaves food on plate on the affected side
[Failure to use the affected side of the body without being reminded to do so]

Desired Outcomes/Evaluation Criteria—Client Will:

- Acknowledge presence of sensory-perceptual impairment.
- Verbalize positive realistic perception of self incorporating the current dysfunction.

Information that appears in brackets has been added by the authors to clarify and enhance the use of nursing diagnoses.

- Identify adaptive/protective measures for individual situation.
- Perform self-care within level of ability.
- Demonstrate behaviors, lifestyle changes necessary to promote physical safety.

Actions/Interventions

NURSING PRIORITY NO. **1.** To assess the extent of altered perception and the related degree of disability:

- Measure visual acuity and field of vision.
- Assess sensory awareness (e.g., response to stimulus of hot/cold, dull/sharp); note problems with awareness of motion and proprioception.
- Observe client's behavior **to determine the extent of impairment.**
- Assess ability to distinguish between right and left.
- Note physical signs of neglect (e.g., disregard for position of affected limb(s), skin irritation/injury).
- Observe ability to function within limits of impairment. Compare with client's perception of own abilities.
- Explore and encourage verbalization of feelings **to identify meaning of loss/dysfunction/change to the client and impact it may have on assuming ADLs.**

NURSING PRIORITY NO. **2.** To promote optimal comfort and safety for the client in the environment:

- Approach client from the unaffected side during acute phase. Explain to client that one side is being neglected; repeat as needed.
- Orient to physical environment.
- Remove excess stimuli from the environment when working with the client.
- Encourage client to turn head and eyes in full rotation and "scan" the environment **to compensate for visual field loss.**
- Position bedside table and objects (such as call bell, tissues) within functional field of vision.
- Position furniture and equipment so travel path is not obstructed. Keep doors wide open or completely closed.
- Remove articles in the environment that may create a safety hazard (e.g., footstool, throw rug).
- Ensure adequate lighting in the environment.
- Monitor affected body part(s) for positioning/anatomic alignment, pressure points/skin irritation/injury, and dependent edema. **(Increased risk of injury/ulcer formation necessitates close observation and timely intervention.)**
- Protect affected body part(s) from pressure/injury/burns, and help client learn to assume this responsibility.

NURSING PRIORITY NO. **3**. To promote wellness (Teaching/ Discharge Considerations):

- Increase the amount of touch in providing client care.
- Encourage the client to look at and handle affected side to stimulate awareness.
- Bring the affected limb across the midline for the client to visualize during care.
- Provide tactile stimuli to the affected side by touching/ manipulating, stroking, and communicating about the affected side by itself rather than stimulating both sides simultaneously.
- Provide objects of various weight, texture, and size for the client to handle.
- Assist the client to position the affected extremity carefully and teach to routinely visualize placement of the extremity. Remind with visual cues. If the client completely ignores one side of the body, use positioning to improve perception (e.g., position client facing/looking at the affected side).
- Encourage client to accept affected limb/side as part of self even when it no longer feels like it belongs.
- Use a mirror to help the client adjust position by visualizing both sides of the body.
- Use descriptive terms to identify body parts rather than "left" and "right"; for example, "Lift this leg" (point to leg) or "Lift your affected leg."
- Describe where affected areas of body are when moving the client.
- Acknowledge and accept feelings of despondency, grief, and anger. (When feelings are openly expressed, client can deal with them and move forward.)
- Reinforce to client the reality of the dysfunction and need to compensate.
- Avoid participating in the client's use of denial.
- Encourage family members and SO(s) to treat client normally and not as an invalid, including client in family activities.
- Assist with ADLs, maximizing self-care potential. Help client to bathe, apply lotion, and so forth to affected side.
- Place nonessential items (e.g., TV, pictures, hairbrush) on affected side during postacute phase once client begins to cross midline to encourage continuation of behavior.
- Refer to/encourage client to use rehabilitative services to enhance independence in functioning.
- Identify additional resources to meet individual needs (e.g., Meals on Wheels, home-care services) to maximize independence, allow client to return to community setting.

Documentation Focus

ASSESSMENT/REASSESSMENT

- Individual findings, including extent of altered perception, degree of disability, effect on independence/participation in ADLs.

PLANNING

- Plan of care and who is involved in the planning.
- Teaching plan.

IMPLEMENTATION/EVALUATION

- Responses to intervention/teaching and actions performed.
- Attainment/progress toward desired outcome(s).
- Modifications to plan of care.

DISCHARGE PLANNING

- Long-term needs and who is responsible for actions to be taken.
- Available resources, specific referrals made.

SAMPLE NURSING OUTCOMES & INTERVENTIONS CLASSIFICATIONS (NOC/NIC)

NOC—Self-Care: Activities of Daily Living (ADL)
NIC—Unilateral Neglect Management

Urinary Elimination, impaired

Taxonomy II: Elimination—Class 1 Urinary System
(00016)
[Diagnostic Division: Elimination]
Submitted 1973

Definition: Disturbance in urine elimination

Related Factors

Multiple causality; sensory motor impairment; anatomical obstruction; UTI; [mechanical trauma; fluid/volume states; psychogenic factors; surgical diversion]

Defining Characteristics

SUBJECTIVE

Frequency; urgency
Hesitancy
Dysuria
Nocturia, [enuresis]

Information that appears in brackets has been added by the authors
554 to clarify and enhance the use of nursing diagnoses.

Incontinence
Retention

Desired Outcomes/Evaluation Criteria—Client Will:

- Verbalize understanding of condition.
- Identify causative factors. (Refer to specific NDs for incontinence/retention as appropriate.)
- Achieve normal elimination pattern or participate in measures to correct/compensate for defects.
- Demonstrate behaviors/techniques to prevent urinary infection.
- Manage care of urinary catheter, or stoma and appliance following urinary diversion.

Actions/Interventions

NURSING PRIORITY NO. 1. To assess causative/contributing factors:

- Identify physical diagnoses that may be involved, such as surgery (including urinary diversion); neurologic deficits, such as MS, paraplegia/tetraplegia; mental/emotional dysfunction; prostate disease; recent/multiple pregnancies; cardiovascular disease; pelvic trauma; use of penile clamps (may result in urethral trauma).
- Determine whether problem is due to loss of neurologic functioning or disorientation (e.g., Alzheimer's disease).
- Determine pathology of bladder dysfunction relative to medical diagnosis identified. (For example, in neurologic/demyelinating diseases, such as MS, problem may be failure to store urine, empty bladder, or both.)
- Inspect stoma of urinary diversion for edema, scarring, presence of congealed mucus.
- Review drug regimen. Note use of drugs that may be nephrotoxic (e.g., aminoglycosides, tetracyclines), especially in clients who are immunosuppressed. Also note those that may result in retention (e.g., atropine, belladonna).
- Note age and sex of client. (UTIs are more prevalent in women and older men.)
- Rule out gonorrhea in men when urethritis with a penile discharge is present and there are no bacteria in the urine.
- Assist with antibody-coated bacteria assay to diagnose bacterial infection of the kidney or prostate.
- Review laboratory tests for hyperparathyroidism, changes in renal function, presence of infection.

• Strain all urine for calculi and describe stones expelled and/or send to laboratory for analysis.

NURSING PRIORITY NO. 2. To assess degree of interference/ disability:

• Determine client's previous pattern of elimination and compare with current situation. Note reports of frequency, urgency, burning, incontinence, nocturia/enuresis, size and force of urinary stream.
• Palpate bladder **to assess retention.**
• Investigate pain, noting location, duration, intensity; presence of bladder spasms, back or flank pain, and so forth.
• Determine client's usual daily fluid intake (both amount and beverage choices/use of caffeine). Note condition of skin and mucous membranes, color of urine **to help determine level of hydration.**

NURSING PRIORITY NO. 3. To assist in treating/preventing urinary alteration:

• Refer to specific NDs Incontinence (specify), Urinary Retention.
• Encourage fluid intake up to 3000 to 4000 mL/day (within cardiac tolerance), including cranberry juice, **to help maintain renal function, prevent infection and formation of urinary stones, avoid encrustation around catheter, or to flush urinary diversion appliance.**
• Assist with developing toileting routines as appropriate.
• Encourage client to void in sitz bath after surgical procedures of the perineal area. (**Warm water helps relax muscles and soothe sore tissues, facilitating voiding.**)
• Observe for signs of infection—cloudy, foul odor; bloody urine. Send urine (midstream clean-voided specimen) for culture and sensitivities as indicated.
• Encourage client to verbalize fear/concerns (e.g., disruption in sexual activity, inability to work). **Open expression allows client to deal with feelings and begin problem solving.**
• Monitor medication regimen, antimicrobials (single-dose is frequently being used for UTI), sulfonamides, antispasmodics, and so on **to note client's response, need to modify treatment.**
• Discuss surgical procedures and review medical regimen for client with benign prostatic hypertrophy bladder/prostatic cancer, and so forth.

NURSING PRIORITY NO. 4. To assist in management of long-term urinary alterations:

• Keep bladder deflated by use of an indwelling catheter

connected to closed drainage. Investigate alternatives when possible (e.g., intermittent catheterization, surgical interventions, urinary drugs, voiding maneuvers, condom catheter).

- Provide latex-free catheter and care supplies **to reduce risk of latex sensitivity.**
- Check frequently for bladder distention and observe for overflow **to reduce risk of infection and/or autonomic hyperreflexia.**
- Maintain acidic environment of the bladder by the use of agents, such as vitamin C, Mandelamine when appropriate **to discourage bacterial growth.**
- Adhere to a regular bladder/diversion appliance emptying schedule **to avoid accidents.**
- Provide for routine diversion appliance care, and assist client to recognize and deal with problems such as alkaline salt encrustation, ill-fitting appliance, malodorous urine, infection, and so forth.

NURSING PRIORITY NO. **5.** To promote wellness (Teaching/Discharge Considerations):

- Emphasize importance of keeping area clean and dry **to reduce risk of infection and/or skin breakdown.**
- Instruct female clients with UTI to drink large amounts of fluid, void immediately after intercourse, wipe from front to back, promptly treat vaginal infections, and take showers rather than tub baths **to limit risk/avoid reinfection.**
- Encourage SO(s) who participate in routine care to recognize complications (including latex allergy) necessitating medical interventions.
- Instruct in proper application and care of appliance for urinary diversion. Encourage liberal fluid intake, avoidance of foods/medications that produce strong odor, use of white vinegar or deodorizer in pouch **to promote odor control.**
- Identify sources for supplies, programs/agencies providing financial assistance **to obtain needed equipment.**
- Recommend avoidance of gas-forming foods in presence of ureterosigmoidostomy **as flatus can cause urinary incontinence.**
- Recommend use of silicone catheter when permanent/long-term catheterization is required.
- Demonstrate proper positioning of catheter drainage tubing and bag **to facilitate drainage/prevent reflux.**
- Refer client/SO(s) to appropriate community resources such as ostomy specialist, support group, sex therapist, psychiatric clinical nurse specialist, and so on **to deal with changes in body image/function when indicated.**

Documentation Focus

ASSESSMENT/REASSESSMENT

- Individual findings, including previous and current pattern of voiding, nature of problem, effect on desired lifestyle.

PLANNING

- Plan of care and who is involved in planning.
- Teaching plan.

IMPLEMENTATION/EVALUATION

- Response to interventions/teaching and actions performed.
- Attainment/progress toward desired outcome(s).
- Modifications to plan of care.

DISCHARGE PLANNING

- Long-term needs and who is responsible for actions to be taken.
- Available resources/specific referrals made.
- Individual equipment needs and sources.

SAMPLE NURSING OUTCOMES & INTERVENTIONS CLASSIFICATIONS (NOC/NIC)

NOC—Urinary Elimination
NIC—Urinary Elimination Management

Urinary Elimination, readiness for enhanced

Taxonomy II: Elimination—Class 1 Urinary System (00166)
[Diagnostic Division: Elimination]
Submitted 2002

Definition: A pattern of urinary functions that is sufficient for meeting eliminatory needs and can be strengthened

Related Factors

To be developed

Defining Characteristics

SUBJECTIVE

Expresses willingness to enhance urinary elimination
Positions self for emptying of bladder

Information that appears in brackets has been added by the authors
558 to clarify and enhance the use of nursing diagnoses.

OBJECTIVE

Urine is straw colored with no odor
Specific gravity is within normal limits
Amount of output is within normal limits for age and other factors
Fluid intake is adequate for daily needs

Desired Outcomes/Evaluation Criteria—Client Will:

- Verbalize understanding of condition that has potential for altering elimination.
- Achieve normal elimination pattern, voiding in appropriate amounts.
- Alter environment to accommodate individual needs.

Actions/Interventions

NURSING PRIORITY NO. 1. To assess status and adaptive skills being used by client:

- Identify physical diagnoses (e.g., surgery, childbirth, recent/ multiple pregnancies, pelvic trauma, stroke, mental/emotional dysfunction, prostate disease) **that may have impacted client's elimination patterns.**
- Determine client's previous pattern of elimination and compare with current situation. Review voiding diary if available. **Provides baseline for future comparison.**
- Observe voiding patterns, time, color, and amount voided if indicated (e.g., postsurgical or postpartum client) **to document normalization of elimination.**
- Ascertain methods of self-management (e.g., limiting or increasing liquid intake, regular voiding schedule).
- Determine client's usual daily fluid intake. **Both amount and beverage choices are important in managing elimination.**
- Note condition of skin and mucous membranes, color of urine **to help determine level of hydration.**

NURSING PRIORITY NO. 2. To assist client to improve management of urinary elimination:

- Encourage fluid intake, including water and cranberry juice, **to help maintain renal function, prevent infection.**
- Regulate liquid intake at prescheduled times **to promote predictable voiding pattern.** Restrict fluid intake 2 to 3 hours before bedtime **to reduce voiding during the night.**
- Assist with modifying current routines as appropriate. **Client may benefit from additional information in enhancing success, such as regarding cues/urge to void; adjusting schedule of voiding (shorter or longer); relaxation and/or distraction techniques, standing or sitting upright during voiding to**

ensure that bladder is completely empty, and/or practicing pelvic muscle strengthening exercises.
- Provide assistance/devices as indicated (e.g., provide means of summoning assistance; place bedside commode, urinal, or bedpan within client's reach; elevated toilet seats; mobility devices) when client is frail or mobility impaired.
- Modify/recommend diet changes if indicated. For example, reduction of caffeine, because of its bladder irritant effect; or weight reduction may help reduce overactive bladder symptoms and incontinence with decreased pressure on the bladder.
- Modify medication regimens as appropriate (e.g., administer prescribed diuretics in the morning to lessen nighttime voiding). Reduce or eliminate use of hypnotics if possible as client may be too sedated to recognize/respond to urge to void.

NURSING PRIORITY NO. 3. To promote optimum wellness:

- Encourage continuation of successful toileting program and identify possible alterations to meet individual needs (e.g., use of adult briefs for extended outing or travel with limited access to toilet). Promotes proactive problem solving and supports normalization of activities.
- Instruct client/SO(s)/caregivers in cues that client needs, such as voiding on routine schedule, showing client location of the bathroom, providing adequate room lighting, signs, color coding of door, to assist client in continued continence especially when in unfamiliar surroundings.
- Review signs/symptoms of urinary complications and need for medical follow-up. Promotes timely intervention to limit or prevent adverse events.

Documentation Focus

ASSESSMENT/REASSESSMENT

- Findings/adaptive skills being used.

PLANNING

- Plan of care and who is involved in planning.
- Teaching plan.

IMPLEMENTATION/EVALUATION

- Responses to treatment plan/interventions and actions performed.
- Attainment/progress toward desired outcome(s).
- Modifications to plan of care.

DISCHARGE PLANNING

- Available resources, equipment needs/sources.

NOC—Urinary Elimination
NIC—Urinary Elimination Management

Urinary Incontinence, functional

Taxonomy II: Elimination—Class 1 Urinary System
(00020)
[Diagnostic Division: Elimination]
Submitted 1986; Nursing Diagnosis Extension and
Classification (NDEC) Revision 1998

Definition: Inability of usually continent person to
reach toilet in time to avoid unintentional loss of urine

Related Factors

Altered environmental factors [e.g., poor lighting or inability to locate
 bathroom]
Neuromuscular limitations
Weakened supporting pelvic structures
Impaired vision/cognition
Psychological factors; [reluctance to use call light or bedpan]
[Increased urine production]

Defining Characteristics

SUBJECTIVE

Senses need to void
[Voiding in large amounts]

OBJECTIVE

Loss of urine before reaching toilet; amount of time required to reach
 toilet exceeds length of time between sensing urge and uncontrolled
 voiding
Able to completely empty bladder
May only be incontinent in early morning

Desired Outcomes/Evaluation
Criteria—Client Will:

- Verbalize understanding of condition and identify interven-
  tions to prevent incontinence.
- Alter environment to accommodate individual needs.
- Report voiding in individually appropriate amounts.
- Urinate at acceptable times and places.

Information that appears in brackets has been added by the authors
to clarify and enhance the use of nursing diagnoses.

Actions/Interventions

NURSING PRIORITY NO. **1**. To assess causative/contributing factors:

- Determine if client is voluntarily postponing urination.
- Review history for disease, use of medication/substances known to increase urine output and/or alter bladder tone (e.g., diabetes mellitus, prolapsed bladder, diuretics, alcohol, caffeine).
- Test urine with Chemstix to note presence of glucose, **which can cause polyuria and result in overdistention of the bladder.**
- Determine the difference between the time it takes to get to the bathroom/remove clothing and the time between urge and involuntary loss of urine.
- Review disease process and medications. **Could affect mental status/orientation to place, recognition of urge to void, and/ or its significance.**
- Identify environmental conditions that interfere with timely access to bathroom/successful toileting process. **Factors such as unfamiliar surroundings, dexterity problems, poor lighting, improperly fitted chair walker, low toilet seat, absence of safety bars, and travel distance to toilet may affect self-care ability.**

NURSING PRIORITY NO. **2**. To assess degree of interference/ disability:

- Assist client to keep voiding diary. Determine the frequency and timing of continent/incontinent voids.
- Measure/estimate amount of urine voided or lost with incontinence.
- Examine urine for signs of bacteriuria (e.g., cloudy/hazy).
- Ascertain effect on lifestyle (including socialization and sexuality) and self-esteem.

NURSING PRIORITY NO. **3**. To assist in treating/preventing incontinence:

- Administer prescribed diuretics in the morning **to lessen nighttime voidings.**
- Reduce or eliminate use of hypnotics if possible, **as client may be too sedated to recognize/respond to urge to void.**
- Provide means of summoning assistance (e.g., call light or bell).
- Adapt clothes for quick removal: Velcro fasteners, full skirts, crotchless panties or no panties, suspenders or elastic waists instead of belts on pants. **Facilitates toileting once urge to void is noted.**
- Use night-lights **to mark bathroom location.**

- Provide cues, such as adequate room lighting, signs, color coding of door, **to assist client who is disoriented to find the bathroom.**
- Remove throw rugs, excess furniture in travel path to bathroom.
- Raise chair and/or toilet seat.
- Provide bedside commode, urinal, or bedpan as indicated.
- Schedule voiding for every 3 hours **to minimize bladder pressure.**
- Restrict fluid intake 2 to 3 hours before bedtime **to reduce voiding during the night.**
- Instruct in pelvic floor strengthening exercises as appropriate.
- Implement bladder training program as indicated.
- Include physical/occupational therapist in determining ways to alter environment, appropriate assistive devices to meet client's individual needs.

NURSING PRIORITY NO. 4. To promote wellness (Teaching/Discharge Considerations):

- Discuss need to respond immediately to urge to void.
- Suggest limiting intake of coffee, tea, and alcohol **because of diuretic effect and impact on voiding pattern.**
- Review use/intake of foods, fluids, and supplements containing potassium. **Potassium deficiency can negatively affect bladder tone.**
- Emphasize importance of perineal care following voiding.
- Maintain positive regard **to reduce embarrassment associated with incontinence, need for assistance, use of bedpan.**
- Promote participation in developing long-term plan of care.
- Refer to NDs Urinary Incontinence, reflex; Urinary Incontinence, stress; Urinary Incontinence, total; Urinary Incontinence, urge.

Documentation Focus

ASSESSMENT/REASSESSMENT

- Current elimination pattern/assessment findings and effect on lifestyle and self-esteem.

PLANNING

- Plan of care and who is involved in planning.
- Teaching plan.

IMPLEMENTATION/EVALUATION

- Response to interventions/teaching and actions performed.
- Attainment/progress toward desired outcome(s).
- Modifications to plan of care.

DISCHARGE PLANNING

- Long-term needs and who is responsible for actions to be taken.
- Specific referrals made.

SAMPLE NURSING OUTCOMES & INTERVENTIONS CLASSIFICATIONS (NOC/NIC)

NOC—Urinary Continence
NIC—Prompted Voiding

Urinary Incontinence, reflex

Taxonomy II: Elimination—Class 1 Urinary System (00018)
[Diagnostic Division: Elimination]
Submitted 1986; Nursing Diagnosis Extension and Classification (NDEC) Revision 1998

Definition: Involuntary loss of urine at somewhat predictable intervals when a specific bladder volume is reached

Related Factors

Tissue damage from radiation cystitis, inflammatory bladder conditions, or radical pelvic surgery
Neurological impairment above level of sacral or pontine micturition center

Defining Characteristics

SUBJECTIVE

No sensation of bladder fullness/urge to void/voiding
Sensation of urgency without voluntary inhibition of bladder contraction
Sensations associated with full bladder such as sweating, restlessness, and abdominal discomfort

OBJECTIVE

Predictable pattern of voiding
Inability to voluntarily inhibit or initiate voiding
Complete emptying with [brain] lesion above pontine micturition center
Incomplete emptying with [spinal cord] lesion above sacral micturition center

---

Information that appears in brackets has been added by the authors to clarify and enhance the use of nursing diagnoses.

Desired Outcomes/Evaluation Criteria—Client Will:

- Verbalize understanding of condition/contributing factors.
- Establish bladder regimen appropriate for individual situation.
- Demonstrate behaviors/techniques to control condition and prevent complications.
- Urinate at acceptable times and places.

Actions/Interventions

NURSING PRIORITY NO. 1. To assess degree of interference/disability:

- Note causative/disease process as listed in Related Factors.
- Evaluate for concomitant urinary retention.
- Assess ability to sense bladder fullness, awareness of incontinence.
- Review voiding diary if available or record frequency and time of urination. Compare timing of voidings, particularly in relation to liquid intake and medications.
- Measure amount of each voiding, **because incontinence often occurs once a specific bladder volume is achieved.**
- Evaluate ability to manipulate/use urinary collection device or catheter.
- Refer to urologist/appropriate specialist for testing of sphincter control and volumes.

NURSING PRIORITY NO. 2. To assist in managing incontinence:

- Encourage minimum of 1500 to 2000 mL of fluid intake daily. **Regulate liquid intake at prescheduled times (with and between meals) to promote predictable voiding pattern.**
- Restrict fluids 2 to 3 hours before bedtime **to reduce voiding during sleep.**
- Instruct client, or take to toilet before the expected time of incontinence, **in an attempt to stimulate the reflex for voiding.**
- Instruct in measures such as pouring warm water over perineum, running water in sink, stimulating/massaging skin of lower abdomen, thighs, and so on **to stimulate voiding reflexes.**
- Set alarm to awaken during night **to maintain schedule,** or use external catheter as appropriate.
- Demonstrate application of external collection device or intermittent self-catheterization using small-lumen straight catheter if condition indicates.

- Establish intermittent catheterization schedule based on client's activity schedule as indicated.
- Measure postvoid residuals/catheterization volumes. **Determines frequency for emptying bladder.**

NURSING PRIORITY NO. **3**. To promote wellness (Teaching/Discharge Considerations):

- Encourage continuation of regular toileting program.
- Suggest use of incontinence pads/pants during day and social contact, if appropriate, dependent on client's activity level, amount of urine loss, manual dexterity, and cognitive ability.
- Stress importance of perineal care following voiding and frequent changing of incontinence pads if used.
- Encourage limited intake of coffee, tea, and alcohol **because of diuretic effect, which may affect predictability of voiding pattern.**
- Instruct in proper care of catheter and clean techniques **to reduce risk of infection.**
- Review signs/symptoms of urinary complications and need for medical follow-up.

Documentation Focus

ASSESSMENT/REASSESSMENT

- Findings/degree of disability and effect on lifestyle.

PLANNING

- Plan of care and who is involved in planning.
- Teaching plan.

IMPLEMENTATION/EVALUATION

- Responses to treatment plan/interventions and actions performed.
- Attainment/progress toward desired outcome(s).
- Modifications to plan of care.

DISCHARGE PLANNING

- Long-term needs and who is responsible for actions to be taken.
- Available resources, equipment needs/sources.

SAMPLE NURSING OUTCOMES & INTERVENTIONS CLASSIFICATIONS (NOC/NIC)

NOC—Urinary Continence
NIC—Urinary Bladder Training

Urinary Incontinence, stress

Taxonomy II: Elimination—Class 1 Urinary System
(00017)
[Diagnostic Division: Elimination]
Submitted 1986

Definition: Loss of less than 50 mL of urine occurring
with increased abdominal pressure

Related Factors

Degenerative changes in pelvic muscles and structural supports associ-
ated with increased age [e.g., poor closure of urethral sphincter,
estrogen deficiency]
High intra-abdominal pressure (e.g., obesity, gravid uterus)
Incompetent bladder outlet; overdistention between voidings
Weak pelvic muscles and structural supports [e.g., straining with
chronic constipation]
[Neural degeneration, vascular deficits, surgery, radiation therapy]

Defining Characteristics

SUBJECTIVE

Reported dribbling with increased abdominal pressure [e.g., coughing,
sneezing, lifting, impact aerobics, changing position]
Urinary urgency; frequency (more often than every 2 hours)

OBJECTIVE

Observed dribbling with increased abdominal pressure

Desired Outcomes/Evaluation
Criteria—Client Will:

- Verbalize understanding of condition and interventions for
  bladder conditioning.
- Demonstrate behaviors/techniques to strengthen pelvic floor
  musculature.
- Remain continent even with increased intra-abdominal
  pressure.

Actions/Interventions

NURSING PRIORITY NO. 1. To assess causative/contributing
factors:

- Identify physiologic causes of increased intra-abdominal
  pressure (e.g., obesity, gravid uterus). Note contributing
  history such as multiple births, bladder or pelvic trauma/
  repairs.
- Assess for urine loss with coughing or sneezing, relaxed pelvic

---

Information that appears in brackets has been added by the authors
to clarify and enhance the use of nursing diagnoses.

musculature and support, noting inability to start/stop stream while voiding, bulging of perineum when bearing down. Refer to urologic specialists **for sphincter weakness or hypermobility testing.**

- Perform ultrasound or catheterize as indicated **to rule out the possibility of postvoid residuals.**

NURSING PRIORITY NO. **2.** To assess degree of interference/disability:

- Observe voiding patterns, time and amount voided, and stimulus provoking incontinence. Review voiding diary if available.
- Prepare for/assist with appropriate testing (e.g., cystoscopy, cystometrogram).
- Determine effect on lifestyle (including socialization and sexuality) and self-esteem.
- Ascertain methods of self-management (e.g., limiting liquid intake, using undergarment protection).
- Assess for concomitant urge or functional incontinence, noting whether bladder irritability, reduced bladder capacity, or voluntary overdistention is present. (Refer to appropriate NDs.)

NURSING PRIORITY NO. **3.** To assist in treating/preventing incontinence:

- Assist with medical treatment of underlying urologic condition as indicated (surgery, medications, biofeedback, etc.).
- Suggest starting and stopping stream 2 or 3 times during voiding **to isolate muscles involved in voiding process for exercise training.**
- Encourage regular pelvic floor strengthening exercises (Kegel exercises or use of vaginal cones). Combine activity with biofeedback as appropriate **to enhance training.**
- Incorporate "bent-knee sit-ups" into exercise program **to increase abdominal muscle tone.**
- Suggest that client urinate at least every 3 hours during the day **to reduce bladder pressure.** Recommend consciously delaying voiding as appropriate **to slowly achieve desired 3- to 4-hour intervals between voids.**
- Restrict intake 2 to 3 hours prior to bedtime **to decrease incontinence during sleep.**

NURSING PRIORITY NO. **4.** To promote wellness (Teaching/Discharge Considerations):

- Encourage limiting use of coffee/tea and alcohol **because of diuretic effect, which may lead to bladder distention, increasing likelihood of incontinence.**

- Suggest use of incontinence pads/pants as needed. Consider client's activity level, amount of urine loss, physical size, manual dexterity, and cognitive ability **to determine specific product choices best suited to individual situation and needs.**
- Stress importance of perineal care following voiding and frequent changing of incontinence pads **to prevent irritation and infection.** Recommend application of oil-based emollient **to protect skin from irritation.**
- Avoid/limit participation in activities, such as heavy lifting, impact aerobics, **that increase intra-abdominal pressure.** Substitute swimming, bicycling, or low-impact exercise.
- Refer to weight-loss program/support group **when obesity is a contributing factor.**
- Review use of sympathomimetic drugs, if prescribed, **to improve resting tone of the bladder neck and proximal urethra.**

Documentation Focus

ASSESSMENT/REASSESSMENT

- Findings/pattern of incontinence and physical factors present.
- Effect on lifestyle and self-esteem.
- Client understanding of condition.

PLANNING

- Plan of care and who is involved in the planning.
- Teaching plan.

IMPLEMENTATION/EVALUATION

- Responses to interventions/teaching, actions performed, and changes that are identified.
- Attainment/progress toward desired outcome(s).
- Modifications to plan of care.

DISCHARGE PLANNING

- Long-term needs/referrals and who is responsible for specific actions.
- Specific referrals made.

SAMPLE NURSING OUTCOMES & INTERVENTIONS CLASSIFICATIONS (NOC/NIC)

NOC—Urinary Continence
NIC—Pelvic Muscle Exercise

Urinary Incontinence, total

Taxonomy II: Elimination—Class 1 Urinary System
(00021)
[Diagnostic Division: Elimination]
Submitted 1986

Definition: Continuous and unpredictable loss of urine

Related Factors

Neuropathy preventing transmission of reflex [signals to the reflex arc]
indicating bladder fullness
Neurological dysfunction [e.g., cerebral lesions] causing triggering of
micturition at unpredictable times
Independent contraction of detrusor reflex due to surgery
Trauma or disease affecting spinal cord nerves [destruction of sensory
or motor neurons below the injury level]
Anatomic (fistula)

Defining Characteristics

SUBJECTIVE

Constant flow of urine at unpredictable times without uninhibited
bladder contractions/spasm or distention
Nocturia
Lack of perineal or bladder filling awareness
Unawareness of incontinence

OBJECTIVE

Unsuccessful incontinence refractory treatments

Desired Outcomes/Evaluation Criteria—Client/Caregiver Will:

- Verbalize awareness of causative/contributing factors.
- Establish bladder regimen for individual situation.
- Demonstrate behaviors, techniques to manage condition and
to prevent complications.
- Manage incontinence so that social functioning is regained/
maintained.

Actions/Interventions

NURSING PRIORITY NO. 1. To assess causative/contributing
factors:

- Determine if client is aware of incontinence.
- Be aware of/note effect of medical history of global neurologic
impairment, neuromuscular trauma after surgery/radiation
therapy, or presence of fistula.
- Determine concomitant chronic retention (e.g., palpate bladder, ultrasound scan/catheterize for residual).

Information that appears in brackets has been added by the authors
570 to clarify and enhance the use of nursing diagnoses.

- Carry out/assist with procedures/tests (e.g., cystoscopy, cystogram) **to establish diagnosis/identify appropriateness of surgical repair.**

NURSING PRIORITY NO. 2. To assess degree of interference/ disability:
- Toilet client every 2 hours and note time of voiding and incontinence **to determine pattern of urination.**
- Ascertain effect of condition on lifestyle and self-esteem.
- Inspect skin **for areas of erythema/excoriation.**
- Review history for past interventions regarding alterations in urinary elimination.

NURSING PRIORITY NO. 3. assist in preventing/managing incontinence:
- Encourage at least 1500 to 2000 mL liquid intake per day. Regulate liquid intake at prescheduled times (with and between meals) **to promote predictable voiding pattern.**
- Restrict intake 2 to 3 hours before bedtime **to reduce voiding during sleep.**
- Establish voiding schedule by toileting at same time as recorded voidings and 30 minutes earlier than recorded time of incontinence.
- Encourage measures such as pouring warm water over perineum, running water in sink, massaging lower abdomen **to stimulate voiding.** (**Note:** This may not be successful if reflex is not intact.)
- Adjust schedule, once continent, by increasing voiding time in 30-minute increments **to achieve desired 3- to 4-hour intervals between voids.**
- Use condom catheter or female cone during the day and pad the bed during the night if external device is not tolerated.
- Establish intermittent catheterization schedule if condition requires.

NURSING PRIORITY NO. 4. To promote wellness (Teaching/ Discharge Considerations):
- Assist client to identify regular period of time for voiding **to establish elimination program.**
- Suggest use of adult briefs as indicated (e.g., during social contacts) **for extra protection and to enhance confidence.**
- Stress importance of pericare after each voiding (using alcohol-free products) and application of oil-based emollient **to protect the skin from irritation.**
- Demonstrate techniques of clean intermittent self-catheterization (CISC) using small-lumen straight catheter (or Mitrofanoff continent urinary channel for clients not able to catheterize themselves) as indicated.

- Instruct in proper care of catheter and clean technique **to prevent infection.**
- Recommend use of silicone catheter when long-term/continuous placement is indicated after other measures/bladder training have failed.
- Encourage self-monitoring of catheter patency and avoidance of reflux of urine. **Reduces risk of infection.**
- Suggest intake of acidifying juices **to discourage bacterial growth/adherence to bladder wall.**

Documentation Focus

ASSESSMENT/REASSESSMENT

- Current elimination pattern.
- Assessment findings including effect on lifestyle and self-esteem.

PLANNING

- Plan of care/interventions, including who is involved in planning.
- Teaching plan.

IMPLEMENTATION/EVALUATION

- Response to interventions/teaching and actions performed.
- Attainment/progress toward desired outcome(s).
- Modifications to plan of care.

DISCHARGE PLANNING

- Discharge plan/long-term needs and who is responsible for actions to be taken.
- Specific referrals made.

SAMPLE NURSING OUTCOMES & INTERVENTIONS CLASSIFICATIONS (NOC/NIC)

NOC—Urinary Continence
NIC—Urinary Incontinence Care

Urinary Incontinence, urge

Taxonomy II: Elimination—Class 1 Urinary System
(00019)
[Diagnostic Division: Elimination]
Submitted 1986

Definition: Involuntary passage of urine occurring soon after a strong sense of urgency to void

Information that appears in brackets has been added by the authors
572 to clarify and enhance the use of nursing diagnoses.

Related Factors

Decreased bladder capacity (e.g., history of pelvic inflammatory disease—PID, abdominal surgeries, indwelling urinary catheter)

Irritation of bladder stretch receptors causing spasm (e.g., bladder infection, [atrophic urethritis, vaginitis]; alcohol, caffeine, increased fluids; increased urine concentration; overdistention of bladder

[Medication use, such as diuretics, sedatives, anticholinergic agents]

[Constipation/stool impaction]

[Restricted mobility; psychological disorder such as depression, change in mentation/confusional state, e.g., stroke, dementia, Parkinson's disease]

Defining Characteristics

SUBJECTIVE

Urinary urgency
Frequency (voiding more often than every 2 hours)
Bladder contracture/spasm
Nocturia (more than 2 times per night)

OBJECTIVE

Inability to reach toilet in time
Voiding in small amounts (less than 100 cc) or in large amounts (greater than 550 cc)

Desired Outcomes/Evaluation Criteria—Client Will:

- Verbalize understanding of condition.
- Demonstrate behaviors/techniques to control/correct situation.
- Report increase in interval between urge and involuntary loss of urine.
- Void every 3 to 4 hours in individually appropriate amounts.

Actions/Interventions

NURSING PRIORITY NO. 1. To assess causative/contributing factors:

- Assess for signs and symptoms of bladder infection (e.g., cloudy, odorous urine; bacteriuria).
- Determine use/presence of bladder irritants (e.g., significant intake of alcohol or caffeine, resulting in increased output or concentrated urine).
- Determine whether there is a history of long-standing habits or medical conditions that may reduce bladder capacity (e.g., severe PID, abdominal surgeries, recent/lengthy use of indwelling urinary catheter, or frequent voluntary voiding).
- Note factors that may affect ability to respond to urge to void (e.g., impaired mobility, use of sedation).

- Clinitest urine for glucose. **Presence of glucose in urine causes polyuria, resulting in overdistention of the bladder.**
- Assess for concomitant functional incontinence. Refer to ND Urinary Incontinence, functional.
- Palpate bladder for overdistention. Rule out high postvoid residuals via palpation/ultrasound/catheterization.
- Prepare for/assist with appropriate testing (e.g., urinalysis, cystometrogram).

NURSING PRIORITY NO. **2.** To assess degree of interference/ disability:

- Measure amount of urine voided, especially noting amounts less than 100 cc or greater than 550 cc.
- Record frequency and degree of urgency.
- Note length of warning time between initial urge and loss of urine.
- Ascertain effect on lifestyle (including socialization and sexuality) and self-esteem.

NURSING PRIORITY NO. **3.** To assist in treating/preventing incontinence:

- Increase fluid intake to 1500 to 2000 mL/day.
- Regulate liquid intake at prescheduled times (with and between meals) **to promote predictable voiding pattern.**
- Provide assistance/devices as indicated for clients who are mobility impaired (e.g., provide means of summoning assistance; place bedside commode, urinal, or bedpan within client's reach).
- Establish schedule for voiding (habit training) based on client's usual voiding pattern.
- Instruct client to tighten pelvic floor muscles before arising from bed. **Helps prevent loss of urine as abdominal pressure changes.**
- Suggest starting and stopping stream two or more times during voiding **to isolate muscles involved in voiding process for exercise training.**
- Encourage regular pelvic floor strengthening exercise (Kegel exercises or use of vaginal cones). Combine activity with bio-feedback as appropriate **to enhance effectiveness of training.**
- Set alarm to awaken during night if indicated, **to continue voiding schedule.**
- Recommend consciously delaying voiding **to gradually increase intervals between voiding to every 2 to 4 hours.**

NURSING PRIORITY NO. **4.** To promote wellness (Teaching/ Discharge Considerations):

- Suggest limiting intake of coffee/tea and alcohol **because of irritating effect on the bladder.**
- Recommend use of incontinence pads/pants if necessary, considering client's level of activity, amount of urine loss, physical size, manual dexterity, and cognitive ability.
- Suggest wearing loose-fitting or especially adapted clothing **to facilitate response to voiding urge.**
- Emphasize importance of perineal care after each voiding **to prevent skin irritation.**
- Identify signs/symptoms indicating urinary complications and need for medical follow-up.
- Review use of anticholinergics, if prescribed, **to increase warning time by blocking impulses within the sacral reflex arc.**
- Discuss possible surgical intervention or use of electronic stimulation therapy **to induce bladder contraction/inhibit detrusor overactivity as appropriate.**

Documentation Focus

ASSESSMENT/REASSESSMENT

- Individual findings, including pattern of incontinence, effect on lifestyle, and self-esteem.

PLANNING

- Plan of care/interventions and who is involved in planning.
- Teaching plan.

IMPLEMENTATION/EVALUATION

- Response to interventions/teaching and actions performed.
- Attainment/progress toward desired outcome(s).
- Modifications to plan of care.

DISCHARGE PLANNING

- Discharge needs/referrals and who is responsible for actions to be taken.
- Specific referrals made.

SAMPLE NURSING OUTCOMES & INTERVENTIONS CLASSIFICATIONS (NOC/NIC)

NOC—Urinary Continence
NIC—Urinary Habit Training

Urinary Incontinence, risk for urge

Taxonomy II: Elimination—Class 1 Urinary System
(00022)
[Diagnostic Division: Elimination]
Submitted 1998; Nursing Diagnosis Extension and
Classification (NDEC) Submission 1998

Definition: At risk for an involuntary loss of urine associated with a sudden, strong sensation or urinary
urgency

Risk Factors

Effects of medications; caffeine; alcohol
Detrusor hyperreflexia from cystitis, urethritis, tumors, renal calculi,
    CNS disorders above pontine micturition center
Detrusor muscle instability with impaired contractility; involuntary
    sphincter relaxation
Ineffective toileting habits
Small bladder capacity

NOTE: A risk diagnosis is not evidenced by signs and symptoms, as
the problem has not occurred and nursing interventions are
directed at prevention.

Desired Outcomes/Evaluation
Criteria—Client Will:

- Identify individual risk factors and appropriate interventions.
- Demonstrate behaviors or lifestyle changes to prevent development of problem.

Actions/Interventions

NURSING PRIORITY NO. 1. To assess potential for developing
incontinence:

- Determine use/presence of bladder irritants (e.g., significant
  intake of alcohol or caffeine, resulting in increased output or
  concentrated urine).
- Review history for long-standing habits or medical conditions
  that may reduce bladder capacity, (e.g., impaired mobility, use
  of sedation).
- Note factors that may affect ability to respond to urge to void
  (e.g., impaired mobility, use of sedation).
- Prepare for/assist with appropriate testing (e.g., urinalysis,
  cystometrogram) to evaluate voiding pattern, identify
  pathology.

NURSING PRIORITY NO. 2. To prevent occurrence of problem:

- Measure amount of urine voided, especially noting amounts
  less than 100 mL or greater than 550 mL.

Information that appears in brackets has been added by the authors
to clarify and enhance the use of nursing diagnoses.

- Record intake and frequency/degree of urgency of voiding.
- Ascertain client's awareness/concerns about developing problem and whether lifestyle is affected (e.g., socialization, sexual patterns).
- Regulate liquid intake at prescheduled times (with and between meals) **to promote predictable voiding pattern.**
- Establish schedule for voiding (habit training) based on client's usual voiding pattern.
- Provide assistance/devices as indicated for clients who are mobility impaired (e.g., provide means of summoning assistance; place bedside commode, urinal, or bedpan within client's reach).
- Instruct client to tighten pelvic floor muscles before arising from bed. **Helps prevent loss of urine as abdominal pressure changes.**
- Suggest starting and stopping stream two or more times during voiding **to isolate muscles involved in voiding process for exercise training.**
- Encourage regular pelvic floor strengthening exercise (Kegel exercises or use of vaginal cones). Combine activity with biofeedback, as appropriate, **to enhance effectiveness of training.**

NURSING PRIORITY NO. **3.** To promote wellness (Teaching/Discharge Considerations):

- Recommend limiting intake of coffee/tea and alcohol **because of their irritating effect on the bladder.**
- Suggest wearing loose-fitting or especially adapted clothing **to facilitate response to voiding urge.**
- Emphasize importance of perineal care after each voiding **to reduce risk of ascending infection.**
- Discuss use of hormone (conjugated estrogens—Premarin) creme vaginally **to strengthen urethral tissues as appropriate.**

Documentation Focus

ASSESSMENT/REASSESSMENT

- Individual findings, including specific risk factors and pattern of voiding.

PLANNING

- Plan of care/interventions and who is involved in planning.
- Teaching plan.

IMPLEMENTATION/EVALUATION

- Response to interventions/teaching and actions performed.
- Attainment/progress toward desired outcome(s).
- Modifications to plan of care.

DISCHARGE PLANNING

- Discharge needs/referrals and who is responsible for actions to be taken.
- Specific referrals made.

SAMPLE NURSING OUTCOMES & INTERVENTIONS CLASSIFICATIONS (NOC/NIC)

NOC—Urinary Continence
NIC—Urinary Habit Training

Urinary Retention [acute/chronic]

Taxonomy II: Elimination—Class 1 Urinary System (00023)
[Diagnostic Division: Elimination]
Submitted 1986

Definition: Incomplete emptying of the bladder

Related Factors

High urethral pressure caused by weak[/absent] detrusor
Inhibition of reflex arc
Strong sphincter; blockage [e.g., benign prostatic hypertrophy-BPH, perineal swelling]
[Habituation of reflex arc]
[Infections]
[Neurological diseases/trauma]
[Use of medications with side effect of retention (e.g., atropine, belladonna, psychotropics, antihistamines, opiates)]

Defining Characteristics

SUBJECTIVE

Sensation of bladder fullness
Dribbling
Dysuria

OBJECTIVE

Bladder distention
Small, frequent voiding or absence of urine output
Residual urine [150 mL or more]
Overflow incontinence
[Reduced stream]

Desired Outcomes/Evaluation Criteria—Client Will:

- Verbalize understanding of causative factors and appropriate interventions for individual situation.

Information that appears in brackets has been added by the authors
578 to clarify and enhance the use of nursing diagnoses.

- Demonstrate techniques/behaviors to alleviate/prevent retention.
- Void in sufficient amounts with no palpable bladder distention; experience no postvoid residuals greater than 50 mL; have no dribbling/overflow.

Actions/Interventions

ACUTE

NURSING PRIORITY NO. **1**. To assess causative/contributing factors:

- Note presence of pathological conditions (**e.g., neurologic disease, infection, stone formation**).
- Assess for effects of medication, such as psychotropics, anesthesia, opiates, sedatives, antihistamines.
- Determine anxiety level (e.g., **client may be too embarrassed to void in presence of others**).
- Examine for fecal impaction, surgical site swelling, postpartal edema, vaginal or rectal packing, enlarged prostate, or other "mechanical" factors **that may produce a blockage of the urethra.**
- Evaluate general hydration status.

NURSING PRIORITY NO. **2**. To determine degree of interference/disability:

- Determine if there has been any significant urine output in the last 6 to 8 hours.
- Palpate height of the bladder.
- Note recent amount/type of fluid intake.
- Ascertain whether client has sensation of bladder fullness, level of discomfort.

NURSING PRIORITY NO. **3**. To assist in treating/preventing retention:

- Relieve pain by administering appropriate medications and measures **to reduce swelling/treat underlying cause.**
- Sit upright on bedpan/commode or stand **to provide functional position of voiding.**
- Provide privacy.
- Use ice techniques, spirits of wintergreen, stroking inner thigh, running water in sink or warm water over perineum **to stimulate reflex arc.**
- Remove blockage if possible (e.g., vaginal packing, bowel impaction). Prepare for more aggressive intervention (e.g., surgery/prostatectomy).
- Catheterize with intermittent or indwelling catheter **to resolve acute retention.**
- Drain bladder slowly with straight catheter in increments of

200 mL at a time **to prevent possibility of occurrence of hematuria, syncope.**

- Observe for signs of infection/send urine to laboratory for culture as indicated.
- Reduce recurrences by controlling causative/contributing factors when possible (e.g., ice to perineum, use of stool softeners/laxatives, change of medication/dosage).

NURSING PRIORITY NO. 4. To promote wellness (Teaching/Discharge Considerations):

- Encourage client to report problems immediately **so treatment can be instituted promptly.**
- Emphasize need for adequate fluid intake.

CHRONIC

NURSING PRIORITY NO. 1. To assess causative/contributing factors:

- Review medical history for diagnoses, such as prostatic hypertrophy, scarring, recurrent stone formation, **that may suggest detrusor muscle atrophy and/or chronic overdistention because of outlet obstruction.**
- Determine presence of weak or absent sensory and/or motor impulses (as with CVAs, spinal injury, or diabetes).
- Evaluate customary fluid intake.
- Assess for effects of psychotropics, antihistamines, atropine, belladonna, and so forth.
- Strain urine **for presence of stones/calculi.**

NURSING PRIORITY NO. 2. To determine degree of interference/disability:

- Measure amount voided and postvoid residuals.
- Determine frequency and timing of dribbling and/or voiding.
- Note size and force of urinary stream.
- Palpate height of bladder.
- Determine presence of bladder spasms.
- Ascertain effect of condition on functioning/lifestyle.

NURSING PRIORITY NO. 3. To assist in treating/preventing retention:

- Recommend client void on timed schedule.
- Demonstrate and instruct client/SO(s) in use of Credé's maneuver **to facilitate emptying of the bladder.**
- Encourage client to use Valsalva's maneuver if appropriate **to increase intra-abdominal pressure.**
- Establish regular voiding/self-catheterization program **to prevent reflux and increased renal pressures.**

NURSING PRIORITY NO. 4. To promote wellness (Teaching/Discharge Considerations):

- Establish regular schedule for bladder emptying whether voiding or using catheter.
- Stress need for adequate fluid intake, including use of acidifying fruit juices or ingestion of vitamin C/Mandelamine **to discourage bacterial growth and stone formation.**
- Instruct client/SO(s) in clean intermittent catheterization (CIC) techniques.
- Review signs/symptoms of complications requiring medical evaluation/intervention.

Documentation Focus

ASSESSMENT/REASSESSMENT

- Individual findings, including nature of problem, degree of impairment, and whether client is incontinent.

PLANNING

- Plan of care and who is involved in planning.
- Teaching plan.

IMPLEMENTATION/EVALUATION

- Response to interventions.
- Attainment/progress toward desired outcome(s).
- Modifications to plan of care.

DISCHARGE PLANNING

- Long-term needs/referrals and who is responsible for actions to be taken.
- Specific referrals made.

SAMPLE NURSING OUTCOMES & INTERVENTIONS CLASSIFICATIONS (NOC/NIC)

NOC—Urinary Elimination
NIC—Urinary Retention Care

Ventilation, impaired spontaneous

Taxonomy II: Activity/Rest—Class 2
Cardiovascular/Pulmonary Response (00033)
[Diagnostic Division: Respiration]
Submitted 1992

Definition: Decreased energy reserves results in an individual's inability to maintain breathing adequate to support life

Information that appears in brackets has been added by the authors to clarify and enhance the use of nursing diagnoses.

Related Factors

Metabolic factors; [hypermetabolic state (e.g., infection), nutritional deficits/depletion of energy stores]
Respiratory muscle fatigue
[Airway size/resistance; problems with secretion management]

Defining Characteristics

SUBJECTIVE

Dyspnea
Apprehension

OBJECTIVE

Increased metabolic rate
Increased heart rate
Increased restlessness
Decreased cooperation
Increased use of accessory muscles
Decreased tidal volume
Decreased Po_2; Sao_2
Increased Pco_2

Desired Outcomes/Evaluation Criteria—Client Will:

- Reestablish/maintain effective respiratory pattern via ventilator with absence of retractions/use of accessory muscles, cyanosis, or other signs of hypoxia; and with ABGs/Sao2 within acceptable range.
- Participate in efforts to wean (as appropriate) within individual ability.

Caregiver Will:

- Demonstrate behaviors necessary to maintain respiratory function.

Actions/Interventions

NURSING PRIORITY NO. 1. To determine degree of impairment:

- Investigate etiology of respiratory failure **to determine client's future capabilities, ventilation needs, and most appropriate type of ventilatory support.**
- Assess spontaneous respiratory pattern, noting rate, depth, rhythm, symmetry of chest movement, use of accessory muscles **to measure work of breathing.**
- Auscultate breath sounds, noting presence/absence and equality of breath sounds, adventitious breath sounds.
- Obtain ABGs, pulmonary function studies as appropriate.

- Review chest x-ray and magnetic resonance imaging (MRI)/CT scan results if done.
- Note response to respiratory therapy (e.g., bronchodilators, supplemental oxygen, IPPB treatments).

NURSING PRIORITY NO. 2. To provide/maintain ventilatory support:

- Observe overall breathing pattern, distinguishing between spontaneous respirations and ventilator breaths.
- Administer sedation as required **to synchronize respirations and reduce work of breathing/energy expenditure.**
- Count client's respirations for 1 full minute and compare to desired/ventilator set rate.
- Verify that client's respirations are in phase with the ventilator. **Decreases work of breathing, maximizes O_2 delivery.**
- Inflate tracheal/endotracheal tube cuff properly using minimal leak/occlusive technique. Check cuff inflation every 4 to 8 hours and whenever cuff is deflated/reinflated **to prevent risk associated with under/overinflation.**
- Check tubing for obstruction (e.g., kinking or accumulation of water). Drain tubing as indicated; avoid draining toward the client, or back into the reservoir **resulting in contamination/providing medium for growth of bacteria.**
- Check ventilator alarms for proper functioning. Do not turn off alarms, even for suctioning. Remove from ventilator and ventilate manually if source of ventilator alarm cannot be quickly identified and rectified. Verify that alarms can be heard in the nurses' station by care providers.
- Assess ventilator settings routinely and readjust as indicated according to client's primary disease and results of diagnostic testing.
- Verify that oxygen line is in proper outlet/tank; monitor inline oxygen analyzer or perform periodic oxygen analysis.
- Note tidal volume (10 to 15 mL/kg). Verify proper function of spirometer, bellows, or computer readout of delivered volume. Note alterations from desired volume delivery **to determine alteration in lung compliance or leakage through machine/around tube cuff (if used).**
- Monitor airway pressure **for developing complications/equipment problems.**
- Monitor inspiratory and expiratory (I:E) ratio.
- Promote maximal ventilation of alveoli; check sigh rate intervals (usually $1\frac{1}{2}$ to 2 times tidal volume). **Reduces risk of atelectasis, helps mobilize secretions.**
- Note inspired humidity and temperature; maintain hydration **to liquefy secretions facilitating removal.**
- Auscultate breath sounds periodically. Note frequent crackles or rhonchi that do not clear with coughing/suctioning

because they may indicate developing complications (atelectasis, pneumonia, acute bronchospasm, pulmonary edema).
- Suction as needed **to clear secretions.**
- Note changes in chest symmetry. **May indicate improper placement of ET tube, development of barotrauma.**
- Keep resuscitation bag at bedside and ventilate manually whenever indicated (e.g., if client is removed from ventilator or troubleshooting equipment problems).
- Administer and monitor response to medications that promote airway patency and gas exchange.

NURSING PRIORITY NO. **3.** To prepare for/assist with weaning process if appropriate:

- Determine physical/psychological readiness to wean, including specific respiratory parameters; presence/absence of infection, cardiac failure, nutritional status.
- Explain weaning activities/techniques, individual plan and expectations. **Reduces fear of unknown.**
- Elevate head of bed/place in orthopedic chair if possible, or position **to alleviate dyspnea and facilitate oxygenation.**
- Assist client in "taking control" of breathing if weaning is attempted or ventilatory support is interrupted during procedure/activity.
- Coach client to take slower, deeper breaths, practice abdominal/pursed-lip breathing, assume position of comfort, and use relaxation techniques **to maximize respiratory function.**
- Assist client to practice effective coughing, secretion management.
- Provide quiet environment, calm approach, undivided attention of nurse. **Promotes relaxation decreasing energy/oxygen requirements.**
- Involve family/SO(s) as appropriate. Provide diversional activity. **Helps client focus on something other than breathing.**
- Instruct client in use of energy-saving techniques during care activities **to limit oxygen consumption/fatigue.**
- Acknowledge and provide ongoing encouragement for client's efforts. Communicate hope for successful weaning response (even partial). **Enhances commitment to continue activity, maximizing outcomes.**

NURSING PRIORITY NO. **4.** To prepare for discharge on ventilator when indicated:

- Ascertain plan for discharge placement (e.g., return home, short-term/permanent placement in long-term care—LTC).
- Determine specific equipment needs. Identify resources for equipment needs/maintenance and arrange for delivery prior to client discharge.

- Review layout of home, noting size of rooms, doorways; placement of furniture, number/type of electrical outlets to identify necessary changes.
- Obtain no-smoking signs to be posted in home. Encourage family members to refrain from smoking.
- Have family/SO(s) notify utilities company and fire department of presence of ventilator in home.
- Review and provide written materials regarding proper ventilator management, maintenance, and safety for reference in home setting, enhancing client's/SO's level of comfort.
- Demonstrate airway management techniques and proper equipment cleaning practices.
- Instruct SO(s)/care provider in other pulmonary physiotherapy measures as indicated (e.g., chest physiotherapy—CPT).
- Allow sufficient opportunity for SO(s)/family to practice new skills. Role-play potential crisis situations to enhance confidence in ability to handle client's needs.
- Identify signs/symptoms requiring prompt medical evaluation/intervention. Timely treatment may prevent progression of problem.
- Provide positive feedback and encouragement for efforts of SO(s)/family. Promotes continuation of desired behaviors.
- List names and phone numbers for identified contact persons/resources. Refer to individual(s) who have managed home ventilation. Round-the-clock availability reduces sense of isolation and enhances likelihood of obtaining appropriate information when needed.

NURSING PRIORITY NO. 5. To promote wellness (Teaching/Discharge Considerations):

- Discuss impact of specific activities on respiratory status and problem-solve solutions to maximize weaning effort.
- Engage client in specialized exercise program to enhance respiratory muscle strength and general endurance.
- Protect client from sources of infection (e.g., monitor health of visitors, roommate, staff involved in care).
- Recommend involvement in support group; introduce to individuals dealing with similar problems to provide role models, assistance for problem solving.
- Encourage time-out for care providers so they may attend to personal needs, wellness, and growth.
- Provide opportunities for client/SO(s) to discuss termination of therapy/end-of-life decisions.
- Identify ventilator-dependent individuals who are successfully managing condition to encourage hope for the future.
- Refer to additional resources (e.g., spiritual advisor, counselor).

Documentation Focus

ASSESSMENT/REASSESSMENT

- Baseline findings, subsequent alterations in respiratory function.
- Results of diagnostic testing.
- Individual risk factors/concerns.

PLANNING

- Plan of care and who is involved in planning.
- Teaching plan.

IMPLEMENTATION/EVALUATION

- Client's/SO's responses to interventions, teaching, and actions performed.
- Skill level/assistance needs of SO(s)/family.
- Attainment, progress toward desired outcome(s).
- Modifications to plan of care.

DISCHARGE PLANNING

- Discharge plan, including appropriate referrals, action taken, and who is responsible for each action.
- Equipment needs and source.
- Resources for support persons/home care providers.

SAMPLE NURSING OUTCOMES & INTERVENTIONS CLASSIFICATIONS (NOC/NIC)

NOC—Respiratory Status: Ventilation
NIC—Mechanical Ventilation

Ventilatory Weaning Response, dysfunctional

Taxonomy II: Activity/Rest—Class 4
Cardiovascular/Pulmonary Responses (00034)
[Diagnostic Division: Respiration]
Submitted 1992

Definition: Inability to adjust to lowered levels of mechanical ventilator support that interrupts and prolongs the weaning process

Related Factors

PHYSICAL

Ineffective airway clearance
Sleep pattern disturbance

Information that appears in brackets has been added by the authors

to clarify and enhance the use of nursing diagnoses.

Inadequate nutrition
Uncontrolled pain or discomfort
[Muscle weakness/fatigue, inability to control respiratory muscles;
   immobility]

PSYCHOLOGICAL

Knowledge deficit of the weaning process, client's role
Client's perceived inefficacy about the ability to wean
Decreased motivation
Decreased self-esteem
Anxiety (moderate, severe); fear; insufficient trust in the nurse
Hopelessness; powerlessness
[Unprepared for weaning attempt]

SITUATIONAL

Uncontrolled episodic energy demands or problems
Inappropriate pacing of diminished ventilator support
Inadequate social support
Adverse environment (noisy, active environment, negative events in
   the room, low nurse-client ratio; extended nurse absence from
   bedside, unfamiliar nursing staff)
History of ventilator dependence greater than 1 week
History of multiple unsuccessful weaning attempts

Defining Characteristics

Responds to lowered levels of mechanical ventilator support with:

MILD DVWR

Subjective
Expressed feelings of increased need for O_2; breathing discomfort;
   fatigue, warmth
Queries about possible machine malfunction
Objective
Restlessness
Slight increased respiratory rate from baseline
Increased concentration on breathing

MODERATE DVWR

Subjective
Apprehension
Objective
Slight increase from baseline blood pressure (<20 mm Hg)
Slight increase from baseline heart rate (<20 beats/min)
Baseline increase in respiratory rate (<5 breaths/min)
Hypervigilance to activities
Inability to respond to coaching/cooperate
Diaphoresis
Eye widening, "wide-eyed look"
Decreased air entry on auscultation
Color changes; pale, slight cyanosis
Slight respiratory accessory muscle use

SEVERE DVWR

Objective

Agitation

Deterioration in ABGs from current baseline

Increase from baseline BP (>20 mm Hg)

Increase from baseline heart rate (>20 beats/min)

Respiratory rate increases significantly from baseline

Profuse diaphoresis

Full respiratory accessory muscle use; shallow, gasping breaths; paradoxical abdominal breathing

Discoordinated breathing with the ventilator

Decreased level of consciousness

Adventitious breath sounds, audible airway secretions

Cyanosis

Desired Outcomes/Evaluation Criteria—Client Will:

- Actively participate in the weaning process.
- Reestablish independent respiration with ABGs within client's normal range and be free of signs of respiratory failure.
- Demonstrate increased tolerance for activity/participate in self-care within level of ability.

Actions/Interventions

NURSING PRIORITY NO. 1. To identify contributing factors/degree of dysfunction:

- Note length of ventilator dependence. Review previous episodes of dependence/weaning.
- Assess physical factors involved in weaning (e.g., stability of vital signs, hydration status, presence of fever/pain; nutritional intake and muscle strength).
- Ascertain client's understanding of weaning process, expectations, and concerns.
- Determine psychologic readiness, presence/degree of anxiety.
- Review laboratory studies reflecting number/integrity of red blood cells (O_2 transport) and nutritional status (sufficient energy to meet demands of weaning).
- Review chest x-ray/pulse oximetry and ABGs.

NURSING PRIORITY NO. 2. To support weaning process:

- Consult with dietitian, nutritional support team for adjustments of composition of diet **to prevent excessive production of CO_2, which could alter respiratory drive.**
- Explain weaning techniques, e.g., T-piece, SIMV, CPAP, pressure support. Discuss individual plan and expectations. **Reduces fear of unknown, enhances sense of trust.**
- Introduce client to individual who has shared similar experiences with successful outcome.

- Provide undisturbed rest/sleep periods. Avoid stressful procedures/situations or nonessential activities.
- Time medications during weaning efforts **to minimize sedative effects.**
- Provide quiet room; calm approach, undivided attention of nurse. **Enhances relaxation, conserving energy.**
- Involve SO(s)/family as appropriate (e.g., sit at bedside, provide encouragement, and help monitor client status).
- Provide diversional activity (e.g., watching TV, reading aloud) **to focus attention away from breathing.**
- Note response to activity/client care during weaning and limit as indicated **to prevent excessive O_2 consumption/demand with increased possibility of failure.**
- Auscultate breath sounds periodically; suction airway as indicated.
- Acknowledge and provide ongoing encouragement for client's efforts.
- Minimize setbacks, focus client attention on gains and progress to date **to reduce frustration that may further impair progress.**
- Suspend weaning (take a "holiday") periodically as individually appropriate (e.g., initially may "rest" 45 or 50 minutes each hour, progressing to a 20-minute rest every 4 hours, then weaning during daytime and resting during night).

NURSING PRIORITY NO. **3.** To promote wellness (Teaching/Discharge Considerations):

- Discuss impact of specific activities on respiratory status and problem-solve solutions to maximize weaning effort.
- Engage in rehabilitation program **to enhance respiratory muscle strength and general endurance.**
- Teach client/SO(s) how to protect client from sources of infection (e.g., monitor health of visitors, persons involved in care; avoid crowds during flu season).
- Identify conditions requiring immediate medical intervention **to prevent respiratory failure.**

Documentation Focus

ASSESSMENT/REASSESSMENT

- Baseline findings and subsequent alterations.
- Results of diagnostic testing/procedures.
- Individual risk factors.

PLANNING

- Plan of care/interventions and who is involved in the planning.
- Teaching plan.

IMPLEMENTATION/EVALUATION

- Client response to interventions.
- Attainment of/progress toward desired outcome(s).
- Modifications to plan of care.

DISCHARGE PLANNING

- Status at discharge, long-term needs and referrals, indicating who is to be responsible for each action.
- Equipment needs/supplier.

SAMPLE NURSING OUTCOMES & INTERVENTIONS CLASSIFICATIONS (NOC/NIC)

NOC—Respiratory Status: Ventilation
NIC—Mechanical Ventilatory Weaning

NANDA has separated the diagnosis of Violence into its two elements: "directed at others" and "self-directed." However, the interventions in general address both situations and have been left in one block following the definition and supporting data of the two diagnoses.

Violence, [actual/] risk for other-directed

Taxonomy II: Safety/Protection—Class 3 Violence (00138)
[Diagnostic Division: Safety]

Definition: At risk for behaviors in which an individual demonstrates that he or she can be physically, emotionally, and/or sexually harmful to others

Risk Factors/[Indicators]*

HISTORY OF VIOLENCE:

Against others (e.g., hitting, kicking, scratching, biting or spitting, or throwing objects at someone; attempted rape, rape, sexual molestation; urinating/defecating on a person)

Threats (e.g., verbal threats against property/person, social threats, cursing, threatening notes/letters or gestures, sexual threats)

Antisocial behavior (e.g., stealing, insistent borrowing, insistent demands for privileges, insistent interruption of meetings; refusal to eat or to take medication, ignoring instructions)

---

* Note: Although a risk diagnosis does not have defining characteristics (signs and symptoms), the factors identified here can be used to denote an actual diagnosis or as indicators of risk for/escalation of violence.

Information that appears in brackets has been added by the authors to clarify and enhance the use of nursing diagnoses.

Indirect (e.g., tearing off clothes, urinating/defecating on floor, stamping feet, temper tantrum; running in corridors, yelling, writing on walls, ripping objects off walls, throwing objects, breaking a window, slamming doors; sexual advances).

OTHER FACTORS:

Neurological impairment (e.g., positive EEG, CT, or MRI; head trauma; positive neurological findings; seizure disorders, [temporal lobe epilepsy])

Cognitive impairment (e.g., learning disabilities, attention deficit disorder, decreased intellectual functioning); [organic brain syndrome]

History of childhood abuse/witnessing family violence, [negative role modeling]; cruelty to animals; firesetting

Prenatal and perinatal complications/abnormalities

History of drug/alcohol abuse; pathological intoxication, [toxic reaction to medication]

Psychotic symptomatology (e.g., auditory, visual, command hallucinations; paranoid delusions; loose, rambling, or illogical thought processes); [panic states; rage reactions; catatonic/manic excitement]

Motor vehicle offenses (e.g., frequent traffic violations, use of motor vehicle to release anger)

Suicidal behavior; impulsivity; availability and/or possession of weapon(s)

Body language: rigid posture, clenching of fists and jaw, hyperactivity, pacing, breathlessness, threatening stances

[Hormonal imbalance (e.g., premenstrual syndrome—PMS, postpartal depression/psychosis)]

[Expressed intent/desire to harm others directly or indirectly]

[Almost continuous thoughts of violence]

Violence, [actual/] risk for self-directed

Taxonomy II: Safety/Protection—Class 3 Violence (00140) [Diagnostic Division: Safety]

Definition: At risk for behaviors in which an individual demonstrates that he or she can be physically, emotionally, and/or sexually harmful to self

Risk Factors/[Indicators]*

Ages 15 to 19; over age 45
Marital status (single, widowed, divorced)

---

* Note: Although a risk diagnosis does not have defining characteristics (signs and symptoms), the factors identified here can be used to denote an actual diagnosis or as indicators of risk for/escalation of violence.

Information that appears in brackets has been added by the authors to clarify and enhance the use of nursing diagnoses.

Employment (unemployed, recent job loss/failure); occupation (executive, administrator/owner of business, professional, semiskilled
worker)

Conflictual interpersonal relationships

Family background (chaotic or conflictual, history of suicide)

Sexual orientation: bisexual (active), homosexual (inactive)

Physical health (hypochondriac, chronic or terminal illness)

Mental health (severe depression, psychosis, severe personality disorder, alcoholism, or drug abuse)

Emotional status (hopelessness, [lifting of depressed mood], despair,
increased anxiety, panic, anger, hostility); history of multiple suicide
attempts; suicidal ideation (frequent, intense prolonged); suicide
plan (clear and specific; lethality, method and availability of
destructive means)

Personal resources (poor achievement, poor insight, affect unavailable
and poorly controlled)

Social resources (poor rapport, socially isolated, unresponsive family)

Verbal clues (e.g., talking about death, "better off without me," asking
questions about lethal dosages of drugs)

Behavioral clues (e.g., writing forlorn love notes, directing angry
messages at an SO who has rejected the person, giving away
personal items, taking out a large life insurance policy), people who
engage in autoerotic sexual acts [e.g., asphyxiation]

Desired Outcomes/Evaluation Criteria
[for directed at others/self-
directed]—Client Will:

* Acknowledge realities of the situation.
* Verbalize understanding of why behavior occurs.
* Identify precipitating factors.
* Express realistic self-evaluation and increased sense of self-
esteem.
* Participate in care and meet own needs in an assertive
manner.
* Demonstrate self-control as evidenced by relaxed posture,
nonviolent behavior.
* Use resources and support systems in an effective manner.

Actions/Interventions

(Address both "directed at others" and "self-directed")

NURSING PRIORITY NO. 1. To assess causative/contributing
factors:

* Determine underlying dynamics as listed in the Risk
Factors.
* Ascertain client's perception of self/situation. Note use of
defense mechanisms (e.g., denial, projection).
* Observe/listen for early cues of distress/increasing anxiety

(e.g., irritability, lack of cooperation, demanding behavior, body posture/expression).
- Identify conditions such as acute/chronic brain syndrome; panic state; hormonal imbalance (e.g., PMS, postpartal psychosis, drug-induced, postsurgical/postseizure confusion; psychomotor seizure activity) that may interfere with ability to control own behavior.
- Review laboratory findings (e.g., blood alcohol, blood glucose, ABGs, electrolytes, renal function tests).
- Observe for signs of suicidal/homicidal intent (e.g., perceived morbid or anxious feeling while with the client; warning from the client, "It doesn't matter," "I'd/They'd be better off dead"; mood swings; "accident-prone"/self-destructive behavior; suicidal attempts, possession of alcohol and/or other drug(s) in known substance abuser).
- Note family history of suicidal/homicidal behavior.
- Ask directly if the person is thinking of acting on thoughts/feelings to determine violent intent.
- Determine availability of suicidal/homicidal means.
- Assess client coping behaviors already present. (Note: Client believes there are no alternatives other than violence.)
- Identify risk factors and assess for indicators of child abuse/neglect: unexplained/frequent injuries, failure to thrive, and so forth.

NURSING PRIORITY NO. 2. To assist client to accept responsibility for impulsive behavior and potential for violence:

- Develop therapeutic nurse-client relationship. Provide consistent caregiver when possible. Promotes sense of trust, allowing client to discuss feelings openly.
- Maintain straightforward communication to avoid reinforcing manipulative behavior.
- Note motivation for change (e.g., failing relationships, job loss, involvement with judicial system). Crisis situation can provide impetus for change but requires timely therapeutic intervention to sustain efforts.
- Help client recognize that own actions may be in response to own fear (may be afraid of own behavior, loss of control), dependency, and feeling of powerlessness.
- Make time to listen to expressions of feelings. Acknowledge reality of client's feelings and that feelings are OK. (Refer to ND Self-Esteem, [specify].)
- Confront client's tendency to minimize situation/behavior.
- Identify factors (feelings/events) involved in precipitating violent behavior.
- Discuss impact of behavior on others/consequences of actions.

- Acknowledge reality of suicide/homicide as an option. Discuss consequences of actions if they were to follow through on intent. Ask how it will help client to resolve problems.
- Accept client's anger without reacting on emotional basis. Give permission to express angry feelings in acceptable ways and let client know that staff will be available to assist in maintaining control. **Promotes acceptance and sense of safety.**
- Help client identify more appropriate solutions/behaviors (e.g., motor activities/exercise) **to lessen sense of anxiety and associated physical manifestations.**
- Provide directions for actions client can take, avoiding negatives, such as "do nots."

NURSING PRIORITY NO. 3. To assist client in controlling behavior:

- Contract with client regarding safety of self/others.
- Give client as much control as possible within constraints of individual situation. **Enhances self-esteem, promotes confidence in ability to change behavior.**
- Be truthful when giving information and dealing with client. **Builds trust, enhancing therapeutic relationship.**
- Identify current/past successes and strengths. Discuss effectiveness of coping techniques used and possible changes. (Refer to ND Coping, ineffective.) **Client is often not aware of positive aspects of life, and once recognized, they can be used as a basis for change.**
- Assist client to distinguish between reality and hallucinations/delusions.
- Approach in positive manner, acting as if the client has control and is responsible for own behavior. Be aware, though, that the client may not have control, especially if under the influence of drugs (including alcohol).
- Maintain distance and do not touch client when situation indicates client does not tolerate such closeness (e.g., posttrauma response).
- Remain calm and state limits on inappropriate behavior (including consequences) in a firm manner.
- Direct client to stay in view of staff.
- Administer prescribed medications (e.g., antianxiety/antipsychotic), taking care not to oversedate client.
- Monitor for possible drug interactions, cumulative effects of drug regimen (e.g., anticonvulsants/antidepressants).
- Give positive reinforcement for client's efforts. **Encourages continuation of desired behaviors.**
- Explore death fantasies when expressed (e.g., "I'll look down and watch them suffer; they'll be sorry," "They'll be glad to get rid of me") or the idea that death is not final (e.g., "I can come back").

NURSING PRIORITY NO. 4. To assist client/SO(s) to correct/deal with existing situation:

- Gear interventions to individual(s) involved, based on age, relationship, and so forth.
- Maintain calm, matter-of-fact, nonjudgmental attitude. **Decreases defensive response.**
- Notify potential victims in the presence of serious homicidal threat in accordance with legal/ethical guidelines.
- Discuss situation with abused/battered person, providing accurate information about choices and effective actions that can be taken.
- Assist individual to understand that angry, vengeful feelings are appropriate in the situation, need to be expressed and not acted on. (Refer to ND Post-Trauma Syndrome, as psychologic responses may be very similar.)
- Identify resources available for assistance (e.g., battered women's shelter, social services).

NURSING PRIORITY NO. 5. To promote safety in event of violent behavior:

- Provide a safe, quiet environment and remove items from the client's environment that could be used to inflict harm to self/others.
- Maintain distance from client who is striking out/hitting and take evasive/controlling actions as indicated.
- Call for additional staff/security personnel.
- Approach aggressive/attacking client from the front, just out of reach, in a commanding posture with palms down.
- Tell client to stop. **This may be sufficient to help client control own actions.**
- Maintain direct/constant eye contact when appropriate.
- Speak in a low, commanding voice.
- Provide client with a sense that caregiver is in control of the situation **to provide feeling of safety.**
- Maintain clear route for staff and client and be prepared to move quickly.
- Hold client, using restraints or seclusion when necessary until client regains self-control. Administer medication as indicated.

NURSING PRIORITY NO. 6. To promote wellness (Teaching/Discharge Considerations):

- Promote client involvement in planning care within limits of situation, allowing for meeting own needs for enjoyment. **Individuals often believe they are not entitled to pleasure and good things in their lives and need to learn how to meet these needs.**

- Assist client to learn assertive rather than manipulative, nonassertive/aggressive behavior.
- Discuss reasons for client's behavior with SO(s). Determine desire/commitment of involved parties to sustain current relationships.
- Develop strategies to help parents learn more effective parenting skills (e.g., parenting classes, appropriate ways of dealing with frustrations).
- Identify support systems (e.g., family/friends, clergy).
- Refer to formal resources as indicated (e.g., individual/group psychotherapy, substance abuse treatment program, social services, safe house facility).
- Refer to NDs Parenting, impaired; Coping, family [specify]; Post-Trauma Syndrome.

Documentation Focus

ASSESSMENT/REASSESSMENT

- Individual findings, including nature of concern (e.g., suicidal/homicidal), behavioral risk factors and level of impulse control, plan of action/means to carry out plan.
- Client's perception of situation, motivation for change.

PLANNING

- Plan of care and who is involved in the planning.
- Details of contract regarding violence to self/others.
- Teaching plan.

IMPLEMENTATION/EVALUATION

- Actions taken to promote safety, including notification of parties at risk.
- Response to interventions/teaching and actions performed.
- Attainment/progress toward desired outcome(s).
- Modifications to plan of care.

DISCHARGE PLANNING

- Long-range needs and who is responsible for actions to be taken.
- Available resources, specific referrals made.

SAMPLE NURSING OUTCOMES & INTERVENTIONS CLASSIFICATIONS (NOC/NIC)

NOC—Aggression Control
NIC—Anger Control Assistance

Walking, impaired

Taxonomy II: Activity/Rest—Class 2 Activity/Exercise
(00088)
[Diagnostic Division: Activity/Rest]

Definition: Limitation of independent movement within
the environment on foot

Related Factors

To be developed
[Condition affecting muscles/joints impairing ability to walk]

Defining Characteristics

SUBJECTIVE OR OBJECTIVE

Impaired ability to walk required distances, walk on an incline/decline,
or on uneven surfaces, to navigate curbs, climb stairs
[Specify level of independence—refer to ND Mobility, impaired physical, for suggested functional level classification]

Desired Outcomes/Evaluation
Criteria—Client Will:

- Be able to move about within environment as needed/desired
within limits of ability or with appropriate adjuncts.
- Verbalize understanding of situation/risk factors and safety
measures.

Actions/Interventions

NURSING PRIORITY NO. 1. To assess causative/contributing
factors:

- Identify condition/diagnoses that contribute to difficulty
walking (e.g., advanced age, acute illness, weakness/chronic
illness, recent surgery, trauma, arthritis, brain injury, vision
impairments, pain, fatigue, cognitive dysfunction).
- Determine ability to follow directions, and note emotional/
behavioral responses that may be affecting the situation.

NURSING PRIORITY NO. 2. To assess functional ability:

- Determine degree of impairment in relation to suggested
functional scale (0 to 4), noting that impairment can be either
temporary/permanent or progressive.
- Note emotional/behavioral responses of client/SO to problems of mobility.

Information that appears in brackets has been added by the authors
to clarify and enhance the use of nursing diagnoses.

NURSING PRIORITY NO. 3. To promote safe, optimal level of independence in walking:

- Assist with treatment of underlying condition causing dysfunction as needed/indicated by individual situation.
- Consult with PT/OT **to develop individual mobility/walking program and identify appropriate adjunctive devices.**
- Demonstrate use of adjunctive devices (e.g., walker, cane, crutches, prosthesis).
- Schedule walking/exercise activities interspersed with adequate rest periods **to reduce fatigue.** Provide ample time to perform mobility-related tasks. Advance levels of exercise as able.
- Provide safety measures as indicated, including environmental management/fall prevention.

NURSING PRIORITY NO. 4. To promote wellness (Teaching/Discharge Considerations):

- Involve client/SO in care, assisting them to learn ways of managing deficits **to enhance safety for client and SO(s)/caregivers.**
- Identify appropriate resources for obtaining and maintaining appliances, equipment, and environmental modifications **to promote mobility.**
- Instruct client/SO in safety measures as individually indicated (e.g., maintaining safe travel pathway, proper lighting/handrails on stairs, etc.) **to reduce risk of falls.**

Documentation Focus

ASSESSMENT/REASSESSMENT

- Individual findings, including level of function/ability to participate in specific/desired activities.

PLANNING

- Plan of care and who is involved in the planning.
- Teaching plan.

IMPLEMENTATION/EVALUATION

- Responses to interventions/teaching and actions performed.
- Attainment/progress toward desired outcome(s).
- Modifications to plan of care.

DISCHARGE PLANNING

- Discharge/long-range needs, noting who is responsible for each action to be taken.
- Specific referrals made.
- Sources of/maintenance for assistive devices.

SAMPLE NURSING OUTCOMES
& INTERVENTIONS CLASSIFICATIONS (NOC/NIC)

NOC—Ambulation: Walking
NIC—Exercise Therapy: Ambulation

Wandering [specify sporadic or continuous]

Taxonomy II: Activity/Rest—Class 2 Activity/Exercise
(00154)
[Diagnostic Division: Safety]
Submitted 2000

Definition: Meandering, aimless, or repetitive locomotion that exposes the individual to harm; frequently incongruent with boundaries, limits, or obstacles

Related Factors

Cognitive impairment, specifically memory and recall deficits, disorientation, poor visuoconstructive (or visuospatial) ability, language (primarily expressive) defects
Cortical atrophy
Premorbid behavior (e.g., outgoing, sociable personality; premorbid dementia)
Separation from familiar people and places
Emotional state, especially frustration, anxiety, boredom, or depression (agitation)
Physiological state or need (e.g., hunger/thirst, pain, urination, constipation)
Over/understimulating social or physical environment; sedation
Time of day

Defining Characteristics

OBJECTIVE

Frequent or continuous movement from place to place, often revisiting the same destinations
Persistent locomotion in search of "missing" or unattainable people or places; scanning, seeking, or searching behaviors
Haphazard locomotion; fretful locomotion or pacing; long periods of locomotion without an apparent destination
Locomotion into unauthorized or private spaces; trespassing
Locomotion resulting in unintended leaving of a premise
Inability to locate significant landmarks in a familiar setting; getting lost
Locomotion that cannot be easily dissuaded or redirected; following behind or shadowing a caregiver's locomotion

---

Information that appears in brackets has been added by the authors to clarify and enhance the use of nursing diagnoses.

Hyperactivity

Periods of locomotion interspersed with periods of nonlocomotion
(e.g., sitting, standing, sleeping)

Desired Outcomes/Evaluation Criteria—Client Will:

• Be free of injury, or unplanned exits.

Caregiver(s) Will:

• Modify environment as indicated to enhance safety.
• Provide for maximal independence of client.

Actions/Interventions

NURSING PRIORITY NO. 1. To assess degree of impairment/stage of disease process:

• Ascertain history of client's memory loss and cognitive changes.
• Note results of diagnostic testing, confirming diagnosis and type of dementia.
• Evaluate client's mental status during daytime and nighttime, noting when client's confusion is most pronounced, and when client sleeps.
• Monitor client's use/need for assistive devices such as glasses, hearing aids, cane, and so forth.
• Assess frequency and pattern of wandering behavior **to determine individual risks/safety needs.**
• Identify client's reason for wandering if possible (e.g., looking for lost item, desire to go home, boredom, need for activity, hunger, thirst, or discomfort).
• Ascertain if client has delusions due to shadows, lights, and noises.

NURSING PRIORITY NO. 2. To assist client/caregiver to deal with situations:

• Provide a structured daily routine. **Decreases wandering behavior and minimizes caregiver stress.**
• Encourage participation in family activities and familiar routines such as folding laundry, listening to music, walking outdoors. **Activities and exercises may reduce anxiety and restlessness.**
• Bring client to bathroom on a regular schedule.
• Provide safe place for client to wander, away from safety hazards (e.g., hot water/kitchen stove, open stairway) and other noisy clients. Arrange furniture and other items **to accommodate wandering.**
• Make sure that doors have alarms and that alarms are turned

on. Provide door and window locks that are not easily opened **to prevent unsafe exits.**

- Provide 24-hour reality orientation. (**Client can be awake at any time and fail to recognize day/night routines.**)
- Sit with client and talk. Provide TV/radio/music.
- Avoid overstimulation from activities or new partners/room-mate during rest periods when client is in a facility.
- Use pressure-sensitive bed/chair alarms **to alert caregivers of movement.**
- Avoid using physical or chemical restraints (sedatives) to control wandering behavior. **May increase agitation, sensory deprivation, and falls, and may contribute to wandering behavior.**
- Provide consistent staff as much as possible.
- Provide room near monitoring station; check client location on frequent basis.

NURSING PRIORITY NO. 3. To Promote Wellness (Teaching/ Discharge Considerations):

- Identify problems that are remediable and assist client/SO to seek appropriate assistance and access resources. (**Encourages problem solving to improve condition rather than accept the status quo.**)
- Notify neighbors about client's condition and request that they contact client's family or local police if they see client outside alone. **Community awareness can prevent/reduce risk of client being lost or hurt.**
- Use community resources, such as Alzheimer's Association Safe Return Program, **to assist in identification, location, and safe return of individual with wandering behaviors.**
- Help client/SO develop plan of care when problem is progressive.
- Refer to community resources such as day care programs, support groups, and so forth.
- Refer to NDs: Confusion, acute; Sensory Perception, disturbed (specify: visual, auditory, kinesthetic, gustatory, tactile, olfactory); Injury, risk for; Falls, risk for.

Documentation Focus

ASSESSMENT/REASSESSMENT

- Assessment findings, including individual concerns, family involvement, and support factors/availability of resources.

PLANNING

- Plan of care and who is involved in planning.
- Teaching plan.

IMPLEMENTATION/EVALUATION

- Responses of client/SO(s) to plan interventions and actions performed.
- Attainment/progress toward desired outcome(s).
- Modifications to plan of care.

DISCHARGE PLANNING

- Long-range needs and who is responsible for actions to be taken.
- Specific referrals made.

SAMPLE NURSING OUTCOMES
& INTERVENTIONS CLASSIFICATIONS (NOC/NIC)

NOC—Risk Control
NIC—Elopement Precautions

CHAPTER 5

Health Conditions and Client Concerns with Associated Nursing Diagnoses

This chapter presents over 400 disorders/health conditions reflecting all specialty areas, with associated nursing diagnoses written as client problem/need statements that include "related to" and "evidenced by" statements.

This section will facilitate and help validate the assessment and diagnosis steps of the nursing process. Because the nursing process is perpetual and ongoing, other nursing diagnoses may be appropriate based on changing individual situations. Therefore, the nurse must continually assess, identify, and validate new client needs and evaluate subsequent care. Once the appropriate nursing diagnoses have been selected from this chapter, the reader may refer to Chapter 4, which lists the 167 NANDA diagnoses, and review the diagnostic definition, defining characteristics, and related or risk factors for further validation. This step is necessary to determine if the nursing diagnosis statement is an accurate match, if more data are required, or if another diagnosis needs to be investigated.

To facilitate access to the health conditions/concerns and nursing diagnoses, the client needs have been listed alphabetically and coded to identify nursing specialty areas.

MS: Medical-Surgical
PED: Pediatric
OB: Obstetric
CH: Community/Home
PSY: Psychiatric/Behavioral
GYN: Gynecological

A separate category for geriatric has not been made because geriatric concerns/conditions actually are subsumed under the other specialty areas, because elderly persons are susceptible to the majority of these problems.

Abdominal hysterectomy   **MS**
(Refer to Hysterectomy)

Abdominal perineal resection   MS
(Also refer to Surgery, general)

disturbed Body Image may be related to presence of surgical wounds possibly evidenced by verbalizations of feelings/perceptions, fear of reaction by others, preoccupation with change.

risk for Constipation: risk factors may include decreased physical activity/gastric motility, abdominal muscle weakness, insufficient fluid intake, change in usual foods/eating pattern.*

risk for Sexual Dysfunction: risk factors may include altered body structure/function, radical resection/treatment procedures, vulnerability/psychologic concern about response of significant other(s), and disruption of sexual response pattern (e.g., erection difficulty).*

Abortion, elective termination   OB

risk for Decisional Conflict: risk factors may include unclear personal values/beliefs, lack of experience or interference with decision making, information from divergent sources, deficient support system.*

deficient Knowledge [Learning Need] regarding reproduction, contraception, self-care, Rh factor may be related to lack of exposure/recall or misinterpretation of information possibly evidenced by request for information, statement of misconception, inaccurate follow-through of instructions, development of preventable events/complications.

risk for Spiritual Distress: risk factors may include perception of moral/ethical implications of therapeutic procedure.*

Anxiety [specify level] may be related to situational/maturational crises, unmet needs, unconscious conflict about essential values/beliefs possibly evidenced by increased tension, apprehension, fear of unspecific consequences, sympathetic stimulation, focus on self.

acute Pain/[Discomfort] may be related to after effects of procedure/drug effect possibly evidenced by verbal report, distraction behaviors, changes in muscle tone, autonomic responses/changes in vital signs.

risk for maternal Injury: risk factors may include surgical procedure, effects of anesthesia/medications.*

Abortion, spontaneous termination   OB

deficient Fluid Volume [isotonic] may be related to excessive blood loss, possibly evidenced by decreased pulse volume and pressure, delayed capillary refill, or changes in sensorium.

risk for Spiritual Distress: risk factors may include need to adhere to personal religious beliefs/practices, blame for loss directed at self or God.*

deficient Knowledge [Learning Need] regarding cause of abortion, self-care, contraception/future pregnancy may be related to lack of familiarity with new self/healthcare needs, sources for support, possibly evidenced by requests for information and statement of concern/misconceptions, development of preventable complications.

---

*A risk diagnosis is not evidenced by signs and symptoms, as the problem has not occurred and nursing interventions are directed at prevention.

Grieving [expected] related to perinatal loss, possibly evidenced by crying, expressions of sorrow, or changes in eating habits/sleep patterns.

risk for ineffective Sexuality Patterns: risk factors may include increasing fear of pregnancy and/or repeat loss, impaired relationship with significant other(s), self-doubt regarding own femininity.*

Abruptio placentae   OB

deficient Fluid Volume [isotonic] may be related to excessive blood loss, possibly evidenced by hypotension, increased heart rate, decreased pulse volume and pressure, delayed capillary refill, or changes in sensorium.

Fear related to threat of death (perceived or actual) to fetus/self, possibly evidenced by verbalization of specific concerns, increased tension, sympathetic stimulation.

acute Pain may be related to collection of blood between uterine wall and placenta, possibly evidenced by verbal reports, abdominal guarding, muscle tension, or alterations in vital signs.

impaired fetal Gas Exchange may be related to altered uteroplacental O_2 transfer, possibly evidenced by alterations in fetal heart rate and movement.

Abscess, brain (acute)   MS

acute Pain may be related to inflammation, edema of tissues, possibly evidenced by reports of headache, restlessness, irritability, and moaning.

risk for Hyperthermia: risk factors may include inflammatory process/hypermetabolic state and dehydration.*

acute Confusion may be related to physiologic changes (e.g., cerebral edema/altered perfusion, fever), possibly evidenced by fluctuation in cognition/level of consciousness, increased agitation/restlessness, hallucinations.

risk for Suffocation/Trauma: risk factors may include development of clonic/tonic muscle activity and changes in consciousness (seizure activity).*

Abscess, skin/tissue   CH/MS

impaired Skin/Tissue Integrity may be related to immunologic deficit/infection possibly evidenced by disruption of skin, destruction of skin layers/tissues, invasion of body structures.

risk for Infection [spread]: risk factors may include broken skin/traumatized tissues, chronic disease, malnutrition, insufficient knowledge.*

Abuse   CM
(Also refer to Battered child syndrome)
risk for Trauma: risk factors may include vulnerable client, recipient of verbal threats, history of physical abuse.*

---

*A risk diagnosis is not evidenced by signs and symptoms, as the problem has not occurred and nursing interventions are directed at prevention.

<u>Powerlessness</u> may be related to abusive relationship, lifestyle of help-lessness as evidenced by verbal expressions of having no control, reluctance to express true feelings, apathy, passivity.

<u>chronic low Self-Esteem</u> may be related to continual negative evaluation of self/capabilities, personal vulnerability, willingness to tolerate possible life-threatening domestic violence as evidenced by self-negative verbalization, evaluates self as unable to deal with events, rationalizes away/rejects positive feedback.

Achalasia (cardiac sphincter)   MS

<u>impaired Swallowing</u> may be related to neuromuscular impairment, possibly evidenced by observed difficulty in swallowing or regurgitation.

<u>imbalanced Nutrition: less than body requirements</u> may be related to inability and/or reluctance to ingest adequate nutrients to meet metabolic demands/nutritional needs, possibly evidenced by reported/observed inadequate intake, weight loss, and pale conjunctiva and mucous membranes.

<u>acute Pain</u> may be related to spasm of the lower esophageal sphincter, possibly evidenced by reports of substernal pressure, recurrent heartburn, or gastric fullness (gas pains).

<u>Anxiety [specify level]/Fear</u> may be related to recurrent pain, choking sensation, altered health status, possibly evidenced by verbalizations of distress, apprehension, restlessness, or insomnia.

<u>risk for Aspiration:</u> risk factors may include regurgitation/spillover of esophageal contents.*

<u>deficient Knowledge [Learning Need] regarding condition, prognosis, self-care and treatment needs</u> may be related to lack of familiarity with pathology and treatment of condition, possibly evidenced by requests for information, statement of concern, or development of preventable complications.

Acidosis, metabolic   MS

(Refer to Diabetic ketoacidosis)

Acidosis, respiratory   MS

(Also refer to underlying cause/condition)

<u>impaired Gas Exchange</u> may be related to ventilation perfusion imbalance (decreased oxygen-carrying capacity of blood, altered oxygen-supply, alveolar-capillary membrane changes) possibly evidenced by dyspnea with exertion, tachypnea, changes in mentation, irritability, tachycardia, hypoxia, hypercapnia.

Acne   CH/PED

<u>impaired Skin Integrity</u> may be related to secretions, infectious process as evidenced by disruptions of skin surface.

<u>disturbed Body Image</u> may be related to change in visual appearance as evidenced by fear of rejection of others, focus on past appearance, negative feelings about body, change in social involvement.

---

*A risk diagnosis is not evidenced by signs and symptoms, as the problem has not occurred and nursing interventions are directed at prevention.

---

situational low Self-Esteem may be related to adolescence, negative perception of appearance as evidenced by self-negating verbalizations, expressions of helplessness.

Acquired immune deficiency syndrome CH
(Refer to AIDS)

Acromegaly CH
chronic Pain may be related to soft tissue swelling, joint degeneration, peripheral nerve compression possibly evidenced by verbal reports, altered ability to continue previous activities, changes in sleep pattern, fatigue.

disturbed Body Image may be related to biophysical illness/changes possibly evidenced by verbalization of feelings/concerns, fear of rejection or of reaction of others, negative comments about body, actual change in structure/appearance, change in social involvement.

risk for Sexual Dysfunction: risk factors may include altered body structure, changes in libido.*

Acute respiratory distress syndrome (ARDS) MS
ineffective Airway Clearance may be related to loss of ciliary action, increased amount and viscosity of secretions, and increased airway resistance, possibly evidenced by presence of dyspnea, changes in depth/rate of respiration, use of accessory muscles for breathing, wheezes/crackles, cough with or without sputum production.

impaired Gas Exchange may be related to changes in pulmonary capillary permeability with edema formation, alveolar hypoventilation and collapse, with intrapulmonary shunting; possibly evidenced by tachypnea, use of accessory muscles, cyanosis, hypoxia per arterial blood gases (ABGs)/oximetry; anxiety and changes in mentation.

risk for deficient Fluid Volume: risk factors may include active loss from diuretic use and restricted intake.*

risk for decreased Cardiac Output: risk factors may include alteration in preload (hypovolemia, vascular pooling, diuretic therapy, and increased intrathoracic pressure/use of ventilator/positive end-expiratory pressure–PEEP).*

Anxiety [specify level]/Fear may be related to physiologic factors (effects of hypoxemia); situational crisis, change in health status/threat of death; possibly evidenced by increased tension, apprehension, restlessness, focus on self, and sympathetic stimulation.

risk for barotrauma Injury: risk factors may include increased airway pressure associated with mechanical ventilation (PEEP).*

Adams-Stokes syndrome CH
(Refer to Dysrhythmia)

ADD PEDS
(Refer to Attention deficit disorder)

---

*A risk diagnosis is not evidenced by signs and symptoms, as the problem has not occurred and nursing interventions are directed at prevention.

Addiction CH/PSY

(Refer to specific substances; Substance dependence/abuse rehabilitation)

Addison's disease

deficient Fluid Volume [hypotonic] may be related to vomiting, diarrhea, increased renal losses, possibly evidenced by delayed capillary refill, poor skin turgor, dry mucous membranes, report of thirst.

decreased Cardiac Output may be related to hypovolemia and altered electrical conduction (dysrhythmias) and/or diminished cardiac muscle mass, possibly evidenced by alterations in vital signs, changes in mentation, and irregular pulse or pulse deficit.

CH

Fatigue may be related to decreased metabolic energy production, altered body chemistry (fluid, electrolyte, and glucose imbalance), possibly evidenced by unremitting overwhelming lack of energy, inability to maintain usual routines, decreased performance, impaired ability to concentrate, lethargy, and disinterest in surroundings.

disturbed Body Image may be related to changes in skin pigmentation, mucous membranes, loss of axillary/pubic hair, possibly evidenced by verbalization of negative feelings about body and decreased social involvement.

risk for impaired physical Mobility: risk factors may include neuromuscular impairment (muscle wasting/weakness) and dizziness/syncope.*

imbalanced Nutrition: less than body requirements may be related to glucocorticoid deficiency; abnormal fat, protein, and carbohydrate metabolism; nausea, vomiting, anorexia, possibly evidenced by weight loss, muscle wasting, abdominal cramps, diarrhea, and severe hypoglycemia.

risk for impaired Home Maintenance: risk factors may include effects of disease process, impaired cognitive functioning, and inadequate support systems.*

Adenoidectomy PED/MS

Anxiety [specify level]/Fear may be related to separation from supportive others, unfamiliar surroundings, and perceived threat of injury/abandonment, possibly evidenced by crying, apprehension, trembling, and sympathetic stimulation (pupil dilation, increased heart rate).

risk for ineffective Airway Clearance: risk factors may include sedation, collection of secretions/blood in oropharynx, and vomiting.*

risk for deficient Fluid Volume: risk factors may include operative trauma to highly vascular site/hemorrhage.*

acute Pain may be related to physical trauma to oronasopharynx, presence of packing, possibly evidenced by restlessness, crying, and facial mask of pain.

---

*A risk diagnosis is not evidenced by signs and symptoms, as the problem has not occurred and nursing interventions are directed at prevention.

Adjustment disorder PSY

moderate to severe Anxiety may be related to situational/maturational crisis, threat to self-concept, unmet needs, fear of failure, dysfunctional family system, fixation in earlier level of development possibly evidenced by overexcitement/restlessness, increased tension, insomnia, feelings of inadequacy, focus on self, difficulty concentrating, continuous attention-seeking behaviors, numerous physical complaints.

risk for self/other-directed Violence: risk factors may include depressed mood, hopelessness, powerlessness, inability to tolerate frustration, rage reactions, unmet needs, negative role modeling, substance use/abuse, history of suicide attempt.*

ineffective Coping may be related to situational/maturational crisis, dysfunctional family system, negative role modeling, unmet dependency needs, retarded ego development possibly evidenced by inability to problem-solve, chronic worry, depressed/anxious mood, manipulation of others, destructive behaviors, increased dependency, refusal to follow rules.

dysfunctional Grieving may be related to real or perceived loss of any concept of value to individual, bereavement overload/cumulative grief, thwarted grieving response, feelings of guilt generated by ambivalent relationship with the lost concept/person possibly evidenced by difficulty in expressing/denial of loss, excessive/inappropriately expressed anger, labile affect, developmental regression, changes in concentration/pursuit of tasks.

Hopelessness may be related to lifestyle of helplessness (repeated failures, dependency), incomplete grief work of losses in life, lost belief in transcendent values/God possibly evidenced by verbal cues/despondent content, apathy/passivity, decreased response to stimuli, lack of initiative, nonparticipation in care or decision-making.

Adoption/loss of child custody PSY

risk for dysfunctional Grieving: risk factors may include actual loss of child, expectations for future of child/self, thwarted grieving response to loss.*

risk for Powerlessness: risk factors may include perceived lack of options, no input into decision process, no control over outcome.*

Adrenal crisis, acute MS

(Also refer to Addison's disease; Shock)

deficient Fluid Volume [hypotonic] may be related to failure of regulatory mechanism (damage to/suppression of adrenal gland), inability to concentrate urine possibly evidenced by decreased venous filling/pulse volume and pressure, hypotension, dry mucous membranes, changes in mentation, decreased serum sodium.

acute Pain may be related to effects of disease process/metabolic imbalances, decreased tissue perfusion, possibly evidenced by reports of severe pain in abdomen, lower back, or legs.

---

*A risk diagnosis is not evidenced by signs and symptoms, as the problem has not occurred and nursing interventions are directed at prevention.

impaired physical Mobility may be related to neuromuscular impairment, decreased muscle strength/control possibly evidenced by generalized weakness, inability to perform desired activities/movements.

risk for Hyperthermia: risk factors may include presence of illness/infectious process, dehydration.*

risk for ineffective Protection: risk factors may include hormone deficiency, drug therapy, nutritional/metabolic deficiencies.*

Adrenalectomy   MS

altered Tissue Perfusion (specify) may be related to hypovolemia and vascular pooling (vasodilation), possibly evidenced by diminished pulse, pallor/cyanosis, hypotension, and changes in mentation.

risk for Infection: risk factors may include inadequate primary defenses (incision, traumatized tissues), suppressed inflammatory response, invasive procedures.*

deficient Knowledge [Learning Need] regarding condition, prognosis, self-care and treatment needs may be related to unfamiliarity with long-term therapy requirements, possibly evidenced by request for information and statement of concern/misconceptions.

Adrenal insufficiency   CH
(Refer to Addison's disease)

Affective disorder   PSY
(Refer to Bipolar disorder; Depressive disorders, major)

Affective disorder, seasonal   PSY
(Also refer to Depressive disorders, major)

intermittent ineffective Coping may be related to situational crisis (fall/winter season), disturbance in pattern of tension release, and inadequate resources available possibly evidenced by verbalizations of inability to cope, changes in sleep pattern (too little or too much), reports of lack of energy/fatigue, lack of resolution of problem, behavioral changes (irritability, discouragement).

risk for imbalanced Nutrition: more/less than body requirements: risk factors may include eating in response to internal cues other than hunger, alteration in usual coping patterns, change in usual activity level, decreased appetite, lack of energy/interest to prepare food.*

Agoraphobia   PSY
(Also refer to Phobia)

Anxiety [panic] may be related to contact with feared situation (public place/crowds) possibly evidenced by tachycardia, chest pain, dyspnea, gastrointestinal distress, faintness, sense of impending doom.

Agranulocytosis   MS
risk for infection: risk factors may include suppressed inflammatory response.*

---

*A risk diagnosis is not evidenced by signs and symptoms, as the problem has not occurred and nursing interventions are directed at prevention.

risk for impaired Oral Mucous Membrane: risk factors may include infection.*

risk for imbalanced Nutrition: less than body requirements: risk factors may include inability to ingest food/fluids (lesions of oral cavity).*

AIDS (acquired immunodeficiency syndrome)   MS
(Also refer to HIV positive)

risk for Infection, [progression to sepsis/onset of new opportunistic infection]: risk factors may include depressed immune system, use of antimicrobial agents, inadequate primary defenses; broken skin, traumatized tissue; malnutrition, and chronic disease processes.*

risk for deficient Fluid Volume: risk factors may include excessive losses: copious diarrhea, profuse sweating, vomiting, hypermetabolic state or fever, and restriction intake (nausea, anorexia, lethargy).*

acute/chronic Pain may be related to tissue inflammation/destruction: infections, internal/external cutaneous lesions, rectal excoriation, malignancies, necrosis, peripheral neuropathies, myalgias and arthralgias, possibly evidenced by verbal reports, self-focusing/narrowed focus, alteration in muscle tone, paresthesias, paralysis, guarding behaviors, changes in vital signs (acute), autonomic responses, and restlessness.

CH

imbalanced Nutrition: less than body requirements may be related to altered ability to ingest, digest, and/or absorb nutrients (nausea/vomiting, hyperactive gag reflex, intestinal disturbances); increased metabolic activity/nutritional needs (fever, infection), possibly evidenced by weight loss, decreased subcutaneous fat/muscle mass; lack of interest in food/aversion to eating, altered taste sensation; abdominal cramping, hyperactive bowel sounds, diarrhea, sore and inflamed buccal cavity.

Fatigue may be related to decreased metabolic energy production, increased energy requirements (hypermetabolic state), overwhelming psychological/emotional demands; altered body chemistry (side effects of medication, chemotherapy), possibly evidenced by unremitting/overwhelming lack of energy, inability to maintain usual routines, decreased performance; impaired ability to concentrate, lethargy/restlessness, and disinterest in surroundings.

ineffective Protection may be related to chronic disease affecting immune and neurologic systems, inadequate nutrition, drug therapies, possibly evidenced by deficient immunity, impaired healing, neurosensory alterations, maladaptive stress response, fatigue, anorexia, disorientation.

PSY

Social Isolation may be related to changes in physical appearance/mental status, state of wellness, perceptions of unacceptable social or sexual behavior/values, physical isolation, phobic fear of others

---

*A risk diagnosis is not evidenced by signs and symptoms, as the problem has not occurred and nursing interventions are directed at prevention.

(transmission of disease); possibly evidenced by expressed feelings of aloneness/rejection, absence of supportive significant other(s)—SO(s), and withdrawal from usual activities.

disturbed Thought Processes/chronic Confusion may be related to physiologic changes (hypoxemia, central nervous system—CNS—infection by HIV, brain malignancies, and/or disseminated systemic opportunistic infection); altered drug metabolism/excretion, accumulation of toxic elements (renal failure, severe electrolyte imbalance, hepatic insufficiency), possibly evidenced by clinical evidence of organic impairment, altered attention span, distractibility, memory deficit, disorientation, cognitive dissonance, delusional thinking, impaired ability to make decisions/problem-solve, inability to follow complex commands/mental tasks, loss of impulse control and altered personality.

AIDS dementia   CH

(Also refer to Dementia, presenile/senile)

impaired Environmental Interpretation Syndrome may be related to dementia, depression, possibly evidenced by consistent disorientation, inability to follow simple directions/instructions, loss of social functioning from memory decline.

ineffective Protection may be related to chronic disease affecting immune and neurologic systems, inadequate nutrition, drug therapies, possibly evidenced by deficient immunity, impaired healing, neurosensory alterations, maladaptive stress response, fatigue, anorexia, disorientation.

Alcohol abuse/withdrawal   CH/MS/PSY

(Refer to Drug overdose, acute [depressants]; Delirium tremens; Substance dependency/abuse rehabilitation)

Alcohol intoxication, acute   MS

(Also refer to Delirium tremens)

acute Confusion may be related to substance abuse, hypoxemia possibly evidenced by hallucinations, exaggerated emotional response, fluctuation in cognition/level of consciousness, increased agitation.

risk for ineffective Breathing Pattern: risk factors may include neuromuscular impairment/CNS depression.*

risk for Aspiration: risk factors may include reduced level of consciousness, depressed cough/gag reflexes, delayed gastric emptying.*

Aldosteronism, primary   MS

deficient Fluid Volume [isotonic] may be related to increased urinary losses, possibly evidenced by dry mucous membranes, poor skin turgor, dilute urine, excessive thirst, weight loss.

impaired physical Mobility may be related to neuromuscular impairment, weakness, and pain, possibly evidenced by impaired coordination, decreased muscle strength, paralysis, and positive Chvostek's and Trousseau's signs.

---

*A risk diagnosis is not evidenced by signs and symptoms, as the problem has not occurred and nursing interventions are directed at prevention.

risk for decreased Cardiac Output: risk factors may include hypovolemia and altered electrical conduction/dysrhythmias.*

Alkalosis, respiratory   MS
(Also refer to underlying cause/condition)

impaired Gas Exchange may be related to ventilation perfusion imbalance (decreased oxygen-carrying capacity of blood, altered oxygensupply, alveolar-capillary membrane changes) possibly evidenced by dyspnea, tachypnea, changes in mentation, tachycardia, hypoxia, hypocapnia.

Allergies, seasonal   CH
(Refer to Hay fever)

Alopecia   CH
disturbed Body Image may be related to effects of illness/therapy or aging process, change in appearance possibly evidenced by verbalization of feelings/concerns, fear of rejection/reaction of others, focus on past appearance, preoccupation with change, feelings of helplessness.

ALS   CH
(Refer to Amyotrophic lateral sclerosis)

Alzheimer's disease   CH
(Also refer to Dementia, presenile/senile)

risk for Injury/Trauma: risk factors may include inability to recognize/identify danger in environment, disorientation, confusion, impaired judgment, weakness, muscular incoordination, balancing difficulties, and altered perception.*

chronic Confusion related to physiologic changes (neuronal degeneration); possibly evidenced by inaccurate interpretation of/response to stimuli, progressive/long-standing cognitive impairment, short-term memory deficit, impaired socialization, altered personality, and clinical evidence of organic impairment.

disturbed Sensory Perception (specify) may be related to altered sensory reception, transmission, and/or integration (neurologic disease/deficit), socially restricted environment (homebound/institutionalized), sleep deprivation possibly evidenced by changes in usual response to stimuli, change in problem-solving abilities, exaggerated emotional responses (anxiety, paranoia, hallucinations), inability to tell position of body parts, diminished/altered sense of taste.

disturbed Sleep Pattern may be related to sensory impairment, changes in activity patterns, psychologic stress (neurologic impairment), possibly evidenced by wakefulness, disorientation (day/night reversal); increased aimless wandering, inability to identify need/time for sleeping, changes in behavior/performance, lethargy; dark circles under eyes, and frequent yawning.

---

*A risk diagnosis is not evidenced by signs and symptoms, as the problem has not occurred and nursing interventions are directed at prevention.

<u>ineffective Health Maintenance</u> may be related to deterioration affecting ability in all areas, including coordination/communication, cognitive impairment; ineffective individual/family coping, possibly evidenced by reported or observed inability to take responsibility for meeting basic health practices, lack of equipment/financial or other resources, and impairment of personal support system.

PSY

<u>compromised family Coping/Caregiver Role Strain</u> may be related to family disorganization, role changes, family/caregiver isolation, long-term illness/complexity and amount of homecare needs exhausting supportive/financial capabilities of family member(s), lack of respite; possibly evidenced by verbalizations of frustrations in dealing with day-to-day care, reports of conflict, feelings of depression, expressed anger/guilt directed toward client, and withdrawal from interaction with client/social contacts.

<u>risk for Relocation Stress Syndrome:</u> risk factors may include little or no preparation for transfer to a new setting, changes in daily routine, sensory impairment, physical deterioration, separation from support systems.*

Amphetamine abuse
PSY

(Refer to Stimulant abuse)

Amputation
MS

<u>risk for ineffective peripheral Tissue Perfusion:</u> risk factors may include reduced arterial/venous blood flow; tissue edema, hematoma formation; hypovolemia.*

<u>acute Pain</u> may be related to tissue and nerve trauma, psychologic impact of loss of body part, possibly evidenced by reports of incisional/phantom pain, guarding/protective behavior, narrowed/self-focus, and autonomic responses.

<u>impaired physical Mobility</u> may be related to loss of limb (primarily lower extremity), altered sense of balance, pain/discomfort, possibly evidenced by reluctance to attempt movement, impaired coordination; decreased muscle strength, control, and mass.

<u>disturbed Body Image</u> may be related to loss of a body part, possibly evidenced by verbalization of feelings of powerlessness, grief, preoccupation with loss, and unwillingness to look at/touch stump.

Amyotrophic lateral sclerosis (ALS)
MS

<u>impaired physical Mobility</u> may be related to muscle wasting/weakness, possibly evidenced by impaired coordination, limited range of motion, and impaired purposeful movement.

<u>ineffective Breathing Pattern/impaired spontaneous Ventilation</u> may be related to neuromuscular impairment, decreased energy, fatigue,

---

*A risk diagnosis is not evidenced by signs and symptoms, as the problem has not occurred and nursing interventions are directed at prevention.

tracheobronchial obstruction, possibly evidenced by shortness of breath, fremitus, respiratory depth changes, and reduced vital capacity.

impaired Swallowing may be related to muscle wasting and fatigue, possibly evidenced by recurrent coughing/choking and signs of aspiration.

PSY

Powerlessness [specify level] may be related to chronic/debilitating nature of illness, lack of control over outcome, possibly evidenced by expressions of frustration about inability to care for self and depression over physical deterioration.

anticipatory Grieving may be related to perceived potential loss of self/physiopsychosocial well-being, possibly evidenced by sorrow, choked feelings, expression of distress, changes in eating habits, sleeping patterns, and altered communication patterns/ libido.

CH

impaired verbal Communication may be related to physical barrier (neuromuscular impairment), possibly evidenced by impaired articulation, inability to speak in sentences, and use of nonverbal cues (changes in facial expression).

risk for Caregiver Role Strain: risk factors may include illness severity of care receiver, complexity and amount of home-care needs, duration of caregiving required, caregiver is spouse, family/caregiver isolation, lack of respite/recreation for caregiver.*

Anaphylaxis   CH

(Also refer to Shock)

ineffective Airway Clearance may be related to airway spasm (bronchial), laryngeal edema possibly evidenced by diminished/ adventitious breath sounds, cough ineffective or absent, difficulty vocalizing, wide-eyed.

decreased Cardiac Output may be related to decreased preload-increased capillary permeability (third spacing) and vasodilation possibly evidenced by tachycardia/palpitations, changes in blood pressure (BP), anxiety, restlessness.

Anemia   CH

Activity Intolerance may be related to imbalance between O_2 supply (delivery) and demand, possibly evidenced by reports of fatigue and weakness, abnormal heart rate or BP response, decreased exercise/ activity level, and exertional discomfort or dyspnea.

imbalanced Nutrition: less than body requirements may be related to failure to ingest/inability to digest food or absorb nutrients necessary for formation of normal red blood cells (RBCs); possibly evidenced by weight loss/weight below normal for age, height, body build; decreased triceps skinfold measurement, changes in gums/oral

---

*A risk diagnosis is not evidenced by signs and symptoms, as the problem has not occurred and nursing interventions are directed at prevention.

mucous membranes; decreased tolerance for activity, weakness, and loss of muscle tone.

deficient Knowledge [Learning Need] regarding condition, prognosis, self-care and treatment needs may be related to inadequate understanding or misinterpretation of dietary/physiologic needs, possibly evidenced by inadequate dietary intake, request for information, and development of preventable complications.

Anemia, sickle cell   MS

impaired Gas Exchange may be related to decreased O_2-carrying capacity of blood, reduced RBC life span, abnormal RBC structure, increased blood viscosity, predisposition to bacterial pneumonia/pulmonary infarcts, possibly evidenced by dyspnea, use of accessory muscles, cyanosis/signs of hypoxia, tachycardia, changes in mentation, and restlessness.

ineffective Tissue Perfusion: (specify) may be related to stasis, vaso-occlusive nature of sickling, inflammatory response, atrioventricular (AV) shunts in pulmonary and peripheral circulation, myocardial damage (small infarcts, iron deposits, fibrosis), possibly evidenced by signs and symptoms dependent on system involved, for example: renal: decreased specific gravity and pale urine in face of dehydration; cerebral: paralysis and visual disturbances; peripheral: distal ischemia, tissue infarctions, ulcerations, bone pain; cardiopulmonary: angina, palpitations.

                                                          CH

acute/chronic Pain may be related to intravascular sickling with localized vascular stasis, occlusion, infarction/necrosis and deprivation of O_2 and nutrients, accumulation of noxious metabolites, possibly evidenced by reports of localized, generalized, or migratory joint and/or abdominal/back pain; guarding and distraction behaviors (moaning, crying, restlessness), facial grimacing, narrowed focus, and autonomic responses.

deficient Knowledge [Learning Need] regarding disease process, genetic factors, prognosis, self-care and treatment needs may be related to lack of exposure/recall, misinterpretation of information, unfamiliarity with resources, possibly evidenced by questions, statement of concern/misconceptions, exacerbation of condition, inadequate follow-through of therapy instructions, and development of preventable complications.

delayed Growth and Development may be related to effects of physical condition, possibly evidenced by altered physical growth and delay/difficulty performing skills typical of age group.

compromised family Coping may be related to chronic nature of disease/disability, family disorganization, presence of other crises/situations impacting significant person/parent, lifestyle restrictions, possibly evidenced by significant person/parent expressing preoccupation with own reaction and displaying protective behavior disproportionate to client's ability or need for autonomy.

Aneurysm, abdominal aortic (AAA)   MS
(Refer to Aortic aneurysm, abdominal)

Angina pectoris   MS

acute Pain may be related to decreased myocardial blood flow, increased cardiac workload/O_2 consumption, possibly evidenced by verbal reports, narrowed focus, distraction behaviors (restlessness, moaning), and autonomic responses (diaphoresis, changes in vital signs).

decreased Cardiac Output may be related to inotropic changes (transient/prolonged myocardial ischemia, effects of medications), alterations in rate/rhythm and electrical conduction, possibly evidenced by changes in hemodynamic readings, dyspnea, restlessness, decreased tolerance for activity, fatigue, diminished peripheral pulses, cool/pale skin, changes in mental status, and continued chest pain.

Anxiety [specify level] may be related to situational crises, change in health status and/or threat of death, negative self-talk possibly evidenced by verbalized apprehension, facial tension, extraneous movements, and focus on self.

CH

Activity Intolerance may be related to imbalance between O_2 supply and demand, possibly evidenced by exertional dyspnea, abnormal pulse/BP response to activity, and electrocardiogram (ECG) changes.

deficient Knowledge [Learning Need] regarding condition, prognosis, self-care and treatment needs may be related to lack of exposure, inaccurate/misinterpretation of information, possibly evidenced by questions, request for information, statement of concern, and inaccurate follow-through of instructions.

risk for impaired Adjustment: risk factors may include condition requiring long-term therapy/change in lifestyle, assault to self-concept, and altered locus of control.*

Anorexia nervosa   MS

imbalanced Nutrition: less than body requirements may be related to psychologic restrictions of food intake and/or excessive activity, self-induced vomiting, laxative abuse, possibly evidenced by weight loss, poor skin turgor/muscle tone, denial of hunger, unusual hoarding or handling of food, amenorrhea, electrolyte imbalance, cardiac irregularities, hypotension.

risk for deficient Fluid Volume: risk factors may include inadequate intake of food and liquids, chronic/excessive laxative or diuretic use, self-induced vomiting.*

PSY

disturbed Thought Processes may be related to severe malnutrition/ electrolyte imbalance, psychologic conflicts; possibly evidenced by impaired ability to make decisions, problem-solve, nonreality-based verbalizations, ideas of reference, altered sleep patterns, altered attention span/distractibility; perceptual disturbances with failure to recognize hunger, fatigue, anxiety, and depression.

---

*A risk diagnosis is not evidenced by signs and symptoms, as the problem has not occurred and nursing interventions are directed at prevention.

disturbed Body Image/chronic low Self-Esteem may be related to altered
perception of body, perceived loss of control in some aspect of life,
unmet dependency needs, personal vulnerability, dysfunctional
family system, possibly evidenced by negative feelings, distorted view
of body, use of denial, feeling powerless to prevent/make changes,
expressions of shame/guilt, overly conforming, dependent on others'
opinions.

interrupted Family Processes may be related to ambivalent family relationships and ways of transacting issues of control, situational/matu-
rational crises possibly evidenced by enmeshed family, dissonance
among family members, family developmental tasks not being met,
family members acting as enablers.

Antisocial personality disorder   PSY

risk for other-directed Violence: risk factors may include contempt for
authority/rights of others, inability to tolerate frustration, need for
immediate gratification, easy agitation, vulnerable self-concept,
inability to verbalize feelings, use of maladjusted coping mechanisms
including substance use.*

ineffective Coping may be related to very low tolerance for external
stress, lack of experience of internal anxiety (e.g., guilt/shame),
personal vulnerability, unmet expectations, multiple life changes
possibly evidenced by choice of aggression and manipulation to
handle problems/conflicts, inappropriate use of defense mechanisms
(e.g., denial, projection), chronic worry, anxiety, destructive behaviors, high rate of accidents.

chronic low Self-Esteem may be related to lack of positive and/or
repeated negative feedback, unmet dependency needs, retarded ego
development, dysfunctional family system possibly evidenced by
acting-out behaviors (e.g., substance abuse, sexual promiscuity, feelings of inadequacy, nonparticipation in therapy.

compromised/disabling family Coping may be related to family disor-
ganization/role changes, highly ambivalent family relationships,
client providing little support in turn for the primary person(s),
history of abuse/neglect in the home possibly evidenced by expressions of concern or complaints, preoccupation of primary person
with own reactions to situation, display of protective behaviors
disproportionate to client's abilities or need for autonomy.

impaired Social Interaction may be related to inadequate personal
resources (shallow feelings), immature interests, underdeveloped
conscious, unaccepted social values possibly evidenced by difficulty
meeting expectations of others, lack of belief that rules pertain to self,
sense of emptiness/inadequacy covered by expressions of self-
conceit/arrogance/contempt, behavior unaccepted by dominant
cultural group.

Anxiety disorder, generalized   PSY

Anxiety [specify level]/Powerlessness may be related to real or perceived
threat to physical integrity or self-concept (may or may not be able

---

*A risk diagnosis is not evidenced by signs and symptoms, as the
problem has not occurred and nursing interventions are directed at
prevention.

to identify the threat), unconscious conflict about essential values/beliefs and goals of life, unmet needs, negative self-talk, possibly evidenced by sympathetic stimulation, extraneous movements (foot shuffling, hand/arm fidgeting, rocking movements, restlessness), persistent feelings of apprehension and uneasiness, a general anxious feeling that client has difficulty alleviating, poor eye contact, focus on self, impaired functioning, free-floating anxiety, impaired functioning, and nonparticipation in decision making.

ineffective Coping may be related to level of anxiety being experienced by the client, personal vulnerability; unmet expectations/unrealistic perceptions, inadequate coping methods and/or support systems possibly evidenced by verbalization of inability to cope/problem-solve, excessive compulsive behaviors (e.g., smoking, drinking), and emotional/muscle tension, alteration in societal participation, high rate of accidents.

disturbed Sleep Pattern may be related to psychologic stress, repetitive thoughts, possibly evidenced by reports of difficulty in falling asleep/awakening earlier or later than desired, reports of not feeling rested, dark circles under eyes, and frequent yawning.

risk for compromised family Coping: risk factors may include inadequate/incorrect information or understanding by a primary person, temporary family disorganization and role changes, prolonged disability that exhausts the supportive capacity of significant other(s).*

impaired Social Interaction/Social Isolation may be related to low self-concept, inadequate personal resources, misinterpretation of internal/external stimuli, hypervigilance possibly evidenced by discomfort in social situations, withdrawal from or reported change in pattern of interactions, dysfunctional interactions; expressed feelings of difference from others; sad, dull affect.

Anxiolytic abuse   PSY
(Refer to Depressant abuse)

Aortic aneurysm, abdominal (AAA)   MS
risk for ineffective peripheral Tissue Perfusion: risk factors may include interruption of arterial blood flow [embolus formation, spontaneous blockage of aorta].*

risk for Infection: risk factors may include turbulent blood flow through arteriosclerotic lesion.*

acute Pain may be related to vascular enlargement-dissection/rupture possibly evidenced by verbal coded reports, guarding behavior, facial mask, change in abdominal muscle tone.

Aortic aneurysm repair, abdominal   MS
(Also refer to Surgery, general)
Fear related to threat of injury/death, surgical intervention possibly evidenced by verbal reports, apprehension, decreased self-assurance, increased tension, changes in vital signs.

*A risk diagnosis is not evidenced by signs and symptoms, as the problem has not occurred and nursing interventions are directed at prevention.

risk for deficient Fluid Volume: risk factors may include weakening of vascular wall, failure of vascular repair.*

risk for ineffective renal/peripheral Tissue Perfusion: risk factors may include interruption of arterial blood flow, hypovolemia.*

Aortic stenosis   MS

decreased Cardiac Output may be related to structural changes of heart valve, left ventricular outflow obstruction, alteration of afterload (increased left ventricular end-diastolic pressure and systemic vascular resistance—SVR), alteration in preload/increased atrial pressure and venous congestion, alteration in electrical conduction, possibly evidenced by fatigue, dyspnea, changes in vital signs/hemodynamic parameters, and syncope.

risk for impaired Gas Exchange: risk factors may include alveolar-capillary membrane changes/congestion.*

CH

risk for acute Pain: risk factors may include episodic ischemia of myocardial tissues and stretching of left atrium.*

Activity Intolerance may be related to imbalance between O_2 supply and demand (decreased/fixed cardiac output), possibly evidenced by exertional dyspnea, reported fatigue/weakness, and abnormal blood pressure or ECG changes/dysrhythmias in response to activity.

Aplastic anemia   CH

(Also refer to Anemia)

risk for ineffective Protection: risk factors may include abnormal blood profile (leukopenia, thrombocytopenia), drug therapies (antineoplastics, antibiotics, NSAIDs [nonsteroidal anti-inflammatory drugs], anticonvulsants).*

Fatigue may be related to anemia, disease states, malnutrition possibly evidenced by verbalization of overwhelming lack of energy, inability to maintain usual routines/level of physical activity, tired, decreased libido, lethargy, increase in physical complaints.

Appendicitis   MS

acute Pain may be related to distention of intestinal tissues by inflammation, possibly evidenced by verbal reports, guarding behavior, narrowed focus, and autonomic responses (diaphoresis, changes in vital signs).

risk for deficient Fluid Volume: risk factors may include nausea, vomiting, anorexia, and hypermetabolic state.*

risk for Infection: risk factors may include release of pathogenic organisms into peritoneal cavity.*

ARDS   MS

(Refer to Acute respiratory distress syndrome)

Arrhythmia, cardiac   MS/CH

(Refer to Dysrhythmia, cardiac)

---

*A risk diagnosis is not evidenced by signs and symptoms, as the problem has not occurred and nursing interventions are directed at prevention.

Arterial occlusive disease, peripheral   CH

ineffective peripheral Tissue Perfusion may be related to decreased arterial blood flow possibly evidenced by skin discolorations, temperature changes, altered sensation, claudication, delayed healing.

risk for impaired Walking: risk factors may include presence of circulatory problems, pain with activity.*

risk for impaired Skin/Tissue Integrity: risk factors may include altered circulation/sensation.*

Arthritis, juvenile rheumatoid   PED/CH
   (Also refer to Arthritis, rheumatoid)

risk for delayed Development: risk factors may include effects of physical disability and required therapy.*

risk for Social Isolation: risk factors may include delay in accomplishing developmental task, altered state of wellness, and changes in physical appearance.*

Arthritis, rheumatoid   CH

acute/chronic Pain, may be related to accumulation of fluid/inflammatory process, degeneration of joint, and deformity, possibly evidenced by verbal reports, narrowed focus, guarding/protective behaviors, and physical and social withdrawal.

impaired physical Mobility may be related to musculoskeletal deformity, pain/discomfort, decreased muscle strength, possibly evidenced by limited range of motion, impaired coordination, reluctance to attempt movement, and decreased muscle strength/control and mass.

Self-Care Deficit [specify] may be related to musculoskeletal impairment, decreased strength/endurance and range of motion, pain on movement, possibly evidenced by inability to manage activities of daily living (ADLs).

disturbed Body Image/Role Performance ineffective may be related to change in body structure/function, impaired mobility/ability to perform usual tasks, focus on past strength/function/appearance, possibly evidenced by negative self-talk, feelings of helplessness, change in lifestyle/physical abilities, dependence on others for assistance, decreased social involvement.

Arthritis, septic   CH

acute Pain may be related to joint inflammation possibly evidenced by verbal/coded reports, guarding behaviors, restlessness, narrowed focus.

impaired physical Mobility may be related to joint stiffness, pain/discomfort, reluctance to initiate movement possibly evidenced by limited range of motion, slowed movement.

Self-Care Deficit [specify] may be related to musculoskeletal impairment, pain/discomfort, decreased strength, impaired coordination possibly evidenced by inability to perform desired ADLs.

risk for Infection [spread]: risk factors may include presence of infectious process, chronic disease states, invasive procedures.*

---

*A risk diagnosis is not evidenced by signs and symptoms, as the problem has not occurred and nursing interventions are directed at prevention.

Arthroplasty MS

risk for Infection: risk factors may include breach of primary defenses (surgical incision), stasis of body fluids at operative site, and altered inflammatory response.*

risk for deficient Fluid Volume [isotonic]: risk factors may include surgical procedure/trauma to vascular area.*

impaired physical Mobility may be related to decreased strength, pain, musculoskeletal changes, possibly evidenced by impaired coordination and reluctance to attempt movement.

acute Pain may be related to tissue trauma, local edema, possibly evidenced by verbal reports, narrowed focus, guarded movement, and autonomic responses (diaphoresis, changes in vital signs).

Arthroscopy MS

deficient Knowledge [Learning Need] regarding procedure/outcomes and self-care needs may be related to unfamiliarity with information/resources, misinterpretations, possibly evidenced by questions and requests for information, misconceptions.

risk for impaired Walking: risk factors may include joint stiffness, discomfort, prescribed movement restrictions, use of assistive devices/crutches for ambulation.*

Asthma MS
(Also refer to Emphysema)

ineffective Airway Clearance, may be related to increased production/retained pulmonary secretions, bronchospasm, decreased energy/fatigue, possibly evidenced by wheezing, difficulty breathing, changes in depth/rate of respirations, use of accessory muscles, and persistent ineffective cough with or without sputum production.

impaired Gas Exchange may be related to altered delivery of inspired O_2/air trapping, possibly evidenced by dyspnea, restlessness, reduced tolerance for activity, cyanosis, and changes in ABGs and vital signs.

Anxiety [specify level] may be related to perceived threat of death, possibly evidenced by apprehension, fearful expression, and extraneous movements.

CH

Activity Intolerance may be related to imbalance between O_2 supply and demand, possibly evidenced by fatigue and exertional dyspnea.

Athlete's foot CH

impaired Skin Integrity may be related to fungal invasion, humidity, secretions, possibly evidenced by disruption of skin surface, reports of painful itching.

risk for Infection [spread]: risk factors may include multiple breaks in skin, exposure to moist/warm environment.*

Atrial fibrillation CH
(Refer to Dysrhythmias)

---

*A risk diagnosis is not evidenced by signs and symptoms, as the problem has not occurred and nursing interventions are directed at prevention.

Atrial flutter   **CH**
(Refer to Dysrhythmias)

Atrial tachycardia   **CH**
(Refer to Dysrhythmias)

Attention deficit disorder (ADD)   **PED/PSY**
ineffective Coping may be related to situational/maturational crisis, retarded ego development, low self-concept possibly evidenced by easy distraction by extraneous stimuli, shifting between uncompleted activities.

chronic low Self-Esteem may be related to retarded ego development, lack of positive/repeated negative feedback, negative role models possibly evidenced by lack of eye contact, derogatory self comments, hesitance to try new tasks, inadequate level of confidence.

deficient Knowledge regarding condition, prognosis, therapy may be related to misinformation/misinterpretations, unfamiliarity with resources possibly evidenced by verbalization of problems/misconceptions, poor school performance, unrealistic expectations of medication regimen.

Autistic disorder   **PED/PSY**
impaired Social Interaction may be related to abnormal response to sensory input/inadequate sensory stimulation, organic brain dysfunction; delayed development of secure attachment/trust, lack of intuitive skills to comprehend and accurately respond to social cues, disturbance in self-concept, possibly evidenced by lack of responsiveness to others, lack of eye contact or facial responsiveness, treating persons as objects, lack of awareness of feelings in others, indifference/aversion to comfort, affection, or physical contact; failure to develop cooperative social play and peer friendships in childhood.

impaired verbal Communication may be related to inability to trust others, withdrawal into self, organic brain dysfunction, abnormal interpretation/response to and/or inadequate sensory stimulation, possibly evidenced by lack of interactive communication mode, no use of gestures or spoken language, absent or abnormal nonverbal communication; lack of eye contact or facial expression; peculiar patterns of speech (form, content, or speech production), and impaired ability to initiate or sustain conversation despite adequate speech.

risk for Self-Mutilation: risk factors may include organic brain dysfunction, inability to trust others, disturbance in self-concept, inadequate sensory stimulation or abnormal response to sensory input (sensory overload); history of physical, emotional, or sexual abuse; and response to demands of therapy, realization of severity of condition.*

disturbed Personal Identity may be related to organic brain dysfunction, lack of development of trust, maternal deprivation, fixation at presymbiotic phase of development, possibly evidenced by lack of

---

*A risk diagnosis is not evidenced by signs and symptoms, as the problem has not occurred and nursing interventions are directed at prevention.

awareness of the feelings or existence of others, increased anxiety resulting from physical contact with others, absent or impaired imitation of others, repeating what others say, persistent preoccupation with parts of objects, obsessive attachment to objects, marked distress over changes in environment; autoerotic/ritualistic behaviors, self-touching, rocking, swaying.

compromised/disabling family Coping may be related to family members unable to express feelings; excessive guilt, anger, or blaming among family members regarding child's condition; ambivalent or dissonant family relationships, prolonged coping with problem exhausting supportive ability of family members, possibly evidenced by denial of existence or severity of disturbed behaviors, preoccupation with personal emotional reaction to situation, rationalization that problem will be outgrown, attempts to intervene with child are achieving increasingly ineffective results, family withdraws from or becomes overly protective of child.

Barbiturate abuse   CH/PSY

(Refer to Depressant abuse)

Battered child syndrome   PED/CH

(Also refer to Abuse)

risk for Trauma: risk factors may include dependent position in relationship(s), vulnerability (e.g., congenital problems/chronic illness), history of previous abuse/neglect, lack/nonuse of support systems by caregiver(s).*

interrupted Family Processes/impaired Parenting may be related to poor role model/identity, unrealistic expectations, presence of stressors, and lack of support, possibly evidenced by verbalization of negative feelings, inappropriate caretaking behaviors, and evidence of physical/psychological trauma to child.

PSY

chronic low Self-Esteem may be related to deprivation and negative feedback of family members, personal vulnerability, feelings of abandonment, possibly evidenced by lack of eye contact, withdrawal from social contacts, discounting own needs, nonassertive/passive, indecisive, or overly conforming behaviors.

Post-Trauma Syndrome may be related to sustained/recurrent physical or emotional abuse; possibly evidenced by acting-out behavior, development of phobias, poor impulse control, and emotional numbness.

ineffective Coping may be related to situational or maturational crisis, overwhelming threat to self, personal vulnerability, inadequate support systems, possibly evidenced by verbalized concern about ability to deal with current situation, chronic worry, anxiety, depression, poor self-esteem, inability to problem-solve, high illness rate, destructive behavior toward self/others.

---

*A risk diagnosis is not evidenced by signs and symptoms, as the problem has not occurred and nursing interventions are directed at prevention.

Benign prostatic hyperplasia   CH/MS

[acute/chronic] Urinary Retention may be related to mechanical obstruction (enlarged prostate), decompensation of detrusor musculature, inability of bladder to contract adequately, possibly evidenced by frequency, hesitancy, inability to empty bladder completely, incontinence/dribbling, bladder distention, residual urine.

acute Pain may be related to mucosal irritation, bladder distention, colic, urinary infection, and radiation therapy, possibly evidenced by verbal reports (bladder/rectal spasm), narrowed focus, altered muscle tone, grimacing, distraction behaviors, restlessness, and autonomic responses.

risk for deficient Fluid Volume: risk factors may include postobstructive diuresis, endocrine/electrolyte imbalances.*

Fear/Anxiety [specify level] may be related to change in health status (possibility of surgical procedure/malignancy); embarrassment/loss of dignity associated with genital exposure before, during, and after treatment, and concern about sexual ability, possibly evidenced by increased tension, apprehension, worry, expressed concerns regarding perceived changes, and fear of unspecific consequences.

Bipolar disorder   PSY

risk for other-directed Violence: risk factors may include irritability, impulsive behavior; delusional thinking; angry response when ideas are refuted or wishes denied; manic excitement, with possible indicators of threatening body language/verbalizations, increased motor activity, overt and aggressive acts; hostility.*

imbalanced Nutrition: less than body requirements may be related to inadequate intake in relation to metabolic expenditures, possibly evidenced by body weight 20% or more below ideal weight, observed inadequate intake, inattention to mealtimes, and distraction from task of eating; laboratory evidence of nutritional deficits/imbalances.

risk for Poisoning [lithium toxicity]: risk factors may include narrow therapeutic range of drug, client's ability (or lack of) to follow through with medication regimen and monitoring, and denial of need for information/therapy.*

disturbed Sleep Pattern may be related to psychologic stress, lack of recognition of fatigue/need to sleep, hyperactivity, possibly evidenced by denial of need to sleep, interrupted nighttime sleep, one or more nights without sleep, changes in behavior and performance, increasing irritability/restlessness, and dark circles under eyes.

disturbed Sensory Perception (specify) [overload] may be related to decrease in sensory threshold, endogenous chemical alteration, psychologic stress, sleep deprivation, possibly evidenced by increased distractibility and agitation, anxiety, disorientation, poor concentration, auditory/visual hallucination, bizarre thinking, and motor incoordination.

interrupted Family Processes may be related to situational crises (illness,

---

*A risk diagnosis is not evidenced by signs and symptoms, as the problem has not occurred and nursing interventions are directed at prevention.

economics, change in roles); euphoric mood and grandiose ideas/actions of client, manipulative behavior and limit testing, client's refusal to accept responsibility for own actions, possibly evidenced by statements of difficulty coping with situation, lack of adaptation to change or not dealing constructively with illness; ineffective family decision-making process, failure to send and to receive clear messages, and inappropriate boundary maintenance.

Bone cancer   MS/CH

(Also refer to Myeloma, multiple; Amputation)

acute Pain may be related to bone destruction, pressure on nerves possibly evidenced by verbal or coded report, protective behavior, autonomic responses.

risk for Trauma: risk factors may include increased bone fragility, general weakness, balancing difficulties.*

Borderline personality disorder   PSY

risk for self/other-directed Violence/Self-Mutilation: risk factors may include use of projection as a major defense mechanism, pervasive problems with negative transference, feelings of guilt/need to "punish" self, distorted sense of self, inability to cope with increased psychologic/physiologic tension in a healthy manner.*

Anxiety [severe to panic] may be related to unconscious conflicts (experience of extreme stress), perceived threat to self-concept, unmet needs, possibly evidenced by easy frustration and feelings of hurt, abuse of alcohol/other drugs, transient psychotic symptoms and performance of self-mutilating acts.

chronic low Self-Esteem/disturbed Personal Identity may be related to lack of positive feedback, unmet dependency needs, retarded ego development/fixation at an earlier level of development, possibly evidenced by difficulty identifying self or defining self-boundaries, feelings of depersonalization, extreme mood changes, lack of tolerance of rejection or of being alone, unhappiness with self, striking out at others, performance of ritualistic self-damaging acts, and belief that punishing self is necessary.

Social Isolation may be related to immature interests, unaccepted social behavior, inadequate personal resources, and inability to engage in satisfying personal relationships, possibly evidenced by alternating clinging and distancing behaviors, difficulty meeting expectations of others, experiencing feelings of difference from others, expressing interests inappropriate to developmental age, and exhibiting behavior unaccepted by dominant cultural group.

Botulism (food borne)   MS

deficient Fluid Volume [isotonic] may be related to active losses—vomiting, diarrhea; decreased intake—nausea, dysphagia, possibly evidenced by reports of thirst; dry skin/mucous membranes, decreased BP and urine output, change in mental state, increased hematocrit (Hct).

---

*A risk diagnosis is not evidenced by signs and symptoms, as the problem has not occurred and nursing interventions are directed at prevention.

impaired physical Mobility may be related to neuromuscular impairment possibly evidenced by limited ability to perform gross/fine motor skills.

Anxiety [specify level]/Fear may be related to threat of death, interpersonal transmission possibly evidenced by expressed concerns, apprehension, awareness of physiologic symptoms, focus on self.

risk for impaired spontaneous Ventilation: risk factors may include neuromuscular impairment, presence of infectious process.*

CH

risk for Poisoning: risk factors may include lack of proper precautions in food storage/preparation.*

Brain tumor   MS

acute Pain may be related to pressure on brain tissues, possibly evidenced by reports of headache, facial mask of pain, narrowed focus, and autonomic responses (changes in vital signs).

disturbed Thought Processes may be related to altered circulation to and/or destruction of brain tissue, possibly evidenced by memory loss, personality changes, impaired ability to make decisions/conceptualize, and inaccurate interpretation of environment.

disturbed Sensory Perception (specify) may be related to compression/displacement of brain tissue, disruption of neuronal conduction, possibly evidenced by changes in visual acuity, alterations in sense of balance/gait disturbance, and paresthesia.

risk for deficient Fluid Volume: risk factors may include recurrent vomiting from irritation of vagal center in medulla and decreased intake.*

Self-Care Deficit [specify] may be related to sensory/neuromuscular impairment interfering with ability to perform tasks, possibly evidenced by unkempt/disheveled appearance, body odor, and verbalization/observation of inability to perform activities of daily living.

Breast cancer   MS/CH
(Also refer to Cancer)

Anxiety [specify level] may be related to change in health status, threat of death, stress, interpersonal transmission possibly evidenced by expressed concerns, apprehension, uncertainty, focus on self, diminished productivity.

deficient Knowledge regarding diagnosis, prognosis, and treatment options may be related to lack of exposure/unfamiliarity with information resources, information misinterpretation, cognitive limitation/anxiety possibly evidenced by verbalizations, statements of misconceptions, inappropriate behaviors.

risk for disturbed Body Image: risk factors may include significance of body part with regard to sexual perceptions.*

risk for ineffective Sexual Patterns: risk factors may include health-related changes, medical treatments, concern about relationship with SO.*

---

*A risk diagnosis is not evidenced by signs and symptoms, as the problem has not occurred and nursing interventions are directed at prevention.

Bronchitis

ineffective Airway Clearance may be related to excessive, thickened mucous secretions, possibly evidenced by presence of rhonchi, tachypnea, and ineffective cough.

Activity Intolerance [specify level] may be related to imbalance between O_2 supply and demand, possibly evidenced by reports of fatigue, dyspnea, and abnormal vital sign response to activity.

acute Pain may be related to localized inflammation, persistent cough, aching associated with fever, possibly evidenced by reports of discomfort, distraction behavior, and facial mask of pain.

Bronchopneumonia

(Also refer to Bronchitis)

ineffective Airway Clearance may be related to tracheal bronchial inflammation, edema formation, increased sputum production, pleuritic pain, decreased energy, fatigue, possibly evidenced by changes in rate/depth of respirations, abnormal breath sounds, use of accessory muscles, dyspnea, cyanosis, effective/ineffective cough—with or without sputum production.

impaired Gas Exchange may be related to inflammatory process, collection of secretions affecting O_2 exchange across alveolar membrane, and hypoventilation, possibly evidenced by restlessness/changes in mentation, dyspnea, tachycardia, pallor, cyanosis, and ABGs/oximetry evidence of hypoxia.

risk for Infection [spread]: risk factors may include decreased ciliary action, stasis of secretions, presence of existing infection.*

Bulimia nervosa

(Also refer to Anorexia nervosa)

impaired Dentition may be related to dietary habits, poor oral hygiene, chronic vomiting possibly evidenced by erosion of tooth enamel, multiple caries, abraded teeth.

impaired Oral Mucous Membrane may be related to malnutrition or vitamin deficiency, poor oral hygiene, chronic vomiting possibly evidenced by sore, inflamed buccal mucosa; swollen salivary glands, ulcerations of mucosa, reports of constant sore mouth/throat.

risk for deficient Fluid Volume: risk factors may include consistent self-induced vomiting, chronic/excessive laxative/diuretic use, esophageal erosion or tear (Mallory-Weiss syndrome).*

deficient Knowledge [Learning Need] regarding condition, prognosis, complication, treatment may be related to lack of exposure to/unfamiliarity with information about condition, learned maladaptive coping skills possibly evidenced by verbalization of misconception of relationship of current situation and behaviors, distortion of body image, binging and purging behaviors, verbalized need for information/desire to change behaviors.

---

*A risk diagnosis is not evidenced by signs and symptoms, as the problem has not occurred and nursing interventions are directed at prevention.

Burn (dependent on type, degree, and severity of the injury)   MS/CH

risk for deficient Fluid Volume: risk factors may include loss of fluids through wounds, capillary damage and evaporation, hypermetabolic state, insufficient intake, hemorrhagic losses.*

risk for ineffective Airway Clearance: risk factors may include mucosal edema and loss of ciliary action (smoke inhalation), direct upper airway injury by flame, steam, chemicals.*

risk for Infection: risk factors may include loss of protective dermal barrier, traumatized/necrotic tissue, decreased hemoglobin, suppressed inflammatory response, environmental exposure/invasive procedures.*

acute/chronic Pain may be related to destruction of/trauma to tissue and nerves, edema formation, and manipulation of impaired tissues, possibly evidenced by verbal reports, narrowed focus, distraction and guarding behaviors, facial mask of pain, and autonomic responses (changes in vital signs).

risk for imbalanced Nutrition: less than body requirements: risk factors may include hypermetabolic state in response to burn injury/stress, inadequate intake, protein catabolism.*

Post-Trauma Syndrome may be related to life-threatening event, possibly evidenced by reexperiencing the event, repetitive dreams/nightmares, psychic/emotional numbness, and sleep disturbance.

ineffective Protection may be related to extremes of age, inadequate nutrition, anemia, impaired immune system, possibly evidenced by impaired healing, deficient immunity, fatigue, anorexia.

PED

deficient Diversional Activity may be related to long-term hospitalization, frequent lengthy treatments, and physical limitations, possibly evidenced by expressions of boredom, restlessness, withdrawal, and requests for something to do.

risk for delayed Development: risk factors may include effects of physical disability, separation from SO(s), and environmental deficiencies.*

Bursitis   CH

acute/chronic Pain may be related to inflammation of affected joint, possibly evidenced by verbal reports, guarding behavior, and narrowed focus.

impaired physical Mobility may be related to inflammation and swelling of joint, and pain, possibly evidenced by diminished range of motion, reluctance to attempt movement, and imposed restriction of movement by medical treatment.

Calculi, urinary   CH/MS

acute Pain may be related to increased frequency/force of ureteral contractions, tissue distention/trauma and edema formation, cellular

---

*A risk diagnosis is not evidenced by signs and symptoms, as the problem has not occurred and nursing interventions are directed at prevention.

ischemia possibly evidenced by reports of sudden, severe, colicky pains; guarding and distraction behaviors, self focus, and autonomic responses.

impaired Urinary Elimination may be related to stimulation of the bladder by calculi, renal or ureteral irritation, mechanical obstruction of urinary flow, edema formation, inflammation possibly evidenced by urgency and frequency; oliguria (retention); hematuria.

risk for deficient Fluid Volume: risk factors may include stimulation of renal-intestinal reflexes causing nausea, vomiting, and diarrhea; changes in urinary output, postoperative diuresis; and decreased intake.*

risk for Infection: risk factors may include stasis of urine.*

deficient Knowledge [Learning Need] regarding condition, prognosis, self-care and treatment needs may be related to lack of exposure/recall and information misinterpretation, possibly evidenced by requests for information, statements of concern, and recurrence/development of preventable complications.

Cancer   MS

(Also refer to Chemotherapy; Radiation therapy)

Fear/death Anxiety may be related to situational crises, threat to/change in health/socioeconomic status, role functioning, interaction patterns; threat of death, separation from family, interpersonal transmission of feelings, possibly evidenced by expressed concerns, feelings of inadequacy/helplessness, insomnia; increased tension, restlessness, focus on self, sympathetic stimulation.

anticipatory Grieving may be related to potential loss of physiologic well-being (body part/function), perceived separation from SO(s)/lifestyle (death), possibly evidenced by anger, sadness, withdrawal, choked feelings, changes in eating/sleep patterns, activity level, libido, and communication patterns.

acute/chronic Pain may be related to the disease process (compression of nerve tissue, infiltration of nerves or their vascular supply, obstruction of a nerve pathway, inflammation), or side effects of therapeutic agents, possibly evidenced by verbal reports, self-focusing/narrowed focus, alteration in muscle tone, facial mask of pain, distraction/guarding behaviors, autonomic responses, and restlessness.

Fatigue may be related to decreased metabolic energy production, increased energy requirements (hypermetabolic state), overwhelming psychological/emotional demands, and altered body chemistry (side effects of medications, chemotherapy), possibly evidenced by unremitting/overwhelming lack of energy, inability to maintain usual routines, decreased performance, impaired ability to concentrate, lethargy/listlessness, and disinterest in surroundings.

impaired Home Maintenance may be related to debilitation, lack of resources, and/or inadequate support systems, possibly evidenced by verbalization of problem, request for assistance, and lack of necessary equipment or aids.

---

*A risk diagnosis is not evidenced by signs and symptoms, as the problem has not occurred and nursing interventions are directed at prevention.

compromised/disabled family Coping may be related to chronic nature of disease and disability, ongoing treatment needs, parental supervision, and lifestyle restrictions, possibly evidenced by expression of denial/despair, depression, and protective behavior disproportionate to client's abilities or need for autonomy.

readiness for enhanced family Coping may be related to the fact that the individual's needs are being sufficiently gratified and adaptive tasks effectively addressed, enabling goals of self-actualization to surface, possibly evidenced by verbalizations of impact of crisis on own values, priorities, goals, or relationships.

Candidiasis   CH

(Also refer to Thrush)

impaired Skin/Tissue Integrity may be related to infectious lesions possibly evidenced by disruption of skin surfaces/mucous membranes.

acute Pain/[Discomfort] may be related to exposure of irritated skin/mucous membranes to excretions (urine/feces) possibly evidenced by verbal/coded reports, restlessness, guarding behaviors.

risk for Sexual Dysfunction: risk factors include presence of infectious process/vaginal discomfort.*

Cannabis abuse   CH

(Refer to Stimulant abuse)

Cardiac surgery   MS/PED

Anxiety [specify level]/Fear may be related to change in health status and threat to self-concept/of death, possibly evidenced by sympathetic stimulation, increased tension, and apprehension.

risk for decreased Cardiac Output: risk factors may include decreased preload (hypovolemia), depressed myocardial contractility, changes in SVR (afterload), and alterations in electrical conduction (dysrhythmias).*

deficient Fluid Volume [isotonic] may be related to intraoperative bleeding with inadequate blood replacement; bleeding related to insufficient heparin reversal, fibrinolysis, or platelet destruction; or volume depletion effects of intraoperative/postoperative diuretic therapy, possibly evidenced by increased pulse rate, decreased pulse volume/pressure, decreased urine output, hemoconcentration.

risk for impaired Gas Exchange: risk factors may include alveolar-capillary membrane changes (atelectasis), intestinal edema, inadequate function or premature discontinuation of chest tubes, and diminished oxygen-carrying capacity of the blood.*

acute Pain/[Discomfort] may be related to tissue inflammation/trauma, edema formation, intraoperative nerve trauma, and myocardial ischemia, possibly evidenced by reports of incisional discomfort/pain in chest and donor site; paresthesia/pain in hand, arm, shoulder,

*A risk diagnosis is not evidenced by signs and symptoms, as the problem has not occurred and nursing interventions are directed at prevention.

anxiety, restlessness, irritability; distraction behaviors, and autonomic responses.

impaired Skin/Tissue Integrity related to mechanical trauma (surgical incisions, puncture wounds) and edema evidenced by disruption of skin surface/tissues.

Cardiogenic shock   MS
(Refer to Shock, cardiogenic)

Cardiomyopathy   CH/MS
decreased Cardiac Output may be related to altered contractility possibly evidenced dyspnea, fatigue, chest pain, dizziness, syncope.

Activity Intolerance may be related to imbalance between oxygen supply and demand possibly evidenced by weakness/fatigue, dyspnea, abnormal heart rate/BP response to activity, ECG changes.

ineffective Role Performance may be related to changes in physical health, stress, demands of job/life possibly evidenced by change in usual patterns of responsibility, role strain, change in capacity to resume role.

Carpal tunnel syndrome   CH/MS
acute/chronic Pain may be related to pressure on median nerve, possibly evidenced by verbal reports, reluctance to use affected extremity, guarding behaviors, expressed fear of reinjury, altered ability to continue previous activities.

impaired physical Mobility may be related to neuromuscular impairment and pain, possibly evidenced by decreased hand strength, weakness, limited range of motion, and reluctance to attempt movement.

risk for Peripheral Neurovascular Dysfunction: risk factors may include mechanical compression (e.g., brace, repetitive tasks/motions), immobilization.*

deficient Knowledge [Learning Need] regarding condition, prognosis and treatment/safety needs may be related to lack of exposure/recall, information misinterpretation, possibly evidenced by questions, statements of concern, request for information, inaccurate follow-through of instructions/development of preventable complications.

Casts   CH/MS
(Also refer to Fractures)

risk for Peripheral Neurovascular Dysfunction: risk factors may include presence of fracture(s), mechanical compression (cast), tissue trauma, immobilization, vascular obstruction.*

risk for impaired Skin Integrity: risk factors may include pressure of cast, moisture/debris under cast, objects inserted under cast to relieve itching, and/or altered sensation/circulation.*

Self-Care Deficit [specify] may be related to impaired ability to perform self-care tasks, possibly evidenced by statements of need for assistance and observed difficulty in performing activities of daily living.

---

*A risk diagnosis is not evidenced by signs and symptoms, as the problem has not occurred and nursing interventions are directed at prevention.

disturbed visual Sensory Perception may be related to altered sensory reception/status of sense organs, and therapeutically restricted environment (surgical procedure, patching), possibly evidenced by diminished acuity, visual distortions, and change in usual response to stimuli.

risk for Trauma: risk factors may include poor vision, reduced hand/eye coordination.*

Anxiety [specify level]/Fear may be related to alteration in visual acuity, threat of permanent loss of vision/independence, possibly evidenced by expressed concerns, apprehension, and feelings of uncertainty.

deficient Knowledge [Learning Need] regarding ways of coping with altered abilities, therapy choices, lifestyle changes may be related to lack of exposure/recall, misinterpretation, or cognitive limitations, possibly evidenced by requests for information, statement of concern, inaccurate follow-through of instructions/development of preventable complications.

Cat scratch disease   **CH**

acute Pain may be related to effects of circulating toxins (fever, headache, and lymphadenitis), possibly evidenced by verbal reports, guarding behavior, and autonomic response (changes in vital signs).

Hyperthermia may be related to inflammatory process, possibly evidenced by increased body temperature, flushed warm skin, tachypnea and tachycardia.

Cerebrovascular accident (CVA)   **MS**

ineffective cerebral Tissue Perfusion may be related to interruption of blood flow (occlusive disorder, hemorrhage, cerebral vasospasm/edema), possibly evidenced by altered level of consciousness, changes in vital signs, changes in motor/sensory responses, restlessness, memory loss; sensory, language, intellectual, and emotional deficits.

impaired physical Mobility may be related to neuromuscular involvement (weakness, paresthesia, flaccid/hypotonic paralysis, spastic paralysis), perceptual/cognitive impairment, possibly evidenced by inability to purposefully move involved body parts/limited range of motion; impaired coordination, and/or decreased muscle strength/control.

impaired verbal [and/or written] Communication may be related to impaired cerebral circulation, neuromuscular impairment, loss of facial/oral muscle tone and control; generalized weakness/fatigue, possibly evidenced by impaired articulation, does not/cannot speak (dysarthria); inability to modulate speech, find and/or name words, identify objects and/or inability to comprehend written/spoken language; inability to produce written communication.

Self-Care Deficit [specify] may be related to neuromuscular impairment, decreased strength/endurance, loss of muscle control/coordination, perceptual/cognitive impairment, pain/discomfort, and

---

*A risk diagnosis is not evidenced by signs and symptoms, as the problem has not occurred and nursing interventions are directed at prevention.

depression, possibly evidenced by stated/observed inability to perform ADLs, requests for assistance, disheveled appearance, and incontinence.

risk for impaired Swallowing: risk factors may include muscle paralysis and perceptual impairment.*

risk for Unilateral Neglect: risk factors may include sensory loss of part of visual field with perceptual loss of corresponding body segment.*

CH

impaired Home Maintenance may be related to condition of individual family member, insufficient finances/family organization or planning, unfamiliarity with resources, and inadequate support systems, possibly evidenced by members expressing difficulty in managing home in a comfortable manner/requesting assistance with home maintenance, disorderly surroundings, and overtaxed family members.

situational low Self-Esteem/disturbed Body Image/ineffective Role Performance may be related to biophysical, psychosocial, and cognitive/perceptual changes, possibly evidenced by actual change in structure and/or function, change in usual patterns of responsibility/physical capacity to resume role; and verbal/nonverbal response to actual or perceived change.

Cervix, dysfunctional OB

(Refer to Dilation of cervix, premature)

Cesarean birth, postpartal OB

(Also refer to Postpartal period)

risk for impaired parent/infant Attachment: risk factors may include developmental transition/gain of a family member, situational crisis (e.g., surgical intervention, physical complications interfering with initial acquaintance/interaction, negative self-appraisal).*

acute Pain/[Discomfort] may be related to surgical trauma, effects of anesthesia, hormonal effects, bladder/abdominal distention possibly evidenced by verbal reports (e.g., incisional pain, cramping/after-pains, spinal headache), guarding/distraction behaviors, irritability, facial mask of pain.

risk for situational low Self-Esteem: risk factors may include perceived "failure" at life event, maturational transition, perceived loss of control in unplanned delivery.*

risk for Injury: risk factors may include biochemical or regulatory functions (e.g., orthostatic hypotension, development of PIH or eclampsia), effects of anesthesia, thromboembolism, abnormal blood profile (anemia/excessive blood loss, rubella sensitivity, Rh incompatibility), tissue trauma.*

risk for Infection: risk factors may include tissue trauma/broken skin, decreased Hb, invasive procedures and/or increased environmental exposure, prolongs rupture of amniotic membranes, malnutrition.*

---

*A risk diagnosis is not evidenced by signs and symptoms, as the problem has not occurred and nursing interventions are directed at prevention.

Self-Care Deficit (specify) may be related to effects of anesthesia, decreased strength and endurance, physical discomfort possibly evidenced by verbalization of inability to perform desired ADL(s).

Cesarean birth, unplanned OB

(Also refer to Cesarean birth, postpartal)

deficient Knowledge [Learning Need] regarding underlying procedure, pathophysiology, and self-care needs may be related to incomplete/inadequate information, possibly evidenced by request for information, verbalization of concerns/misconceptions and inappropriate/exaggerated behavior.

Anxiety [specify level] may be related to actual/perceived threat to mother/fetus, emotional threat to self-esteem, unmet needs/expectations, interpersonal transmission, possibly evidenced by increased tension, apprehension, feelings of inadequacy, sympathetic stimulation, and narrowed focus, restlessness.

Powerlessness may be related to interpersonal interaction, perception of illness-related regimen, lifestyle of helplessness possibly evidenced by verbalization of lack of control, lack of participation in care or decision making, passivity.

risk for impaired fetal Gas Exchange: risk factors may include altered blood flow to placenta and/or through umbilical cord.*

risk for acute Pain: risk factors may include increased/prolonged contractions, psychologic reaction.*

risk for Infection: risk factors may include invasive procedures, rupture of amniotic membranes, break in skin, decreased hemoglobin, exposure to pathogens.*

Chemotherapy MS/CH

(Also refer to Cancer)

risk for deficient Fluid Volume: risk factors may include gastrointestinal losses (vomiting), interference with adequate intake (stomatitis/anorexia), losses through abnormal routes (indwelling tubes, wounds, fistulas), hypermetabolic state.*

imbalanced Nutrition: less than body requirements may be related to inability to ingest adequate nutrients (nausea, stomatitis, and fatigue), hypermetabolic state, possibly evidenced by weight loss (wasting), aversion to eating, reported altered taste sensation, sore, inflamed buccal cavity; diarrhea and/or constipation.

impaired Oral Mucous Membrane may be related to side effects of therapeutic agents/radiation, dehydration, and malnutrition, possibly evidenced by ulcerations, leukoplakia, decreased salivation, and reports of pain.

disturbed Body Image may be related to anatomical/structural changes; loss of hair and weight, possibly evidenced by negative feelings about body, preoccupation with change, feelings of helplessness/hopelessness, and change in social environment.

---

*A risk diagnosis is not evidenced by signs and symptoms, as the problem has not occurred and nursing interventions are directed at prevention.

ineffective Protection may be related to inadequate nutrition, drug ther-
apy/radiation, abnormal blood profile, disease state (cancer), possibly
evidenced by impaired healing, deficient immunity, anorexia,
fatigue.

Cholecystectomy   MS

acute Pain may be related to interruption in skin/tissue layers with
mechanical closure (sutures/staples) and invasive procedures (including T-tube/nasogastric—NG—tube), possibly evidenced by verbal
reports, guarding/distraction behaviors, and autonomic responses
(changes in vital signs).

ineffective Breathing Pattern may be related to decreased lung expansion (pain and muscle weakness), decreased energy/fatigue, ineffective cough, possibly evidenced by fremitus, tachypnea, and decreased
respiratory depth/vital capacity.

risk for deficient Fluid Volume: risk factors may include vomiting/NG
aspiration, medically restricted intake, altered coagulation.*

Cholelithiasis   CH

acute Pain may be related to inflammation and distortion of tissues,
ductal spasm, possibly evidenced by verbal reports, guarding/distrac-
tion behaviors, and autonomic responses (changes in vital signs).

imbalanced Nutrition: less than body requirements may be related to
inability to ingest/absorb adequate nutrients (food intolerance/pain,
nausea/vomiting, anorexia), possibly evidenced by aversion to
food/decreased intake and weight loss.

deficient Knowledge [Learning Need] regarding pathophysiology, therapy choices, and self-care needs may be related to lack of information,
misinterpretation, possibly evidenced by verbalization of concerns,
questions, and recurrence of condition.

Chronic obstructive lung disease   CH/MS

impaired Gas Exchange may be related to altered O_2 delivery (obstruction of airways by secretions/bronchospasm, air trapping) and alveoli
destruction, possibly evidenced by dyspnea, restlessness, confusion,
abnormal ABG values, and reduced tolerance for activity.

ineffective Airway Clearance may be related to bronchospasm, increased
production of tenacious secretions, retained secretions, and
decreased energy/fatigue, possibly evidenced by presence of wheezes,
crackles, tachypnea, dyspnea, changes in depth of respirations, use of
accessory muscles, cough (persistent), and chest x-ray findings.

Activity Intolerance may be related to imbalance between O_2 supply
and demand, and generalized weakness, possibly evidenced by
verbal reports of fatigue, exertional dyspnea, and abnormal vital sign
response.

imbalanced Nutrition: less than body requirements may be related to
inability to ingest adequate nutrients (dyspnea, fatigue, medication
side effects, sputum production, anorexia), possibly evidenced by

---

*A risk diagnosis is not evidenced by signs and symptoms, as the
problem has not occurred and nursing interventions are directed at
prevention.

weight loss, reported altered taste sensation, decreased muscle mass/subcutaneous fat, poor muscle tone, and aversion to eating/lack of interest in food.

risk for Infection: risk factors may include decreased ciliary action, stasis of secretions, and debilitated state/malnutrition.*

Circumcision PEDS

deficient Knowledge [Learning Need] regarding surgical procedure, prognosis, and treatment may be related to lack of exposure, misinterpretation, unfamiliarity with information resources possibly evidenced by request for information, verbalization of concern/misconceptions, inaccurate follow-through of instructions.

acute Pain may be related to trauma to/edema of tender tissues possibly evidenced by crying, changes in sleep pattern, refusal to eat.

impaired urinary Elimination may be related to tissue injury/inflammation, or development of urethral fistula possibly evidenced by edema, difficulty voiding.

risk for Injury [hemorrhage]: risk factors may include decreased clotting factors immediately after birth, previously undiagnosed problems with bleeding/clotting.*

risk for Infection: risk factors may include immature immune system, invasive procedure/tissue trauma, environmental exposure.*

Cirrhosis MS/CH

(Also refer to Substance dependence/abuse rehabilitation; Hepatitis, acute viral)

imbalanced Nutrition: less than body requirements may be related to inability to ingest/absorb nutrients (anorexia, nausea, indigestion, early satiety), abnormal bowel function, impaired storage of vitamins, possibly evidenced by aversion to eating, observed lack of intake, muscle wasting, weight loss, and imbalances in nutritional studies.

excess Fluid Volume may be related to compromised regulatory mechanism (e.g., syndrome of inappropriate antidiuretic hormone—SIADH, decreased plasma proteins/malnutrition) and excess sodium/fluid intake, possibly evidenced by generalized or abdominal edema, weight gain, dyspnea, BP changes, positive hepatojugular reflex, change in mentation, altered electrolytes, changes in urine specific gravity, and pleural effusion.

risk for impaired Skin Integrity: risk factors may include altered circulation/metabolic state, poor skin turgor, skeletal prominence, and presence of edema/ascites, accumulation of bile salts in skin.*

risk for acute Confusion: risk factors may include alcohol abuse, increased serum ammonia level, and inability of liver to detoxify certain enzymes/drugs.*

situational low Self-Esteem/disturbed Body Image may be related to biophysical changes/altered physical appearance, uncertainty of prognosis, changes in role function, personal vulnerability, self-destructive

---

*A risk diagnosis is not evidenced by signs and symptoms, as the problem has not occurred and nursing interventions are directed at prevention.

behavior (alcohol-induced disease), possibly evidenced by verbalization of changes in lifestyle, fear of rejection/reaction of others, negative feelings about body/abilities, and feelings of helplessness/hopelessness/powerlessness.

risk for Injury [hemorrhage]: risk factors may include abnormal blood profile (altered clotting factors), portal hypertension/development of esophageal varices.*

Cocaine hydrochloride
poisoning, acute   MS

(Also refer to Stimulant abuse; Substance dependence/abuse rehabilitation)

ineffective Breathing Pattern may be related to pharmacologic effects on respiratory center of the brain, possibly evidenced by tachypnea, altered depth of respiration, shortness of breath, and abnormal ABGs.

risk for decreased Cardiac Output: risk factors may include drug effect on myocardium (degree dependent on drug purity/quality used), alterations in electrical rate/rhythm/conduction, preexisting myocardiopathy.*

                                                                   CH

imbalanced Nutrition: less than body requirements may be related to anorexia, insufficient/inappropriate use of financial resources, possibly evidenced by reported inadequate intake, weight loss/less than normal weight gain; lack of interest in food, poor muscle tone, signs/laboratory evidence of vitamin deficiencies.

risk for Infection: risk factors may include injection techniques, impurities of drugs; localized trauma/nasal septum damage, malnutrition, altered immune state.*

                                                                   PSY

ineffective Coping may be related to personal vulnerability, negative role modeling, inadequate support systems; ineffective/inadequate coping skills with substitution of drug, possibly evidenced by use of harmful substance despite evidence of undesirable consequences.

disturbed Sensory Perception (specify) may be related to exogenous chemical, altered sensory reception/transmission/integration (hallucination), altered status of sense organs, possibly evidenced by responding to internal stimuli from hallucinatory experiences, bizarre thinking, anxiety/panic changes in sensory acuity (sense of smell/taste).

Coccidioidomycosis (San   CH
Joaquin/Valley Fever)

acute Pain may be related to inflammation, possibly evidenced by verbal reports, distraction behaviors, and narrowed focus.

---

*A risk diagnosis is not evidenced by signs and symptoms, as the problem has not occurred and nursing interventions are directed at prevention.

<u>Fatigue</u> may be related to decreased energy production; states of discomfort, possibly evidenced by reports of overwhelming lack of energy, inability to maintain usual routine, emotional lability/irritability, impaired ability to concentrate, and decreased endurance/libido.

<u>deficient Knowledge [Learning Need] regarding nature/course of disease, therapy and self-care needs</u> may be related to lack of information, possibly evidenced by statements of concern and questions.

Colitis, ulcerative   MS

<u>Diarrhea</u> may be related to inflammation or malabsorption of the bowel, presence of toxins and/or segmental narrowing of the lumen, possibly evidenced by increased bowel sounds/peristalsis, urgency, frequency/watery stools (acute phase), changes in stool color, and abdominal pain/cramping.

<u>acute/chronic Pain</u> may be related to inflammation of the intestines/hyperperistalsis and anal/rectal irritation, possibly evidenced by verbal reports, guarding/distraction behaviors.

<u>risk for deficient Fluid Volume:</u> risk factors may include continued GI losses (diarrhea, vomiting, capillary plasma loss), altered intake, hypermetabolic state.*

CH

<u>imbalanced Nutrition: less than body requirements</u> may be related to altered intake/absorption of nutrients (medically restricted intake, fear that eating may cause diarrhea) and hypermetabolic state, possibly evidenced by weight loss, decreased subcutaneous fat/muscle mass, poor muscle tone, hyperactive bowel sounds, steatorrhea, pale conjunctiva and mucous membranes, and aversion to eating.

<u>ineffective Coping</u> may be related to chronic nature and indefinite outcome of disease, multiple stressors (repeated over time), personal vulnerability, severe pain, inadequate sleep, lack of/ineffective support systems, possibly evidenced by verbalization of inability to cope, discouragement, anxiety; preoccupation with physical self, chronic worry, emotional tension; depression, and recurrent exacerbation of symptoms.

<u>risk for Powerlessness:</u> risk factors may include unresolved dependency conflicts, feelings of insecurity/resentment, repression of anger and aggressive feelings, lacking a sense of control in stressful situations, sacrificing own wishes for others, and retreat from aggression or frustration.*

Colostomy   MS

<u>risk for impaired Skin Integrity:</u> risk factors may include absence of sphincter at stoma and chemical irritation from caustic bowel contents, reaction to product/removal of adhesive, and improperly fitting appliance.*

---

*A risk diagnosis is not evidenced by signs and symptoms, as the problem has not occurred and nursing interventions are directed at prevention.

risk for Diarrhea/Constipation: risk factors may include interruption/ alteration of normal bowel function (placement of ostomy), changes in dietary/fluid intake, and effects of medication.*

CH

deficient Knowledge [Learning Need] regarding changes in physiologic function and self-care/treatment needs may be related to lack of exposure/recall, information misinterpretation, possibly evidenced by questions, statement of concern, and inaccurate follow-through of instruction/development of preventable complications.

disturbed Body Image may be related to biophysical changes (presence of stoma; loss of control of bowel elimination) and psychosocial factors (altered body structure, disease process/associated treatment regimen, e.g., cancer, colitis), possibly evidenced by verbalization of change in perception of self, negative feelings about body, fear of rejection/reaction of others, not touching/looking at stoma, and refusal to participate in care.

impaired Social Interaction may be related to fear of embarrassing situation secondary to altered bowel control with loss of contents, odor, possibly evidenced by reduced participation and verbalized/observed discomfort in social situations.

risk for Sexual dysfunction: risk factors may include altered body structure/function, radical resection/treatment procedures, vulnerability/psychologic concern about response of significant other(s), and disruption of sexual response pattern (e.g., erection difficulty).*

Coma, diabetic   MS
(Refer to Diabetic ketoacidosis; Unconsciousness)

Concussion, brain   CH
acute Pain may be related to trauma to/edema of cerebral tissue, possibly evidenced by reports of headache, guarding/distraction behaviors, and narrowed focus.

risk for deficient Fluid Volume: risk factors may include vomiting, decreased intake, and hypermetabolic state (fever).*

risk for disturbed Thought Processes: risk factors may include trauma to/edema of cerebral tissue.*

deficient Knowledge [Learning Need] regarding condition, treatment/ safety needs, and potential complications may be related to lack of recall, misinterpretation, cognitive limitation, possibly evidenced by questions/statement of concerns, development of preventable complications.

Conduct disorder (childhood,   PSY/PED
adolescence)
risk for self/other-directed Violence: risk factors may include retarded ego development, antisocial character, poor impulse control, dysfunctional family system, loss of significant relationships, history of suicidal/acting-out behaviors.*

---

*A risk diagnosis is not evidenced by signs and symptoms, as the problem has not occurred and nursing interventions are directed at prevention.

defensive Coping may be related to inadequate coping strategies, maturational crisis, multiple life changes/losses, lack of control of impulsive actions, and personal vulnerability, possibly evidenced by inappropriate use of defense mechanisms, inability to meet role expectations, poor self-esteem, failure to assume responsibility for own actions, hypersensitivity to slight or criticism, and excessive smoking/drinking/drug use.

disturbed Thought Processes may be related to physiologic changes, lack of appropriate psychologic conflict, biochemical changes, as evidenced by tendency to interpret the intentions/actions of others as blaming and hostile; deficits in problem-solving skills, with physical aggression the solution most often chosen.

chronic low Self-Esteem may be related to life choices perpetuating failure, personal vulnerability, possibly evidenced by self-negating verbalizations, anger, rejection of positive feedback, frequent lack of success in life events.

CH

compromised/disabled family Coping may be related to excessive guilt, anger, or blaming among family members regarding child's behavior; parental inconsistencies; disagreements regarding discipline, limit setting, and approaches; and exhaustion of parental resources (prolonged coping with disruptive child), possibly evidenced by unrealistic parental expectations, rejection or overprotection of child; and exaggerated expressions of anger, disappointment, or despair regarding child's behavior or ability to improve or change.

impaired Social Interaction may be related to retarded ego development, developmental state (adolescence), lack of social skills, low self-concept, dysfunctional family system, and neurologic impairment, possibly evidenced by dysfunctional interaction with others (difficulty waiting turn in games or group situations, not seeming to listen to what is being said), difficulty playing quietly and maintaining attention to task or play activity, often shifting from one activity to another and interrupting or intruding on others.

Congestive heart failure   MS
(Refer to Heart failure, chronic)

Conn's syndrome   MS/CH
(Refer to Aldosteronism, primary)

Constipation   CH
Constipation may be related to weak abdominal musculature, GI obstructive lesions, pain on defecation, diagnostic procedures, pregnancy, possibly evidenced by change in character/frequency of stools, feeling of abdominal/rectal fullness or pressure, changes in bowel sounds, abdominal distention.

acute Pain may be related to abdominal fullness/pressure, straining to defecate, and trauma to delicate tissues, possibly evidenced by verbal reports, reluctance to defecate, and distraction behaviors.

deficient Knowledge [Learning Need] regarding dietary needs, bowel function, and medication effect may be related to lack of information/misconceptions, possibly evidenced by development of problem and verbalization of concerns/questions.

Coronary artery bypass surgery   MS

risk for decreased Cardiac Output: risk factors may include decreased myocardial contractility, diminished circulating volume (preload), alterations in electrical conduction, and increased SVR (afterload).*

acute Pain may be related to direct chest tissue/bone trauma, invasive tubes/lines, donor site incision, tissue inflammation/edema formation, intraoperative nerve trauma, possibly evidenced by verbal reports, autonomic responses (changes in vital signs), and distraction behaviors/(restlessness), irritability.

disturbed Sensory Perception (specify) may be related to restricted environment (postoperative/acute), sleep deprivation, effects of medications; continuous environmental sounds/activities, and psychologic stress of procedure, possibly evidenced by disorientation, alterations in behavior, exaggerated emotional responses, and visual/auditory distortions.

CH

ineffective Role Performance may be related to situational crises (dependent role)/recuperative process, uncertainty about future, possibly evidenced by delay/alteration in physical capacity to resume role, change in usual role or responsibility, change in self/others' perception of role.

Crohn's disease   MS/CH

(Also refer to Colitis, ulcerative)

imbalanced Nutrition: less than body requirements may be related to intestinal pain after eating; and decreased transit time through bowel, possibly evidenced by weight loss, aversion to eating, and observed lack of intake.

Diarrhea may be related to inflammation of small intestines, presence of toxins, particular dietary intake, possibly evidenced by hyperactive bowel sounds, cramping, and frequent loose liquid stools.

deficient Knowledge [Learning Need] regarding condition, nutritional needs, and prevention of recurrence may be related to insufficient information/misinterpretation, unfamiliarity with resources, possibly evidenced by statements of concern/questions, inaccurate follow-through of instructions, and development of preventable complications/exacerbation of condition.

Croup   PED/CH

ineffective Airway Clearance may be related to presence of thick, tenacious mucus and swelling/spasms of the epiglottis, possibly evidenced by harsh/brassy cough, tachypnea, use of accessory breathing muscles, and presence of wheezes.

---

*A risk diagnosis is not evidenced by signs and symptoms, as the problem has not occurred and nursing interventions are directed at prevention.

deficient Fluid Volume [isotonic] may be related to decreased ability/ aversion to swallowing, presence of fever, and increased respiratory losses, possibly evidenced by dry mucous membranes, poor skin turgor, and scanty/concentrated urine.

Croup membranous   PED/CH

(Also refer to Croup)

risk for Suffocation: risk factors may include inflammation of larynx with formation of false membrane.*

Anxiety [specify level]/Fear may be related to change in environment, perceived threat to self (difficulty breathing), and transmission of anxiety of adults, possibly evidenced by restlessness, facial tension, glancing about, and sympathetic stimulation.

C-Section   OB

(Refer to Cesarean birth, unplanned)

Cushing's syndrome   CH/MS

risk for excess Fluid Volume: risk factors may include compromised regulatory mechanism (fluid/sodium retention).*

risk for Infection: risk factors may include immunosuppressed inflammatory response, skin and capillary fragility, and negative nitrogen balance.*

imbalanced Nutrition: less than body requirements may be related to inability to utilize nutrients (disturbance of carbohydrate metabolism), possibly evidenced by decreased muscle mass and increased resistance to insulin.

Self-Care Deficit [specify] may be related to muscle wasting, generalized weakness, fatigue, and demineralization of bones, possibly evidenced by statements of/observed inability to complete or perform ADLs.

disturbed Body Image may be related to change in structure/appearance (effects of disease process, drug therapy), possibly evidenced by negative feelings about body, feelings of helplessness, and changes in social involvement.

Sexual Dysfunction may be related to loss of libido, impotence, and cessation of menses, possibly evidenced by verbalization of concerns and/or dissatisfaction with and alteration in relationship with significant other.

risk for Trauma [fractures]: risk factors may include increased protein breakdown, negative protein balance, demineralization of bones.*

CVA   MS/CH

(Refer to Cerebrovascular accident)

Cystic fibrosis   CH/PED

ineffective Airway Clearance may be related to excessive production of thick mucus and decreased ciliary action, possibly evidenced by abnormal breath sounds, ineffective cough, cyanosis, and altered respiratory rate/depth.

---

*A risk diagnosis is not evidenced by signs and symptoms, as the problem has not occurred and nursing interventions are directed at prevention.

risk for Infection: risk factors may include stasis of respiratory secretions and development of atelectasis.*

imbalanced Nutrition: less than body requirements may be related to impaired digestive process and absorption of nutrients, possibly evidenced by failure to gain weight, muscle wasting, and retarded physical growth.

deficient Knowledge [Learning Need] regarding pathophysiology of condition, medical management, and available community resources may be related to insufficient information/misconceptions, possibly evidenced by statements of concern, questions; inaccurate follow-through of instructions, development of preventable complications.

compromised family Coping may be related to chronic nature of disease and disability, inadequate/incorrect information or understanding by a primary person, and possibly evidenced by significant person attempting assistive or supportive behaviors with less than satisfactory results, protective behavior disproportionate to client's abilities or need for autonomy.

Cystitis   CH

acute Pain may be related to inflammation and bladder spasms, possibly evidenced by verbal reports, distraction behaviors, and narrowed focus.

impaired Urinary Elimination may be related to inflammation/irritation of bladder, possibly evidenced by frequency, nocturia, and dysuria.

deficient Knowledge [Learning Need] regarding condition, treatment, and prevention of recurrence may be related to inadequate information/misconceptions, possibly evidenced by statements of concern and questions; recurrent infections.

Cytomegalic inclusion disease   CH
(Refer to Cytomegalovirus infection)

Cytomegalovirus (CMV) infection   CH

risk for disturbed visual Sensory Perception: risk factors may include inflammation of the retina.*

risk for fetal Infection: risk factors may include transplacental exposure, contact with blood/body fluids.*

Deep Vein Thrombosis (DVT)   CH/MS
(Refer to Thrombophlebitis)

Degenerative joint disease   CH
(Refer to Arthritis, rheumatoid)

Dehiscence (abdominal)   MS

impaired Skin Integrity may be related to altered circulation, altered nutritional state (obesity/malnutrition), and physical stress on incision, possibly evidenced by poor/delayed wound healing and disruption of skin surface/wound closure.

---

*A risk diagnosis is not evidenced by signs and symptoms, as the problem has not occurred and nursing interventions are directed at prevention.

risk for Infection: risk factors may include inadequate primary defenses (separation of incision, traumatized intestines, environmental exposure).*

risk for impaired Tissue Integrity: risk factors may include exposure of abdominal contents to external environment.*

Fear/[severe] Anxiety may be related to crises, perceived threat of death, possibly evidenced by fearfulness, restless behaviors, and sympathetic stimulation.

deficient Knowledge [Learning Need] regarding condition/prognosis and treatment needs may be related to lack of information/recall and misinterpretation of information, possibly evidenced by development of preventable complication, requests for information, and statement of concern.

Dehydration   PED

deficient Fluid Volume [specify] may be related to etiology as defined by specific situation, possibly evidenced by dry mucous membranes, poor skin turgor, decreased pulse volume/pressure, and thirst.

risk for impaired Oral Mucous Membrane: risk factors may include dehydration and decreased salivation.*

deficient Knowledge [Learning Need] regarding fluid needs may be related to lack of information/misinterpretation, possibly evidenced by questions, statement of concern, and inadequate follow-through of instructions/development of preventable complications.

Delirium tremens (acute   MS/PSY
alcohol withdrawal)

Anxiety [severe/panic]/Fear may be related to cessation of alcohol intake/physiologic withdrawal, threat to self-concept, perceived threat of death, possibly evidenced by increased tension, apprehension, fear of unspecified consequences; identifies object of fear.

disturbed Sensory Perception (specify) may be related to exogenous (alcohol consumption/sudden cessation)/endogenous (electrolyte imbalance, elevated ammonia and blood urea nitrogen—BUN) chemical alterations, sleep deprivation, and psychologic stress, possibly evidenced by disorientation, restlessness, irritability, exaggerated emotional responses, bizarre thinking, and visual and auditory distortions/hallucinations.

risk for decreased Cardiac Output: risk factors may include direct effect of alcohol on heart muscle, altered SVR, presence of dysrhythmias.*

risk for Trauma: risk factors may include alterations in balance, reduced muscle coordination, cognitive impairment, and involuntary clonic/tonic muscle activity.*

imbalanced Nutrition: less than body requirements may be related to poor dietary intake, effects of alcohol on organs involved in digestion, interference with absorption/metabolism of nutrients and amino acids, possibly evidenced by reports of inadequate food intake, altered taste sensation, lack of interest in food, debilitated state, decreased

---

*A risk diagnosis is not evidenced by signs and symptoms, as the problem has not occurred and nursing interventions are directed at prevention.

subcutaneous fat/muscle mass, signs of mineral/electrolyte deficiency including abnormal laboratory findings.

Delivery, precipitous/out of hospital — OB
(Also refer to Labor, precipitous; Labor stages I–II)

risk for deficient Fluid Volume: risk factors may include presence of nausea/vomiting, lack of intake, excessive vascular loss.*

risk for Infection: risk factors may include broken/traumatized tissue, increased environmental exposure, rupture of amniotic membranes.*

risk for fetal Injury: risk factors may include rapid descent/pressure changes, compromised circulation, environmental exposure.*

Delusional disorder — PSY

risk for self/other-directed Violence: risk factors may include perceived threats of danger, increased feelings of anxiety, acting out in an irrational manner.*

[severe] Anxiety may be related to inability to trust possibly evidenced by rigid delusional system, frightened of other people and own hostility.

Powerlessness may be related to lifestyle of helplessness, feelings of inadequacy, interpersonal interaction possibly evidenced by verbal expressions of no control/influence over situation(s), use of paranoid delusions, aggressive behavior to compensate for lack of control.

disturbed Thought Processes may be related to psychologic conflicts, increasing anxiety/fear possibly evidenced by interference with ability to think clearly/logically, fragmentation and autistic thinking, delusions, beliefs and behaviors of suspicion/violence.

impaired Social Interaction may be related to mistrust of others/delusional thinking, lack of knowledge/skills to enhance mutuality possibly evidenced by discomfort in social situations, difficulty in establishing relationships with others, expression of feelings of rejection, no sense of belonging.

Dementia, presenile/senile — CH/PSY
(Also refer to Alzheimer's disease)

impaired Memory may be related to neurologic disturbances, possibly evidenced by observed experiences of forgetting, inability to determine if a behavior was performed, inability to perform previously learned skills, inability to recall factual information or recent/past events.

Fear may be related to decreases in functional abilities, public disclosure of disabilities, further mental/physical deterioration possibly evidenced by social isolation, apprehension, irritability, defensiveness, suspiciousness, aggressive behavior.

Self-Care Deficit [specify] may be related to cognitive decline, physical limitations, frustration over loss of independence, depression, possibly evidenced by impaired ability to perform ADLs.

risk for Trauma: risk factors may include changes in muscle coordination/balance, impaired judgment, seizure activity.*

---

*A risk diagnosis is not evidenced by signs and symptoms, as the problem has not occurred and nursing interventions are directed at prevention.

risk for Caregiver Role Strain: risk factors may include illness severity of care receiver, duration of caregiving required, care receiver exhibiting deviant/bizarre behavior; family/caregiver isolation, lack of respite/recreation, spouse is caregiver.*

Depressant abuse   CH/PSY

(Also refer to Drug overdose, acute [depressants])

ineffective Denial may be related to weak underdeveloped ego, unmet self-needs possibly evidenced by inability to admit impact of condition on life, minimizes symptoms/problem, refuses healthcare attention.

ineffective Coping may be related to weak ego possibly evidenced by abuse of chemical agents, lack of goal-directed behavior, inadequate problem solving, destructive behavior toward self.

imbalanced Nutrition: less than body requirements may be related to use of substance in place of nutritional food possibly evidenced by loss of weight, pale conjunctiva and mucous membranes, electrolyte imbalances, anemias.

risk for Injury: risk factors may include changes in sleep, decreased concentration, loss of inhibitions.*

Depressive disorders, major   PSY
depression, dysthymia

risk for self-directed Violence: risk factors may include depressed mood and feeling of worthlessness and hopelessness.*

[moderate to severe] Anxiety/disturbed Thought Processes may be related to psychologic conflicts, unconscious conflict about essential values/goals of life, unmet needs, threat to self-concept, sleep deprivation, interpersonal transmission/contagion, possibly evidenced by reports of nervousness or fearfulness, feelings of inadequacy; agitation, angry/tearful outbursts, rambling/discoordinated speech, restlessness, hand rubbing or wringing, tremulousness; poor memory/concentration, decreased ability to grasp ideas, inability to follow/impaired ability to make decisions, numerous/repetitious physical complaints without organic cause, ideas of reference, hallucinations/delusions.

disturbed Sleep Pattern may be related to biochemical alterations (decreased serotonin), unresolved fears and anxieties, and inactivity, possibly evidenced by difficulty in falling/remaining asleep, early morning awakening/awakening later than desired, reports of not feeling rested, physical signs (e.g., dark circles under eyes, excessive yawning); hypersomnia (using sleep as an escape).

Social Isolation/impaired Social Interaction may be related to alterations in mental status/thought processes (depressed mood), inadequate personal resources, decreased energy/inertia, difficulty engaging in satisfying personal relationships, feelings of worthlessness/low self-concept, inadequacy in or absence of significant purpose in life, and knowledge/skill deficit about social interactions, possibly evidenced by decreased involvement with others, expressed

---

*A risk diagnosis is not evidenced by signs and symptoms, as the problem has not occurred and nursing interventions are directed at prevention.

feelings of difference from others, remaining in home/room/bed, refusing invitations/suggestions of social involvement, and dysfunctional interaction with peers, family, and/or others.

interrupted Family Processes may be related to situational crises of illness of family member with change in roles/responsibilities, developmental crises (e.g., loss of family member/relationship), possibly evidenced by statements of difficulty coping with situation, family system not meeting needs of its members, difficulty accepting or receiving help appropriately, ineffective family decision-making process, and failure to send and to receive clear messages.

risk for Injury [effects of electroconvulsive therapy (ECT)]: risk factors may include effects of therapy on the cardiovascular, respiratory, musculoskeletal, and nervous systems; and pharmacologic effects of anesthesia.*

Dermatitis seborrheic   CH

impaired Skin Integrity may be related to chronic inflammatory condition of the skin, possibly evidenced by disruption of skin surface with dry or moist scales, yellowish crusts, erythema, and fissures.

Diabetes mellitus   CH/PED

deficient Knowledge [Learning Need] regarding disease process/treatment and individual care needs may be related to unfamiliarity with information/lack of recall, misinterpretation, possibly evidenced by requests for information, statements of concern/misconceptions, inadequate follow-through of instructions, and development of preventable complications.

imbalanced Nutrition: less than body requirements may be related to inability to utilize nutrients (imbalance between intake and utilization of glucose) to meet metabolic needs, possibly evidenced by change in weight, muscle weakness, increased thirst/urination, and hyperglycemia.

risk for impaired Adjustment: risk factors may include all-encompassing change in lifestyle, self-concept requiring lifelong adherence to therapeutic regimen and internal/altered locus of control.*

risk for Infection: risk factors may include decreased leukocyte function, circulatory changes, and delayed healing.*

risk for disturbed Sensory Perception (specify) risk factors may include endogenous chemical alteration (glucose/insulin and/or electrolyte imbalance).*

compromised family Coping may be related to inadequate or incorrect information or understanding by primary person(s), other situational/developmental crises or situations the significant person(s) may be facing, lifelong condition requiring behavioral changes impacting family, possibly evidenced by family expressions of confusion about what to do, verbalizations that they are having difficulty coping with situation; family does not meet physical/emotional needs of its members; SO(s) preoccupied with personal reaction (e.g., guilt,

*A risk diagnosis is not evidenced by signs and symptoms, as the problem has not occurred and nursing interventions are directed at prevention.

fear), display protective behavior disproportionate (too little/too much) to client's abilities or need for autonomy.

Diabetic ketoacidosis   CH/MS

deficient Fluid Volume [specify] may be related to hyperosmolar urinary losses, gastric losses and inadequate intake, possibly evidenced by increased urinary output/dilute urine; reports of weakness, thirst; sudden weight loss, hypotension, tachycardia, delayed capillary refill, dry mucous membranes, poor skin turgor.

imbalanced Nutrition: less than body requirements that may be related to inadequate utilization of nutrients (insulin deficiency), decreased oral intake, hypermetabolic state, possibly evidenced by recent weight loss, reports of weakness, lack of interest in food, gastric fullness/abdominal pain, and increased ketones, imbalance between glucose/insulin levels.

Fatigue may be related to decreased metabolic energy production, altered body chemistry (insufficient insulin), increased energy demands (hypermetabolic state/infection), possibly evidenced by overwhelming lack of energy, inability to maintain usual routines, decreased performance, impaired ability to concentrate, listlessness.

risk for Infection: risk factors may include high glucose levels, decreased leukocyte function, stasis of body fluids, invasive procedures, alteration in circulation/perfusion.*

Dialysis, general   CH

(Also refer to Dialysis, peritoneal; Hemodialysis)

imbalanced Nutrition: less than body requirements may be related to inadequate ingestion of nutrients (dietary restrictions, anorexia, nausea/vomiting, stomatitis), loss of peptides and amino acids (building blocks for proteins) during procedure, possibly evidenced by reported inadequate intake, aversion to eating, altered taste sensation, poor muscle tone/weakness, sore/inflamed buccal cavity, pale conjunctiva/mucous membranes.

anticipatory Grieving may be related to actual or perceived loss, chronic and/or fatal illness, and thwarted grieving response to a loss, possibly evidenced by verbal expression of distress/unresolved issues, denial of loss; altered eating habits, sleep and dream patterns, activity levels, libido; crying, labile affect; feelings of sorrow, guilt, and anger.

disturbed Body Image/situational low Self-Esteem may be related to situational crisis and chronic illness with changes in usual roles/body image, possibly evidenced by verbalization of changes in lifestyle, focus on past function, negative feelings about body, feelings of helplessness/powerlessness, extension of body boundary to incorporate environmental objects (e.g., dialysis setup), change in social involvement, overdependence on others for care, not taking responsibility for self-care/lack of follow-through, and self-destructive behavior.

---

*A risk diagnosis is not evidenced by signs and symptoms, as the problem has not occurred and nursing interventions are directed at prevention.

Self-Care Deficit [specify] may be related to perceptual/cognitive impairment (accumulated toxins); intolerance to activity, decreased strength and endurance; pain/discomfort, possibly evidenced by reported inability to perform ADLs, disheveled/unkempt appearance, strong body odor.

Powerlessness may be related to illness-related regimen and healthcare environment, possibly evidenced by verbal expression of having no control, depression over physical deterioration, nonparticipation in care, anger, and passivity.

compromised/disabled family Coping may be related to inadequate or incorrect information or understanding by a primary person, temporary family disorganization and role changes, client providing little support in turn for the primary person, and prolonged disease/disability progression that exhausts the supportive capacity of significant persons, possibly evidenced by expressions of concern or reports about response of SO(s)/family to client's health problem, preoccupation of SO(s) with own personal reactions, display of intolerance/rejection, and protective behavior disproportionate (too little or too much) to client's abilities or need for autonomy.

Dialysis, peritoneal   MS/CH

(Also refer to Dialysis, general)

risk for excess Fluid Volume: risk factors may include inadequate osmotic gradient of dialysate, fluid retention (dialysate drainage problems/inappropriate osmotic gradient of solution, bowel distention), excessive PO/IV intake.*

risk for Trauma: risk factors may include improper placement during insertion or manipulation of catheter.*

acute Pain may be related to procedural factors (catheter irritation, improper catheter placement), presence of edema/abdominal distention, inflammation, or infection, rapid infusion/infusion of cold or acidic dialysate, possibly evidenced by verbal reports, guarding/distraction behaviors, and self-focus.

risk for Infection [peritonitis]: risk factors may include contamination of catheter/infusion system, skin contaminants, sterile peritonitis (response to composition of dialysate).*

risk for ineffective Breathing Pattern: risk factors may include increased abdominal pressure with restricted diaphragmatic excursion, rapid infusion of dialysate, pain/discomfort, inflammatory process (e.g., atelectasis/pneumonia).*

Diaper rash   PED

(Refer to Candidiasis)

Diarrhea   PED/CH

deficient Knowledge [Learning Need] regarding causative/contributing factors and therapeutic needs may be related to lack of information/misconceptions, possibly evidenced by statements of concern, questions, and development of preventable complications.

---

*A risk diagnosis is not evidenced by signs and symptoms, as the problem has not occurred and nursing interventions are directed at prevention.

risk for deficient Fluid Volume: risk factors may include excessive losses
through GI tract, altered intake.*

acute Pain may be related to abdominal cramping and irritation/excoriation of skin, possibly evidenced by verbal reports, facial grimacing,
and autonomic responses.

impaired Skin Integrity may be related to effects of excretions on delicate tissues, possibly evidenced by reports of discomfort and disruption of skin surface/destruction of skin layers.

Digitalis toxicity   MS/CH

decreased Cardiac Output may be related to altered myocardial contractility/electrical conduction, properties of digitalis (long half-life and
narrow therapeutic range), concurrent medications, age/general
health status and electrolyte/acid-base balance, possibly evidenced by
changes in rate/rhythm/conduction (development/worsening of
dysrhythmias), changes in mentation, worsening of heart failure,
elevated serum drug levels.

risk for imbalanced Fluid Volume: risk factors may include excessive
losses from vomiting/diarrhea, decreased intake/nausea, decreased
plasma proteins, malnutrition, continued use of diuretics; excess
sodium/fluid retention.*

deficient Knowledge [Learning Need] regarding condition/therapy
and self-care needs may be related to information misinterpretation and lack of recall, possibly evidenced by inaccurate
follow-through of instructions and development of preventable
complications.

risk for disturbed Thought Processes: risk factors may include physiologic effects of toxicity/reduced cerebral perfusion.*

Dilation and curettage (D and C)   OB/GYN

(Also refer to Abortion, elective or spontaneous termination)

deficient Knowledge [Learning Need] regarding surgical procedure,
possible postprocedural complications, and therapeutic needs may be
related to lack of exposure/unfamiliarity with information, possibly
evidenced by requests for information and statements of concern/
misconceptions.

Dilation of cervix, premature   OB

(Also refer to Labor, preterm)

Anxiety [specify level] may be related to situational crisis, threat of
death/fetal loss possibly evidenced by increased tension, apprehension, feelings of inadequacy, sympathic stimulation, and repetitive
questioning.

risk for maternal Injury: risk factors may include surgical intervention,
use of tocolytic drugs.*

risk for fetal Injury: risk factors may include premature delivery, surgical procedure.*

---

*A risk diagnosis is not evidenced by signs and symptoms, as the
problem has not occurred and nursing interventions are directed at
prevention.

anticipatory Grieving may be related to perceived potential fetal loss possibly evidenced by expression of distress, guilt, anger, chocked feelings.

Dislocation/subluxation of joint   CH

acute Pain may be related to lack of continuity of bone/joint, muscle spasms, edema possibly evidenced by verbal or coded reports, guarded/protective behaviors, narrowed focus, autonomic responses.

risk for Injury: risk factors may include nerve impingement, improper fitting of splint device.*

impaired physical Mobility may be related to immobilization device/activity restrictions, pain, edema, decreased muscle strength possibly evidenced by limited range of motion, limited ability to perform motor skills, gait changes.

Disseminated intravascular coagulation (DIC)   MS

risk for deficient Fluid Volume: risk factors may include failure of regulatory mechanism (coagulation process) and active loss/hemorrhage.*

ineffective Tissue Perfusion (specify) may be related to alteration of arterial/venous flow (microemboli throughout circulatory system, and hypovolemia), possibly evidenced by changes in respiratory rate and depth, changes in mentation, decreased urinary output, and development of acral cyanosis/focal gangrene.

Anxiety [specify level]/Fear may be related to sudden change in health status/threat of death, interpersonal transmission/contagion, possibly evidenced by sympathetic stimulation, restlessness, focus on self, and apprehension.

risk for impaired Gas Exchange: risk factors may include reduced oxygen-carrying capacity, development of acidosis, fibrin deposition in microcirculation, and ischemic damage of lung parenchyma.*

acute Pain may be related to bleeding into joints/muscles, with hematoma formation, and ischemic tissues with areas of acral cyanosis/focal gangrene, possibly evidenced by verbal reports, narrowed focus, alteration in muscle tone, guarding/distraction behaviors, restlessness, autonomic responses.

Dissociative disorders   PSY

Anxiety [severe/panic]/Fear may be related to a maladaptation or ineffective coping continuing from early life, unconscious conflict(s), threat to self-concept, unmet needs, or phobic stimulus, possibly evidenced by maladaptive response to stress (e.g., dissociating self/fragmentation of the personality), increased tension, feelings of inadequacy, and focus on self, projection of personal perceptions onto the environment.

risk for self/other-directed Violence: risk factors may include dissociative state/conflicting personalities, depressed mood, panic states, and suicidal/homicidal behaviors.*

*A risk diagnosis is not evidenced by signs and symptoms, as the problem has not occurred and nursing interventions are directed at prevention.

disturbed Personal Identity may be related to psychologic conflicts (dissociative state), childhood trauma/abuse, threat to physical integrity/self-concept, and underdeveloped ego, possibly evidenced by alteration in perception or experience of the self, loss of one's own sense of reality/the external world, poorly differentiated ego boundaries, confusion about sense of self, purpose or direction in life; memory loss, presence of more than one personality within the individual.

compromised family Coping may be related to multiple stressors repeated over time, prolonged progression of disorder that exhausts the supportive capacity of significant person(s), family disorganization and role changes, high-risk family situation possibly evidenced by family/SO(s) describing inadequate understanding or knowledge that interferes with assistive or supportive behaviors; relationship and marital conflict.

Diverticulitis   CH

acute Pain may be related to inflammation of intestinal mucosa, abdominal cramping, and presence of fever/chills, possibly evidenced by verbal reports, guarding/distraction behaviors, autonomic responses, and narrowed focus.

Diarrhea/Constipation may be related to altered structure/function and presence of inflammation, possibly evidenced by signs and symptoms dependent on specific problem (e.g., increase/decrease in frequency of stools and change in consistency).

deficient Knowledge [Learning Need] regarding disease process, potential complications, therapeutic and self-care needs may be related to lack of information/misconceptions, possibly evidenced by statements of concern, request for information, and development of preventable complications.

risk for Powerlessness: risk factors may include chronic nature of disease process and recurrent episodes despite cooperation with medical regimen.*

Down syndrome   PED/CH
(Also refer to Mental retardation)

delayed Growth and Development may be related to effects of physical/mental disability, possibly evidenced by altered physical growth; delay/inability in performing skills and self-care/self-control activities appropriate for age.

risk for Trauma: risk factors may include cognitive difficulties and poor muscle tone/coordination, weakness.*

imbalanced Nutrition: less than body requirements may be related to poor muscle tone and protruding tongue, possibly evidenced by weak and ineffective sucking/swallowing and observed lack of adequate intake with weight loss/failure to gain.

interrupted Family Processes may be related to situational/maturational crises requiring incorporation of new skills into family dynamics, possibly evidenced by confusion about what to do, verbalized difficulty coping with situation, unexamined family myths.

*A risk diagnosis is not evidenced by signs and symptoms, as the problem has not occurred and nursing interventions are directed at prevention.

<u>risk for dysfunctional Grieving:</u> risk factors may include loss of "the perfect child," chronic condition requiring long-term care, and unresolved feelings.*

<u>risk for impaired parent/infant/child Attachment:</u> risk factors may include ill infant/child who is unable to effectively initiate parental contact due to altered behavioral organization, inability of parents to meet the personal needs.*

<u>risk for Social Isolation:</u> risk factors may include withdrawal from usual social interactions and activities, assumption of total child care, and becoming overindulgent/overprotective.*

Drug overdose, acute (depressants)   MS/PSY
(Also refer to Substance dependence/abuse rehabilitation)

<u>ineffective Breathing Pattern/impaired Gas Exchange</u> may be related to neuromuscular impairment/CNS depression, decreased lung expansion, possibly evidenced by changes in respirations, cyanosis, and abnormal ABGs.

<u>risk for Trauma/Suffocation/Poisoning:</u> risk factors may include CNS depression/agitation, hypersensitivity to the drug(s), psychologic stress.*

<u>risk for self/other-directed Violence:</u> risk factors may include suicidal behaviors, toxic reactions to drug(s).*

<u>risk for Infection:</u> risk factors may include drug injection techniques, impurities in injected drugs, localized trauma; malnutrition, altered immune state.*

Duchenne's muscular dystrophy   PED/CH
(Refer to Muscular dystrophy [Duchenne's])

DVT   CH/MS
(Refer to Thrombophlebitis)

Dysmenorrhea   GYN
<u>acute Pain</u> may be related to exaggerated uterine contractibility, possibly evidenced by verbal reports, guarding/distraction behaviors, narrowed focus, and autonomic responses (changes in vital signs).

<u>risk for Activity Intolerance:</u> risk factors may include severity of pain and presence of secondary symptoms (nausea, vomiting, syncope, chills), depression.*

<u>ineffective Coping</u> may be related to chronic, recurrent nature of problem; anticipatory anxiety, and inadequate coping methods, possibly evidenced by muscular tension, headaches, general irritability, chronic depression, and verbalization of inability to cope, report of poor self-concept.

Dysrhythmia, cardiac   MS
<u>risk for decreased Cardiac Output:</u> risk factors may include altered electrical conduction and reduced myocardial contractility.*

---

*A risk diagnosis is not evidenced by signs and symptoms, as the problem has not occurred and nursing interventions are directed at prevention.

Anxiety [specify level] may be related to perceived threat of death, possibly evidenced by increased tension, apprehension, and expressed concerns.

deficient Knowledge [Learning Need] regarding medical condition/therapy needs may be related to lack of information/misinterpretation and unfamiliarity with information resources, possibly evidenced by questions, statement of misconception, failure to improve on previous regimen, and development of preventable complications.

risk for Activity Intolerance: risk factors may include imbalance between myocardial O_2 supply and demand, and cardiac depressant effects of certain drugs (β-blockers, antidysrhythmics).*

risk for Poisoning, [digitalis toxicity]: risk factors may include limited range of therapeutic effectiveness, lack of education/proper precautions, reduced vision/cognitive limitations.*

Eating disorders   CH/PSY
(Refer to Anorexia nervosa; Bulimia nervosa)

Eclampsia   OB
(Refer to Pregnancy-induced hypertension)

Ectopic pregnancy (tubal)   OB
(Also refer to Abortion, spontaneous termination)

acute Pain may be related to distention/rupture of fallopian tube, possibly evidenced by verbal reports, guarding/distraction behaviors, facial mask of pain, and autonomic responses (diaphoresis, changes in vital signs).

risk for deficient Fluid Volume [isotonic]: risk factors may include hemorrhagic losses and decreased/restricted intake.*

Anxiety [specify level]/Fear may be related to threat of death and possible loss of ability to conceive, possibly evidenced by increased tension, apprehension, sympathetic stimulation, restlessness, and focus on self.

Eczema (dermatitis)   CH
Pain/[Discomfort] may be related to cutaneous inflammation and irritation, possibly evidenced by verbal reports, irritability, and scratching.

risk for Infection: risk factors may include broken skin and tissue trauma.*

Social Isolation may be related to alterations in physical appearance, possibly evidenced by expressed feelings of rejection and decreased interaction with peers.

Edema, pulmonary   MS
excess Fluid Volume may be related to decreased cardiac functioning, excessive fluid/sodium intake, possibly evidenced by dyspnea, presence of crackles (rales), pulmonary congestion on x ray, restlessness,

---

*A risk diagnosis is not evidenced by signs and symptoms, as the problem has not occurred and nursing interventions are directed at prevention.

anxiety, and increased central venous pressure (CVP)/pulmonary pressures.

impaired Gas Exchange may be related to altered blood flow and decreased alveolar/capillary exchange (fluid collection/shifts into interstitial space/alveoli), possibly evidenced by hypoxia, restlessness, and confusion.

Anxiety [specify level]/Fear may be related to perceived threat of death (inability to breathe), possibly evidenced by responses ranging from apprehension to panic state, restlessness, and focus on self.

Emphysema   CH/MS

impaired Gas Exchange may be related to alveolar capillary membrane changes/destruction, possibly evidenced by dyspnea, restlessness, changes in mentation, abnormal ABG values.

ineffective Airway Clearance may be related to increased production/ retained tenacious secretions, decreased energy level, and muscle wasting, possibly evidenced by abnormal breath sounds (rhonchi), ineffective cough, changes in rate/depth of respirations, and dyspnea.

Activity Intolerance may be related to imbalance between O_2 supply and demand, possibly evidenced by reports of fatigue/weakness, exertional dyspnea, and abnormal vital sign response to activity.

imbalanced Nutrition: less than body requirements may be related to inability to ingest food (shortness of breath, anorexia, generalized weakness, medication side effects), possibly evidenced by lack of interest in food, reported altered taste, loss of muscle mass and tone, fatigue, and weight loss.

risk for Infection: risk factors may include inadequate primary defenses (stasis of body fluids, decreased ciliary action), chronic disease process, and malnutrition.*

Powerlessness may be related to illness-related regimen and healthcare environment, possibly evidenced by verbal expression of having no control, depression over physical deterioration, nonparticipation in therapeutic regimen; anger, and passivity.

Encephalitis   MS

risk for ineffective cerebral Tissue Perfusion: risk factors may include cerebral edema altering/interrupting cerebral arterial/venous blood flow, hypovolemia, exchange problems at cellular level (acidosis).*

Hyperthermia may be related to increased metabolic rate, illness, and dehydration, possibly evidenced by increased body temperature, flushed/warm skin, and increased pulse and respiratory rates.

acute Pain may be related to inflammation/irritation of the brain and cerebral edema, possibly evidenced by verbal reports of headache, photophobia, distraction behaviors, restlessness, and autonomic response (changes in vital signs).

risk for Trauma/Suffocation: risk factors may include restlessness, clonic/tonic activity, altered sensorium, cognitive impairment; generalized weakness, ataxia, vertigo.*

---

*A risk diagnosis is not evidenced by signs and symptoms, as the problem has not occurred and nursing interventions are directed at prevention.

risk for decreased Cardiac Output: risk factors may include inflammation of lining of heart and structural change in valve leaflets.*

Anxiety [specify level] may be related to change in health status and threat of death, possibly evidenced by apprehension, expressed concerns, and focus on self.

acute Pain may be related to generalized inflammatory process and effects of embolic phenomena, possibly evidenced by verbal reports, narrowed focus, distraction behaviors, and autonomic responses (changes in vital signs).

risk for Activity Intolerance: risk factors may include imbalance between O_2 supply and demand, debilitating condition.*

risk for ineffective Tissue Perfusion (specify): risk factors may include embolic interruption of arterial flow (embolization of thrombi/valvular vegetations).*

Endometriosis GYN

acute/chronic Pain may be related to pressure of concealed bleeding/formation of adhesions, possibly evidenced by verbal reports (pain between/with menstruation), guarding/distraction behaviors, and narrowed focus.

Sexual Dysfunction may be related to pain secondary to presence of adhesions, possibly evidenced by verbalization of problem, and altered relationship with partner.

deficient Knowledge [Learning Need] regarding pathophysiology of condition and therapy needs may be related to lack of information/misinterpretations, possibly evidenced by statements of concern and misconceptions.

Enteritis MS/CH

(Refer to Colitis, ulcerative; Crohn's disease)

Epididymitis MS

acute Pain may be related to inflammation, edema formation, and tension on the spermatic cord, possibly evidenced by verbal reports, guarding/distraction behaviors (restlessness), and autonomic responses (changes in vital signs).

risk for Infection, [spread]: risk factors may include presence of inflammation/infectious process, insufficient knowledge to avoid spread of infection.*

deficient Knowledge [Learning Need] regarding pathophysiology, outcome, and self-care needs may be related to lack of information/misinterpretations, possibly evidenced by statements of concern, misconceptions, and questions.

Epilepsy CH

(Refer to Seizure disorder)

---

*A risk diagnosis is not evidenced by signs and symptoms, as the problem has not occurred and nursing interventions are directed at prevention.

Erectile dysfunction   CH

Sexual Dysfunction may be related to altered body function possibly evidenced by reports of disruption of sexual response pattern, inability to achieve desired satisfaction.

situational low Self-Esteem may be related to functional impairment; rejection of other(s).

Failure to thrive   PED

imbalanced Nutrition: less than body requirements may be related to inability to ingest/digest/absorb nutrients (defects in organ function/metabolism, genetic factors), physical deprivation/psychosocial factors, possibly evidenced by lack of appropriate weight gain/weight loss, poor muscle tone, pale conjunctiva, and laboratory tests reflecting nutritional deficiency.

delayed Growth and Development may be related to inadequate caretaking (physical/emotional neglect or abuse); indifference, inconsistent responsiveness, multiple caretakers; environmental and stimulation deficiencies, possibly evidenced by altered physical growth, flat affect, listlessness, decreased response; delay or difficulty in performing skills or self-control activities appropriate for age group.

risk for impaired Parenting: risk factors may include lack of knowledge, inadequate bonding, unrealistic expectations for self/infant, and lack of appropriate response of child to relationship.*

deficient Knowledge [Learning Need] regarding pathophysiology of condition, nutritional needs, growth/development expectations, and parenting skills may be related to lack of information/misinformation or misinterpretation, possibly evidenced by verbalization of concerns, questions, misconceptions; or development of preventable complications.

Fatigue syndrome, chronic   CH

Fatigue may be related to disease state, inadequate sleep, possibly evidenced by verbalization of unremitting/overwhelming lack of energy, inability to maintain usual routines, listless, compromised concentration.

chronic Pain may be related to chronic physical disability possibly evidenced by verbal reports of headache, sore throat, arthralgias, abdominal pain, muscle aches; altered ability to continue previous activities, changes in sleep pattern.

Self-Care Deficit [specify] may be related to tiredness, pain/discomfort possibly evidenced by reports of inability to perform desired ADLs.

risk for ineffective Role Performance: risk factors may include health alterations, stress.*

Fetal alcohol syndrome   PED

risk for Injury [CNS damage]: risk factors may include external chemical factors (alcohol intake by mother), placental insufficiency, fetal drug withdrawal in utero/postpartum and prematurity.*

---

*A risk diagnosis is not evidenced by signs and symptoms, as the problem has not occurred and nursing interventions are directed at prevention.

---

disorganized Infant Behavior may be related to prematurity, environmental overstimulation, lack of containment/boundaries, possibly evidenced by change from baseline physiologic measures; tremors, startles, twitches, hyperextension of arms/legs, deficient self-regulatory behaviors, deficient response to visual/auditory stimuli.

risk for impaired Parenting: risk factors may include mental and/or physical illness, inability of mother to assume the overwhelming task of unselfish giving and nurturing, presence of stressors (financial/legal problems), lack of available or ineffective role model, interruption of bonding process, lack of appropriate response of child to relationship.*

PSY

ineffective [maternal] Coping may be related to personal vulnerability, low self-esteem, inadequate coping skills, and multiple stressors (repeated over period of time), possibly evidenced by inability to meet basic needs/fulfill role expectations/problem-solve, and excessive use of drug(s).

dysfunctional Family Processes: alcoholism may be related to lack of/insufficient support from others, mother's drug problem and treatment status, together with poor coping skills, lack of family stability/overinvolvement of parents with children and multigenerational addictive behaviors, possibly evidenced by abandonment, rejection, neglectful relationships with family members, and decisions and actions by family that are detrimental.

Fetal demise **OB**

Grieving [expected] may be related to death of fetus/infant (wanted or unwanted), possibly evidenced by verbal expressions of distress, anger, loss; crying; alteration in eating habits or sleep pattern.

situational low Self-Esteem may be related to perceived "failure" at a life event, possibly evidenced by negative self-appraisal in response to life event in a person with a previous positive self-evaluation, verbalization of negative feelings about the self (helplessness, uselessness), difficulty making decisions.

risk for Spiritual Distress: risk factors may include loss of loved one, low self-esteem, poor relationships, challenged belief and value system (birth is supposed to be the beginning of life, not of death) and intense suffering.*

Fractures **MS/CH**

(Also refer to Casts; Traction)

risk for Trauma [additional injury]: risk factors may include loss of skeletal integrity/movement of skeletal fragments, use of traction apparatus, and so on.*

acute Pain may be related to muscle spasms, movement of bone fragments, tissue trauma/edema, traction/immobility device, stress, and anxiety, possibly evidenced by verbal reports, distraction behaviors,

*A risk diagnosis is not evidenced by signs and symptoms, as the problem has not occurred and nursing interventions are directed at prevention.

self-focusing/narrowed focus, facial mask of pain, guarding/protective behavior, alteration in muscle tone, and autonomic responses (changes in vital signs).

risk for Peripheral Neurovascular Dysfunction: risk factors may include reduction/interruption of blood flow (direct vascular injury, tissue trauma, excessive edema, thrombus formation, hypovolemia).*

impaired physical Mobility may be related to neuromuscular/skeletal impairment, pain/discomfort, restrictive therapies (bedrest, extremity immobilization), and psychologic immobility, possibly evidenced by inability to purposefully move within the physical environment, imposed restrictions, reluctance to attempt movement, limited range of motion, and decreased muscle strength/control.

risk for impaired Gas Exchange: risk factors may include altered blood flow, blood/fat emboli, alveolar/capillary membrane changes (interstitial/pulmonary edema, congestion).*

deficient Knowledge [Learning Need] regarding healing process, therapy requirements, potential complications, and self-care needs may be related to lack of exposure, misinterpretation of information, possibly evidenced by statements of concern, questions, and misconceptions.

Frostbite   MS/CH

impaired Tissue Integrity may be related to altered circulation and thermal injury, possibly evidenced by damaged/destroyed tissue.

acute Pain may be related to diminished circulation with tissue ischemia/necrosis and edema formation, possibly evidenced by verbal reports, guarding/distraction behaviors, narrowed focus, and autonomic responses (changes in vital signs).

risk for Infection: risk factors may include traumatized tissue/tissue destruction, altered circulation, and compromised immune response in affected area.*

Gallstones   CH

(Refer to Cholelithiasis)

Gangrene, dry   MS

ineffective peripheral Tissue Perfusion may be related to interruption in arterial flow, possibly evidenced by cool skin temperature, change in color (black), atrophy of affected part, and presence of pain.

acute Pain may be related to tissue hypoxia and necrotic process, possibly evidenced by verbal reports, guarding/distraction behaviors, narrowed focus, and autonomic responses (changes in vital signs).

Gas, lung irritant   MS/CH

ineffective Airway Clearance may be related to irritation/inflammation of airway, possibly evidenced by marked cough, abnormal breath sounds (wheezes), dyspnea, and tachypnea.

risk for impaired Gas Exchange: risk factors may include irritation/inflammation of alveolar membrane (dependent on type of agent, and length of exposure).*

---

*A risk diagnosis is not evidenced by signs and symptoms, as the problem has not occurred and nursing interventions are directed at prevention.

Anxiety [specify level] may be related to change in health status and threat of death, possibly evidenced by verbalizations, increased tension, apprehension, and sympathetic stimulation.

Gastritis, acute · MS

acute Pain may be related to irritation/inflammation of gastric mucosa, possibly evidenced by verbal reports, guarding/distraction behaviors, and autonomic responses (changes in vital signs).

risk for deficient Fluid Volume [isotonic]: risk factors may include excessive losses through vomiting and diarrhea, continued bleeding, reluctance to ingest/restrictions of oral intake.*

Gastritis, chronic · CH

risk for imbalanced Nutrition: less than body requirements: risk factors may include inability to ingest adequate nutrients (prolonged nausea/vomiting, anorexia, epigastric pain).*

deficient Knowledge [Learning Need] regarding pathophysiology, psychologic factors, therapy needs, and potential complications may be related to lack of information/misinterpretation, possibly evidenced by verbalization of concerns, questions, misconceptions, and continuation of problem.

Gastroenteritis · MS

(Refer to Enteritis; Gastritis, chronic)

Gender identity disorder · PSY

(For individuals experiencing persistent and marked distress regarding uncertainty about issues relating to personal identity, e.g., sexual orientation and behavior.)

Anxiety [specify level] may be related to unconscious/conscious conflicts about essential values/beliefs (ego-dystonic gender identification), threat to self-concept, unmet needs, possibly evidenced by increased tension, helplessness, hopelessness, feelings of inadequacy, uncertainty, insomnia and focus on self, and impaired daily functioning.

ineffective Role Performance/disturbed Personal Identity may be related to crisis in development in which person has difficulty knowing/accepting to which sex he or she belongs or is attracted, sense of discomfort and inappropriateness about anatomic sex characteristics, possibly evidenced by confusion about sense of self, purpose or direction in life, sexual identification/preference, verbalization of desire to be/insistence that person is the opposite sex, change in self-perception of role, and conflict in roles.

ineffective Sexuality Patterns may be related to ineffective or absent role models and conflict with sexual orientation and/or preferences, lack of/impaired relationship with an SO, possibly evidenced by verbalizations of discomfort with sexual orientation/role, and lack of information about human sexuality.

---

*A risk diagnosis is not evidenced by signs and symptoms, as the problem has not occurred and nursing interventions are directed at prevention.

risk for compromised/disabled family Coping: risk factors may include inadequate/incorrect information or understanding, significant other unable to perceive or to act effectively in regard to client's needs, temporary family disorganization and role changes, and client providing little support in turn for primary person.*

readiness for enhanced family Coping may be related to individual's basic needs being sufficiently gratified and adaptive tasks effectively addressed to enable goals of self-actualization to surface, possibly evidenced by family member(s) attempts to describe growth/impact of crisis on own values, priorities, goals, or relationships; family member(s) is moving in direction of health-promoting and enriching lifestyle that supports client's search for self; and choosing experiences that optimize wellness.

Genetic disorder CH/OB

Anxiety may be related to presence of specific risk factors (e.g., exposure to teratogens), situational crisis, threat to self-concept, conscious or unconscious conflict about essential values and life goals possibly evidenced by increased tension, apprehension, uncertainty, feelings of inadequacy, expressed concerns.

deficient Knowledge [Learning Need] regarding purpose/process of genetic counseling may be related to lack of awareness of ramifications of diagnosis, process necessary for analyzing available options, and information misinterpretation possibly evidenced by verbalization of concerns, statement of misconceptions, request for information.

risk for interrupted Family Processes: risk factors may include situational crisis, individual/family vulnerability, difficulty reaching agreement regarding options.*

Spiritual Distress may be related to intense inner conflict about the outcome, normal grieving for the loss of the perfect child, anger that is often directed at God/greater power, religious beliefs/moral convictions possibly evidenced by verbalization of inner conflict about beliefs, questioning of the moral and ethical implications of therapeutic choices, viewing situation as punishment, anger, hostility, and crying.

Gigantism CH

(Refer to Acromegaly)

Glaucoma CH

disturbed visual Sensory Perception may be related to altered sensory reception and altered status of sense organ (increased intraocular pressure/atrophy of optic nerve head), possibly evidenced by progressive loss of visual field.

Anxiety [specify level] may be related to change in health status, presence of pain, possibility/reality of loss of vision, unmet needs, and negative self-talk, possibly evidenced by apprehension, uncertainty, and expressed concern regarding changes in life event.

---

*A risk diagnosis is not evidenced by signs and symptoms, as the problem has not occurred and nursing interventions are directed at prevention.

Glomerulonephritis   PED

excess Fluid Volume may be related to failure of regulatory mechanism (inflammation of glomerular membrane inhibiting filtration), possibly evidenced by weight gain, edema/anasarca, intake greater than output, and blood pressure changes.

acute Pain may be related to effects of circulating toxins and edema/distention of renal capsule, possibly evidenced by verbal reports, guarding/distraction behaviors, and autonomic responses (changes in vital signs).

imbalanced Nutrition: less than body requirements may be related to anorexia and dietary restrictions, possibly evidenced by aversion to eating, reported altered taste, weight loss, and decreased intake.

deficient Diversional Activity may be related to treatment modality/restrictions, fatigue, and malaise, possibly evidenced by statements of boredom, restlessness, and irritability.

risk for disproportionate Growth: risk factors may include infection, malnutrition, chronic illness.*

Goiter   CH

disturbed Body Image may be related to visible swelling in neck possibly evidenced by verbalization of feelings, fear of reaction of others, actual change in structure, change in social involvement.

Anxiety may be related to change in health status/progressive growth of mass, perceived threat of death.

risk for imbalanced Nutrition: less than body requirements: risk factors may include decreased ability to ingest/difficulty swallowing.*

risk for ineffective Airway Clearance: risk factors may include tracheal compression/obstruction.*

Gonorrhea   CH

(Also refer to Sexually transmitted disease—STD)

risk for Infection [dissemination/bacteremia]: risk factors may include presence of infectious process in highly vascular area and lack of recognition of disease process.*

acute Pain may be related to irritation/inflammation of mucosa and effects of circulating toxins, possibly evidenced by verbal reports of genital or pharyngeal irritation, perineal/pelvic pain, guarding/distraction behaviors.

deficient Knowledge [Learning Need] regarding disease cause/transmission, therapy, and self-care needs may be related to lack of information/misinterpretation, denial of exposure, possibly evidenced by statements of concern, questions, misconceptions, and inaccurate follow-through of instructions/development of preventable complications.

Gout   CH

acute Pain may be related to inflammation of joint(s), possibly evidenced by verbal reports, guarding/distraction behaviors, and autonomic responses (changes in vital signs).

---

*A risk diagnosis is not evidenced by signs and symptoms, as the problem has not occurred and nursing interventions are directed at prevention.

impaired physical Mobility may be related to joint pain/edema, possibly evidenced by reluctance to attempt movement, limited range of motion, and therapeutic restriction of movement.

deficient Knowledge [Learning Need] regarding cause, treatment, and prevention of condition may be related to lack of information/misinterpretation, possibly evidenced by statements of concern, questions, misconceptions, and inaccurate follow-through of instructions.

Guillain-Barré syndrome (acute polyneuritis)   MS

risk for ineffective Breathing Pattern/Airway Clearance: risk factors may include weakness/paralysis of respiratory muscles, impaired gag/swallow reflexes, decreased energy/fatigue.*

disturbed Sensory Perceptual: (specify) may be related to altered sensory reception/transmission/integration (altered status of sense organs, sleep deprivation), therapeutically restricted environment, endogenous chemical alterations (electrolyte imbalance, hypoxia), and psychologic stress, possibly evidenced by reported or observed change in usual response to stimuli, altered communication patterns, and measured change in sensory acuity and motor coordination.

impaired physical Mobility may be related to neuromuscular impairment, pain/discomfort, possibly evidenced by impaired coordination, partial/complete paralysis, decreased muscle strength/control.

Anxiety [specify level]/Fear may be related to situational crisis, change in health status/threat of death, possibly evidenced by increased tension, restlessness, helplessness, apprehension, uncertainty, fearfulness, focus on self, and sympathetic stimulation.

risk for Disuse Syndrome: risk factors include paralysis and pain.*

Hay fever   CH

Pain/[Discomfort] may be related to irritation/inflammation of upper airway mucous membranes and conjunctiva, possibly evidenced by verbal reports, irritability, and restlessness.

deficient Knowledge [Learning Need] regarding underlying cause, appropriate therapy, and required lifestyle changes may be related to lack of information, possibly evidenced by statements of concern, questions, and misconceptions.

Heart failure, chronic   MS

decreased Cardiac Output may be related to altered myocardial contractility/inotropic changes; alterations in rate, rhythm, and electrical conduction; and structural changes (valvular defects, ventricular aneurysm), possibly evidenced by tachycardia/dysrhythmias, changes in blood pressure, extra heart sounds, decreased urine output, diminished peripheral pulses, cool/ashen skin, orthopnea, crackles; dependent/generalized edema and chest pain.

excess Fluid Volume may be related to reduced glomerular filtration rate/increased ADH production, and sodium/water retention, possibly evidenced by orthopnea and abnormal breath sounds, S_3 heart

---

*A risk diagnosis is not evidenced by signs and symptoms, as the problem has not occurred and nursing interventions are directed at prevention.

sound, jugular vein distention, positive hepatojugular reflex, weight gain, hypertension, oliguria, generalized edema.

risk for impaired Gas Exchange: risk factors may include alveolar-capillary membrane changes (fluid collection/shifts into interstitial space/alveoli).*

CH

Activity Intolerance may be related to imbalance between O_2 supply/demand, generalized weakness, and prolonged bedrest/sedentary lifestyle, possibly evidenced by reported/observed weakness, fatigue; changes in vital signs, presence of dysrhythmias; dyspnea, pallor, and diaphoresis.

deficient Knowledge [Learning Need] regarding cardiac function/disease process, therapy and self-care needs may be related to lack of information/misinterpretation, possibly evidenced by questions, statements of concern/misconceptions; development of preventable complications or exacerbations of condition.

Heatstroke **MS**

Hyperthermia may be related to prolonged exposure to hot environment/vigorous activity with failure of regulating mechanism of the body, possibly evidenced by high body temperature (greater than 105°F/40.6°C), flushed/hot skin, tachycardia, and seizure activity.

decreased Cardiac Output may be related to functional stress of hypermetabolic state, altered circulating volume/venous return, and direct myocardial damage secondary to hyperthermia, possibly evidenced by decreased peripheral pulses, dysrhythmias/tachycardia, and changes in mentation.

Hemodialysis **MS/CH**

(Also refer to Dialysis, general)

risk for Injury, [loss of vascular access]: risk factors may include clotting/thrombosis, infection, disconnection/hemorrhage.*

risk for deficient Fluid Volume: risk factors may include excessive fluid losses/shifts via ultrafiltration, hemorrhage (altered coagulation/disconnection of shunt), and fluid restrictions.*

risk for excess Fluid Volume: risk factors may include excessive fluid intake; rapid IV, blood/plasma expanders/saline given to support BP during procedure.*

ineffective Protection may be related to chronic disease state, drug therapy, abnormal blood profile, inadequate nutrition, possibly evidenced by altered clotting, impaired healing, deficient immunity, fatigue, anorexia.

Hemophilia **PED**

risk for deficient Fluid Volume [isotonic]: risk factors may include impaired coagulation/hemorrhagic losses.*

risk for acute/chronic Pain: risk factors may include nerve compression from hematomas, nerve damage or hemorrhage into joint space.*

---

*A risk diagnosis is not evidenced by signs and symptoms, as the problem has not occurred and nursing interventions are directed at prevention.

risk for impaired physical Mobility: risk factors may include joint hemorrhage, swelling, degenerative changes, and muscle atrophy.*

ineffective Protection may be related to abnormal blood profile, possibly evidenced by altered clotting.

compromised family Coping may be related to prolonged nature of condition that exhausts the supportive capacity of significant person(s), possibly evidenced by protective behaviors disproportionate to client's abilities/need for autonomy.

Hemorrhoidectomy   MS/CH

acute Pain may be related to edema/swelling and tissue trauma, possibly evidenced by verbal reports, guarding/distraction behaviors, focus on self, and autonomic responses (changes in vital signs).

risk for Urinary Retention: risk factors may include perineal trauma, edema/swelling, and pain.*

deficient Knowledge [Learning Need] regarding therapeutic treatment and potential complications may be related to lack of information/misconceptions, possibly evidenced by statements of concern and questions.

Hemorrhoids   CH/OB

acute Pain may be related to inflammation and edema of prolapsed varices, possibly evidenced by verbal reports, and guarding/distraction behaviors.

Constipation may be related to pain on defecation and reluctance to defecate, possibly evidenced by frequency, less than usual pattern and hard/formed stools.

Hemothorax   MS

(Also refer to Pneumothorax)

risk for Trauma/Suffocation: risk factors may include concurrent disease/injury process, dependence on external device (chest drainage system), and lack of safety education/precautions.*

Anxiety [specify level] may be related to change in health status and threat of death, possibly evidenced by increased tension, restlessness, expressed concern, sympathetic stimulation, and focus on self.

Hepatitis, acute viral   MS/CH

Fatigue may be related to decreased metabolic energy production and altered body chemistry, possibly evidenced by reports of lack of energy/inability to maintain usual routines, decreased performance, and increased physical complaints.

imbalanced Nutrition: less than body requirements may be related to inability to ingest adequate nutrients (nausea, vomiting, anorexia); hypermetabolic state, altered absorption and metabolism, possibly evidenced by aversion to eating/lack of interest in food, altered taste sensation, observed lack of intake, and weight loss.

acute Pain/[Discomfort] may be related to inflammation and swelling of the liver, arthralgias, urticarial eruptions, and pruritus, possibly

---

*A risk diagnosis is not evidenced by signs and symptoms, as the problem has not occurred and nursing interventions are directed at prevention.

evidenced by verbal reports, guarding/distraction behaviors, focus on self, and autonomic responses (changes in vital signs).

risk for Infection: risk factors may include inadequate secondary defenses and immunosuppression, malnutrition, insufficient knowledge to avoid exposure to pathogens/spread to others.*

risk for impaired Tissue Integrity: risk factors may include bile salt accumulation in the tissues.*

risk for impaired Home Management: risk factors may include debilitating effects of disease process and inadequate support systems (family, financial, role model).*

deficient Knowledge [Learning Need] regarding disease process/transmission, treatment needs, and future expectations may be related to lack of information/recall, misinterpretation, unfamiliarity with resources, possibly evidenced by questions, statement of concerns/misconceptions, inaccurate follow-through of instructions, and development of preventable complications.

Hernia, hiatal   CH

chronic Pain may be related to regurgitation of acidic gastric contents, possibly evidenced by verbal reports, facial grimacing, and focus on self.

deficient Knowledge [Learning Need] regarding pathophysiology, prevention of complications and self-care needs may be related to lack of information/misconceptions, possibly evidenced by statements of concern, questions, and recurrence of condition.

Herniated nucleus pulposus   CH/MS
(ruptured intervertebral disk)

acute/chronic Pain may be related to nerve compression/irritation and muscle spasms, possibly evidenced by verbal reports, guarding/distraction behaviors, preoccupation with pain, self/narrowed focus, and autonomic responses (changes in vital signs when pain is acute), altered muscle tone/function, changes in eating/sleeping patterns and libido, physical/social withdrawal.

impaired physical Mobility may be related to pain (muscle spasms), therapeutic restrictions (e.g., bedrest, traction/braces), muscular impairment, and depression, possibly evidenced by reports of pain on movement, reluctance to attempt/difficulty with purposeful movement, decreased muscle strength, impaired coordination, and limited range of motion.

deficient Diversional Activity may be related to length of recuperation period and therapy restrictions, physical limitations, pain and depression, possibly evidenced by statements of boredom, disinterest, "nothing to do," and restlessness, irritability, withdrawal.

Herpes, herpes simplex   CH

acute Pain may be related to presence of localized inflammation and open lesions, possibly evidenced by verbal reports, distraction behaviors, and restlessness.

---

*A risk diagnosis is not evidenced by signs and symptoms, as the problem has not occurred and nursing interventions are directed at prevention.

risk for [secondary] Infection: risk factors may include broken/traumatized tissue, altered immune response, and untreated infection/treatment failure.*

risk for ineffective Sexuality Patterns: risk factors may include lack of knowledge, values conflict, and/or fear of transmitting the disease.*

Herpes zoster (shingles)   CH

acute Pain may be related to inflammation/local lesions along sensory nerve(s), possibly evidenced by verbal reports, guarding/distraction behaviors, narrowed focus, and autonomic responses (changes in vital signs).

deficient Knowledge [Learning Need] regarding pathophysiology, therapeutic needs, and potential complications may be related to lack of information/misinterpretation, possibly evidenced by statements of concern, questions, and misconceptions.

High altitude pulmonary edema (HAPE)   MS
(Also refer to Mountain sickness, acute)

impaired Gas Exchange may be related to ventilation perfusion imbalance, alveolar-capillary membrane changes, altered oxygen supply possibly evidenced by dyspnea, confusion, cyanosis, tachycardia, abnormal ABGs.

excess Fluid Volume may be related to compromised regulatory mechanism possibly evidenced by shortness of breath, anxiety, edema, abnormal breath sounds, pulmonary congestion.

High altitude sickness   MS
(Refer to Mountain sickness, acute; High altitude pulmonary edema)

HIV positive   CH
(Also refer to AIDS)

impaired Adjustment may be related to life-threatening, stigmatizing condition/disease; assault to self-esteem, altered locus of control, inadequate support systems, incomplete grieving, medication side effects (fatigue/depression), possibly evidenced by verbalization of nonacceptance/denial of diagnosis, nonexistent or unsuccessful involvement in problem solving/goal setting; extended period of shock and disbelief or anger; lack of future-oriented thinking.

deficient Knowledge [Learning Need] regarding disease, prognosis, and treatment needs may be related to lack of exposure/recall, information misinterpretation, unfamiliarity with information resources, or cognitive limitation, possibly evidenced by statement of misconception/request for information, inappropriate/exaggerated behaviors (hostile, agitated, hysterical, apathetic), inaccurate follow-through of instructions/development of preventable complications.

*A risk diagnosis is not evidenced by signs and symptoms, as the problem has not occurred and nursing interventions are directed at prevention.

Hodgkin's disease

(Also refer to Cancer; Chemotherapy)

Anxiety [specify level]/Fear may be related to threat of self-concept and threat of death, possibly evidenced by apprehension, insomnia, focus on self, and increased tension.

deficient Knowledge [Learning Need] regarding diagnosis, pathophysiology, treatment, and prognosis may be related to lack of information/misinterpretation, possibly evidenced by statements of concern, questions, and misconceptions.

acute Pain/[Discomfort] may be related to manifestations of inflammatory response (fever, chills, night sweats) and pruritus, possibly evidenced by verbal reports, distraction behaviors, and focus on self.

risk for ineffective Breathing Pattern/Airway Clearance: risk factors may include tracheobronchial obstruction (enlarged mediastinal nodes and/or airway edema).*

Hospice/End of life care

CH

acute/chronic Pain may be related to biological, physical, psychological agent possibly evidenced by verbal/coded report, changes in appetite/eating, sleep pattern; protective behavior, restlessness, irritability.

Activity Intolerance/Fatigue may be related to generalized weakness, bedrest/immobility, pain, imbalance between oxygen supply and demand possibly evidenced by inability to maintain usual routine, verbalized lack of desire/interest in activity, decreased performance, lethargy.

anticipatory Grieving/death Anxiety may be related to anticipated loss of physiologic well-being, perceived threat of death.

compromised/disabled family Coping/Caregiver Role Strain may be related to prolonged disease/disability progression, temporary family disorganization and role changes, unrealistic expectations, inadequate or incorrect information or understanding by primary person.

Hydrocephalus

PED/MS

ineffective cerebral Tissue Perfusion may be related to decreased arterial/venous blood flow (compression of brain tissue), possibly evidenced by changes in mentation, restlessness, irritability, reports of headache, pupillary changes, and changes in vital signs.

disturbed visual Sensory Perception may be related to pressure on sensory/motor nerves, possibly evidenced by reports of double vision, development of strabismus, nystagmus, pupillary changes, and optic atrophy.

risk for impaired physical Mobility: risk factors may include neuromuscular impairment, decreased muscle strength, and impaired coordination.*

risk for decreased Intracranial Adaptive Capacity: risk factors may include brain injury, changes in perfusion pressure/intracranial pressure.*

---

*A risk diagnosis is not evidenced by signs and symptoms, as the problem has not occurred and nursing interventions are directed at prevention.

risk for Infection: risk factors may include invasive procedure/presence of shunt.*

deficient Knowledge [Learning Need] regarding condition, prognosis, and long-term therapy needs/medical follow-up may be related to lack of information/misperceptions, possibly evidenced by questions, statement of concern, request for information, and inaccurate follow-through of instruction/development of preventable complications.

Hyperactivity disorder   PED/PSY

defensive Coping may be related to mild neurologic deficits, dysfunctional family system, abuse/neglect possibly evidenced by denial of obvious problems, projection of blame/responsibility, grandiosity, difficulty in reality testing perceptions.

impaired Social Interaction may be related to retarded ego development, negative role models, neurologic impairment possibly evidenced by discomfort in social situations, interrupts/intrudes on others, difficulty waiting turn in games/group activities, difficulty maintaining attention to task.

disabled family Coping may be related to excessive guilt, anger, or blaming among family members, parental inconsistencies, disagreements regarding discipline/limit-setting/approaches, exhaustion of parental expectations possibly evidenced by unrealistic parental expectations, rejection or overprotection of child, exaggerated expression of feelings, despair regarding child's behavior.

Hyperbilirubinemia   PED

risk for Injury [CNS involvement]: risk factors may include prematurity, hemolytic disease, asphyxia, acidosis, hyponatremia, and hypoglycemia.*

risk for Injury [effects of treatment]: risk factors may include physical properties of phototherapy and effects on body regulatory mechanisms, invasive procedure (exchange transfusion), abnormal blood profile, chemical imbalances.*

deficient Knowledge [Learning Need] regarding condition prognosis, treatment/safety needs may be related to lack of exposure/recall and information misinterpretation, possibly evidenced by questions, statement of concern, and inaccurate follow-through of instructions/development of preventable complications.

Hyperemesis gravidarum   OB

deficient Fluid Volume [isotonic] may be related to excessive gastric losses and reduced intake, possibly evidenced by dry mucous membranes, decreased/concentrated urine, decreased pulse volume and pressure, thirst, and hemoconcentration.

imbalanced Nutrition: less than body requirements may be related to inability to ingest/digest/absorb nutrients (prolonged vomiting), possibly evidenced by reported inadequate food intake, lack of interest in food/aversion to eating, and weight loss.

*A risk diagnosis is not evidenced by signs and symptoms, as the problem has not occurred and nursing interventions are directed at prevention.

risk for ineffective Coping: risk factors may include situational/maturational crisis (pregnancy, change in health status, projected role changes, concern about outcome).*

Hypertension CH

deficient Knowledge [Learning Need] regarding condition, therapeutic regimen, and potential complications may be related to lack of information/recall, misinterpretation, cognitive limitations, and/or denial of diagnosis, possibly evidenced by statements of concern/questions, and misconceptions, inaccurate follow-through of instructions, and lack of BP control.

impaired Adjustment may be related to condition requiring change in lifestyle, altered locus of control, and absence of feelings/denial of illness, possibly evidenced by verbalization of nonacceptance of health status change and lack of movement toward independence.

risk for Sexual dysfunction: risk factors may include side effects of medication.*

MS

risk for decreased Cardiac Output: risk factors may include increased afterload (vasoconstriction), fluid shifts/hypovolemia, myocardial ischemia, ventricular hypertrophy/rigidity.*

acute Pain may be related to increased cerebrovascular pressure, possibly evidenced by verbal reports (throbbing pain located in suboccipital region, present on awakening and disappearing spontaneously after being up and about), reluctance to move head, avoidance of bright lights and noise, increased muscle tension.

Hypertension, pulmonary CH/MS

(Refer to Pulmonary hypertension)

Hyperthyroidism CH

(Also refer to Thyrotoxicosis)

Fatigue may be related to hypermetabolic imbalance with increased energy requirements, irritability of CNS, and altered body chemistry, possibly evidenced by verbalization of overwhelming lack of energy to maintain usual routine, decreased performance, emotional lability/irritability, and impaired ability to concentrate.

Anxiety [specify level] may be related to increased stimulation of the CNS (hypermetabolic state, pseudocatecholamine effect of thyroid hormones), possibly evidenced by increased feelings of apprehension, overexcitement/distress, irritability/emotional lability, shakiness, restless movements, tremors.

risk for imbalanced Nutrition: less than body requirements: risk factors may include inability to ingest adequate nutrients for hypermetabolic rate/constant activity, impaired absorption of nutrients (vomiting/diarrhea), hyperglycemia/relative insulin insufficiency.*

risk for impaired Tissue Integrity: risk factors may include altered protective mechanisms of eye related to periorbital edema, reduced

---

*A risk diagnosis is not evidenced by signs and symptoms, as the problem has not occurred and nursing interventions are directed at prevention.

ability to blink, eye discomfort/dryness, and development of corneal abrasion/ulceration.*

Hypoglycemia CH

disturbed Thought Processes may be related to inadequate glucose for cellular brain function and effects of endogenous hormone activity, possibly evidenced by irritability, changes in mentation, memory loss, altered attention span, and emotional lability.

risk for imbalanced Nutrition: less than body requirements: risk factors may include inadequate glucose metabolism and imbalance of glucose/insulin levels.*

deficient Knowledge [Learning Need] regarding pathophysiology of condition and therapy/self-care needs may be related to lack of information/recall, misinterpretations, possibly evidenced by development of hypoglycemia and statements of questions/misconceptions.

Hypoparathyroidism (acute) MS

risk for Injury: risk factors may include neuromuscular excitability/tetany and formation of renal stones.*

acute Pain may be related to recurrent muscle spasms and alteration in reflexes, possibly evidenced by verbal reports, distraction behaviors, and narrowed focus.

risk for ineffective Airway Clearance: risk factors may include spasm of the laryngeal muscles.*

Anxiety [specify level] may be related to threat to, or change in, health status, physiologic responses.

Hypothermia (systemic) CH
   (Also refer to Frostbite)

Hypothermia may be related to exposure to cold environment, inadequate clothing, age extremes (very young/elderly), damage to hypothalamus, consumption of alcohol/medications causing vasodilation, possibly evidenced by reduction in body temperature below normal range, shivering, cool skin, pallor.

deficient Knowledge [Learning Need] regarding risk factors, treatment needs, and prognosis may be related to lack of information/recall, misinterpretation, possibly evidenced by statement of concerns/misconceptions, occurrence of problem, and development of complications.

Hypothyroidism CH
   (Also refer to Myxedema)

impaired physical Mobility may be related to weakness, fatigue, muscle aches, altered reflexes, and mucin deposits in joints and interstitial spaces, possibly evidenced by decreased muscle strength/control and impaired coordination.

Fatigue may be related to decreased metabolic energy production, possibly evidenced by verbalization of unremitting/overwhelming lack of

---

*A risk diagnosis is not evidenced by signs and symptoms, as the problem has not occurred and nursing interventions are directed at prevention.

energy, inability to maintain usual routines, impaired ability to concentrate, decreased libido, irritability, listlessness, decreased performance, increase in physical complaints.

disturbed Sensory Perception (specify) may be related to mucin deposits and nerve compression, possibly evidenced by paresthesias of hands and feet or decreased hearing.

Constipation may be related to decreased peristalsis/physical activity, possibly evidenced by frequency less than usual pattern, decreased bowel sounds, hard dry stools, and development of fecal impaction.

Hysterectomy   GYN/MS

acute Pain may be related to tissue trauma/abdominal incision, edema/hematoma formation, possibly evidenced by verbal reports, guarding/distraction behaviors, and autonomic responses (changes in vital signs).

impaired Urinary Elimination/risk for [acute] Urinary Retention: risk factors may include mechanical trauma, surgical manipulation, presence of localized edema/hematoma, or nerve trauma with temporary bladder atony.*

ineffective Sexuality Patterns/risk for Sexual dysfunction: risk factors may include concerns regarding altered body function/structure, perceived changes in femininity, changes in hormone levels, loss of libido, and changes in sexual response pattern.*

Ileocolitis   MS/CH

(Refer to Crohn's disease)

Ileostomy   MS/CH

(Refer to Colostomy)

Ileus   MS

acute Pain may be related to distention/edema and ischemia of intestinal tissue, possibly evidenced by verbal reports, guarding/distraction behaviors, narrowed focus, and autonomic responses (changes in vital signs).

Diarrhea/Constipation may be related to presence of obstruction/changes in peristalsis, possibly evidenced by changes in frequency and consistency or absence of stool, alterations in bowel sounds, presence of pain, and cramping.

risk for deficient Fluid Volume: risk factors may include increased intestinal losses (vomiting and diarrhea), and decreased intake.*

Impetigo   PED/CH

impaired Skin Integrity may be related to presence of infectious process and pruritus, possibly evidenced by open/crusted lesions.

acute Pain may be related to inflammation and pruritus, possibly evidenced by verbal reports, distraction behaviors, and self-focusing.

risk for [secondary] Infection: risk factors may include broken skin, traumatized tissue, altered immune response, and virulence/contagious nature of causative organism.*

*A risk diagnosis is not evidenced by signs and symptoms, as the problem has not occurred and nursing interventions are directed at prevention.

<u>risk for Infection [transmission]:</u> risk factors may include virulent nature of causative organism, insufficient knowledge to prevent infection of others.*

Infection, prenatal   OB
(Also refer to AIDS)

<u>risk for maternal/fetal Infection:</u> risk factors may include inadequate primary defenses (e.g., broken skin, stasis of body fluids), inadequate secondary defenses (e.g., decreased hemoglobin, immunosuppression), inadequate acquired immunity, environmental exposure, malnutrition, rupture of amniotic membranes.*

<u>deficient Knowledge regarding treatment/prevention, prognosis of condition</u> may be related to lack of exposure to information and/or unfamiliarity with resources, misinterpretation possibly evidenced by verbalization of problem, inaccurate follow-through of instructions, development of preventable complications/continuation of infectious process.

[Discomfort] may be related to body response to infective agent, properties of infection (e.g., skin/tissue irritation, development of lesions) possibly evidenced by verbal reports, restlessness, withdrawal from social contacts.

Inflammatory bowel disease   CH
(Refer to Colitis, ulcerative; Crohn's disease)

Influenza   CH
<u>Pain/[Discomfort]</u> may be related to inflammation and effects of circulating toxins, possibly evidenced by verbal reports, distraction behaviors, and narrowed focus.

<u>risk for deficient Fluid Volume:</u> risk factors may include excessive gastric losses, hypermetabolic state, and altered intake.*

<u>Hyperthermia</u> may be related to effects of circulating toxins and dehydration, possibly evidenced by increased body temperature, warm/flushed skin, and tachycardia.

<u>risk for ineffective Breathing:</u> risk factors may include response to infectious process, decreased energy/fatigue.*

Insulin shock   MS/CH
(Refer to Hypoglycemia)

Intestinal obstruction   MS
(Refer to Ileus)

Irritable bowel syndrome   CH
<u>acute Pain</u> may be related to abnormally strong intestinal contractions, increased sensitivity of intestine to distention, hypersensitivity to hormones gastrin and cholecystokinin, skin/tissue irritation/perirectal excoriation possibly evidenced by verbal reports, guarding behavior, expressive behavior (restlessness, moaning, irritability).

---

*A risk diagnosis is not evidenced by signs and symptoms, as the problem has not occurred and nursing interventions are directed at prevention.

Constipation may be related to motor abnormalities of longitudinal muscles/changes in frequency and amplitude of contractions, dietary restrictions, stress possibly evidenced by change in bowel pattern/decreased frequency, sensation of incomplete evacuation, abdominal pain/distention.

Diarrhea may be related to motor abnormalities of longitudinal muscles/changes in frequency and amplitude of contractions possibly evidenced by precipitous passing of liquid stool on rising or immediately after eating, rectal urgency/incontinence, bloating.

Kawasaki disease   PED

Hyperthermia may be related to increased metabolic rate and dehydration, possibly evidenced by increased body temperature greater than normal range, flushed skin, increased respiratory rate, and tachycardia.

acute Pain may be related to inflammation and edema/swelling of tissues, possibly evidenced by verbal reports, restlessness, guarding behaviors, and narrowed focus.

impaired Skin Integrity may be related to inflammatory process, altered circulation, and edema formation, possibly evidenced by disruption of skin surface including macular rash and desquamation.

impaired Oral Mucous Membrane may be related to inflammatory process, dehydration, and mouth breathing, possibly evidenced by pain, hyperemia, and fissures of lips.

risk for decreased Cardiac Output: risk factors may include structural changes/inflammation of coronary arteries and alterations in rate/rhythm or conduction.*

Kidney stone(s)   CH

(Refer to Calculi, urinary)

Labor, induced/augmented   OB

deficient Knowledge [Learning Need] regarding procedure, treatment needs, and possible outcomes may be related to lack of exposure/recall, information misinterpretation, and unfamiliarity with information resources, possibly evidenced by questions, statement of concern/misconception, and exaggerated behaviors.

risk for maternal Injury: risk factors may include adverse effects/response to therapeutic interventions.*

risk for impaired fetal Gas Exchange: risk factors may include altered placental perfusion/cord prolapse.*

acute Pain may be related to altered characteristics of chemically stimulated contractions, psychologic concerns, possibly evidenced by verbal reports, increased muscle tone, distraction/guarding behaviors, and narrowed focus.

Labor, precipitous   OB

Anxiety [specify level] may be related to situational crisis, threat to self/fetus, interpersonal transmission possibly evidenced by increased tension; scared, fearful, restless/jittery; sympathetic stimulation.

---

*A risk diagnosis is not evidenced by signs and symptoms, as the problem has not occurred and nursing interventions are directed at prevention.

risk for impaired Skin/Tissue Integrity: risk factors may include rapid progress of labor, lack of necessary equipment.*

acute Pain may be related to occurrence of rapid, strong muscle contractions; psychologic issues possibly evidenced by verbalizations of inability to use learned pain-management techniques, sympathetic stimulation, distraction behaviors (e.g., moaning, restlessness).

Labor, preterm   OB/CH

Activity Intolerance may be related to muscle/cellular hypersensitivity, possibly evidenced by continued uterine contractions/irritability.

risk for Poisoning: risk factors may include dose-related toxic/side effects of tocolytics.*

risk for fetal Injury: risk factors may include delivery of premature/immature infant.*

Anxiety [specify level] may be related to situational crisis, perceived or actual threats to self/fetus and inadequate time to prepare for labor, possibly evidenced by increased tension, restlessness, expressions of concern, and autonomic responses (changes in vital signs).

deficient Knowledge [Learning Need] regarding preterm labor treatment needs and prognosis may be related to lack of information and misinterpretation, possibly evidenced by questions, statements of concern, misconceptions, inaccurate follow-through of instruction, and development of preventable complications.

Labor, stage I (active phase)   OB

acute Pain/[Discomfort] may be related to contraction-related hypoxia, dilation of tissues, and pressure on adjacent structures combined with stimulation of both parasympathetic and sympathetic nerve endings, possibly evidenced by verbal reports, guarding/distraction behaviors (restlessness), muscle tension, and narrowed focus.

impaired Urinary Elimination may be related to altered intake/dehydration, fluid shifts, hormonal changes, hemorrhage, severe intrapartal hypertension, mechanical compression of bladder, and effects of regional anesthesia, possibly evidenced by changes in amount/frequency of voiding, urinary retention, slowed progression of labor, and reduced sensation.

risk for ineffective Coping, [Individual/Couple]: risk factors may include situational crises, personal vulnerability, use of ineffective coping mechanisms, inadequate support systems, and pain.*

Labor, stage II (expulsion)   OB

acute Pain may be related to strong uterine contractions, tissue stretching/dilation and compression of nerves by presenting part of the fetus, and bladder distention, possibly evidenced by verbalizations, facial grimacing, guarding/distraction behaviors (restlessness), narrowed focus, and autonomic responses (diaphoresis).

---

*A risk diagnosis is not evidenced by signs and symptoms, as the problem has not occurred and nursing interventions are directed at prevention.

Cardiac Output [fluctuation] may be related to changes in SVR, fluctuations in venous return (repeated/prolonged Valsalva's maneuvers, effects of anesthesia/medications, dorsal recumbent position occluding the inferior vena cava and partially obstructing the aorta), possibly evidenced by decreased venous return, changes in vital signs (BP, pulse), urinary output, fetal bradycardia.

risk for impaired fetal Gas Exchange: risk factors may include mechanical compression of head/cord, maternal position/prolonged labor affecting placental perfusion, and effects of maternal anesthesia, hyperventilation.*

risk for impaired Skin/Tissue Integrity: risk factors may include untoward stretching/lacerations of delicate tissues (precipitous labor, hypertonic contractile pattern, adolescence, large fetus) and application of forceps.*

risk for Fatigue: risk factors may include pregnancy, stress, anxiety, sleep deprivation, increased physical exertion, anemia, humidity/temperature, lights.*

Laminectomy (lumbar)   MS

ineffective Tissue Perfusion (specify) may be related to diminished/interrupted blood flow (dressing, edema/hematoma formation), hypovolemia, possibly evidenced by paresthesia, numbness; decreased range of motion, muscle strength.

risk for [spinal] Trauma: risk factors may include temporary weakness of spinal column, balancing difficulties, changes in muscle tone/coordination.*

acute Pain may be related to traumatized tissues, localized inflammation, and edema, possibly evidenced by altered muscle tone, verbal reports, and distraction/guarding behaviors, autonomic changes.

impaired physical Mobility may be related to imposed therapeutic restrictions, neuromuscular impairment, and pain, possibly evidenced by limited range of motion, decreased muscle strength/control, impaired coordination, and reluctance to attempt movement.

risk for [acute] Urinary Retention: risk factors may include pain and swelling in operative area and reduced mobility/restrictions of position.*

Laryngectomy   MS

(Also refer to Cancer; Chemotherapy)

ineffective Airway Clearance may be related to partial/total removal of the glottis, temporary or permanent change to neck breathing, edema formation, and copious/thick secretions, possibly evidenced by dyspnea/difficulty breathing, changes in rate/depth of respiration, use of accessory respiratory muscles, weak/ineffective cough, abnormal breath sounds, and cyanosis.

impaired Skin/Tissue Integrity may be related to surgical removal of tissues/grafting, effects of radiation or chemotherapeutic agents,

---

*A risk diagnosis is not evidenced by signs and symptoms, as the problem has not occurred and nursing interventions are directed at prevention.

altered circulation/reduced blood supply, compromised nutritional status, edema formation, and pooling/continuous drainage of secretions, possibly evidenced by disruption of skin/tissue surface and destruction of skin/tissue layers.

impaired Oral Mucous Membrane may be related to dehydration/ absence of oral intake, poor/inadequate oral hygiene, patho logical condition (oral cancer), mechanical trauma (oral surgery), decreased saliva production, difficulty swallowing and pooling/drooling of secretions, and nutritional deficits, possibly evidenced by xerostomia (dry mouth), oral discomfort, thick/mucoid saliva, decreased saliva production, dry and crusted/coated tongue, inflamed lips, absent teeth/gums, poor dental health and halitosis.

CH

impaired verbal Communication may be related to anatomic deficit (removal of vocal cords), physical barrier (tracheostomy tube), and required voice rest, possibly evidenced by inability to speak, change in vocal characteristics, and impaired articulation.

risk for Aspiration: risk factors may include impaired swallowing, facial/neck surgery, presence of tracheostomy/feeding tube.*

Laryngitis   CH/PED
(Refer to Croup)

Latex allergy   CH

latex Allergy Response may be related to no immune mechanism response possibly evidenced by contact dermatitis—erythema, blisters; delayed hypersensitivity—eczema, irritation; hypersensitivity— generalized edema, wheezing/bronchospasm, hypotension, cardiac arrest.

Anxiety [specify level]/Fear may be related to threat of death possibly evidenced by expressed concerns, hypervigilance, restlessness, focus on self.

risk for impaired Adjustment: risk factors may include health status requiring change in occupation.*

Lead poisoning, acute   PED/CH
(Also refer to Lead poisoning, chronic)

risk for Trauma: risk factors may include loss of coordination, altered level of consciousness, clonic or tonic muscle activity, neurologic damage.*

risk for deficient Fluid Volume: risk factors may include excessive vomiting, diarrhea, or decreased intake.*

deficient Knowledge [Learning Need] regarding sources of lead and prevention of poisoning may be related to lack of information/misinterpretation, possibly evidenced by statements of concern, questions, and misconceptions.

---

*A risk diagnosis is not evidenced by signs and symptoms, as the problem has not occurred and nursing interventions are directed at prevention.

Lead poisoning, chronic CH

(Also refer to Lead poisoning, acute)

imbalanced Nutrition: less than body requirements may be related to decreased intake (chemically induced changes in the GI tract), possibly evidenced by anorexia, abdominal discomfort, reported metallic taste, and weight loss.

disturbed Thought Processes may be related to deposition of lead in CNS and brain tissue, possibly evidenced by personality changes, learning disabilities, and impaired ability to conceptualize and reason.

chronic Pain may be related to deposition of lead in soft tissues and bone, possibly evidenced by verbal reports, distraction behaviors, and focus on self.

Leukemia, acute MS

(Also refer to Chemotherapy)

risk for Infection: risk factors may include inadequate secondary defenses (alterations in mature white blood cells, increased number of immature lymphocytes, immunosuppression and bone marrow suppression), invasive procedures, and malnutrition.*

Anxiety [specify level]/Fear may be related to change in health status, threat of death, and situational crisis, possibly evidenced by sympathetic stimulation, apprehension, feelings of helplessness, focus on self, and insomnia.

Activity Intolerance [specify level] may be related to reduced energy stores, increased metabolic rate, imbalance between O_2 supply and demand, therapeutic restrictions (bedrest)/effect of drug therapy, possibly evidenced by generalized weakness, reports of fatigue and exertional dyspnea; abnormal heart rate or BP response.

acute Pain may be related to physical agents (infiltration of tissues/organs/CNS, expanding bone marrow) and chemical agents (antileukemic treatments), possibly evidenced by verbal reports (abdominal discomfort, arthralgia, bone pain, headache); distraction behaviors, narrowed focus, and autonomic responses (changes in vital signs).

risk for deficient Fluid Volume: risk factors may include excessive losses (vomiting, hemorrhage, diarrhea), decreased intake (nausea, anorexia), increased fluid need (hypermetabolic state/fever), predisposition for kidney stone formation/tumor lysis syndrome.*

Long-term care CH

(Also refer to condition requiring/contributing to need for facility placement)

Anxiety [specify level]/Fear may be related to change in health status, role functioning, interaction patterns, socioeconomic status, environment; unmet needs, recent life changes, and loss of friends/SO(s), possibly evidenced by apprehension, restlessness, insomnia, repetitive

---

*A risk diagnosis is not evidenced by signs and symptoms, as the problem has not occurred and nursing interventions are directed at prevention.

questioning, pacing, purposeless activity, expressed concern regarding changes in life events, and focus on self.

anticipatory Grieving may be related to perceived/actual or potential loss of physiopsychosocial well-being, personal possessions and significant other(s); as well as cultural beliefs about aging/debilitation, possibly evidenced by denial of feelings, depression, sorrow, guilt; alterations in activity level, sleep patterns, eating habits, and libido.

risk for Poisoning [drug toxicity]: risk factors may include effects of aging (reduced metabolism, impaired circulation, precarious physiologic balance, presence of multiple diseases/organ involvement) and use of multiple prescribed/OTC drugs.*

disturbed Thought Processes may be related to physiologic changes of aging (loss of cells and brain atrophy, decreased blood supply); altered sensory input, pain, effects of medications, and psychologic conflicts (disrupted life pattern), possibly evidenced by slower reaction times, memory loss, altered attention span, disorientation, inability to follow, altered sleep patterns, and personality changes.

disturbed Sleep Pattern may be related to internal factors (illness, psychologic stress, inactivity) and external factors (environmental changes, facility routines), possibly evidenced by reports of difficulty in falling asleep/not feeling rested, interrupted sleep/awakening earlier than desired; change in behavior/performance, increasing irritability, and listlessness.

risk for ineffective Sexuality Patterns: risk factors may include biopsychosocial alteration of sexuality; interference in psychological/physical well-being, self-image, and lack of privacy/SO.*

risk for Relocation Stress Syndrome: risk factors may include multiple losses, feeling of powerlessness, lack of/inappropriate use of support system, changes in psychosocial/physical health status.*

Lupus erythematosus, systemic (SLE) CH

Fatigue may be related to inadequate energy production/increased energy requirements (chronic inflammation), overwhelming psychologic or emotional demands, states of discomfort, and altered body chemistry (including effects of drug therapy), possibly evidenced by reports of unremitting and overwhelming lack of energy/inability to maintain usual routines, decreased performance, lethargy, and decreased libido.

acute Pain may be related to widespread inflammatory process affecting connective tissues, blood vessels, serosal surfaces and mucous membranes, possibly evidenced by verbal reports, guarding/distraction behaviors, self-focusing, and autonomic responses (changes in vital signs).

impaired Skin/Tissue Integrity may be related to chronic inflammation, edema formation, and altered circulation, possibly evidenced by presence of skin rash/lesions, ulcerations of mucous membranes and photosensitivity.

---

*A risk diagnosis is not evidenced by signs and symptoms, as the problem has not occurred and nursing interventions are directed at prevention.

<u>disturbed Body Image</u> may be related to presence of chronic condition with rash, lesions, ulcers, purpura, mottled erythema of hands, alopecia, loss of strength, and altered body function, possibly evidenced by hiding body parts, negative feelings about body, feelings of helplessness, and change in social involvement.

Lyme disease   CH/MS

<u>acute/chronic Pain</u> may be related to systemic effects of toxins, presence of rash, urticaria, and joint swelling/inflammation, possibly evidenced by verbal reports, guarding behaviors, autonomic responses, and narrowed focus.

<u>Fatigue</u> may be related to increased energy requirements, altered body chemistry, and states of discomfort evidenced by reports of overwhelming lack of energy/inability to maintain usual routines, decreased performance, lethargy, and malaise.

<u>risk for decreased Cardiac Output:</u> risk factors may include alteration in cardiac rate/rhythm/conduction.*

Macular degeneration   CH

<u>disturbed visual Sensory Perception</u> may be related to altered sensory reception possibly evidenced by reported/measured change in sensory acuity, change in usual response to stimuli.

<u>Anxiety [specify level]/Fear</u> may be related situational crisis, threat to or change in health status and role function possibly evidenced by expressed concerns, apprehension, feelings of inadequacy, diminished productivity, impaired attention.

<u>risk for impaired Home Maintenance:</u> risk factors may include impaired cognitive functioning, inadequate support systems.*

<u>risk for impaired Social Interaction:</u> risk factors may include limited physical mobility, environmental barriers.*

Mallory-Weiss syndrome   MS

(Also refer to Achalasia)

<u>risk for deficient Fluid Volume [isotonic]:</u> risk factors may include excessive vascular losses, presence of vomiting, and reduced intake.*

<u>deficient Knowledge [Learning Need] regarding causes, treatment, and prevention of condition</u> may be related to lack of information/misinterpretation, possibly evidenced by statements of concern, questions, and recurrence of problem.

Mastectomy   MS

<u>impaired Skin/Tissue Integrity</u> may be related to surgical removal of skin/tissue, altered circulation, drainage, presence of edema, changes in skin elasticity/sensation, and tissue destruction (radiation), possibly evidenced by disruption of skin surface and destruction of skin layers/subcutaneous tissues.

<u>impaired physical Mobility</u> may be related to neuromuscular impairment, pain, and edema formation, possibly evidenced by reluctance to attempt movement, limited range of motion, and decreased muscle mass/strength.

---

*A risk diagnosis is not evidenced by signs and symptoms, as the problem has not occurred and nursing interventions are directed at prevention.

bathing/dressing Self-Care Deficit may be related to temporary loss/altered action of one or both arms, possibly evidenced by statements of inability to perform/complete self-care tasks.

disturbed Body Image may be related to loss of body part denoting femininity, possibly evidenced by not looking at/touching area, negative feelings about body, preoccupation with loss, and change in social involvement/relationship.

Mastitis   OB/GYN

acute Pain may be related to erythema and edema of breast tissues, possibly evidenced by verbal reports, guarding/distraction behaviors, self-focusing, autonomic responses (changes in vital signs).

risk for Infection [spread/abscess formation]: risk factors may include traumatized tissues, stasis of fluids, and insufficient knowledge to prevent complications.*

deficient Knowledge [Learning Need] regarding pathophysiology, treatment, and prevention may be related to lack of information/misinterpretation, possibly evidenced by statements of concern, questions, and misconceptions.

risk for ineffective Breastfeeding: risk factors may include inability to feed on affected side/interruption in breastfeeding.*

Mastoidectomy   PED/MS

risk for Infection [spread]: risk factors may include preexisting infection, surgical trauma, and stasis of body fluids in close proximity to brain.*

acute Pain may be related to inflammation, tissue trauma, and edema formation, possibly evidenced by verbal reports, distraction behaviors, restlessness, self-focusing, and autonomic responses (changes in vital signs).

disturbed auditory Sensory Perception may be related to presence of surgical packing, edema, and surgical disturbance of middle ear structures, possibly evidenced by reported/tested hearing loss in affected ear.

Measles   CH/PED

acute Pain may be related to inflammation of mucous membranes, conjunctiva, and presence of extensive skin rash with pruritus, possibly evidenced by verbal reports, distraction behaviors, self-focusing, and autonomic responses (changes in vital signs).

Hyperthermia may be related to presence of viral toxins and inflammatory response, possibly evidenced by increased body temperature, flushed/warm skin, and tachycardia.

risk for [secondary] Infection: risk factors may include altered immune response and traumatized dermal tissues.*

deficient Knowledge [Learning Need] regarding condition, transmission, and possible complications may be related to lack of information/misinterpretation, possibly evidenced by statements of concern,

---

*A risk diagnosis is not evidenced by signs and symptoms, as the problem has not occurred and nursing interventions are directed at prevention.

questions, misconceptions, and development of preventable complications.

Melanoma, malignant   MS/CH
(Refer to Cancer; Chemotherapy)

Meningitis, acute meningococcal   MS
risk for Infection [spread]: risk factors may include hematogenous dissemination of pathogen, stasis of body fluids, suppressed inflammatory response (medication-induced), and exposure of others to pathogens.*

risk for ineffective cerebral Tissue Perfusion: risk factors may include cerebral edema altering/interrupting cerebral arterial/venous blood flow, hypovolemia, exchange problems at cellular level (acidosis).*

Hyperthermia may be related to infectious process (increased metabolic rate) and dehydration, possibly evidenced by increased body temperature, warm/flushed skin, and tachycardia.

acute Pain may be related to inflammation/irritation of the meninges with spasm of extensor muscles (neck, shoulders, and back), possibly evidenced by verbal reports, guarding/distraction behaviors, narrowed focus, photophobia, and autonomic responses (changes in vital signs).

risk for Trauma/Suffocation: risk factors may include alterations in level of consciousness, possible development of clonic/tonic muscle activity (seizures), and generalized weakness/prostration, ataxia, vertigo.*

Meniscectomy   MS/CH
impaired Walking may be related to pain, joint instability, and imposed medical restrictions of movement, possibly evidenced by impaired ability to move about environment as needed/desired.

deficient Knowledge [Learning Need] regarding postoperative expectations, prevention of complications, and self-care needs may be related to lack of information, possibly evidenced by statements of concern, questions, and misconceptions.

Menopause   GYN
ineffective Thermoregulation may be related to fluctuation of hormonal levels possibly evidenced by skin flushed/warm to touch, diaphoresis, night sweats; cold hands/feet.

Fatigue may be related to change in body chemistry, lack of sleep, depression possibly evidenced by reports of lack of energy, tired, inability to maintain usual routines, decreased performance.

risk for ineffective Sexuality Patterns: risk factors may include perceived altered body function, changes in physical response, myths/inaccurate information, impaired relationship with SO.*

risk for stress urinary Incontinence: risk factors may include degenerative changes in pelvic muscles and structural support.*

---

*A risk diagnosis is not evidenced by signs and symptoms, as the problem has not occurred and nursing interventions are directed at prevention.

Health-Seeking Behaviors: management of life cycle changes may be related to maturational change possibly evidenced by expressed desire for increased control of health practice, demonstrated lack of knowledge in health promotion.

Mental retardation — CH
(Also refer to Down syndrome)

impaired verbal Communication may be related to developmental delay/impairment of cognitive and motor abilities, possibly evidenced by impaired articulation, difficulty with phonation, and inability to modulate speech/find appropriate words (dependent on degree of retardation).

risk for Self-Care Deficit [specify]: risk factors may include impaired cognitive ability and motor skills.*

imbalanced Nutrition: risk for more than body requirements: risk factors may include decreased metabolic rate coupled with impaired cognitive development, dysfunctional eating patterns, and sedentary activity level.*

impaired Social Interaction may be related to impaired thought processes, communication barriers, and knowledge/skill deficit about ways to enhance mutuality, possibly evidenced by dysfunctional interactions with peers, family, and/or SO(s), and verbalized/observed discomfort in social situation.

compromised family Coping may be related to chronic nature of condition and degree of disability that exhausts supportive capacity of SO(s), other situational or developmental crises or situations SO(s) may be facing, unrealistic expectations of SO(s), possibly evidenced by preoccupation of SO with personal reaction, SO(s) withdraw(s) or enter(s) into limited interaction with individual, protective behavior disproportionate (too much or too little) to client's abilities or need for autonomy.

impaired Home Maintenance may be related to impaired cognitive functioning, insufficient finances/family organization or planning, lack of knowledge, and inadequate support systems, possibly evidenced by requests for assistance, expression of difficulty in maintaining home, disorderly surroundings, and overtaxed family members.

risk for Sexual dysfunction: risk factors may include biopsychosocial alteration of sexuality, ineffectual/absent role models, misinformation/lack of knowledge, lack of SO(s), and lack of appropriate behavior control.*

Miscarriage — OB
(Refer to Abortion, spontaneous termination)

Mitral stenosis — MS/CH
Activity Intolerance may be related to imbalance between O_2 supply and demand, possibly evidenced by reports of fatigue, weakness, exertional dyspnea, and tachycardia.

---

*A risk diagnosis is not evidenced by signs and symptoms, as the problem has not occurred and nursing interventions are directed at prevention.

<u>impaired Gas Exchange</u> may be related to altered blood flow, possibly evidenced by restlessness, hypoxia, and cyanosis (orthopnea/paroxysmal nocturnal dyspnea).

<u>decreased Cardiac Output</u> may be related to impeded blood flow as evidenced by jugular vein distention, peripheral/dependent edema, orthopnea/paroxysmal nocturnal dyspnea.

<u>deficient Knowledge [Learning Need] regarding pathophysiology, therapeutic needs, and potential complications</u> may be related to lack of information/recall, misinterpretation, possibly evidenced by statements of concern, questions, inaccurate follow-through of instructions, and development of preventable complications.

Mononucleosis, infectious CH

<u>Fatigue</u> may be related to decreased energy production, states of discomfort, and increased energy requirements (inflammatory process), possibly evidenced by reports of overwhelming lack of energy, inability to maintain usual routines, lethargy, and malaise.

<u>Pain/[Discomfort]</u> may be related to inflammation of lymphoid and organ tissues, irritation of oropharyngeal mucous membranes, and effects of circulating toxins, possibly evidenced by verbal reports, distraction behaviors, and self-focusing.

<u>Hyperthermia</u> may be related to inflammatory process, possibly evidenced by increased body temperature, warm/flushed skin, and tachycardia.

<u>deficient Knowledge [Learning Need] regarding disease transmission, self-care needs, medical therapy, and potential complications</u> may be related to lack of information/misinterpretation, possibly evidenced by statements of concern, misconceptions, and inaccurate follow-through of instructions.

Mood disorders PSY

(Refer to Depressive disorders)

Mountain sickness, acute (AMS) CH/MS

<u>acute Pain</u> may be related to reduced oxygen tension possibly evidenced by reports of headache.

<u>Fatigue</u> may be related to stress, increased physical exertion, sleep deprivation possibly evidenced by overwhelming lack of energy, inability to restore energy even after sleep, compromised concentration, decreased performance.

<u>risk for deficient Fluid Volume:</u> risk factors may include increased water loss (e.g., overbreathing dry air), exertion, altered fluid intake (nausea).*

Multiple personality PSY

(Refer to Dissociative disorders)

Multiple sclerosis CH

<u>Fatigue</u> may be related to decreased energy production/increased energy requirements to perform activities, psychological/emotional

---

*A risk diagnosis is not evidenced by signs and symptoms, as the problem has not occurred and nursing interventions are directed at prevention.

demands, pain/discomfort, medication side effects, possibly evidenced by verbalization of overwhelming lack of energy, inability to maintain usual routine, decreased performance, impaired ability to concentrate, increase in physical complaints.

disturbed visual, kinesthetic, tactile Sensory Perception may be related to delayed/interrupted neuronal transmission, possibly evidenced by impaired vision, diplopia, disturbance of vibratory or position sense, paresthesias, numbness, and blunting of sensation.

impaired physical Mobility may be related to neuromuscular impairment, discomfort/pain, sensoriperceptual impairments, decreased muscle strength, control and/or mass, deconditioning, as evidenced by limited ability to perform motor skills, limited range of motion, gait changes/postural instability.

Powerlessness/Hopelessness may be related to illness-related regimen and lifestyle of helplessness, possibly evidenced by verbal expressions of having no control or influence over the situation, depression over physical deterioration that occurs despite client compliance with regimen, nonparticipation in care or decision making when opportunities are provided, passivity, decreased verbalization/affect.

impaired Home Maintenance may be related to effects of debilitating disease, impaired cognitive and/or emotional functioning, insufficient finances, and inadequate support systems, possibly evidenced by reported difficulty, observed disorderly surroundings, and poor hygienic conditions.

compromised/disabled family Coping may be related to situational crises/temporary family disorganization and role changes, client providing little support in turn for SO(s), prolonged disease/disability progression that exhausts the supportive capacity of SO(s), feelings of guilt, anxiety, hostility, despair, and highly ambivalent family relationships, possibly evidenced by client expressing/confirming concern or report about SO(s) response to client's illness, SO(s) preoccupied with own personal reactions, intolerance, abandonment, neglectful care of the client, and distortion of reality regarding client's illness.

Mumps   PED/CH
acute Pain may be related to presence of inflammation, circulating toxins, and enlargement of salivary glands, possibly evidenced by verbal reports, guarding/distraction behaviors, self-focusing, and autonomic responses (changes in vital signs).

Hyperthermia may be related to inflammatory process (increased metabolic rate) and dehydration, possibly evidenced by increased body temperature, warm/flushed skin, and tachycardia.

risk for deficient Fluid Volume: risk factors may include hypermetabolic state and painful swallowing, with decreased intake.*

Muscular dystrophy (Duchenne's)   PED/CH
impaired physical Mobility may be related to musculoskeletal impairment/weakness, possibly evidenced by decreased muscle strength,

---

*A risk diagnosis is not evidenced by signs and symptoms, as the problem has not occurred and nursing interventions are directed at prevention.

control, and mass; limited range of motion; and impaired coordination.

delayed Growth and Development may be related to effects of physical disability, possibly evidenced by altered physical growth and altered ability to perform self-care/self-control activities appropriate to age.

risk for imbalanced Nutrition: more than body requirements: risk factors may include sedentary lifestyle and dysfunctional eating patterns.*

compromised family Coping may be related to situational crisis/emotional conflicts around issues about hereditary nature of condition and prolonged disease/disability that exhausts supportive capacity of family members, possibly evidenced by preoccupation with personal reactions regarding disability and displaying protective behavior disproportionate (too little/too much) to client's abilities/need for autonomy.

Myasthenia gravis   MS

ineffective Breathing Pattern/Airway Clearance may be related to neuromuscular weakness and decreased energy/fatigue, possibly evidenced by dyspnea, changes in rate/depth of respiration, ineffective cough, and adventitious breath sounds.

impaired verbal Communication may be related to neuromuscular weakness, fatigue, and physical barrier (intubation), possibly evidenced by facial weakness, impaired articulation, hoarseness, and inability to speak.

impaired Swallowing may be related to neuromuscular impairment of laryngeal/pharyngeal muscles and muscular fatigue, possibly evidenced by reported/observed difficulty swallowing, coughing/choking, and evidence of aspiration.

Anxiety [specify level]/Fear may be related to situational crisis, threat to self-concept, change in health/socioeconomic status or role function, separation from support systems, lack of knowledge, and inability to communicate, possibly evidenced by expressed concerns, increased tension, restlessness, apprehension, sympathetic stimulation, crying, focus on self, uncooperative behavior, withdrawal, anger, and noncommunication.

CH

deficient Knowledge [Learning Need] regarding drug therapy, potential for crisis (myasthenic or cholinergic) and self-care management may be related to inadequate information/misinterpretation, possibly evidenced by statements of concern, questions, and misconceptions; development of preventable complications.

impaired physical Mobility may be related to neuromuscular impairment, possibly evidenced by reports of progressive fatigability with repetitive/prolonged muscle use, impaired coordination, and decreased muscle strength/control.

*A risk diagnosis is not evidenced by signs and symptoms, as the problem has not occurred and nursing interventions are directed at prevention.

<u>disturbed visual Sensory Perception</u> may be related to neuromuscular impairment, possibly evidenced by visual distortions (diplopia) and motor incoordination.

Myeloma, multiple   MS/CH
(Also refer to Cancer)

<u>acute/chronic Pain</u> may be related to destruction of tissues/bone, side effects of therapy possibly evidenced by verbal or coded reports, guarding/protective behaviors, changes in appetite/weight, sleep; reduced interaction with others.

<u>impaired physical Mobility</u> may be related to loss of integrity of bone structure, pain, deconditioning, depressed mood possibly evidenced by verbalizations, limited range of motion, slowed movement, gait changes.

<u>risk for ineffective Protection</u>: risk factors may include presence of cancer, drug therapies, radiation treatments, inadequate nutrition.*

Myocardial infarction   MS
(Also refer to Myocarditis)

<u>acute Pain</u> may be related to ischemia of myocardial tissue, possibly evidenced by verbal reports, guarding/distraction behaviors (restlessness), facial mask of pain, self-focusing, and autonomic responses (diaphoresis, changes in vital signs).

<u>Anxiety [specify level]/Fear</u> may be related to threat of death, threat of change of health status/role functioning and lifestyle, interpersonal transmission/contagion, possibly evidenced by increased tension, fearful attitude, apprehension, expressed concerns/uncertainty, restlessness, sympathetic stimulation, and somatic complaints.

<u>risk for decreased Cardiac Output</u>: risk factors may include changes in rate and electrical conduction, reduced preload/increased SVR, and altered muscle contractility/depressant effects of some medications, infarcted/dyskinetic muscle, structural defects.*

Myocarditis   MS
(Also refer to Myocardial infarction)

<u>Activity Intolerance</u> may be related to imbalance in O_2 supply and demand (myocardial inflammation/damage) cardiac depressant effects of certain drugs, and enforced bedrest, possibly evidenced by reports of fatigue, exertional dyspnea, tachycardia/palpitations in response to activity, ECG changes/dysrhythmias, and generalized weakness.

<u>risk for decreased Cardiac Output</u>: risk factors may include degeneration of cardiac muscle.*

<u>deficient Knowledge [Learning Need] regarding pathophysiology of condition/outcomes, treatment, and self-care needs/lifestyle changes</u> may be related to lack of information/misinterpretation, possibly evidenced by statements of concern, misconceptions, inaccurate follow-through of instructions, and development of preventable complications.

*A risk diagnosis is not evidenced by signs and symptoms, as the problem has not occurred and nursing interventions are directed at prevention.

Myringotomy PED/MS
(Refer to Mastoidectomy)

Myxedema CH
(Also refer to Hypothyroidism)

disturbed Body Image may be related to change in structure/function (loss of hair/thickening of skin, masklike facial expression, enlarged tongue, menstrual and reproductive disturbances), possibly evidenced by negative feelings about body, feelings of helplessness, and change in social involvement.

imbalanced Nutrition: more than body requirements may be related to decreased metabolic rate and activity level, possibly evidenced by weight gain greater than ideal for height and frame.

risk for decreased Cardiac Output: risk factors may include altered electrical conduction and myocardial contractility.*

Neglect/Abuse CH/PSY
(Refer to Abuse; Battered child syndrome)

Neonatal, normal newborn PED
risk for impaired Gas Exchange: risk factors may include prenatal or intrapartal stressors, excess production of mucus, or cold stress.*

risk for imbalanced Body Temperature: risk factors may include large body surface in relation to mass, limited amounts of insulating subcutaneous fat, nonrenewable sources of brown fat and few white fat stores, thin epidermis with close proximity of blood vessels to the skin, inability to shiver, and movement from a warm uterine environment to a much cooler environment.*

risk for impaired parent/infant Attachment: risk factors may include developmental transition (gain of a family member), anxiety associated with the parent role, lack of privacy (intrusive family/visitors).*

risk for imbalanced Nutrition: less than body requirements: risk factors may include rapid metabolic rate, high-caloric requirement, increased insensible water losses through pulmonary and cutaneous routes, fatigue, and a potential for inadequate or depleted glucose stores.*

risk for Infection: risk factors may include inadequate secondary defenses (inadequate acquired immunity, e.g., deficiency of neutrophils and specific immunoglobulins), and inadequate primary defenses (e.g., environmental exposure, broken skin, traumatized tissues, decreased ciliary action).*

Neonatal, premature newborn PED
impaired Gas Exchange may be related to alveolar-capillary membrane changes (inadequate surfactant levels), altered blood flow (immaturity of pulmonary arteriole musculature), altered O_2 supply (immaturity of central nervous system and neuromuscular system, tracheobronchial obstruction), altered O_2-carrying capacity of blood (anemia), and cold stress, possibly evidenced by respiratory difficulties, inadequate oxygenation of tissues, and acidemia.

*A risk diagnosis is not evidenced by signs and symptoms, as the problem has not occurred and nursing interventions are directed at prevention.

ineffective Breathing Pattern may be related to immaturity of the respiratory center, poor positioning, drug-related depression and metabolic imbalances, decreased energy/fatigue, possibly evidenced by dyspnea, tachypnea, periods of apnea, nasal flaring/use of accessory muscles, cyanosis, abnormal ABGs, and tachycardia.

risk for ineffective Thermoregulation: risk factors may include immature CNS development (temperature regulation center), decreased ratio of body mass to surface area, decreased subcutaneous fat, limited brown fat stores, inability to shiver or sweat, poor metabolic reserves, muted response to hypothermia, and frequent medical/nursing manipulations and interventions.*

risk for deficit Fluid Volume: risk factors may include extremes of age and weight, excessive fluid losses (thin skin, lack of insulating fat, increased environmental temperature, immature kidney/failure to concentrate urine).*

risk for disorganized Infant Behavior: risk factors may include prematurity (immaturity of CNS system, hypoxia), lack of containment/boundaries, pain, overstimulation, separation from parents.*

Nephrectomy   MS

acute Pain may be related to surgical tissue trauma with mechanical closure (suture), possibly evidenced by verbal reports, guarding/distraction behaviors, self-focusing, and autonomic responses (changes in vital signs).

risk for deficient Fluid Volume: risk factors may include excessive vascular losses and restricted intake.*

ineffective Breathing Pattern may be related to incisional pain with decreased lung expansion, possibly evidenced by tachypnea, fremitus, changes in respiratory depth/chest expansion, and changes in ABGs.

Constipation may be related to reduced dietary intake, decreased mobility, GI obstruction (paralytic ileus), and incisional pain with defecation, possibly evidenced by decreased bowel sounds, reduced frequency/amount of stool, and hard/formed stool.

Nephrolithiasis   MS/CH

(Refer to Calculi, urinary)

Nephrotic syndrome   MS/CH

excess Fluid Volume may be related to compromised regulatory mechanism with changes in hydrostatic/oncotic vascular pressure and increased activation of the renin-angiotensin-aldosterone system, possibly evidenced by edema/anasarca, effusions/ascites, weight gain, intake greater than output, and BP changes.

imbalanced Nutrition: less than body requirements may be related to excessive protein losses and inability to ingest adequate nutrients (anorexia), possibly evidenced by weight loss/muscle wasting (may be difficult to assess due to edema), lack of interest in food, and observed inadequate intake.

risk for Infection: risk factors may include chronic disease and steroidal suppression of inflammatory responses.*

*A risk diagnosis is not evidenced by signs and symptoms, as the problem has not occurred and nursing interventions are directed at prevention.

risk for impaired Skin Integrity: risk factors may include presence of edema and activity restrictions.*

Neuralgia, trigeminal   CH
acute Pain may be related to neuromuscular impairment with sudden violent muscle spasm, possibly evidenced by verbal reports, guarding/distraction behaviors, self-focusing, and autonomic responses (changes in vital signs).
deficient Knowledge [Learning Need] regarding control of recurrent episodes, medical therapies, and self-care needs may be related to lack of information/recall and misinterpretation, possibly evidenced by statements of concern, questions, and exacerbation of condition.

Neuritis   CH
acute/chronic Pain may be related to nerve damage usually associated with a degenerative process, possibly evidenced by verbal reports, guarding/distraction behaviors, self-focusing, and autonomic responses (changes in vital signs).
deficient Knowledge [Learning Need] regarding underlying causative factors, treatment, and prevention may be related to lack of information/misinterpretation, possibly evidenced by statements of concern, questions, and misconceptions.

Obesity   CH/PSY
imbalanced Nutrition: more than body requirements may be related to excessive intake in relation to metabolic needs, possibly evidenced by weight 20% greater than ideal for height and frame, sedentary activity level, reported/observed dysfunctional eating patterns, and excess body fat by triceps skinfold/other measurements.
disturbed Body Image/chronic low Self-Esteem may be related to view of self in contrast to societal values, family/subcultural encouragement of overeating; control, sex, and love issues; possibly evidenced by negative feelings about body, fear of rejection/reaction of others, feeling of hopelessness/powerlessness, and lack of follow-through with treatment plan.
Activity Intolerance may be related to imbalance between oxygen supply and demand, and sedentary lifestyle, possibly evidenced by fatigue or weakness, exertional discomfort, and abnormal heart rate/BP response.
impaired Social Interaction may be related to verbalized/observed discomfort in social situations, self-concept disturbance, possibly evidenced by reluctance to participate in social gatherings, verbalization of a sense of discomfort with others, feelings of rejection, absence of/ineffective supportive SO(s).

Opioid abuse   CH/PSY
(Refer to Depressant abuse)

Organic brain syndrome   CH
(Refer to Alzheimer's disease)

---

*A risk diagnosis is not evidenced by signs and symptoms, as the problem has not occurred and nursing interventions are directed at prevention.

Osteoarthritis (degenerative joint disease)　　　CH

(Refer to Arthritis, rheumatoid)

(Although this is a degenerative process versus the inflammatory process of rheumatoid arthritis, nursing concerns are the same.)

Osteomyelitis　　　MS/CH

acute Pain may be related to inflammation and tissue necrosis, possibly evidenced by verbal reports, guarding/distraction behaviors, self-focus, and autonomic responses (changes in vital signs).

Hyperthermia may be related to increased metabolic rate and infectious process, possibly evidenced by increased body temperature and warm/flushed skin.

ineffective bone Tissue Perfusion may be related to inflammatory reaction with thrombosis of vessels, destruction of tissue, edema, and abscess formation, possibly evidenced by bone necrosis, continuation of infectious process, and delayed healing.

risk for impaired Walking: risk factors may include inflammation and tissue necrosis, pain, joint instability.*

deficient Knowledge [Learning Need] regarding pathophysiology of condition, long-term therapy needs, activity restriction, and prevention of complications may be related to lack of information/misinterpretation, possibly evidenced by statements of concern, questions, and misconceptions, and inaccurate follow-through of instructions.

Osteoporosis　　　CH

risk for Trauma: risk factors may include loss of bone density/integrity increasing risk of fracture with minimal or no stress.*

acute/chronic Pain may be related to vertebral compression on spinal nerve/muscles/ligaments, spontaneous fractures, possibly evidenced by verbal reports, guarding/distraction behaviors, self-focus, and changes in sleep pattern.

impaired physical Mobility may be related to pain and musculoskeletal impairment, possibly evidenced by limited range of motion, reluctance to attempt movement/expressed fear of reinjury, and imposed restrictions/limitations.

Palsy, cerebral (spastic hemiplegia)　　　PED/CH

impaired physical Mobility may be related to muscular weakness/hypertonicity, increased deep tendon reflexes, tendency to contractures, and underdevelopment of affected limbs, possibly evidenced by decreased muscle strength, control, mass; limited range of motion, and impaired coordination.

compromised family Coping may be related to permanent nature of condition, situational crisis, emotional conflicts/temporary family disorganization, and incomplete information/understanding of client's needs, possibly evidenced by verbalized anxiety/guilt regarding client's disability, inadequate understanding and knowledge base,

---

*A risk diagnosis is not evidenced by signs and symptoms, as the problem has not occurred and nursing interventions are directed at prevention.

and displaying protective behaviors disproportionate (too little/too much) to client's abilities or need for autonomy.

delayed Growth and Development may be related to effects of physical disability, possibly evidenced by altered physical growth, delay or difficulty in performing skills (motor, social, expressive), and altered ability to perform self-care/self-control activities appropriate to age.

Pancreatitis   MS

acute Pain may be related to obstruction of pancreatic/biliary ducts, chemical contamination of peritoneal surfaces by pancreatic exudate/autodigestion, extension of inflammation to the retroperitoneal nerve plexus, possibly evidenced by verbal reports, guarding/distraction behaviors, self-focusing, grimacing, autonomic responses (changes in vital signs), and alteration in muscle tone.

risk for deficient Fluid Volume: risk factors may include excessive gastric losses (vomiting, nasogastric suctioning), increase in size of vascular bed (vasodilation, effects of kinins), third-space fluid transudation, ascites formation, alteration of clotting process, hemorrhage.*

imbalanced Nutrition: less than body requirements may be related to vomiting, decreased oral intake as well as altered ability to digest nutrients (loss of digestive enzymes/insulin), possibly evidenced by reported inadequate food intake, aversion to eating, reported altered taste sensation, weight loss, and reduced muscle mass.

risk for Infection: risk factors may include inadequate primary defenses (stasis of body fluids, altered peristalsis, change in pH secretions), immunosuppression, nutritional deficiencies, tissue destruction, and chronic disease.*

Paranoid personality disorder   PSY

risk for other/self-directed Violence: risk factors may include perceived threats of danger, paranoid delusions, and increased feelings of anxiety.*

[severe] Anxiety may be related to inability to trust (has not mastered tasks of trust versus mistrust), possibly evidenced by rigid delusional system (serves to provide relief from stress that justifies the delusion), frightened of other people and own hostility.

Powerlessness may be related to feelings of inadequacy, lifestyle of helplessness, maladaptive interpersonal interactions (e.g., misuse of power, force; abusive relationships), sense of severely impaired self-concept, and belief that individual has no control over situation(s), possibly evidenced by paranoid delusions, use of aggressive behavior to compensate, and expressions of recognition of damage paranoia has caused self and others.

disturbed Thought Processes may be related to psychologic conflicts, increased anxiety, and fear, possibly evidenced by difficulties in the process and character of thought, interference with the ability to think clearly and logically, delusions, fragmentation, and autistic thinking.

*A risk diagnosis is not evidenced by signs and symptoms, as the problem has not occurred and nursing interventions are directed at prevention.

<u>compromised family Coping</u> may be related to temporary or sustained family disorganization/role changes, prolonged progression of condition that exhausts the supportive capacity of SO(s), possibly evidenced by family system not meeting physical/emotional/spiritual needs of its members, inability to express or to accept wide range of feelings, inappropriate boundary maintenance; SO(s) describe(s) preoccupation with personal reactions.

Paraplegia   MS/CH

(Also refer to Quadriplegia)

<u>impaired Transfer Ability</u> may be related to loss of muscle function/control, injury to upper extremity joints (overuse).

<u>disturbed kinesthetic/tactile Sensory Perception:</u> may be related to neurologic deficit with loss of sensory reception and transmission, psychologic stress, possibly evidenced by reported/measured change in sensory acuity and loss of usual response to stimuli.

<u>reflex urinary Incontinence/impaired Urinary Elimination</u> may be related to loss of nerve conduction above the level of the reflex arc, possibly evidenced by lack of awareness of bladder filling/fullness, absence of urge to void, uninhibited bladder contraction, urinary tract infections—UTIs, kidney stone formation.

<u>disturbed Body Image/ineffective Role Performance</u> may be related to loss of body functions, change in physical ability to resume role, perceived loss of self/identity, possibly evidenced by negative feelings about body/self, feelings of helplessness/powerlessness, delay in taking responsibility for self-care/participation in therapy, and change in social involvement.

<u>Sexual Dysfunction</u> may be related to loss of sensation, altered function, and vulnerability, possibly evidenced by seeking of confirmation of desirability, verbalization of concern, alteration in relationship with SO, and change in interest in self/others.

Parathyroidectomy   MS

<u>acute Pain</u> may be related to presence of surgical incision and effects of calcium imbalance (bone pain, tetany), possibly evidenced by verbal reports, guarding/distraction behaviors, self-focus, and autonomic responses (changes in vital signs).

<u>risk for excess Fluid Volume:</u> risk factors may include preoperative renal involvement, stress-induced release of ADH, and changing calcium/electrolyte levels.*

<u>risk for ineffective Airway Clearance:</u> risk factors may include edema formation and laryngeal nerve damage.*

<u>deficient Knowledge [Learning Need] regarding postoperative care/ complications and long-term needs</u> may be related to lack of information/recall, misinterpretation, possibly evidenced by statements of concern, questions, and misconceptions.

Parkinson's disease   CH

<u>impaired Walking</u> may be related to neuromuscular impairment (muscle weakness, tremors, bradykinesia) and musculoskeletal

---

*A risk diagnosis is not evidenced by signs and symptoms, as the problem has not occurred and nursing interventions are directed at prevention.

impairment (joint rigidity), possibly evidenced by inability to move about the environment as desired, increased occurrence of falls.

impaired Swallowing may be related to neuromuscular impairment/ muscle weakness, possibly evidenced by reported/observed difficulty in swallowing, drooling, evidence of aspiration (choking, coughing).

impaired verbal Communication may be related to muscle weakness and incoordination, possibly evidenced by impaired articulation, difficulty with phonation, and changes in rhythm and intonation.

Caregiver Role Strain may be related to illness, severity of care receiver, psychologic/cognitive problems in care receiver, caregiver is spouse, duration of caregiving required, lack of respite/recreation for care- giver, possibly evidenced by feeling stressed, depressed, worried; lack of resources/support, family conflict.

Pelvic inflammatory disease   OB/GYN/CH

risk for Infection [spread]: risk factors may include presence of infec- tious process in highly vascular pelvic structures, delay in seeking treatment.*

acute Pain may be related to inflammation, edema, and congestion of reproductive/pelvic tissues, possibly evidenced by verbal reports, guarding/distraction behaviors, self-focus, and autonomic responses (changes in vital signs).

Hyperthermia may be related to inflammatory process/hypermetabolic state, possibly evidenced by increased body temperature, warm/ flushed skin, and tachycardia.

risk for situational low Self-Esteem: risk factors may include perceived stigma of physical condition (infection of reproductive system).*

deficient Knowledge [Learning Need] regarding cause/complications of condition, therapy needs, and transmission of disease to others may be related to lack of information/misinterpretation, possibly evidenced by statements of concern, questions, misconceptions, and development of preventable complications.

Periarteritis nodosa   MS/CH

(Refer to Polyarteritis [nodosa])

Pericarditis   MS

acute Pain may be related to tissue inflammation and presence of effu- sion, possibly evidenced by verbal reports of pain affected by move- ment/position, guarding/distraction behaviors, self-focus, and autonomic responses (changes in vital signs).

Activity Intolerance may be related to imbalance between O_2 supply and demand (restriction of cardiac filling/ventricular contraction, reduced cardiac output), possibly evidenced by reports of weakness/ fatigue, exertional dyspnea, abnormal heart rate or BP response, and signs of heart failure.

risk for decreased Cardiac Output: risk factors may include accumula- tion of fluid (effusion) restricted cardiac filling/contractility.*

Anxiety [specify level] may be related to change in health status and

---

*A risk diagnosis is not evidenced by signs and symptoms, as the problem has not occurred and nursing interventions are directed at prevention.

perceived threat of death, possibly evidenced by increased tension, apprehension, restlessness, and expressed concerns.

Perinatal loss/death of child   OB/CH

Grieving [expected] may be related to death of fetus/infant possibly evidenced by verbal expressions of distress, anger, loss, guilt; crying, change in eating habits/sleep.

situational low Self-Esteem may be related to perceived failure at a life event, inability to meet personal expectations possibly evidenced by negative self-appraisal in response to situation/personal actions, expressions of helplessness/hopelessness, evaluation of self as unable to deal with situation.

risk for ineffective Role Performance: risk factors may include stress, family conflict, inadequate support system.*

risk for interrupted Family Processes: risk factors may include situational crisis, developmental transition [loss of child], family roles shift.*

risk for Spiritual Distress: risk factors may include blame for loss directed at self/God, intense suffering, alienation from other/support systems.*

Peripheral arterial occlusive disease   CH

(Refer to Arterial occlusive disease)

Peripheral vascular disease (atherosclerosis)   CH

ineffective peripheral Tissue Perfusion may be related to reduction or interruption of arterial/venous blood flow, possibly evidenced by changes in skin temperature/color, lack of hair growth, BP/pulse changes in extremity, presence of bruits, and reports of claudication.

Activity Intolerance may be related to imbalance between O_2 supply and demand, possibly evidenced by reports of muscle fatigue/weakness and exertional discomfort (claudication).

risk for impaired Skin/Tissue Integrity: risk factors may include altered circulation with decreased sensation and impaired healing.*

Peritonitis   MS

risk for Infection [spread/septicemia]: risk factors may include inadequate primary defenses (broken skin, traumatized tissue, altered peristalsis), inadequate secondary defenses (immunosuppression), and invasive procedures.*

deficient Fluid Volume [mixed] may be related to fluid shifts from extracellular, intravascular, and interstitial compartments into intestines and/or peritoneal space, excessive gastric losses (vomiting, diarrhea, NG suction), hypermetabolic state, and restricted intake, possibly evidenced by dry mucous membranes, poor skin turgor, delayed capillary refill, weak peripheral pulses, diminished urinary output, dark/concentrated urine, hypotension, and tachycardia.

---

*A risk diagnosis is not evidenced by signs and symptoms, as the problem has not occurred and nursing interventions are directed at prevention.

acute Pain may be related to chemical irritation of parietal peritoneum, trauma to tissues, accumulation of fluid in abdominal/peritoneal cavity, possibly evidenced by verbal reports, muscle guarding/rebound tenderness, distraction behaviors, facial mask of pain, self-focus, autonomic responses (changes in vital signs).

risk for imbalanced Nutrition: less than body requirements: risk factors may include nausea/vomiting, intestinal dysfunction, metabolic abnormalities, increased metabolic needs.*

Pheochromocytoma   MS

Anxiety [specify level] may be related to excessive physiologic (hormonal) stimulation of the sympathetic nervous system, situational crises, threat to/change in health status, possibly evidenced by apprehension, shakiness, restlessness, focus on self, fearfulness, diaphoresis, and sense of impending doom.

deficient Fluid Volume [mixed] may be related to excessive gastric losses (vomiting/diarrhea), hypermetabolic state, diaphoresis, and hyperosmolar diuresis, possibly evidenced by hemoconcentration, dry mucous membranes, poor skin turgor, thirst, and weight loss.

decreased Cardiac Output/ineffective Tissue Perfusion (specify) may be related to altered preload/decreased blood volume, altered SVR, and increased sympathetic activity (excessive secretion of catecholamines), possibly evidenced by cool/clammy skin, change in BP (hypertension/postural hypotension), visual disturbances, severe headache, and angina.

deficient Knowledge [Learning Need] regarding pathophysiology of condition, outcome, preoperative and postoperative care needs may be related to lack of information/recall, possibly evidenced by statements of concern, questions, and misconceptions.

Phlebitis   CH
(Refer to Thrombophlebitis)

Phobia   PSY
(Also refer to Anxiety disorder, generalized)

Fear may be related to learned irrational response to natural or innate origins (phobic stimulus), unfounded morbid dread of a seemingly harmless object/situation, possibly evidenced by sympathetic stimulation and reactions ranging from apprehension to panic, withdrawal from/total avoidance of situations that place individual in contact with feared object.

impaired Social Interaction may be related to intense fear of encountering feared object/activity or situation and anticipated loss of control, possibly evidenced by reported change of style/pattern of interaction, discomfort in social situations, and avoidance of phobic stimulus.

Placenta previa   OB
risk for deficient Fluid Volume: risk factors may include excessive vascular losses (vessel damage and inadequate vasoconstriction).*

---

*A risk diagnosis is not evidenced by signs and symptoms, as the problem has not occurred and nursing interventions are directed at prevention.

impaired fetal Gas Exchange: may be related to altered blood flow, altered oxygen carrying capacity of blood (maternal anemia), and decreased surface area of gas exchange at site of placental attachment, possibly evidenced by changes in fetal heart rate/activity and release of meconium.

Fear may be related to threat of death (perceived or actual) to self or fetus, possibly evidenced by verbalization of specific concerns, increased tension, sympathetic stimulation.

risk for deficient Diversional Activity: risk factors may include imposed activity restrictions/bedrest.*

Pleurisy   CH

acute Pain may be related to inflammation/irritation of the parietal pleura, possibly evidenced by verbal reports, guarding/distraction behaviors, self-focus, and autonomic responses (changes in vital signs).

ineffective Breathing Pattern may be related to pain on inspiration, possibly evidenced by decreased respiratory depth, tachypnea, and dyspnea.

risk for Infection, [pneumonia]: risk factors may include stasis of pulmonary secretions, decreased lung expansion, and ineffective cough.*

Pneumonia   CH/MS
(Refer to Bronchitis; Bronchopneumonia)

Pneumothorax   MS
(Also refer to Hemothorax)

ineffective Breathing Pattern may be related to decreased lung expansion (fluid/air accumulation), musculoskeletal impairment, pain, inflammatory process, possibly evidenced by dyspnea, tachypnea, altered chest excursion, respiratory depth changes, use of accessory muscles/nasal flaring, cough, cyanosis, and abnormal ABGs.

risk for decreased Cardiac Output: risk factors may include compression/displacement of cardiac structures.*

acute Pain may be related to irritation of nerve endings within pleural space by foreign object (chest tube), possibly evidenced by verbal reports, guarding/distraction behaviors, self-focus, and autonomic responses (changes in vital signs).

Polyarteritis (nodosa)   MS/CH

ineffective Tissue Perfusion (specify) may be related to reduction/interruption of blood flow, possibly evidenced by organ tissue infarctions, changes in organ function, and development of organic psychosis.

Hyperthermia may be related to widespread inflammatory process, possibly evidenced by increased body temperature and warm/flushed skin.

acute Pain may be related to inflammation, tissue ischemia, and necrosis of affected area, possibly evidenced by verbal reports, guarding/distraction behaviors, self-focus, and autonomic responses (changes in vital signs).

*A risk diagnosis is not evidenced by signs and symptoms, as the problem has not occurred and nursing interventions are directed at prevention.

<u>anticipatory Grieving</u> may be related to perceived loss of self, possibly evidenced by expressions of sorrow and anger, altered sleep and/or eating patterns, changes in activity level, and libido.

Polycythemia vera   CH

<u>Activity Intolerance</u> may be related to imbalance between O_2 supply and demand, possibly evidenced by reports of fatigue/weakness.

<u>ineffective Tissue Perfusion (specify)</u> may be related to reduction/interruption of arterial/venous blood flow (insufficiency, thrombosis, or hemorrhage), possibly evidenced by pain in affected area, impaired mental ability, visual disturbances, and color changes of skin/mucous membranes.

Polyradiculitis   MS

(Refer to Guillain-Barré syndrome)

Postoperative recovery period   MS

<u>ineffective Breathing Pattern</u> may be related to neuromuscular and perceptual/cognitive impairment, decreased lung expansion/energy, and tracheobronchial obstruction, possibly evidenced by changes in respiratory rate and depth, reduced vital capacity, apnea, cyanosis, and noisy respirations.

<u>risk for imbalanced Body Temperature:</u> risk factors may include exposure to cool environment, effect of medications/anesthetic agents, extremes of age/weight, and dehydration.*

<u>disturbed Sensory Perception (specify)/disturbed Thought Processes</u> may be related to chemical alteration (use of pharmaceutical agents, hypoxia), therapeutically restricted environment, excessive sensory stimuli and physiologic stress, possibly evidenced by changes in usual response to stimuli, motor incoordination; impaired ability to concentrate, reason, and make decisions; and disorientation to person, place, and time.

<u>risk for deficit Fluid Volume:</u> risk factors may include restriction of oral intake, loss of fluid through abnormal routes (indwelling tubes, drains) and normal routes (vomiting, loss of vascular integrity, changes in clotting ability), extremes of age and weight.*

<u>acute Pain</u> may be related to disruption of skin, tissue, and muscle integrity, musculoskeletal/bone trauma, and presence of tubes and drains, possibly evidenced by verbal reports, alteration in muscle tone, facial mask of pain, distraction/guarding behaviors, narrowed focus, and autonomic responses.

<u>impaired Skin/Tissue Integrity</u> may be related to mechanical interruption of skin/tissues, altered circulation, effects of medication, accumulation of drainage, and altered metabolic state, possibly evidenced by disruption of skin surface/layers and tissues.

<u>risk for Infection:</u> risk factors may include broken skin, traumatized tissues, stasis of body fluids, presence of pathogens/contaminants, environmental exposure, and invasive procedures.*

*A risk diagnosis is not evidenced by signs and symptoms, as the problem has not occurred and nursing interventions are directed at prevention.

risk for impaired parent/infant Attachment/Parenting: risk factors may include lack of support between/from SO(s), ineffective or no role model, anxiety associated with the parental role, unrealistic expectations, presence of stressors (e.g., financial, housing, employment).*

risk for deficient Fluid Volume: risk factors may include excessive blood loss during delivery, reduced intake/inadequate replacement, nausea/vomiting, increased urine output, and insensible losses.*

acute Pain/[Discomfort] may be related to tissue trauma/edema, muscle contractions, bladder fullness, and physical/psychological exhaustion, possibly evidenced by reports of cramping (afterpains), self-focusing, alteration in muscle tone, distraction behaviors, and autonomic responses (changes in vital signs).

impaired Urinary Elimination may be related to hormonal effects (fluid shifts/continued elevation in renal plasma flow), mechanical trauma/tissue edema, and effects of medication/anesthesia, possibly evidenced by frequency, dysuria, urgency, incontinence, or retention.

Constipation may be related to decreased muscle tone associated with diastasis recti, prenatal effects of progesterone, dehydration, excess analgesia or anesthesia, pain (hemorrhoids, episiotomy, or perineal tenderness), prelabor diarrhea and lack of intake, possibly evidenced by frequency less than usual pattern, hard-formed stool, straining at stool, decreased bowel sounds, and abdominal distention.

disturbed Sleep Pattern may be related to pain/discomfort, intense exhilaration/excitement, anxiety, exhausting process of labor/delivery, and needs/demands of family members, possibly evidenced by verbal reports of difficulty in falling asleep/not feeling well-rested, interrupted sleep, frequent yawning, irritability, dark circles under eyes.

Post-traumatic stress disorder **PSY**

Post-Trauma Syndrome related to having experienced a traumatic life event, possibly evidenced by reexperiencing the event, somatic reactions, psychic/emotional numbness, altered lifestyle, impaired sleep, self-destructive behaviors, difficulty with interpersonal relationships, development of phobia, poor impulse control/irritability, and explosiveness.

risk for other-directed Violence: risk factors may include startle reaction, an intrusive memory causing a sudden acting out of a feeling as if the event were occurring; use of alcohol/other drugs to ward off painful effects and produce psychic numbing, breaking through the rage that has been walled of, response to intense anxiety or panic state, and loss of control.*

ineffective Coping may be related to personal vulnerability, inadequate support systems, unrealistic perceptions, unmet expectations, overwhelming threat to self, and multiple stressors repeated over a period of time, possibly evidenced by verbalization of inability to cope or difficulty asking for help, muscular tension/headaches, chronic worry, and emotional tension.

*A risk diagnosis is not evidenced by signs and symptoms, as the problem has not occurred and nursing interventions are directed at prevention.

dysfunctional Grieving may be related to actual/perceived object loss (loss of self as seen before the traumatic incident occurred as well as other losses incurred in/after the incident), loss of physiopsychosocial well-being, thwarted grieving response to a loss, and lack of resolution of previous grieving responses, possibly evidenced by verbal expression of distress at loss, anger, sadness, labile affect; alterations in eating habits, sleep/dream patterns, libido; reliving of past experiences, expression of guilt, and alterations in concentration.

interrupted Family Processes may be related to situational crisis, failure to master developmental transitions, possibly evidenced by expressions of confusion about what to do and that family is having difficulty coping, family system not meeting physical/emotional/spiritual needs of its members, not adapting to change or dealing with traumatic experience constructively, and ineffective family decision-making process.

Pregnancy (prenatal period) 1st trimester   OB/CH

risk for imbalanced Nutrition: less than body requirements: risk factors may include changes in appetite, insufficient intake (nausea/vomiting, inadequate financial resources and nutritional knowledge); meeting increased metabolic demands (increased thyroid activity associated with the growth of fetal and maternal tissues).*

[Discomfort]/acute Pain may be related to hormonal influences, physical changes, possibly evidenced by verbal reports (nausea, breast changes, leg cramps, hemorrhoids, nasal stuffiness), alteration in muscle tone, restlessness, and autonomic responses (changes in vital signs).

risk for fetal Injury: risk factors may include environmental/hereditary factors and problems of maternal well-being that directly affect the developing fetus (e.g., malnutrition, substance use).*

[maximally compensated] Cardiac Output may be related to increased fluid volume/maximal cardiac effort and hormonal effects of progesterone and relaxin (places the client at risk for hypertension and/or circulatory failure), and changes in peripheral resistance (afterload), possibly evidenced by variations in BP and pulse, syncopal episodes, presence of pathological edema.

readiness for enhanced family Coping may be related to situational/maturational crisis with anticipated changes in family structure/roles, needs sufficiently met and adaptive tasks effectively addressed to enable goals of self-actualization to surface, as evidenced by movement toward health-promoting and enriching lifestyle, choosing experiences that optimize pregnancy experience/wellness.

risk for Constipation: risk factors may include changes in dietary/fluid intake, smooth muscle relaxation, decreased peristalsis, and effects of medications (e.g., iron).*

Fatigue/disturbed Sleep Pattern may be related to increased carbohydrate metabolism, altered body chemistry, increased energy requirements to perform ADLs, discomfort, anxiety, inactivity,

---

*A risk diagnosis is not evidenced by signs and symptoms, as the problem has not occurred and nursing interventions are directed at prevention.

possibly evidenced by reports of overwhelming lack of energy/ inability to maintain usual routines, difficulty falling asleep/not feeling well-rested, interrupted sleep, irritability, lethargy, and frequent yawning.

risk for ineffective Role Performance: risk factors may include maturational crisis, developmental level, history of maladaptive coping, absence of support systems.*

deficient Knowledge [Learning Need] regarding normal physiologic/ psychologic changes and self-care needs may be related to lack of information/recall and misinterpretation of normal physiologic/ psychologic changes and their impact on the client/family, possibly evidenced by questions, statements of concern, misconceptions and inaccurate follow-through of instructions/development of preventable complications.

Pregnancy (prenatal period) 2nd trimester   OB/CH
(Also refer to Pregnancy 1st trimester)

risk for disturbed Body Image: risk factors may include perception of biophysical changes, response of others.*

ineffective Breathing Pattern may be related to impingement of the diaphragm by enlarging uterus possibly evidenced by reports of shortness of breath, dyspnea, and changes in respiratory depth.

risk for [decompensated] Cardiac Output: risk factors may include increased circulatory demand, changes in preload (decreased venous return) and afterload (increased peripheral vascular resistance), and ventricular hypertrophy.*

risk for excess Fluid Volume: risk factors may include changes in regulatory mechanisms, sodium/water retention.

ineffective Sexuality Patterns may be related to conflict regarding changes in sexual desire and expectations, fear of physical injury to woman/fetus possibly evidenced by reported difficulties, limitations or changes in sexual behaviors/activities.

Pregnancy (prenatal period) 3rd trimester   OB/CH
(Also refer to Pregnancy 1st and 2nd trimester)

deficient Knowledge [Learning Need] regarding preparation for labor/delivery, infant care may be related to lack of exposure/ experience, misinterpretations of information possibly evidenced by request for information, statement of concerns/misconceptions.

impaired Urinary Elimination may be related to uterine enlargement, increased abdominal pressure, fluctuation of renal blood flow, and glomerular filtration rate (GFR) possibly evidenced by urinary frequency, urgency, dependent edema.

risk for ineffective [individual/] family Coping: risk factors may include situational/maturational crisis, personal vulnerability, unrealistic perceptions, absent/insufficient support systems.*

risk for maternal Injury: risk factors may include presence of hypertension, infection, substance use/abuse, altered immune system, abnormal blood profile, tissue hypoxia, premature rupture of membranes.*

---

*A risk diagnosis is not evidenced by signs and symptoms, as the problem has not occurred and nursing interventions are directed at prevention.

Pregnancy, adolescent   OB/CH

(Also refer to Pregnancy, prenatal period)

interrupted Family Processes may be related to situational/developmental transition (economic, change in roles/gain of a family member), possibly evidenced by family expressing confusion about what to do, unable to meet physical/emotional/spiritual needs of the members, family inability to adapt to change or to deal with traumatic experience constructively; does not demonstrate respect for individuality and autonomy of its members, ineffective family decision-making process, and inappropriate boundary maintenance.

Social Isolation may be related to alterations in physical appearance, perceived unacceptable social behavior, restricted social sphere, stage of adolescence, and interference with accomplishing developmental tasks, possibly evidenced by expressions of feelings of aloneness/rejection/difference from others, uncommunicative, withdrawn, no eye contact, seeking to be alone, unacceptable behavior, and absence of supportive SO(s).

disturbed Body Image/situational/chronic low Self-Esteem may be related to situational/maturational crisis, biophysical changes, and fear of failure at life events, absence of support systems, possibly evidenced by self-negating verbalizations, expressions of shame/guilt, fear of rejection/reaction of other, hypersensitivity to criticism, and lack of follow-through/nonparticipation in prenatal care.

deficient Knowledge [Learning Need] regarding pregnancy, developmental/individual needs, future expectations may be related to lack of exposure, information misinterpretation, unfamiliarity with information resources, lack of interest in learning, possibly evidenced by questions, statement of concern/misconception, sense of vulnerability/denial of reality, inaccurate follow-through of instruction, and development of preventable complications.

risk for impaired Parenting: may be related to chronological age/developmental stage, unmet social/emotional/maturational needs of parenting figures, unrealistic expectation of self/infant/partner, ineffective role model/social support, lack of role identity, and presence of stressors (e.g., financial, social).*

Pregnancy, high-risk   OB/CH

(Also refer to Pregnancy 1st, 2nd, 3rd trimester)

Anxiety [specify level] may be related to situational crisis, threat of maternal/fetal death (perceived or actual), interpersonal transmission/contagion possibly evidenced by increased tension, apprehension, feelings of inadequacy, somatic complaints, difficulty sleeping.

deficient Knowledge [Learning Need] regarding high-risk situation/preterm labor may be related to lack of exposure to/misinterpretation of information, unfamiliarity with individual risks and own role in risk prevention/management possibly evidenced by request for information, statement of concerns/misconceptions, inaccurate follow-through of instructions.

---

*A risk diagnosis is not evidenced by signs and symptoms, as the problem has not occurred and nursing interventions are directed at prevention.

risk of maternal Injury: risk factors may include preexisting medical conditions, complications of pregnancy.*

risk for Activity Intolerance: risk factors may include presence of circulatory/respiratory problems, uterine irritability.*

risk for ineffective individual Therapeutic Regimen Management: risk factors may include client value system, health beliefs/cultural influences, issues of control, presence of anxiety, complexity of therapeutic regimen, economic difficulties, perceived susceptibility.*

Pregnancy-induced hypertension (preeclampsia)   OB/CH

deficient Fluid Volume [isotonic] may be related to a plasma protein loss, decreasing plasma colloid osmotic pressure allowing fluid shifts out of vascular compartment, possibly evidenced by edema formation, sudden weight gain, hemoconcentration, nausea/vomiting, epigastric pain, headaches, visual changes, decreased urine output.

decreased Cardiac Output may be related to hypovolemia/decreased venous return, increased SVR, possibly evidenced by variations in BP/hemodynamic readings, edema, shortness of breath, change in mental status.

ineffective [uteroplacental] Tissue Perfusion: may be related to vasospasm of spiral arteries and relative hypovolemia, possibly evidenced by changes in fetal heart rate/activity, reduced weight gain, and premature delivery/fetal demise.

deficient Knowledge [Learning Need] regarding pathophysiology of condition, therapy, self-care/nutritional needs, and potential complications may be related to lack of information/recall, misinterpretation, possibly evidenced by statements of concern, questions, misconceptions, inaccurate follow-through of instructions/development of preventable complications.

Premenstrual tension syndrome (PMS)   GYN/CH/PSY

chronic/acute Pain may be related to cyclic changes in female hormones affecting other systems (e.g., vascular congestion/spasms), vitamin deficiency, fluid retention, possibly evidenced by increased tension, apprehension, jitteriness, verbal reports, distraction behaviors, somatic complaints, self-focusing, physical and social withdrawal.

excess Fluid Volume may be related to abnormal alterations of hormonal levels, possibly evidenced by edema formation, weight gain, and periodic changes in emotional status/irritability.

Anxiety [specify level] may be related to cyclic changes in female hormones affecting other systems, possibly evidenced by feelings of inability to cope/loss of control, depersonalization, increased tension, apprehension, jitteriness, somatic complaints, and impaired functioning.

---

*A risk diagnosis is not evidenced by signs and symptoms, as the problem has not occurred and nursing interventions are directed at prevention.

---

deficient Knowledge [Learning Need] regarding pathophysiology of condition and self-care/treatment needs may be related to lack of information/misinterpretation, possibly evidenced by statements of concern, questions, misconceptions, and continuation of condition, exacerbating symptoms.

Pressure ulcer or sore   CH
(Also refer to Ulcer, decubitus)

ineffective peripheral Tissue Perfusion may be related to reduced/interrupted blood flow, possibly evidenced by presence of inflamed, necrotic lesion.

deficient Knowledge [Learning Need] regarding cause/prevention of condition and potential complications may be related to lack of information/misinterpretation, possibly evidenced by statements of concern, questions, misconceptions, and inaccurate follow-through of instructions.

Preterm labor   OB/CH
(Refer to Labor, preterm)

Prostatectomy   MS

impaired Urinary Elimination may be related to mechanical obstruction (blood clots, edema, trauma, surgical procedure, pressure/irritation of catheter/balloon) and loss of bladder tone, possibly evidenced by dysuria, frequency, dribbling, incontinence, retention, bladder fullness, suprapubic discomfort.

risk for deficient Fluid Volume: risk factors may include trauma to highly vascular area with excessive vascular losses, restricted intake, postobstructive diuresis.*

acute Pain may be related to irritation of bladder mucosa and tissue trauma/edema, possibly evidenced by verbal reports (bladder spasms), distraction behaviors, self-focus, and autonomic responses (changes in vital signs).

disturbed Body Image may be related to perceived threat of altered body/sexual function, possibly evidenced by preoccupation with change/loss, negative feelings about body, and statements of concern regarding functioning.

CH

risk for Sexual dysfunction: risk factors may include situational crisis (incontinence, leakage of urine after catheter removal, involvement of genital area) and threat to self-concept/change in health status.*

Pruritus   CH

acute Pain may be related to cutaneous hyperesthesia and inflammation, possibly evidenced by verbal reports, distraction behaviors, and self-focus.

risk for impaired Skin Integrity: risk factors may include mechanical

---

*A risk diagnosis is not evidenced by signs and symptoms, as the problem has not occurred and nursing interventions are directed at prevention.

trauma (scratching) and development of vesicles/bullae that may rupture.*

Psoriasis CH

impaired Skin Integrity may be related to increased epidermal cell proliferation and absence of normal protective skin layers, possibly evidenced by scaling papules and plaques.

disturbed Body Image may be related to cosmetically unsightly skin lesions, possibly evidenced by hiding affected body part, negative feelings about body, feelings of helplessness, and change in social involvement.

Pulmonary edema, high altitude MS
(Refer to High altitude pulmonary edema)

Pulmonary embolus MS

ineffective Breathing Pattern may be related to tracheobronchial obstruction (inflammation, copious secretions or active bleeding), decreased lung expansion, inflammatory process, possibly evidenced by changes in depth and/or rate of respiration, dyspnea/use of accessory muscles, altered chest excursion, abnormal breath sounds (crackles, wheezes), and cough (with or without sputum production).

impaired Gas Exchange may be related to altered blood flow to alveoli or to major portions of the lung, alveolar-capillary membrane changes (atelectasis, airway/alveolar collapse, pulmonary edema/effusion, excessive secretions/active bleeding), possibly evidenced by profound dyspnea, restlessness, apprehension, somnolence, cyanosis, and changes in ABGs/pulse oximetry (hypoxemia and hypercapnia).

ineffective cardiopulmonary Tissue Perfusion may be related to interruption of blood flow (arterial/venous), exchange problems at alveolar level or at tissue level (acidotic shifting of the oxyhemoglobin curve), possibly evidenced by radiology/laboratory evidence of ventilation/perfusion mismatch, dyspnea, and central cyanosis.

Fear/Anxiety [specify level] may be related to severe dyspnea/inability to breathe normally, perceived threat of death, threat to/change in health status, physiologic response to hypoxemia/acidosis, and concern regarding unknown outcome of situation, possibly evidenced by restlessness, irritability, withdrawal or attack behavior, sympathetic stimulation (cardiovascular excitation, pupil dilation, sweating, vomiting, diarrhea), crying, voice quivering, and impending sense of doom.

Pulmonary hypertension CH/MS

impaired Gas Exchange may be related to changes in alveolar membrane, increased pulmonary vascular resistance possibly evidenced by dyspnea, irritability, decreased mental acuity, somnolence, abnormal ABGs.

decreased Cardiac Output may be related to increased pulmonary

---

*A risk diagnosis is not evidenced by signs and symptoms, as the problem has not occurred and nursing interventions are directed at prevention.

vascular resistance, decreased blood return to left-side of heart possibly evidenced by increased heart rate, dyspnea, fatigue.

Activity Intolerance may be related to imbalance between oxygen supply and demand possibly evidenced by reports of weakness/fatigue, abnormal vital signs with activity.

Anxiety may be related to change in health status, stress, threat to self-concept possibly evidenced by expressed concerns, uncertainty, anxious, awareness of physiologic symptoms, diminished productivity/ability to problem-solve.

Purpura, idiopathic thrombocytopenic   CH

ineffective Protection may be related to abnormal blood profile, drug therapy (corticosteroids or immunosuppressive agents), possibly evidenced by altered clotting, fatigue, deficient immunity.

Activity Intolerance may be related to decreased oxygen-carrying capacity/imbalance between O_2 supply and demand, possibly evidenced by reports of fatigue/weakness.

deficient Knowledge [Learning Need] regarding therapy choices, outcomes, and self-care needs may be related to lack of information/ misinterpretation, possibly evidenced by statements of concern, questions, and misconceptions.

Pyelonephritis   MS

acute Pain may be related to acute inflammation of renal tissues, possibly evidenced by verbal reports, guarding/distraction behaviors, self-focus, and autonomic responses (changes in vital signs).

Hyperthermia may be related to inflammatory process/increased metabolic rate, possibly evidenced by increase in body temperature, warm/ flushed skin, tachycardia, and chills.

impaired Urinary Elimination may be related to inflammation/irritation of bladder mucosa, possibly evidenced by dysuria, urgency, and frequency.

deficient Knowledge [Learning Need] regarding therapy needs and prevention may be related to lack of information/misinterpretation, possibly evidenced by statements of concern, questions, misconceptions, and recurrence of condition.

Quadriplegia   MS/CH
(Also refer to Paraplegia)

ineffective Breathing Pattern may be related to neuromuscular impairment (diaphragm and intercostal muscle function), reflex abdominal spasms, gastric distention, possibly evidenced by decreased respiratory depth, dyspnea, cyanosis, and abnormal ABGs.

risk for Trauma [additional spinal injury]: risk factors may include temporary weakness/instability of spinal column.*

anticipatory Grieving may be related to perceived loss of self, anticipated alterations in lifestyle and expectations, and limitation of future options/choices, possibly evidenced by expressions of distress, anger, sorrow; choked feelings; and changes in eating habits, sleep, communication patterns.

*A risk diagnosis is not evidenced by signs and symptoms, as the problem has not occurred and nursing interventions are directed at prevention.

total Self-Care Deficit related to neuromuscular impairment, evidenced by inability to perform self-care tasks.

impaired bed/wheelchair Mobility may be related to loss of muscle function/control.

risk for Autonomic Dysreflexia: risk factors may include altered nerve function (spinal cord injury at T6 or above), bladder/bowel/skin stimulation (tactile, pain, thermal).*

impaired Home Maintenance may be related to permanent effects of injury, inadequate/absent support systems and finances, and lack of familiarity with resources, possibly evidenced by expressions of difficulties, requests for information and assistance, outstanding debts/financial crisis, and lack of necessary aids and equipment.

Rape   CH

deficient Knowledge [Learning Need] regarding required medical/legal procedures, prophylactic treatment for individual concerns (STDs, pregnancy), community resources/supports may be related to lack of information, possibly evidenced by statements of concern, questions, misconceptions, and exacerbation of symptoms.

Rape-Trauma Syndrome (acute phase) related to actual or attempted sexual penetration without consent, possibly evidenced by wide range of emotional reactions, including anxiety, fear, anger, embarrassment, and multisystem physical complaints.

risk for impaired Tissue Integrity: risk factors may include forceful sexual penetration and trauma to fragile tissues.*

PSY

ineffective Coping may be related to personal vulnerability, unmet expectations, unrealistic perceptions, inadequate support systems/ coping methods, multiple stressors repeated over time, overwhelming threat to self, possibly evidenced by verbalizations of inability to cope or difficulty asking for help, muscular tension/headaches, emotional tension, chronic worry.

Sexual Dysfunction may be related to biopsychosocial alteration of sexuality (stress of post-trauma response), vulnerability, loss of sexual desire, impaired relationship with SO, possibly evidenced by alteration in achieving sexual satisfaction, change in interest in self/ others, preoccupation with self.

Raynaud's phenomenon   CH

acute/chronic Pain may be related to vasospasm/altered perfusion of affected tissues and ischemia/destruction of tissues, possibly evidenced by verbal reports, guarding of affected parts, self-focusing, and restlessness.

ineffective peripheral Tissue Perfusion may be related to periodic reduction of arterial blood flow to affected areas, possibly evidenced by pallor, cyanosis, coolness, numbness, paresthesia, slow healing of lesions.

---

*A risk diagnosis is not evidenced by signs and symptoms, as the problem has not occurred and nursing interventions are directed at prevention.

<u>deficient Knowledge [Learning Need] regarding pathophysiology of condition, potential for complications, therapy/self-care needs</u> may be related to lack of information/misinterpretation, possibly evidenced by statements of concern, questions, and misconceptions; development of preventable complications.

Reflex sympathetic dystrophy (RSD)   CH

<u>acute/chronic Pain</u> may be related to continued nerve stimulation, possibly evidenced by verbal reports, distraction/guarding behaviors, narrowed focus, changes in sleep patterns, and altered ability to continue previous activities.

<u>ineffective peripheral Tissue Perfusion</u> may be related to reduction of arterial blood flow (arteriole vasoconstriction), possibly evidenced by reports of pain, decreased skin temperature and pallor, diminished arterial pulsations, and tissue swelling.

<u>disturbed tactile Sensory Perception</u> may be related to altered sensory reception (neurologic deficit, pain), possibly evidenced by change in usual response to stimuli/abnormal sensitivity of touch, physiologic anxiety, and irritability.

<u>risk for ineffective Role Performance:</u> risk factors may include situational crisis, chronic disability, debilitating pain.*

<u>risk for compromised family Coping:</u> risk factors may include temporary family disorganization and role changes and prolonged disability that exhausts the supportive capacity of SO(s).*

Regional enteritis   CH
(Refer to Crohn's disease)

Renal failure, acute   MS

<u>excess Fluid Volume</u> may be related to compromised regulatory mechanisms (decreased kidney function), possibly evidenced by weight gain, edema/anasarca, intake greater than output, venous congestion, changes in BP/CVP, and altered electrolyte levels.

<u>imbalanced Nutrition: less than body requirements</u> may be related to inability to ingest/digest adequate nutrients (anorexia, nausea/vomiting, ulcerations of oral mucosa, and increased metabolic needs) in addition to therapeutic dietary restrictions, possibly evidenced by lack of interest in food/aversion to eating, observed inadequate intake, weight loss, loss of muscle mass.

<u>risk for Infection:</u> risk factors may include depression of immunologic defenses, invasive procedures/devices, and changes in dietary intake/malnutrition.*

<u>disturbed Thought Processes</u> may be related to accumulation of toxic waste products and altered cerebral perfusion, possibly evidenced by disorientation, changes in recent memory, apathy, and episodic obtundation.

Renal transplantation   MS

<u>risk for excess Fluid Volume:</u> risk factors may include compromised regulatory mechanism (implantation of new kidney requiring adjustment period for optimal functioning).*

---

*A risk diagnosis is not evidenced by signs and symptoms, as the problem has not occurred and nursing interventions are directed at prevention.

disturbed Body Image may be related to failure and subsequent replacement of body part and medication-induced changes in appearance, possibly evidenced by preoccupation with loss/change, negative feelings about body, and focus on past strength/function.

Fear may be related to potential for transplant rejection/failure and threat of death, possibly evidenced by increased tension, apprehension, concentration on source, and verbalizations of concern.

risk for Infection: risk factors may include broken skin/traumatized tissue, stasis of body fluids, immunosuppression, invasive procedures, nutritional deficits, and chronic disease.*

CH

risk for ineffective Coping/compromised family Coping: risk factors may include situational crises, family disorganization and role changes, prolonged disease exhausting supportive capacity of SO/family, therapeutic restrictions/long-term therapy needs.*

Respiratory distress syndrome (premature infant)   PED

(Also refer to Neonatal, premature newborn)

impaired Gas Exchange may be related to alveolar/capillary membrane changes (inadequate surfactant levels), altered oxygen supply (tracheobronchial obstruction, atelectasis), altered blood flow (immaturity of pulmonary arteriole musculature), altered oxygen-carrying capacity of blood (anemia), and cold stress, possibly evidenced by tachypnea, use of accessory muscles/retractions, expiratory grunting, pallor or cyanosis, abnormal ABGs, and tachycardia.

impaired Spontaneous Ventilation may be related to respiratory muscle fatigue and metabolic factors, possibly evidenced by dyspnea, increased metabolic rate, restlessness, use of accessory muscles, and abnormal ABGs.

risk for Infection: risk factors may include inadequate primary defenses (decreased ciliary action, stasis of body fluids, traumatized tissues), inadequate secondary defenses (deficiency of neutrophils and specific immunoglobulins), invasive procedures, and malnutrition (absence of nutrient stores, increased metabolic demands).*

risk for ineffective gastrointestinal Tissue Perfusion: risk factors may include persistent fetal circulation and exchange problems.*

risk for impaired parent/infant Attachment: risk factors may include premature/ill infant who is unable to effectively initiate parental contact (altered behavioral organization), separation, physical barriers, anxiety associated with the parental role/demands of infant.*

Retinal detachment   CH

disturbed visual Sensory Perception related to decreased sensory reception, possibly evidenced by visual distortions, decreased visual field, and changes in visual acuity.

---

*A risk diagnosis is not evidenced by signs and symptoms, as the problem has not occurred and nursing interventions are directed at prevention.

deficient Knowledge [Learning Need] regarding therapy, prognosis, and self-care needs may be related to lack of information/misconceptions, possibly evidenced by statements of concern and questions.

risk for impaired Home Maintenance: risk factors may include visual limitations/activity/restrictions.*

Reye's syndrome   PED

deficient Fluid Volume [isotonic] may be related to failure of regulatory mechanism (diabetes insipidus), excessive gastric losses (pernicious vomiting), and altered intake, possibly evidenced by increased/dilute urine output, sudden weight loss, decreased venous filling, dry mucous membranes, decreased skin turgor, hypotension, and tachycardia.

ineffective cerebral Tissue Perfusion may be related to diminished arterial/venous blood flow and hypovolemia, possibly evidenced by memory loss, altered consciousness, and restlessness/agitation.

risk for Trauma: risk factors may include generalized weakness, reduced coordination, and cognitive deficits.*

ineffective Breathing Pattern may be related to decreased energy and fatigue, cognitive impairment, tracheobronchial obstruction, and inflammatory process (aspiration pneumonia), possibly evidenced by tachypnea, abnormal ABGs, cough, and use of accessory muscles.

Rheumatic fever   PED

acute Pain may be related to migratory inflammation of joints, possibly evidenced by verbal reports, guarding/distraction behaviors, self-focus, and autonomic responses (changes in vital signs).

Hyperthermia may be related to inflammatory process/hypermetabolic state, possibly evidenced by increased body temperature, warm/flushed skin, and tachycardia.

Activity Intolerance may be related to generalized weakness, joint pain, and medical restrictions/bedrest, possibly evidenced by reports of fatigue, exertional discomfort, and abnormal heart rate in response to activity.

risk for decreased Cardiac Output: risk factors may include cardiac inflammation/enlargement and altered contractility.*

Rickets (osteomalacia)   PED

delayed Growth and Development may be related to dietary deficiencies/indiscretions, malabsorption syndrome, and lack of exposure to sunlight, possibly evidenced by altered physical growth and delay or difficulty in performing motor skills typical for age.

deficient Knowledge [Learning Need] regarding cause, pathophysiology, therapy needs and prevention may be related to lack of information, possibly evidenced by statements of concern, questions, misconceptions, and inaccurate follow-through of instructions.

---

*A risk diagnosis is not evidenced by signs and symptoms, as the problem has not occurred and nursing interventions are directed at prevention.

Ringworm, tinea   **CH**

(Also refer to Athlete's Foot)

impaired Skin Integrity may be related to fungal infection of the dermis, possibly evidenced by disruption of skin surfaces/presence of lesions.

deficient Knowledge [Learning Need] regarding infectious nature, therapy, and self-care needs may be related to lack of information/misinformation, possibly evidenced by statements of concern, questions, and recurrence/spread.

Rubella   **PED/CH**

acute Pain/[Discomfort] may be related to inflammatory effects of viral infection and presence of desquamating rash, possibly evidenced by verbal reports, distraction behaviors/restlessness.

deficient Knowledge [Learning Need] regarding contagious nature, possible complications, and self-care needs may be related to lack of information/misinterpretations, possibly evidenced by statements of concern, questions, and inaccurate follow-through of instructions.

Scabies   **CH**

impaired Skin Integrity may be related to presence of invasive parasite and development of pruritus, possibly evidenced by disruption of skin surface and inflammation.

deficient Knowledge [Learning Need] regarding communicable nature, possible complications, therapy, and self-care needs may be related to lack of information/misinterpretation, possibly evidenced by questions and statements of concern about spread to others.

Scarlet fever   **PED**

Hyperthermia may be related to effects of circulating toxins, possibly evidenced by increased body temperature, warm/flushed skin, and tachycardia.

Pain/[Discomfort] may be related to inflammation of mucous membranes and effects of circulating toxins (malaise, fever), possibly evidenced by verbal reports, distraction behaviors, guarding (decreased swallowing), and self-focus.

risk for deficient Fluid Volume: risk factors may include hypermetabolic state (hyperthermia) and reduced intake.*

Schizophrenia (schizophrenic disorders)   **PSY/CH**

disturbed Thought Processes may be related to disintegration of thinking processes, impaired judgment, presence of psychologic conflicts, disintegrated ego-boundaries, sleep disturbance, ambivalence and concomitant dependence, possibly evidenced by impaired ability to reason/problem-solve, inappropriate affect, presence of delusional system, command hallucinations, obsessions, ideas of reference, cognitive dissonance.

*A risk diagnosis is not evidenced by signs and symptoms, as the problem has not occurred and nursing interventions are directed at prevention.

Social Isolation may be related to alterations in mental status, mistrust of others/delusional thinking, unacceptable social behaviors, inadequate personal resources, and inability to engage in satisfying personal relationships, possibly evidenced by difficulty in establishing relationships with others; dull affect, uncommunicative/withdrawn behavior, seeking to be alone, inadequate/absent significant purpose in life, and expression of feelings of rejection.

ineffective Health Maintenance/impaired Home Maintenance may be related to impaired cognitive/emotional functioning, altered ability to make deliberate and thoughtful judgments, altered communication, and lack/inappropriate use of material resources, possibly evidenced by inability to take responsibility for meeting basic health practices in any or all functional areas and demonstrated lack of adaptive behaviors to internal or external environmental changes, disorderly surroundings, accumulation of dirt/unwashed clothes, repeated hygienic disorders.

risk for self/other-directed Violence: risk factors may include disturbances of thinking/feeling (depression, paranoia, suicidal ideation), lack of development of trust and appropriate interpersonal relationships, catatonic/manic excitement, toxic reactions to drugs (alcohol).*

ineffective Coping may be related to personal vulnerability, inadequate support system(s), unrealistic perceptions, inadequate coping methods, and disintegration of thought processes, possibly evidenced by impaired judgment/cognition and perception, diminished problem-solving/decision-making capacities, poor self-concept, chronic anxiety, depression, inability to perform role expectations, and alteration in social participation.

interrupted Family Processes/disabled family Coping may be related to ambivalent family system/relationships, change of roles, and difficulty of family member in coping effectively with client's maladaptive behaviors, possibly evidenced by deterioration in family functioning, ineffective family decision-making process, difficulty relating to each other, client's expressions of despair at family's lack of reaction/involvement, neglectful relationships with client, extreme distortion regarding client's health problem including denial about its existence/severity or prolonged overconcern.

Self-Care Deficit [specify] may be related to perceptual and cognitive impairment, immobility (withdrawal/isolation and decreased psychomotor activity), and side effects of psychotropic medications, possibly evidenced by inability or difficulty in areas of feeding self, keeping body clean, dressing appropriately, toileting self, and/or changes in bowel/bladder elimination.

Sciatica   CH

acute/chronic Pain may be related to peripheral nerve root compression, possibly evidenced by verbal reports, guarding/distraction behaviors, and self-focus.

impaired physical Mobility may be related to neurologic pain and

*A risk diagnosis is not evidenced by signs and symptoms, as the problem has not occurred and nursing interventions are directed at prevention.

muscular involvement, possibly evidenced by reluctance to attempt movement and decreased muscle strength/mass.

Scleroderma CH

(Also refer to Lupus erythematosus, systemic—SLE)

impaired physical Mobility may be related to musculoskeletal impairment and associated pain, possibly evidenced by decreased strength, decreased range of motion, and reluctance to attempt movement.

ineffective Tissue Perfusion, (specify) may be related to reduced arterial blood flow (arteriolar vasoconstriction), possibly evidenced by changes in skin temperature/color, ulcer formation, and changes in organ function (cardiopulmonary, GI, renal).

imbalanced Nutrition: less than body requirements may be related to inability to ingest/digest/absorb adequate nutrients (sclerosis of the tissues rendering mouth immobile, decreased peristalsis of esophagus/small intestines, atrophy of smooth muscle of colon), possibly evidenced by weight loss, decreased intake/food, and reported/observed difficulty swallowing.

impaired Adjustment may be related to disability requiring change in lifestyle, inadequate support systems, assault to self-concept, and altered locus of control, possibly evidenced by verbalization of nonacceptance of health status change and lack of movement toward independence/future-oriented thinking.

disturbed Body Image may be related to skin changes with induration, atrophy, and fibrosis, loss of hair, and skin and muscle contractures, possibly evidenced by verbalization of negative feelings about body, focus on past strength/function or appearance, fear of rejection/reaction by others, hiding body part, and change in social involvement.

Scoliosis PED

disturbed Body Image may be related to altered body structure, use of therapeutic device(s), and activity restrictions, possibly evidenced by negative feelings about body, change in social involvement, and preoccupation with situation or refusal to acknowledge problem.

deficient Knowledge [Learning Need] regarding pathophysiology of condition, therapy needs, and possible outcomes may be related to lack of information/misinterpretation, possibly evidenced by statements of concern, questions, misconceptions, and inaccurate follow-through of instructions.

impaired Adjustment may be related to lack of comprehension of long-term consequences of behavior, possibly evidenced by failure to adhere to treatment regimen/keep appointments and evidence of failure to improve.

Seizure disorder CH

deficient Knowledge [Learning Need] regarding condition and medication control may be related to lack of information/misinterpretations, scarce financial resources, possibly evidenced by questions, statements of concern/misconceptions, incorrect use of anticonvulsant medication, recurrent episodes/uncontrolled seizures.

chronic low Self-Esteem/disturbed Personal Identity may be related to perceived neurologic functional change/weakness, perception of being out of control, stigma associated with condition, possibly evidenced by negative feelings about "brain"/self, change in social involvement, feelings of helplessness, and preoccupation with perceived change or loss.

impaired Social Interaction may be related to unpredictable nature of condition and self-concept disturbance, possibly evidenced by decreased self-assurance, verbalization of concern, discomfort in social situations, inability to receive/communicate a satisfying sense of belonging/caring, and withdrawal from social contacts/activities.

risk for Trauma/Suffocation: risk factors may include weakness, balancing difficulties, cognitive limitations/altered consciousness, loss of large- or small-muscle coordination (during seizure).*

Sepsis, puerperal   OB
(Also refer to Septicemia)

risk for Infection [spread/septic shock]: risk factors may include presence of infection, broken skin, and/or traumatized tissues, rupture of amniotic membranes, high vascularity of involved area, stasis of body fluids, invasive procedures, and/or increased environmental exposure, chronic disease (e.g., diabetes, anemia, malnutrition), altered immune response, and untoward effect of medications (e.g., opportunistic/secondary infection).*

Hyperthermia may be related to inflammatory process/hypermetabolic state, possibly evidenced by increase in body temperature, warm/flushed skin, and tachycardia.

risk for impaired parent/infant Attachment: risk factors may include interruption in bonding process, physical illness, perceived threat to own survival.*

risk for ineffective peripheral Tissue Perfusion: risk factors may include interruption/reduction of blood flow (presence of infectious thrombi).*

Septicemia   MS
(Also refer to Sepsis, puerperal)

ineffective Tissue Perfusion (specify) may be related to changes in arterial/venous blood flow (selective vasoconstriction, presence of microemboli) and hypovolemia, possibly evidenced by changes in skin temperature/color, changes in blood/pulse pressure; changes in sensorium, and decreased urinary output.

risk for deficient Fluid Volume: risk factors may include marked increase in vascular compartment/massive vasodilation, vascular shifts to interstitial space, and reduced intake.*

risk for decreased Cardiac Output: risk factors may include decreased preload (venous return and circulating volume), altered afterload (increased SVR), negative inotropic effects of hypoxia, complement activation, and lysosomal hydrolase.*

---

*A risk diagnosis is not evidenced by signs and symptoms, as the problem has not occurred and nursing interventions are directed at prevention.

Serum sickness   **CH**

acute Pain may be related to inflammation of the joints and skin eruptions, possibly evidenced by verbal reports, guarding/distraction
behaviors, and self-focus.

deficient Knowledge [Learning Need] regarding nature of condition,
treatment needs, potential complications, and prevention of recurrence may be related to lack of information/misinterpretation, possibly evidenced by statements of concern, questions, misconceptions,
and inaccurate follow-through of instructions.

Sexually transmitted disease (STD)   **GYN/CH**

risk for Infection [transmission]: risk factors may include contagious
nature of infecting agent and insufficient knowledge to avoid exposure to/transmission of pathogens.*

impaired Skin/Tissue Integrity may be related to invasion of/irritation
by pathogenic organism(s), possibly evidenced by disruptions of
skin/tissue and inflammation of mucous membranes.

deficient Knowledge [Learning Need] regarding condition, prognosis/
complications, therapy needs, and transmission may be related to
lack of information/misinterpretation, lack of interest in learning,
possibly evidenced by statements of concern, questions, misconceptions; inaccurate follow-through of instructions, and development of
preventable complications.

Shock   **MS**

(Also refer to Shock, cardiogenic; Shock, hypovolemic/
hemorrhagic)

ineffective Tissue Perfusion (specify) may be related to changes in circulating volume and/or vascular tone, possibly evidenced by changes in
skin color/temperature and pulse pressure, reduced blood pressure,
changes in mentation, and decreased urinary output.

Anxiety [specify level] may be related to change in health status
and threat of death, possibly evidenced by increased tension, apprehension, sympathetic stimulation, restlessness, and expressions of
concern.

Shock, cardiogenic   **MS**

(Also refer to Shock)

decreased Cardiac Output may be related to structural damage,
decreased myocardial contractility, and presence of dysrhythmias,
possibly evidenced by ECG changes, variations in hemodynamic
readings, jugular vein distention, cold/clammy skin, diminished
peripheral pulses, and decreased urinary output.

risk for impaired Gas Exchange: risk factors may include ventilation
perfusion imbalance, alveolar-capillary membrane changes.*

Shock, hypovolemic/hemorrhagic   **MS**

(Also refer to Shock)

deficient Fluid Volume [isotonic] may be related to excessive vascular
loss, inadequate intake/replacement, possibly evidenced by hypoten-

*A risk diagnosis is not evidenced by signs and symptoms, as the
problem has not occurred and nursing interventions are directed at
prevention.

sion, tachycardia, decreased pulse volume and pressure, change in mentation, and decreased/concentrated urine.

Shock, septic MS
(Refer to Septicemia)

Sick sinus syndrome MS
(Also refer to Dysrhythmia, cardiac)

decreased Cardiac Output may be related to alterations in rate, rhythm, and electrical conduction, possibly evidenced by ECG evidence of dysrhythmias, reports of palpitations/weakness, changes in mentation/consciousness, and syncope.

risk for Trauma: risk factors may include changes in cerebral perfusion with altered consciousness/loss of balance.*

SLE CH
(Refer to Lupus erythematosus, systemic)

Smallpox MS
risk of Infection [spread]: risk factors may include contagious nature of organism, inadequate acquired immunity, presence of chronic disease, immunosuppression.*

deficient Fluid Volume may be related to hypermetabolic state, decreased intake (pharyngeal lesions, nausea), increased losses (vomiting), fluid shifts from vascular bed possibly evidenced by reports of thirst, decreased BP, venous filling and urinary output; dry mucous membranes, decreased skin turgor, change in mental state, elevated Hct.

impaired Tissue Integrity may be related to immunologic deficit possibly evidenced by disruption of skin surface, cornea, mucous membranes.

Anxiety[specify level]/Fear may be related to threat of death, interpersonal transmission/contagion, separation from support system possibly evidenced by expressed concerns, apprehension, restlessness, focus on self.

CH

interrupted Family Processes may be related to temporary family disorganization, situational crisis, change in health status of family member possibly evidenced by changes in satisfaction with family, stress-reduction behaviors, mutual support; expression of isolation from community resources.

ineffective community Coping may be related to human-made disaster (bioterrorism), inadequate resources for problem-solving possibly evidenced by deficits of community participation, high illness rate, excessive community conflicts, expressed vulnerability/powerlessness.

Snow blindness CH
disturbed visual Sensory Perception may be related to altered status of sense organ (irritation of the conjunctiva, hyperemia), possibly

*A risk diagnosis is not evidenced by signs and symptoms, as the problem has not occurred and nursing interventions are directed at prevention.

evidenced by intolerance to light (photophobia) and decreased/loss of visual acuity.

acute Pain may be related to irritation/vascular congestion of the conjunctiva, possibly evidenced by verbal reports, guarding/distraction behaviors, and self-focus.

Anxiety [specify level] may be related to situational crisis and threat to/change in health status, possibly evidenced by increased tension, apprehension, uncertainty, worry, restlessness, and focus on self.

Somatoform disorders   PSY

ineffective Coping may be related to severe level of anxiety that is repressed, personal vulnerability, unmet dependency needs, fixation in earlier level of development, retarded ego development, and inadequate coping skills, possibly evidenced by verbalized inability to cope/problem-solve, high illness rate, multiple somatic complaints of several years' duration, decreased functioning in social/occupational settings, narcissistic tendencies with total focus on self/physical symptoms, demanding behaviors, history of "doctor shopping," and refusal to attend therapeutic activities.

chronic Pain may be related to severe level of repressed anxiety, low self-concept, unmet dependency needs, history of self or loved one having experienced a serious illness, possibly evidenced by verbal reports of severe/prolonged pain, guarded movement/protective behaviors, facial mask of pain, fear of reinjury, altered ability to continue previous activities, social withdrawal, demands for therapy/medication.

disturbed Sensory Perception (specify) may be related to psychologic stress (narrowed perceptual fields, expression of stress as physical problems/deficits), poor quality of sleep, presence of chronic pain, possibly evidenced by reported change in voluntary motor or sensory function (paralysis, anosmia, aphonia, deafness, blindness, loss of touch or pain sensation), la belle indifférence (lack of concern over functional loss).

impaired Social Interaction may be related to inability to engage in satisfying personal relationships, preoccupation with self and physical symptoms, altered state of wellness, chronic pain, and rejection by others, possibly evidenced by preoccupation with own thoughts, sad/dull affect, absence of supportive SO(s), uncommunicative/withdrawn behavior, lack of eye contact, and seeking to be alone.

Spinal cord injury (SCI)   MS/CH

(Refer to Paraplegia; Quadriplegia)

Sprain of ankle or foot   CH

acute Pain may be related to trauma to/swelling in joint, possibly evidenced by verbal reports, guarding/distraction behaviors, self-focusing, and autonomic responses (changes in vital signs).

impaired Walking may be related to musculoskeletal injury, pain, and therapeutic restrictions, possibly evidenced by reluctance to attempt movement, inability to move about environment easily.

Stapedectomy   MS

risk for Trauma: risk factors may include increased middle-ear pressure with displacement of prosthesis and balancing difficulties/dizziness.*

risk for Infection: risk factors may include surgically traumatized tissue, invasive procedures, and environmental exposure to upper respiratory infections.*

acute Pain may be related to surgical trauma, edema formation, and presence of packing, possibly evidenced by verbal reports, guarding/distraction behaviors, and self-focus.

STD   CH

(refer to Sexually transmitted disease)

Substance dependence/   PSY/CH
abuse rehabilitation

(following acute detoxification)

ineffective Denial/Coping may be related to personal vulnerability, difficulty handling new situations, learned response patterns, cultural factors, personal/family value systems, possibly evidenced by lack of acceptance that drug use is causing the present situation, use of manipulation to avoid responsibility for self, altered social patterns/ participation, impaired adaptive behavior and problem-solving skills, employment difficulties, financial affairs in disarray, and decreased ability to handle stress of recent events.

Powerlessness may be related to substance addiction with/without periods of abstinence, episodic compulsive indulgence, attempts at recovery, and lifestyle of helplessness, possibly evidenced by ineffective recovery attempts, statements of inability to stop behavior/requests for help, continuous/constant thinking about drug and/or obtaining drug, alteration in personal/occupational and social life.

imbalanced Nutrition: less than body requirements may be related to insufficient dietary intake to meet metabolic needs for psychologic/physiologic/economic reasons, possibly evidenced by weight less than normal for height/body build, decreased subcutaneous fat/muscle mass, reported altered taste sensation, lack of interest in food, poor muscle tone, sore/inflamed buccal cavity, laboratory evidence of protein/vitamin deficiencies.

Sexual Dysfunction may be related to altered body function (neurologic damage and debilitating effects of drug use), changes in appearance, possibly evidenced by progressive interference with sexual functioning, a significant degree of testicular atrophy, gynecomastia, impotence/decreased sperm counts in men; and loss of body hair, thin/soft skin, spider angiomas, and amenorrhea/increase in miscarriages in women.

---

*A risk diagnosis is not evidenced by signs and symptoms, as the problem has not occurred and nursing interventions are directed at prevention.

dysfunctional Family Processes: alcoholism [substance abuse] may be related to abuse/history of alcoholism/drug use, inadequate coping skills/lack of problem-solving skills, genetic predisposition/biochemical influences, possibly evidenced by feelings of anger/frustration/responsibility for alcoholic's behavior, suppressed rage, shame/embarrassment, repressed emotions, guilt, vulnerability; disturbed family dynamics/deterioration in family relationships, family denial/rationalization, closed communication systems, triangulating family relationships, manipulation, blaming, enabling to maintain substance use, inability to accept/receive help.

OB

risk for fetal Injury: risk factors may include drug/alcohol use, exposure to teratogens.*

deficient Knowledge [Learning Need] regarding condition/pregnancy, prognosis, treatment needs may be related to lack/misinterpretation of information, lack of recall, cognitive limitations/interference with learning possibly evidenced by statements of concern, questions/misconceptions, inaccurate follow-through of instructions, development of preventable complications, continued use in spite of complications.

Surgery, general   MS

(Also refer to Postoperative recovery period)

deficient Knowledge [Learning Need] regarding surgical procedure/expectation, postoperative routines/therapy, and self-care needs may be related to lack of information/misinterpretation, possibly evidenced by statements of concern, questions, and misconceptions.

Anxiety [specify level]/Fear may be related to situational crisis, unfamiliarity with environment, change in health status/threat of death and separation from usual support systems, possibly evidenced by increased tension, apprehension, decreased self-assurance, fear of unspecific consequences, focus on self, sympathetic stimulation, and restlessness.

risk for perioperative-positioning Injury: risk factors may include disorientation, immobilization, muscle weakness, obesity/edema.*

risk for ineffective Breathing Pattern: risk factors may include chemically induced muscular relaxation, perception/cognitive impairment, decreased energy.*

risk for deficient Fluid Volume: risk factors may include preoperative fluid deprivation, blood loss, and excessive GI losses (vomiting/gastric suction).*

Synovitis (knee)   CH

acute Pain may be related to inflammation of synovial membrane of the joint with effusion, possibly evidenced by verbal reports, guarding/distraction behaviors, self-focus, and autonomic responses (changes in vital signs).

---

*A risk diagnosis is not evidenced by signs and symptoms, as the problem has not occurred and nursing interventions are directed at prevention.

impaired Walking may be related to pain and decreased strength of joint, possibly evidenced by reluctance to attempt movement, inability to move about environment as desired.

Syphilis, congenital   PED

(Also refer to Sexually transmitted disease—STD)

acute Pain may be related to inflammatory process, edema formation, and development of skin lesions, possibly evidenced by irritability/crying that may be increased with movement of extremities and autonomic responses (changes in vital signs).

impaired Skin/Tissue Integrity may be related to exposure to pathogens during vaginal delivery, possibly evidenced by disruption of skin surfaces and rhinitis.

delayed Growth and Development may be related to effect of infectious process, possibly evidenced by altered physical growth and delay or difficulty performing skills typical of age group.

deficient Knowledge [Learning Need] regarding pathophysiology of condition, transmissibility, therapy needs, expected outcomes, and potential complications may be related to caretaker/parental lack of information, misinterpretation, possibly evidenced by statements of concern, questions, and misconceptions.

Syringomyelia   MS

disturbed Sensory Perception (specify) may be related to altered sensory perception (neurologic lesion), possibly evidenced by change in usual response to stimuli and motor incoordination.

Anxiety [specify level]/Fear may be related to change in health status, threat of change in role functioning and socioeconomic status, and threat to self-concept, possibly evidenced by increased tension, apprehension, uncertainty, focus on self, and expressed concerns.

impaired physical Mobility may be related to neuromuscular and sensory impairment, possibly evidenced by decreased muscle strength, control, and mass; and impaired coordination.

Self-Care Deficit [specify] may be related to neuromuscular and sensory impairments, possibly evidenced by statement of inability to perform care tasks.

Tay-Sachs disease   PED

delayed Growth and Development may be related to effects of physical condition, possibly evidenced by altered physical growth, loss of/failure to acquire skills typical of age, flat affect, and decreased responses.

disturbed visual Sensory Perception may be related to neurologic deterioration of optic nerve, possibly evidenced by loss of visual acuity.

CH

anticipatory family Grieving may be related to expected eventual loss of infant/child, possibly evidenced by expressions of distress, denial, guilt, anger, and sorrow; choked feelings; changes in sleep/eating habits; and altered libido.

family Powerlessness may be related to absence of therapeutic interventions for progressive/fatal disease, possibly evidenced by verbal expressions of having no control over situation/outcome and depression over physical/mental deterioration.

risk for Spiritual Distress: risk factors may include challenged belief and value system by presence of fatal condition with racial/religious connotations and intense suffering.*

compromised family Coping may be related to situational crisis, temporary preoccupation with managing emotional conflicts and personal suffering, family disorganization, and prolonged/progressive disease, possibly evidenced by preoccupations with personal reactions, expressed concern about reactions of other family members, inadequate support of one another, and altered communication patterns.

Thrombophlebitis   CH/MS/OB

ineffective peripheral Tissue Perfusion may be related to interruption of venous blood flow, venous stasis, possibly evidenced by changes in skin color/temperature over affected area, development of edema, pain, diminished peripheral pulses, slow capillary refill.

acute Pain/[Discomfort] may be related to vascular inflammation/irritation and edema formation (accumulation of lactic acid), possibly evidenced by verbal reports, guarding/distraction behaviors, restlessness, and self-focus.

risk for impaired physical Mobility: risk factors may include pain and discomfort and restrictive therapies/safety precautions.*

deficient Knowledge [Learning Need] regarding pathophysiology of condition, therapy/self-care needs, and risk of embolization may be related to lack of information/misinterpretation, possibly evidenced by statements of concern, questions, inaccurate follow-through of instructions, and development of preventable complications.

Thrombosis, venous   MS
(Refer to Thrombophlebitis)

Thrush   CH
impaired Oral Mucous Membrane may be related to presence of infection as evidenced by white patches/plaques, oral discomfort, mucosal irritation, bleeding.

Thyroidectomy   MS
(Also refer to Hyperthyroidism; Hypoparathyroidism; Hypothyroidism)

risk for ineffective Airway Clearance: risk factors may include hematoma/edema formation with tracheal obstruction, laryngeal spasms.*

impaired verbal Communication may be related to tissue edema, pain/discomfort, and vocal cord injury/laryngeal nerve damage, possibly evidenced by impaired articulation, does not/cannot speak, and use of nonverbal cues/gestures.

*A risk diagnosis is not evidenced by signs and symptoms, as the problem has not occurred and nursing interventions are directed at prevention.

risk for Injury [tetany]: risk factors may include chemical imbalance/ excessive CNS stimulation.*

risk for head/neck Trauma: risk factors may include loss of muscle control/support and position of suture line.*

acute Pain may be related to presence of surgical incision/manipulation of tissues/muscles, postoperative edema, possibly evidenced by verbal reports, guarding/distraction behaviors, narrowed focus, and autonomic responses (changes in vital signs).

Thyrotoxicosis   MS

(Also refer to Hyperthyroidism)

risk for decreased Cardiac Output: risk factors may include uncontrolled hypermetabolic state increasing cardiac workload, changes in venous return and SVR; and alterations in rate, rhythm, and electrical conduction.*

Anxiety [specific level] may be related to physiologic factors/CNS stimulation (hypermetabolic state and pseudocatecholamine effect of thyroid hormones), possibly evidenced by increased feelings of apprehension, shakiness, loss of control, panic, changes in cognition, distortion of environmental stimuli, extraneous movements, restlessness, and tremors.

risk for disturbed Thought Processes: risk factors may include physiologic changes (increased CNS stimulation/accelerated mental activity) and altered sleep patterns.*

deficient Knowledge [Learning Needs] regarding condition, treatment needs, and potential for complications/crisis situation may be related to lack of information/recall, misinterpretation, possibly evidenced by statements of concern, questions, misconceptions; and inaccurate follow-through of instructions.

TIA (Transient ischemic attack)   CH

ineffective cerebral Tissue Perfusion may be related to interruption of blood flow (e.g., vasospasm) possibly evidenced by altered mental status, behavioral changes, language deficit, change in motor/sensory response.

Anxiety/Fear may be related to change in health status, threat to self-concept, situational crisis, interpersonal contagion possibly evidenced by expressed concerns, apprehension, restlessness, irritability.

risk for ineffective Denial: risk factors may include change in health status requiring change in lifestyle, fear of consequences, lack of motivation.

Tic douloureux   CH

(Refer to Neuralgia, trigeminal)

Tonsillectomy   PED/MS

(Refer to Adenoidectomy)

---

*A risk diagnosis is not evidenced by signs and symptoms, as the problem has not occurred and nursing interventions are directed at prevention.

Tonsillitis   PED

acute Pain may be related to inflammation of tonsils and effects of circulating toxins, possibly evidenced by verbal reports, guarding/distraction behaviors, reluctance/refusal to swallow, self-focus, and autonomic responses (changes in vital signs).

Hyperthermia may be related to presence of inflammatory process/hypermetabolic state and dehydration, possibly evidenced by increased body temperature, warm/flushed skin, and tachycardia.

deficient Knowledge [Learning Need] regarding cause/transmission, treatment needs, and potential complications may be related to lack of information/misinterpretation, possibly evidenced by statements of concern, questions, inaccurate follow-through of instructions, and recurrence of condition.

Total joint replacement   MS

risk for Infection: risk factors may include inadequate primary defenses (broken skin, exposure of joint), inadequate secondary defenses/immunosuppression (long-term corticosteroid use), invasive procedures/surgical manipulation, implantation of foreign body, and decreased mobility.*

impaired physical Mobility may be related to pain and discomfort, musculoskeletal impairment, and surgery/restrictive therapies, possibly evidenced by reluctance to attempt movement, difficulty purposefully moving within the physical environment, reports of pain/discomfort on movement, limited range of motion, and decreased muscle strength/control.

risk for ineffective peripheral Tissue Perfusion: risk factors may include reduced arterial/venous blood flow, direct trauma to blood vessels, tissue edema, improper location/dislocation of prosthesis, and hypovolemia.*

acute Pain may be related to physical agents (traumatized tissues/surgical intervention, degeneration of joints, muscle spasms) and psychologic factors (anxiety, advanced age), possibly evidenced by verbal reports, guarding/distraction behaviors, self-focus, and autonomic responses (changes in vital signs).

Toxemia of pregnancy   OB
(Refer to Pregnancy-induced hypertension)

Toxic shock syndrome   MS
(Also refer to Septicemia)

Hyperthermia may be related to inflammatory process/hypermetabolic state and dehydration, possibly evidenced by increased body temperature, warm/flushed skin, and tachycardia.

deficient Fluid Volume [isotonic] may be related to increased gastric losses (diarrhea, vomiting), fever/hypermetabolic state, and decreased intake, possibly evidenced by dry mucous membranes, increased pulse, hypotension, delayed venous filling, decreased/concentrated urine, and hemoconcentration.

---

*A risk diagnosis is not evidenced by signs and symptoms, as the problem has not occurred and nursing interventions are directed at prevention.

---

acute Pain may be related to inflammatory process, effects of circulating toxins, and skin disruptions, possibly evidenced by verbal reports, guarding/distraction behaviors, self-focus, and autonomic responses (changes in vital signs).

impaired Skin/Tissue Integrity may be related to effects of circulating toxins and dehydration, possibly evidenced by development of desquamating rash, hyperemia, and inflammation of mucous membranes.

Traction   MS

(Also refer to Casts; Fractures)

acute Pain may be related to direct trauma to tissue/bone, muscle spasms, movement of bone fragments, edema, injury to soft tissue, traction/immobility device, anxiety, possibly evidenced by verbal reports, guarding/distraction behaviors, self-focus, alteration in muscle tone, and autonomic responses (changes in vital signs).

impaired physical Mobility may be related to neuromuscular/skeletal impairment, pain, psychologic immobility, and therapeutic restrictions of movement, possibly evidenced by limited range of motion, inability to move purposefully in environment, reluctance to attempt movement, and decreased muscle strength/control.

risk for Infection: risk factors may include invasive procedures (including insertion of foreign body through skin/bone), presence of traumatized tissue, and reduced activity with stasis of body fluids.*

deficient Diversional Activity may be related to length of hospitalization/therapeutic intervention and environmental lack of usual activity, possibly evidenced by statements of boredom, restlessness, and irritability.

Transfusion reaction, blood   MS

(Also refer to Anaphylaxis)

risk for imbalanced Body Temperature: risk factors may include infusion of cold blood products, systemic response to toxins.*

Anxiety [specify level] may be related to change in health status and threat of death, exposure to toxins possibly evidenced by increased tension, apprehension, sympathetic stimulation, restlessness, and expressions of concern.

risk for impaired Skin Integrity: risk factors may include immunologic response.*

Trichinosis   CH

acute Pain may be related to parasitic invasion of muscle tissues, edema of upper eyelids, small localized hemorrhages, and development of urticaria, possibly evidenced by verbal reports, guarding/distraction behaviors (restlessness), and autonomic responses (changes in vital signs).

deficient Fluid Volume [isotonic] may be related to hypermetabolic state (fever, diaphoresis); excessive gastric losses (vomiting, diarrhea); and decreased intake/difficulty swallowing, possibly evidenced by dry

---

*A risk diagnosis is not evidenced by signs and symptoms, as the problem has not occurred and nursing interventions are directed at prevention.

mucous membranes, decreased skin turgor, hypotension, decreased venous filling, decreased/concentrated urine, and hemoconcentration.

ineffective Breathing Pattern may be related to myositis of the diaphragm and intercostal muscles, possibly evidenced by resulting changes in respiratory depth, tachypnea, dyspnea, and abnormal ABGs.

deficient Knowledge [Learning Need] regarding cause/prevention of condition, therapy needs, and possible complications may be related to lack of information, misinterpretation, possibly evidenced by statements of concern, questions, and misconceptions.

Tuberculosis (pulmonary)   CH

risk for Infection [spread/reactivation]: risk factors may include inadequate primary defenses (decreased ciliary action/stasis of secretions, tissue destruction/extension of infection), lowered resistance/ suppressed inflammatory response, malnutrition, environmental exposure, insufficient knowledge to avoid exposure to pathogens, or inadequate therapeutic intervention.*

ineffective Airway Clearance may be related to thick, viscous or bloody secretions; fatigue/poor cough effort; and tracheal/pharyngeal edema, possibly evidenced by abnormal respiratory rate, rhythm, and depth; adventitious breath sounds (rhonchi, wheezes), stridor and dyspnea.

risk for impaired Gas Exchange: risk factors may include decrease in effective lung surface, atelectasis, destruction of alveolar-capillary membrane, bronchial edema; thick, viscous secretions.*

Activity Intolerance may be related to imbalance between O_2 supply and demand, possibly evidenced by reports of fatigue, weakness, and exertional dyspnea.

imbalanced Nutrition: less than body requirements may be related to inability to ingest adequate nutrients (anorexia, effects of drug therapy, fatigue, insufficient financial resources), possibly evidenced by weight loss, reported lack of interest in food/altered taste sensation, and poor muscle tone.

risk for ineffective Therapeutic Regimen Management: risk factors may include complexity of therapeutic regimen, economic difficulties, family patterns of health care, perceived seriousness/benefits (especially during remission), side effects of therapy.*

Tympanoplasty   MS
(Refer to Stapedectomy)

Typhus (tick-borne/Rocky   CH/MS
Mountain spotted fever)
Hyperthermia may be related to generalized inflammatory process (vasculitis), possibly evidenced by increased body temperature, warm/flushed skin, and tachycardia.

---

*A risk diagnosis is not evidenced by signs and symptoms, as the problem has not occurred and nursing interventions are directed at prevention.

acute Pain may be related to generalized vasculitis and edema formation, possibly evidenced by verbal reports, guarding/distraction
behaviors, self-focus, and autonomic responses (changes in vital
signs).

ineffective Tissue Perfusion (specify) may be related to reduction/inter-
ruption of blood flow (generalized vasculitis/thrombi formation),
possibly evidenced by reports of headache/abdominal pain, changes
in mentation, and areas of peripheral ulceration/necrosis.

Ulcer, decubitus   CH/MS

impaired Skin/Tissue Integrity may be related to altered circulation,
nutritional deficit, fluid imbalance, impaired physical mobility, irritation of body excretions/secretions, and sensory impairments,
evidenced by tissue damage/destruction.

acute Pain may be related to destruction of protective skin layers and
exposure of nerves, possibly evidenced by verbal reports, distraction
behaviors, and self-focus.

risk for Infection: risk factors may include broken/traumatized tissue,
increased environmental exposure, and nutritional deficits.*

Ulcer, peptic (acute)   MS/CH

deficient Fluid Volume [isotonic] may be related to vascular losses
(hemorrhage), possibly evidenced by hypotension, tachycardia, delayed capillary refill, changes in mentation, restlessness,
concentrated/decreased urine, pallor, diaphoresis, and hemoconcentration.

risk for ineffective Tissue Perfusion (specify): risk factors may include
hypovolemia.*

Fear/Anxiety [specify level] may be related to change in health status
and threat of death, possibly evidenced by increased tension, restlessness, irritability, fearfulness, trembling, tachycardia, diaphoresis, lack
of eye contact, focus on self, verbalization of concerns, withdrawal,
and panic or attack behavior.

acute Pain may be related to caustic irritation/destruction of gastric
tissues, possibly evidenced by verbal reports, distraction behaviors,
self-focus, and autonomic responses (changes in vital signs).

deficient Knowledge [Learning Need] regarding condition, therapy/
self-care needs, and potential complications may be related to lack
of information/recall, misinterpretation, possibly evidenced by
statements of concern, questions, misconceptions; inaccurate follow-
through of instructions, and development of preventable complica-
tions/recurrence of condition.

Unconsciousness (coma)   MS

risk for Suffocation: risk factors may include cognitive impairment/loss
of protective reflexes and purposeful movement.*

risk for deficient Fluid Volume/imbalanced Nutrition: less than body
requirements: risk factors may include inability to ingest food/fluids,
increased needs/hypermetabolic state.*

*A risk diagnosis is not evidenced by signs and symptoms, as the
problem has not occurred and nursing interventions are directed at
prevention.

<u>total Self-Care Deficit</u> may be related to cognitive impairment and absence of purposeful activity, evidenced by inability to perform ADLs.

<u>risk for ineffective cerebral Tissue Perfusion:</u> risk factors may include reduced or interrupted arterial/venous blood flow (direct injury, edema formation, space-occupying lesions), metabolic alterations, effects of drug/alcohol overdose, hypoxia/anoxia.*

<u>risk for Infection:</u> risk factors may include stasis of body fluids (oral, pulmonary, urinary), invasive procedures, and nutritional deficits.*

Urinary diversion   MS/CH

<u>risk for impaired Skin Integrity:</u> risk factors may include absence of sphincter at stoma, character/flow of urine from stoma, reaction to product/chemicals, and improperly fitting appliance or removal of adhesive.*

<u>disturbed Body Image,</u> related factors may include biophysical factors, (presence of stoma, loss of control of urine flow), and psychosocial factors (altered body structure, disease process/associated treatment regimen, such as cancer), possibly evidenced by verbalization of change in body image, fear of rejection/reaction of others, negative feelings about body, not touching/looking at stoma, refusal to participate in care.

<u>acute Pain</u> may be related to physical factors (disruption of skin/tissues, presence of incisions/drains), biological factors (activity of disease process, such as cancer, trauma), and psychologic factors (fear, anxiety), possibly evidenced by verbal reports, self-focusing, guarding/distraction behaviors, restlessness, and autonomic responses (changes in vital signs).

<u>impaired Urinary Elimination</u> may be related to surgical diversion, tissue trauma, and postoperative edema, possibly evidenced by loss of continence, changes in amount and character of urine, and urinary retention.

Urolithiasis   MS/CH

(Refer to Calculi, urinary)

Uterine bleeding, abnormal   GYN/MS

<u>Anxiety [specify level]</u> may be related to perceived change in health status and unknown etiology, possibly evidenced by apprehension, uncertainty, fear of unspecified consequences, expressed concerns, and focus on self.

<u>Activity Intolerance</u> may be related to imbalance between oxygen supply and demand/decreased oxygen-carrying capacity of blood (anemia), possibly evidenced by reports of fatigue/weakness.

Uterus, rupture of, in pregnancy   OB

<u>deficient Fluid Volume [isotonic]</u> may be related to excessive vascular losses, possibly evidenced by hypotension, increased pulse rate, decreased venous filling, and decreased urine output.

*A risk diagnosis is not evidenced by signs and symptoms, as the problem has not occurred and nursing interventions are directed at prevention.

decreased Cardiac Output, may be related to decreased preload (hypovolemia), possibly evidenced by cold/clammy skin, decreased peripheral pulses, variations in hemodynamic readings, tachycardia, and cyanosis.

acute Pain may be related to tissue trauma and irritation of accumulating blood, possibly evidenced by verbal reports, guarding/distraction behaviors, self-focus, and autonomic responses (changes in vital signs).

Anxiety [specify level] may be related to threat of death of self/fetus, interpersonal contagion, physiologic response (release of catecholamines), possibly evidenced by fearful/scared affect, sympathetic stimulation, stated fear of unspecified consequences, and expressed concerns.

Vaginismus   GYN/CH

acute Pain may be related to muscle spasm and hyperesthesia of the nerve supply to vaginal mucous membrane, possibly evidenced by verbal reports, distraction behaviors, and self-focus.

Sexual Dysfunction may be related to physical and/or psychological alteration in function (severe spasms of vaginal muscles), possibly evidenced by verbalization of problem, inability to achieve desired satisfaction, and alteration in relationship with significant other.

Vaginitis   GYN/CH

impaired Tissue Integrity may be related to irritation/inflammation and mechanical trauma (scratching) of sensitive tissues, possibly evidenced by damaged/destroyed tissue, presence of lesions.

acute Pain may be related to localized inflammation and tissue trauma, possibly evidenced by verbal reports, distraction behaviors, and self-focus.

deficient Knowledge [Learning Need] regarding hygienic/therapy needs and sexual behaviors/transmission of organisms may be related to lack of information/misinterpretation, possibly evidenced by statements of concern, questions, and misconceptions.

Varices, esophageal   MS

(Also refer to Ulcer, peptic [acute])

deficient Fluid Volume [isotonic] may be related to excessive vascular loss, reduced intake, and gastric losses (vomiting), possibly evidenced by hypotension, tachycardia, decreased venous filling, and decreased/concentrated urine.

Anxiety [specify level]/Fear may be related to change in health status and threat of death, possibly evidenced by increased tension/apprehension, sympathetic stimulation, restlessness, focus on self, and expressed concerns.

Varicose veins   CH

chronic Pain may be related to venous insufficiency and stasis, possibly evidenced by verbal reports.

disturbed Body Image may be related to change in structure (presence of enlarged, discolored tortuous superficial leg veins) possibly evidenced by hiding affected parts and negative feelings about body.

risk for impaired Skin/Tissue Integrity: risk factors may include altered circulation/venous stasis and edema formation.*

Venereal disease   CH
(Refer to Sexually transmitted disease—STD)

Ventricular fibrillation   MS
(Refer to Dysrhythmias)

Ventricular tachycardia   MS
(Refer to Dysrhythmias)

West Nile fever   CH/MS
Hyperthermia may be related to infectious process possibly evidenced by elevated body temperature, skin flushed/warm to touch, tachycardia, increased respiratory rate.

acute Pain may be related to infectious process/circulating toxins possibly evidenced by reports of headache, myalgia, eye pain, abdominal discomfort.

risk for deficient Fluid Volume: risk factors may include hypermetabolic state, decreased intake anorexia, nausea, losses from normal routes (vomiting, diarrhea).*

risk for impaired Skin Integrity: risk factors may include hyperthermia, decreased fluid intake, alterations in skin turgor, bedrest, circulating toxins.*

Wilms' tumor   PED
(Also refer to Cancer; Chemotherapy)

Anxiety [specify level]/Fear may be related to change in environment and interaction patterns with family members and threat of death with family transmission and contagion of concerns, possibly evidenced by fearful/scared affect, distress, crying, insomnia, and sympathetic stimulation.

risk for Injury: risk factors may include nature of tumor (vascular, mushy with very thin covering) with increased danger of metastasis when manipulated.*

interrupted Family Processes, may be related to situational crisis of life-threatening illness, possibly evidenced by a family system that has difficulty meeting physical, emotional, and spiritual needs of its members, and inability to deal with traumatic experience effectively.

deficient Diversional Activity may be related to environmental lack of age-appropriate activity (including activity restrictions) and length of hospitalization/treatment, possibly evidenced by restlessness, crying, lethargy, and acting-out behavior.

Wound, gunshot   MS
(Depends on site and speed/character of bullet)

risk for deficient Fluid Volume: risk factors may include excessive vascular losses, altered intake/restrictions.*

---

*A risk diagnosis is not evidenced by signs and symptoms, as the problem has not occurred and nursing interventions are directed at prevention.

acute Pain may be related to destruction of tissue (including organ and musculoskeletal), surgical repair, and therapeutic interventions, possibly evidenced by verbal reports, guarding/distraction behaviors, self-focus, and autonomic responses (changes in vital signs).

impaired Tissue Integrity may be related to mechanical factors (yaw of projectile and muzzle blast), possibly evidenced by damaged or destroyed tissue.

risk for Infection: risk factors may include tissue destruction and increased environmental exposure, invasive procedures, and decreased hemoglobin.*

CH

risk for Post-Trauma Syndrome: risk factors may include nature of incident (catastrophic accident, assault, suicide attempt) and possibly injury/death of other(s) involved.*

---

*A risk diagnosis is not evidenced by signs and symptoms, as the problem has not occurred and nursing interventions are directed at prevention.

NANDA's Taxonomy II

The 13 domains and their classes are:

Domain 1 Health Promotion: The awareness of well-being or normality of function and the strategies used to maintain control of and enhance that well-being or normality of function

> **Class 1 Health Awareness: Recognition of normal function and well-being**
> **Class 2 Health Management: Identifying, controlling, performing, and integrating activities to maintain health and well-being**

Domain 2 Nutrition: The activities of taking in, assimilating, and using nutrients for the purposes of tissue maintenance, tissue repair, and the production of energy

> **Class 1 Ingestion: Taking food or nutrients into the body**
> **Class 2 Digestion: The physical and chemical activities that convert foodstuffs into substances suitable for absorption and assimilation**
> **Class 3 Absorption: The act of taking up nutrients through body tissues**
> **Class 4 Metabolism: The chemical and physical processes occurring in living organisms and cells for the development and use of protoplasm production of waste and energy, with the release of energy for all vital processes**
> **Class 5 Hydration: The taking in and absorption of fluids and electrolytes**

Domain 3 Elimination: Secretion and excretion of waste products from the body

> **Class 1 Urinary System: The process of secretion and excretion of urine**
> **Class 2 Gastrointestinal System: Excretion and expulsion of waste products from the bowel**
> **Class 3 Integumentary System: Process of secretion and excretion through the skin**
> **Class 4 Pulmonary System: Removal of byproducts of metabolic products, secretions, and foreign material from the lung or bronchi**

Domain 4 Activity/Rest: The production, conservation, expenditure, or balance of energy resources

Class 1 Sleep/Rest: Slumber, repose, ease, or inactivity

Class 2 Activity/Exercise: Moving parts of the body (mobility), doing work, or performing actions often (but not always) against resistance

Class 3 Energy Balance: A dynamic state of harmony between intake and expenditure of resources

Class 4 Cardiovascular/Pulmonary Responses: Cardiopulmonary mechanisms that support activity/rest

Domain 5 Perception/Cognition: The human information processing system including attention, orientation, sensation, perception, cognition, and communication

Class 1 Attention: Mental readiness to notice or observe

Class 2 Orientation: Awareness of time, place, and person

Class 3 Sensation/Perception: Receiving information through the senses of touch, taste, smell, vision, hearing, and kinesthesia and the comprehension of sense data resulting in naming, associating, and/or pattern recognition

Class 4 Cognition: Use of memory, learning, thinking, problem solving, abstraction, judgment, insight, intellectual capacity, calculation, and language

Class 5 Communication: Sending and receiving verbal and nonverbal information

Domain 6 Self-Perception: Awareness about the self

Class 1 Self-Concept: The perception(s) about the total self

Class 2 Self-Esteem: Assessment of one's own worth, capability, significance, and success

Class 3 Body Image: A mental image of one's own body

Domain 7 Role Relationships: The positive and negative connections or associations between persons or groups of persons and the means by which those connections are demonstrated

Class 1 Caregiving Roles: Socially expected behavior patterns by persons providing care who are not healthcare professionals

Class 2 Family Relationships: Associations of people who are biologically related or related by choice

> **Class 3 Role Performance: Quality of functioning in socially expected behavior patterns**

Domain 8 Sexuality: Sexual identity, sexual function, and reproduction

> **Class 1 Sexual Identity: The state of being a specific person in regard to sexuality and/or gender**
> **Class 2 Sexual Function: The capacity or ability to participate in sexual activities**
> **Class 3 Reproduction: Any process by which new individuals (people) are produced**

Domain 9 Coping/Stress Tolerance: Contending with life events/life processes

> **Class 1 Post-Trauma Responses: Reactions occurring after physical or psychological trauma**
> **Class 2 Coping Responses: The process of managing environmental stress**
> **Class 3 Neurobehavioral Stress: Behavioral responses reflecting nerve and brain function**

Domain 10 Life Principles: Principles underlying conduct, thought, and behavior about acts, customs, or institutions viewed as being true or having intrinsic worth

> **Class 1 Values: The identification and ranking of preferred mode of conduct or end states**
> **Class 2 Beliefs: Opinions, expectations, or judgments about acts, customs, or institutions viewed as being true or having intrinsic worth**
> **Class 3 Value/Belief/Action Congruence: The correspondence or balance achieved between values, beliefs, and actions**

Domain 11 Safety/Protection: Freedom from danger, physical injury, or immune system damage; preservation from loss; and protection of safety and security

> **Class 1 Infection: Host responses following pathogenic invasion**
> **Class 2 Physical Injury: Bodily harm or hurt**
> **Class 3 Violence: The exertion of excessive force or power so as to cause injury or abuse**
> **Class 4 Environmental Hazards: Sources of danger in the surroundings**
> **Class 5 Defensive Processes: The processes by which the self protects itself from the nonself**
> **Class 6 Thermoregulation: The physiologic process of regulating heat and energy within the body for purposes of protecting the organism**

Domain 12 Comfort: Sense of mental, physical, or social well-being or ease

Class 1 Physical Comfort: Sense of well-being or ease
Class 2 Environmental Comfort: Sense of well-being or ease in/with one's environment
Class 3 Social Comfort: Sense of well-being or ease with one's social situations

Domain 13 Growth/Development: Age-appropriate increases in physical dimensions, organ systems, and/or attainment of developmental milestones

Class 1 Growth: Increases in physical dimensions or maturity of organ systems
Class 2 Development: Attainment, lack of attainment, or loss of developmental milestones

Definitions of Taxonomy II Axes

Axis 1 The Diagnostic Concept: Defined as the principal element or the fundamental and essential part, the root, of the diagnostic statement.

Axis 2 Time: Defined as the duration of a period or interval.

> ***Acute:*** **Less that 6 months**
> ***Chronic:*** **More than 6 months**
> ***Intermittent:*** **Stopping or starting again at intervals, periodic, cyclic**
> ***Continuous:*** **Uninterrupted, going on without stops**

Axis 3 The Unit of Care: Defined as the distinct population for which a nursing diagnosis is determined. Values are:

> ***Individual:*** **A single human being distinct from others, a person**
> ***Family:*** **Two or more people having continuous or sustained relationships, perceiving reciprocal obligations, sensing common meaning, and sharing certain obligations toward others; related by blood or choice**
> ***Group:*** **Individuals gathered, classified, or acting together**
> ***Community:*** **" 'A group of people living in the same locale under the same government.' Examples include neighborhoods, cities, census tracts, and populations at risk." (Craft Rosenberg, 1999, p. 127) When the unit of care is not explicitly stated, it becomes the individual by default.**

Axis 4 Age: Defined as the length of time or interval during which an individual has existed. Values are:

Fetus	Adolescent
Neonate	Young adult
Infant	Middle-age adult
Toddler	Young-old adult
Pre-school child	Middle-old adult
School-age child	Old-old adult

Axis 5 Health Status: Defined as the position or rank on the health continuum. Values are:

Wellness: The quality or state of being healthy, especially as a result of deliberate effort
Risk: Vulnerability, especially as a result of exposure to factors that increase the chance of injury or loss
Actual: Existing in fact or reality, existing at the present time.

Axis 6 Descriptor: Defined as a judgment that limits or specifies the meaning of a nursing diagnosis. Values are:

Ability: Capacity to do or act
Anticipatory: To realize beforehand, foresee
Balance: State of equilibrium
Compromised: To make vulnerable to threat
Decreased: Lessened; lesser in size, amount or degree
Deficient: Inadequate in amount, quality, or degree; not sufficient; incomplete
Defensive: To feel constantly under attack and the need to quickly justify on actions
Delayed: To postpone, impede, and retard
Depleted: Emptied wholly or in part, exhausted of
Disabling: To make unable or unfit, to incapacitate
Disorganized: To destroy the systematic arrangement
Disproportionate: Not consistent with a standard
Disturbed: Agitated or interrupted, interfered with
Dysfunctional: Abnormal, incomplete functioning
Effective: Producing the intended or expected effect
Excessive: Characterized by the amount or quantity that is greater than necessary, desirable, or useful
Functional: Normal, complete functioning
Imbalanced: State of disequilibrium
Impaired: Made worse, weakened, damaged, reduced, deteriorated
Inability: Incapacity to do or act
Increased: Greater in size, amount, or degree
Ineffective: Not producing the desired effect
Interrupted: To break the continuity or uniformity
Low: Containing less than normal amount of some usual element
Organized: To form as into a systematic arrangement
Perceived: To become aware of by means of the senses; assignment of meaning
Readiness for enhanced (for use with wellness diagnoses): To make greater, to increase in quality, to attain the more desired

Axis 7 Topology: Consists of parts/regions of the body—all tissues, organs, anatomical sites, or structures. Values are:

Auditory	Olfactory
Bowel	Peripheral neurovascular
Cardiopulmonary	Peripheral vascular
Cerebral	Renal
Gastrointestinal	Skin
Gustatory	Tactile
Intracranial	Urinary
Mucous membranes	Visual
Oral	

(NANDA: Nursing Diagnoses: Definitions & Classification 2001-2002, Philadelphia, 2001.)

Bibliography

Books

Acute Pain Management: Operative or Medical Procedures and Trauma: Clinical Practice Guideline. US Department of Health and Human Services, Public Health Service Agency for Health Care Policy and Research, Rockville, MD, Feb 1992.

American Nurses' Association: Nursing's Social Policy Statement. Washington, DC, 1995.

American Nurses' Association: Standards of Clinical Nursing Practice. Kansas City, MO, 1991.

Androwich, I, Burkhart, L, and Gettrust, KV: Community and Home Health Nursing. Delmar, Albany, NY, 1996.

Beers, MH, and Berkow, R: The Merck Manual of Diagnosis and Therapy, ed. 17. Merck Research Laboratories, Whitehouse Station, NJ, 1999.

Carey, CF, Lee, HH, and Woeltje, KF (eds): The Washington Manual of Medical Therapeutics, ed. 29. Lippincott-Raven, Philadelphia, 1998.

Cassileth, BR: The Alternative Medicine Handbook: The Complete Reference Guide to Alternative and Complementary Therapies. WW Norton & Co, New York, 1998.

Cataract in Adults: Management of Functional Impairment. AHCPR Pub 93-0542, US Department of Health and Human Services, Public Health Agency for Health Care Policy and Research, Rockville, MD, 1993.

The Colorado SIDS Program, Inc, 6825 East Tennessee Ave, Suite 300, Denver, CO 80224-1631.

Condon, RE, and Nyhus, LM (eds): Manual of Surgical Therapeutics, ed. 9. Little, Brown & Co., Boston, 1996.

Cox, H, et al: Clinical Applications of Nursing Diagnosis: Adult, Child, Women's Psychiatric, Gerontic, and Home Health Considerations, ed. 4. F.A. Davis, Philadelphia, 2002.

Deglin, J, and Vallerand, A: Davis's Drug Guide for Nurses, ed. 6. F.A. Davis, Philadelphia, 1999.

Depression in Primary Care, Vol. 1, Detection and Diagnosis. AHCPR Pub 93-0550, US Department of Health and Human Services, Public Health Service Agency for Health Care Policy and Research, Rockville, MD, April 1993.

Depression in Primary Care, Vol. 2, Treatment of Major Depression. AHCPR Pub 93-0551, US Department of Health and Human Services, Public Health Service Agency for Health Care Policy and Research, Rockville, MD, April 1993.

Doenges, M, Moorhouse, M, and Geissler-Murr, A: Nursing Care Plans: Nursing Diagnoses in Patient Care, ed. 6. F.A. Davis, Philadelphia, 2002.

Doenges, M, Townsend, M, and Moorhouse, M: Psychiatric Care Plans: Guidelines for Planning and Documenting Client Care, ed. 3. F.A. Davis, Philadelphia, 1999.

Early Identification of Alzheimer's Disease and Related Dementias: Clinical Practice Guideline, US Department of Health and Human Services, Public Health Service Agency for Health Care Policy and Research, Rockville, MD, Nov 1996.

Engel, J: Pocket Guide to Pediatric Assessment, ed. 4. Mosby, St. Louis, 2002.

Gordon, M: Manual of Nursing Diagnosis. Mosby, St. Louis, 1997.

Gordon, T: Parent Effectiveness Training. Three Rivers Press, New York, 2000.

Gordon, T: Teaching Children Self-Discipline: At Home and At School. Random House, New York, 1989.

Gorman, L, Sultan, D, and Raines, M: Davis's Manual of Psychosocial Nursing for General Patient Care. F.A. Davis, Philadelphia, 1996.

Harkulich, JT, et al: Teacher's Guide: A Manual for Caregivers of Alzheimer's Disease in Long-Term Care. Embassy Printing, Cleveland Heights, Ohio, Copyright pending.

Higgs, ZR, and Gustafson, DD: Community as a Client: Assessment and Diagnosis. F.A. Davis, Philadelphia, 1985.

Jaffe, MS, and McVan, BF: Laboratory and Diagnostic Test Handbook. F.A. Davis, Philadelphia, 1997.

Johnson, M, and Maas, M: Nursing Outcomes Classification (NOC), ed. 2. Mosby, St. Louis, 2000.

Kuhn, MA: Pharmacotherapeutics: A Nursing Process Approach, ed. 4. F.A. Davis, Philadelphia, 1998.

Lampe, S: Focus Charting, ed. 7. Creative Healthcare Management, Inc., Minneapolis, 1997.

Lee, D, Barrett, C, and Ignatavicius, D: Fluids and Electrolytes: A Practical Approach, ed. 4. F.A. Davis, Philadelphia, 1996.

Leiniger, MM: Transcultural Nursing: Theories, Research and Practices, ed. 3. McGraw-Hill, Hilliard, OH, 1996.

Lipson, JG, et al: Culture and Nursing Care: A Pocket Guide. UCSF Nursing Press, University of California, San Francisco, 1996.

Management of Cancer Pain. AHCPR Pub 93-0592, US Department of Health and Human Services, Public Health Agency for Health Care Policy and Research, Rockville, MD, 1994.

McCance, KL, and Huether, SE: Pathophysiology: The Biologic Basis for Disease in Adults and Children, ed. 3. Mosby, St. Louis, 1997.

McCloskey, JC, and Bulechek, GM (eds): Nursing Interventions Classification, ed. 3. Mosby, St. Louis, 2000.

Mentgen, J, and Bulbrook, MJT: Healing Touch, Level I Notebook. Healing Touch, Lakewood, CO, 1994.

NANDA Nursing Diagnoses: Definitions and Classification 2003–2004. International, Philadelphia, 2003.

Olds, SB, London, ML, Ladewig, PW: Maternity-Newborn Nursing: A Family-Centered Approach, ed. 6. Prentice Hall, Upper Saddle River, NJ, 1999.

Phillips, CR: Family-Centered Maternity and Newborn Care, ed. 4. Mosby, St. Louis, MO, 1996.

Post-Stroke Rehabilitation: Assessment, Referral, and Patient

Management. AHCPR Pub 95-0663, US Department of Health and Human Services, Public Health Service Agency for Health Care Policy and Research, Rockville, MD, 1995.

Pressure Ulcers in Adults: Prediction and Prevention. AHCPR Pub 92-0047, US Department of Health and Human Services, Public Health Service Agency for Health Care Policy and Research, Rockville, MD, 1992.

Purnell, LD, and Paulanka, BJ: Transcultural Health Care: A Culturally Competent Approach. F.A. Davis, Philadelphia, 1998.

Shore, LS: Nursing Diagnosis: What It Is and How to Do It: A Programmed Text. Medical College of Virginia Hospitals, Richmond, VA, 1988.

Sickle Cell Disease: Screening, Diagnosis, Management, and Counseling in Newborns and Infants. AHCPR Pub 93-0562, US Department of Health and Human Services, Public Health Service Agency for Health Care Policy and Research, Rockville, MD, April 1993.

Sommers, MS, and Johnson, SA: Davis Manual of Nursing Therapeutics for Disease and Disorders. F.A. Davis, Philadelphia, 1997.

Sparks, SM, and Taylor, CM: Nursing Diagnoses Reference Manual, ed. 5. Springhouse, Springhouse, PA, 2001.

Stanley, M, and Beare, PG: Gerontological Nursing: A Health Promotion/Protection Approach, ed. 2. F.A. Davis, Philadelphia, 1999.

Townsend, M: Nursing Diagnoses in Psychiatric Nursing: A Pocket Guide for Care Plan Construction, ed. 4. F.A. Davis, Philadelphia, 1997.

Townsend, M: Psychiatric Mental Health Nursing: Concepts of Care, ed. 2. F.A. Davis, Philadelphia, 1996.

Traumatic Brain Injury Medical Treatment Guidelines. State of Colorado Labor and Employment, Division of Worker's Compensation, Denver, March 15, 1998.

Urinary Incontinence in Adults: Clinical Practice Guideline. AHCPR Pub 92-0038, US Department of Health and Human Services, Public Health Service Agency for Health Care Policy and Research, Rockville, MD, March 1992.

Venes, D, and Thomas, CL (eds): Taber's Cyclopedic Medical Dictionary, ed. 19. F.A. Davis, Philadelphia, 2001.

Articles

Ackerman, MH, and Mick, DJ: Instillation of normal saline before suctioning patients with pulmonary infections: A prospective randomized controlled trial. Am J Crit Care 7(4):261, 1998.

Acute Confusion/Delirium. Research Dissemination Core, University of Iowa Gerontological Nursing Interventions Research Center (GNIRC). Iowa City, IA, 1998.

Albert, N: Heart failure: The physiologic basis for current therapeutic concepts. Crit Care Nurse (Suppl), June, 1999.

Allen, LA: Treating agitation without drugs. Am J Nurs 99(4):36, 1999.

American Academy of Pediatrics, Task Force on Sleep Position and SIDS: Changing concepts of sudden infant death syndrome:

Implications for infant sleeping environment and sleep position. Pediatrics 105:650, 2000.

Angelucci, PA: Caring for patients with benign prostatic hyperplasia. Nursing 27(11):34, 1997.

Armstrong, ML, and Murphy, KP: A look at adolescent tattooing. School Health Reporter, Summer 1999.

Augustus, LJ: Nutritional care for patients with HIV. Am J Nurs 97(10):62, 1997.

Barry, J, McQuade, C, and Livingstone, T: Using nurse case management to promote self-efficiency in individuals with rheumatoid arthritis. Rehabil Nurs 23(6):300, 1998.

Bergen, AF: Heads up: A 20-year tale in several parts. Team Rehabilitation Report 9(9):45, 1998.

Berkowitz, C: Epidural pain control: Your job, too. RN 60(8):22, 1997.

Bermingham, J: Discharge planning: Charting patient progress. Contin Care 16(1):13, 1997.

Birkett, DP: What is the relationship between stroke and depression? Harv Ment Health Lett 14(12):8, 1998.

Blank, CA, and Reid, PC: Taking the tension out of traumatic pneumothoraxes. Nursing 29(4):41, 1999.

Bone, LA: Restoring electrolyte balance: Calcium and phosphorus. RN 59(3):47, 1996.

Boon, T: Don't forget the hospice option. RN 61(2):32, 1998.

Borton, D: Isolation precautions: Clearing up the confusion. Nursing 27(1):49, 1997.

Boucher, MA: When laryngectomy complicates care. RN 59(88):40, 1996.

Bradley, M, and Pupiales, M: Essential elements of ostomy care. Am J Nurs 97(7):38, 1997.

Branski, SH: Delirium in hospitalized geriatric patients. Am J Nurs 97(4):161, 1998.

Brown, KA: Malignant hyperthermia. Am J Nurs 97(10):33, 1997.

Buckle, J: Alternative/complementary therapies. Crit Care Nurse 18(5):54, 1998.

Burgio, KL, et al: Behavioral training for post-prostatectomy urinary incontinence. J Urol 141(2):303, 1989.

Burt, S: What you need to know about latex allergy. Nursing 28(10):33, 1998.

Calcium in kidney stones. Harv Health Lett 22(8):8, 1997.

Canales, MAP: Asthma management, putting your patient on the team. Nursing 27(12):33, 1997.

Capili, B, and Anastasi, JK: A symptom review: Nausea and vomiting in HIV. JANAC 9(6):47, 1998.

Carbone, IM: An interdisciplinary approach to the rehabilitation of open-heart surgical patients. Rehabil Nurs 24(2):55, 1999.

Carlson, EV, Kemp, MG, and Short, S: Predicting the risk of pressure ulcers in critically ill patients. Am J Crit Care 8(4):262, 1999.

Carroll, P: Closing in on safer suctioning. RN 61(5):22, 1998.

Carroll, P: Preventing nosocomial pneumonia. RN 61(6):44, 1998.

Carroll, P: Pulse oximetry: At your fingertips. RN 60(2):22, 1997.

Cataldo, R: Decoding the mystery: Evaluating complementary and alternative medicine. Rehab Manag 12(2):42, 1999.

Cavendish, R: Clinical snapshot: Periodontal disease. Am J Nurs 99(3):36, 1999.

Chatterton, R, et al: Suicides in an Australian inpatient environment. J Psychosoc Nurs Ment Health Serv 37(6):34, 1999.

Chilton, BA: Recognizing spirituality. Image J Nurs Sch 30(4):400, 1998.

Cirolia, B: Understanding edema: When fluid balance fails. Nursing 26(2):66, 1996.

Clark, CC: Posttraumatic stress disorder: How to support healing. Am J Nurs 97(8):26, 1996.

Consult Stat: Chest tubes: When you don't need a seal. RN 61(3):67, 1998.

Cook, L: The value of lab values. Am J Nurs 99(5):66, 1999.

Crigger, N, and Forbes, W: Assessing neurologic function in older patients. Am J Nurs 97(3):37, 1997.

Crow, S: Combating infection: Your guide to gloves. Nursing 27(3):26, 1997.

DeJong, MJ: Emergency! Hyponatremia. Am J Nurs 98(12):36, 1998.

Dennison, RD: Nurse's guide to common postoperative complications. Nursing 27(11):56, 1997.

Dossey, BM, and Dossey, L: Body-Mind-Spirit: Attending to holistic care. Am J Nurs 98(8):35, 1998.

Dossey, BM: Holistic modalities and healing moments. Am J Nurs 98(6):44, 1998.

Drugs that bring erections down. Sex & Health Institute, p. 5, May 1998.

Dunne, D: Common questions about ileoanal reservoirs. Am J Nurs 97(11):67, 1997.

Edmond, M: Combating infection: Tackling disease transmission. Nursing 27(7):65, 1997.

Edwards-Beckett, J, and King, H: The impact of spinal pathology on bowel control in children. Rehabil Nurs 21(6):292, 1996.

Epps, CK: The delicate business of ostomy care. RN 5(11):32, 1996.

Faries, J: Easing your patient's postoperative pain. Nursing 28(6):58, 1998.

Ferrin, MS: Restoring electrolyte balance: Magnesium. RN 59(5):31, 1996.

Fish, KB: Suicide awareness at the elementary school level. J of Psychosoc Nurs Ment Health Serv, 38(7):20, 2000.

Fishman, TD, Freedline, AD, and Kahn, D: Putting the best foot forward. Nursing 26(1):58, 1996.

Flannery, J: Using the levels of cognitive functioning assessment scale with traumatic brain injury in an acute care setting. Rehabil Nurs 23(2):88, 1998.

Focazio, B: Clinical snapshot: Mucositis. Am J Nurs 97(12):48, 1997.

Garnett, LR: Is obesity all in the genes? Harv Health Lett 21(6):1, 1996.

Goshorn, J: Clinical snapshot: Kidney stones. Am J Nurs 96(9):40, 1996.

Grandjean, CK, and Gibbons, SW: Assessing ambulatory geriatric sleep complaints. Nurse Pract 25(9):25, 2000.

Gregory, CM: Caring for caregivers: Proactive planning eases burdens on caregivers. Lifelines 1(2):51, 1997.

Greifzu, S: Fighting cancer fatigue. RN 61(8):41, 1998.

Gritter, M: The latex threat. Am J Nurs 98(9):26, 1998.

Grzankowski, JA: Altered thought processes related to traumatic brain injury and their nursing implications. Rehabil Nurs 22(1):24, 1997.

Hahn, J: Cueing in to client language. Reflections 25(1):8–11, 1999.

Halpin-Landry, JE, and Goldsmith, S: Feet first: Diabetes care. Am J Nurs 99(2):26, 1999.

Hanson, MJS: Caring for a patient with COPD. Nursing 27(12):39, 1997.

Harvey, C, Dixon, M, and Padberg, N: Support group for families of trauma patients: A unique approach. Crit Care Nurse 15(4):59, 1995.

Hayes, DD: Bradycardia. Keeping the current flowing. Nursing 27(6):50, 1997.

Hayn, MA, and Fisher, TR: Stroke rehabilitation: Salvaging ability after the storm. Nursing 27(3):40, 1997.

Hernandez, D: Microvascular complications of diabetes nursing assessment and interventions. Am J Nurs 98(6):16, 1998.

Herson, L, et al: Rehabil Nurs 24(4):148, 1999.

Hess, CT: Caring for a diabetic ulcer. Nursing 29(5):70, 1999.

Hess, CT: Wound care. Nursing 28(3):18, 1998.

Hoffman, J: Tuning in to the power of music. RN 60(6):52, 1997.

Holcomb, SS: Understanding the ins and outs of diuretic therapy. Nursing 27(2):34, 1997.

Hunt, R: Community-based nursing. Am J Nurs 98(10):44, 1998.

Huston, CJ: Emergency! Dental luxation and avulsion. Am J Nurs 97(9):48, 1997.

Hutchison, CP: Healing touch: An energetic approach. Am J Nurs 99(4):43, 1999.

Isaacs, A: Depression and your patient. Am J Nurs 98(7):26, 1998.

It's probably not Alzheimer's: New insights on memory loss. Focus on Healthy Aging 2(7):1, 1999.

Iyasu, S, et al: Risk factors for sudden infant death syndrome among Northern Plains Indians. JAMA, 288(21):2717, 2002.

Jaempf, G, and Goralski, VJ: Monitoring postop patients. RN 59(7):30, 1996.

Jennings, LM: Latex allergy: Another real Y2K issue. Rehabil Nurs 24(4):140, 1999.

Jirovec, MM, Wyman, JF, and Wells, TJ: Addressing urinary incontinence with educational continence-care competencies. Image J Nurs Sch 30(4):375, 1998.

Johnson, J, Pearson, V, and McDivitt, L: Stroke rehabilitation: Assessing stroke survivors' long-term learning needs. Rehabil Nurs 22(5):243, 1997.

Kachourbos, MJ: Relief at last: An implanted bladder control system helps people control their bodily functions. Team Rehabilitation Reports, p. 31, Aug 1997.

Kanachki, L: How to guide ventilator-dependent patients from hospital to home. Am J Nurs 97(2):37, 1997.

Keegan, L: Getting comfortable with alternative and complementary therapies. Nursing 28(4):50, 1998.

King, B: Preserving renal function. RN 60(8):34, 1997.

Kinloch, D: Instillation of normal saline during endotracheal suctioning: Effects on mixed venous oxygen saturation. Am J Crit Care 8(4):231, 1999.

Kirshblum, S, and O'Connor, K: The problem of pain: A common condition of people with SCI. Team Rehabilitation Reports, p. 15, Aug 1997.

Klonowski, EI, and Masodi, JE: The patient with Crohn's disease. RN 62(3):32, 1999.

Korinko, A, and Yurick, A: Maintaining skin integrity during radiation therapy. Am J Nurs 97(2):40, 1997.

Kumasaka, L, and Miles, A: "My pain is God's will." Am J Nurs 96(6):45, 1996.

Kurtz, MJ, Van Zandt, DK, and Sapp, LR: A new technique in independent intermittent catheterization: The Mitrofanoff catheterizable channel. Rehabil Nurs 21(6):311, 1996.

Lai, SC, and Cohen, MN: Promoting lifestyle changes. Am J Nurs 99(4):63, 1999.

Larsen, LS: Effectiveness of a counseling intervention to assist family caregivers of chronically ill relatives. J Psychosoc Nurs Ment Health Serv 36(8):26, 1998.

Lewis, ML, and Dehn, DS: Violence against nurses in outpatient mental health settings. J Psychosoc Nurs Ment Health Serv 37(6):28, 1999.

Linch, SH: Elder abuse: What to look for, how to intervene. Am J Nurs 97(1):26, 1997.

Loeb, JL: Pain management in long-term care. Am J Nurs 99(2):48, 1999.

Loughrey, L: Taking a sensitive approach to urinary incontinence. Nursing 29(5):60, 1999.

MacNeill, D, and Weis, T: Case study: Coordinating care. Contin Care 17(4):78, 1998.

Matthews, PJ: Ventilator-associated infections. I. Reducing the risks. Nursing 27(2):59, 1997.

McCaffery, M: Pain management handbook. Nursing 27(4):42, 1997.

McCaffery, M, and Ferrell, BR: Opioids and pain management: What do nurses know? Nursing 29(3):48, 1999.

McCain, D, and Sutherland, S: Nursing essentials: Skin grafts for patients with burns. Am J Nurs 98(7):34, 1998.

McClave, SA, et al: Are patients fed appropriately according to their caloric requirements? JPEN 22(6):375, 1998.

McConnel, E: Preventing transient increases in intracranial pressure. Nursing 28(4):66, 1998.

McHale, JM, et al: Expert nursing knowledge in the care of patients at risk of impaired swallowing. Image J Nurs Sch 30(2):137, 1998.

McKinley, LL, and Zasler, CP: Weaving a plan of care. Contin Care 17(7):38, 1998.

Mendez-Eastman, S: When wounds won't heal. RN 51(1):20, 1998.

Metheny, N, et al: Testing feeding tube placement: Auscultation vs pH method. Am J Nurs 98(5):37, 1998.

Mohr, WK: Cross-ethnic variations in the care of psychiatric patients: A review of contributing factors and practice considerations. J Psychosoc Nurs Ment Health Serv 36(5):16, 1998.

Nunnelee, JD: Healing venous ulcers. RN 60(11):38, 1997.

O'Donnell, M: Addisonian crisis. Am J Nurs 97(3):41, 1997.

O'Neil, C, Avila, JR, and Fetrow, CW: Herbal medicines, getting beyond the hype. Nursing 29(4):58, 1999.

Parkman, CA, and Calfee, BE: Advance directives, honoring your patient's end-of-life wishes. Nursing 27(4):48, 1997.

Phillips, JK: Actionstat: Wound dehiscence. Nursing 28(3):33, 1998.

Pierce, LL: Barriers to access: Frustrations of people who use a wheelchair for full-time mobility. Rehabil Nurs 23(3):120, 1998.

Pignone, MP, et al: Counseling to promote a healthy diet in adults: A summary of the evidence for the US Preventive Services Task Force. Am J Prev Med. 24(1):75, 2003.

Powers, J, and Bennett, SJ: Measurement of dyspnea in patients treated with mechanical ventilation. Am J Crit Care 8(4):254, 1999.

Pronitis-Ruotolo, D: Surviving the night shift: Making Zeitgeber work for you. Am J Nurs 101(7):63, 2001.

Rawsky, E: Review of the literature on falls among the elderly. Image J Nurs Sch 30(1):47, 1998.

Robinson, AW: Getting to the heart of denial. Am J Nurs 99(5):38, 1999.

Rogers, S, Ryan, M, and Slepoy, L: Successful ventilator weaning: A collaborative effort. Rehabil Nurs 23(5):265, 1998.

Sampselle, CM: Behavioral interventions in young and middle-age women. Am J Nurs 103(3):9, 2003. (Suppl) State of the Science on Urinary Incontinence.

Scanlon, C: Defining standards for end-of-life care. Am J Nurs 97(11):58, 1997.

Schaffer, DB: Closed suction wound drainage. Nursing 27(11):62, 1997.

Scheck, A: Therapists on the team: Diabetic wound prevention is everybody's business. Rehabil Nurs 16(7):18, 1999.

Schiweiger, JL, and Huey, RA: Alzheimer's disease. Nursing 29(6):34, 1999.

Schraeder, C, et al: Community nursing organizations: A new frontier. Am J Nurs 97(1):63, 1997.

Schulmeister, L: Pacemakers and environmental safety: What your patient needs to know. Nursing 28(7):58, 1998.

Short stature and growth hormone: A delicate balance. Practice Update (newsletter). The Children's Hospital, Denver, Summer, 1999.

Sinacore, DR: Managing the diabetic foot. Rehab Manag 11(4):60, 1998.

Smatlak, P, and Knebel, AR: Clinical evaluation of noninvasive monitoring of oxygen saturation in critically ill patients. Am J Crit Care 7(5):370, 1998.

Smith, AM, and Schwirian, PM: The relationship between caregiver burden and TBI survivors' cognition and functional ability after discharge. Rehabil Nurs 23(5):252, 1998.

Smochek, MR, et al: Interventions for risk for suicide and risk for violence. Nurs Diagn. The International Journal of Nursing Language and Classification 11(2):60, April–June 2000.

Stockert, PA: Getting UTI patients back on track. RN 62(3):49, 1999.

Strimike, CL, Wojcik, JM, and Stark, BA: Incision care that really cuts it. RN 60(7):22, 1997.

Summer, CH: Recognizing and responding to spiritual distress. Am J Nurs 98(1):26, 1998.

Szymanski, L and King, B: (1999). Practice parameters for the assessment and treatment of children, adolescents, and adults with mental retardation and comorbid mental disorders. J Am Acad Child Adolesc Psychiatry, Dec 38 (12 suppl).

Travers, PL: Autonomic dysreflexia: A clinical rehabilitation problem. Rehabil Nurs 24(1):19, 1997.

Travers, PL: Poststroke dysphagia: Implications for nurses. Rehabil Nurs 24(2):69, 1999.

Ufema, J: Reflections on death and dying. Nursing 29(6):96, 1999.

Vigilance pays off in preventing falls. Harv Health Lett 24(6):1, 1999.

Walker, BL: Preventing falls. RN 61(5):40, 1998.

Walker, D: Back to basics: Choosing the correct wound dressing. Am J Nurs 96(9):35, 1996.

Watson, R, et al: The relationship between caregiver burden and self-care deficits in former rehabilitation patients. Rehabil Nurs 23(5):258, 1998.

Weeks, SM: Caring for patients with heart failure. Nursing 26(3):52, 1996.

Wehling-Weepie, AK, and MCarthy, A: A healthy lifestyle program: Promoting child health in schools. J School Nurs 18(6):322, 2002.

Whittle, H, et al: Nursing management of pressure ulcers using a hydrogel dressing protocol: Four case studies. Rehabil Nurs 21(5):237, 1996.

Williams, AM, and Deaton, SB: Phantom limb pain: Elusive, yet real. Rehabil Nurs 22(2):73, 1997.

Wyman, JF, et al: Comparative efficacy of behavioral interventions in the management of female urinary incontinence. Am J Obstet Gynecol 179(4):999, 1998.

Wyman, JF: Treatment of urinary incontinence in men and older women. Am J Nurs 103(3):26, 2003. (Suppl) State of the Science on Urinary Incontinence.

Electronic Resources

Brain basics: Understanding sleep, National Institute of Neurological Disorders and Stroke (NINDS), retrieved August 15, 2003. http://www.ninds.nih.gov.

Enslein, J, et al: (2002). Evidence-based protocol. Interpreter facilitation for persons with limited English proficiency. University of Iowa Gerontological Nursing Interventions Research center Web Site. Retrieved from National Guidelines Clearinghouse, June 2003. http://www.guideline.gov.

Lyons, SS, and Specht, JKP: (1999). Prompted voiding for persons with urinary incontinence. Iowa City (IA): University of Iowa Gerontological Nursing Interventions Research Center Web Site. Retrieved from the National Guidelines Clearinghouse [NGC: 950], June 29, 2003. http://www.guideline.gov.

Noise. Information Sheet. American Speech-Language-Hearing Association (ASHA). Web site, retrieved, June 2003. www.asha.org.

Older Americans Month. Food & Nutrition Information. American Dietetic Association Web site, retrieved 6/27/03. http://www.eatright.org/Public/Nutritioninformation/92_12402.cfm.

Questions/Answers about Voice Problems. Information Sheet. American Speech-Language-Hearing Association (ASHA). Web site, retrieved June 2003. www.asha.org.

Speech for Clients with Tracheostomies or Ventilators. Information Sheet. American Speech-Language-Hearing Association (ASHA). Web site, retrieved June 2003. www.asha.org.

What is Language? What is Speech? Information Sheet. American Speech-Language-Hearing Association (ASHA). Web site, retrieved August 3, 2003. http://www.asha.org/public/speech/development.

Index

Gigantism. *See* Acromegaly
Glaucoma, 662
Glomerulonephritis, 663
Goiter, 663
Gonorrhea, 663
   See also Sexually transmitted disease—STD
Gordon's Functional Health Patterns, 5–9
Gout, 663–664
Grieving
   anticipatory, 260–263
   dysfunctional, 263–266
Growth and development, delayed, 266–271
Growth, risk for disproportionate, 271–275
Growth/development domain, 735
Guillain-Barré syndrome (acute polyneuritis), 664
Gunshot wound, 730–731

H

Hay fever, 664
Healthcare settings, 2
Health maintenance, ineffective, 275–278
Health maintenance organizations (HMOs), 2
Health promotion domain, 732
Health-seeking behaviors, 278–281
Health status axis, 736
Heart
   angina pectoris, 617
   aortic stenosis, 620
   coronary artery bypass surgery, 642
   dysrhythmia, cardiac, 654–655
   endocarditis, 657
   failure, chronic, 664–665
   myocardial infarction, 688
   myocarditis, 688
   pericarditis, 695–696
   surgery, 720
Heatstroke, 665
Hemodialysis, 665
   See also Dialysis, general
Hemophilia, 665–666
Hemorrhoidectomy, 666
Hemorrhoids, 666
Hemothorax, 666
   See also Pneumothorax
Hepatitis, acute viral, 666–667
Hernia, hiatal, 667
Herniated nucleus pulposus (ruptured intervertebral disk), 667
Herpes infections
   simplex, 667–668
   zoster (shingles), 668

Intestinal obstruction. *See* Ileus
Intracranial adaptive capacity, decreased, 316–319
Intrapartal assessment tool, 31–32
Irritable bowel syndrome, 674–675
Isotonic fluid volume. *See* Fluid volume, isotonic